Advanced Reconstruction Hip

American Academy of Orthopaedic Surgeons

Advanced Reconstruction Hip

Edited by

Jay R. Lieberman, MD
Professor of Orthopaedic Surgery
David Geffen School of Medicine at UCLA
Los Angeles, California

Daniel J. Berry, MD
Professor and Chairman
Department of Orthopaedic Surgery, Mayo Clinic
Rochester, Minnesota

Developed by
The Hip Society

Published by the
American Academy of Orthopaedic Surgeons
6300 North River Road
Rosemont, IL 60018

Advanced Reconstruction Foot and Ankle

American Academy of Orthopaedic Surgeons

First Edition

Copyright © 2005 by the American Academy of Orthopaedic Surgeons

ISBN 0-89203-346-0

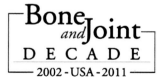

Acknowledgments

Editorial Board
Jay R. Lieberman, MD
Daniel J. Berry, MD

The Hip Society

Board of Directors, 2005

James D' Antonio, MD
President

John Callaghan, MD
First Vice President

Lawrence Dorr, MD
Second Vice President

William Maloney, MD
Secretary-Treasurer

Paul Lachiewicz, MD
Member at Large

William Maloney, MD
Chairman, Education Committee

Richard White, MD
Immediate Past President

American Academy of Orthopaedic Surgeons

Board of Directors, 2005

Stuart L. Weinstein, MD
President

Richard F. Kyle, MD
First Vice President

James H. Beaty, MD
Second Vice President

Edward A. Toriello, MD
Treasurer

Robert W. Bucholz, MD
James H. Herndon, MD
Gordon M. Aamoth, MD
Oheneba Boachie-Adjei, MD
Frances A. Farley, MD
Kristy Weber, MD
Frank B. Kelly, MD
Dwight W. Burney III, MD
Matthew S. Shapiro, MD
Mark C. Gebhardt, MD
Andrew N. Pollak, MD
Joseph C. McCarthy, MD
Leslie L. Altick
William L. Healy, MD
Karen L. Hackett, FACHE, CAE (Ex Officio)

Staff

Mark Wieting, Chief Education Officer
Marilyn L. Fox, PhD, Director, Department of Publications
Lynne Roby Shindoll, Managing Editor
Joan Abern, Senior Editor
Kathleen Reyes, Medical Editor
Mary Steermann, Manager, Production and Archives
Sophie Tosta, Assistant Production Manager
Susan Morritz Baim, Production Coordinator
Michael Bujewski, Database Coordinator
Courtney Astle, Production Assistant
Karen Danca, Production Assistant

Contributors

Michael J. Archibeck, MD
New Mexico Center for Joint
　Replacement Surgery
New Mexico Orthopaedics
Albuquerque, New Mexico

Sanjeev Agarwal, FRCS
Arthroplasty Fellow
Department of Orthopaedic Surgery
Massachusetts General Hospital
Boston, Massachusetts

Mathew S. Austin, MD
Attending Orthopaedic Surgeon
Cooper Bone and Joint Institute
University of Medicine and Dentistry
　of New Jersey
Camden, New Jersey

Robert L. Barrack, MD
Charles F. and Joanne Knight
　Distinguished Professor of
　Orthopaedic Surgery
Department of Orthopaedic Surgery
Washington University School of
　Medicine
St. Louis, Missouri

William P. Barrett, MD
Associate Clinical Professor
Department of Orthopedics
University of Washington School of
　Medicine
Seattle, Washington

Keith R. Berend, MD
Clinical Assistant Professor
Director, Division of Adult
　Reconstruction
Department of Orthopaedics
The Ohio State University
Columbus, Ohio

Richard A. Berger, MD
Assistant Professor of Orthopaedics
Department of Orthopaedics
Rush Medical Center
Chicago, Illinois

James V. Bono, MD
Associate Clinical Professor of
　Orthopaedic Surgery
Tufts University School of Medicine
Attending Orthopedic Surgeon
New England Baptist Hospital
Boston, Massachusetts

Robert B. Bourne, MD
Professor and Chair of Orthopedic
　Surgery
Division of Orthopaedic Surgery
The University of Western Ontario
London Health Sciences Centre
London, Ontario, Canada

Martha Brinson, MSN
Southern Joint Replacement Institute
Nashville, Tennessee

R. Stephen J. Burnett, MD, FRCSC
Clinical Fellow
Division of Orthopedic Surgery
The University of Western Ontario
London Health Sciences Center
London, Ontario, Canada

Miguel E. Cabanela, MD
Professor of Orthopedic Surgery
Mayo Clinic College of Medicine
Department of Orthopedic Surgery,
　Mayo Clinic
Rochester, Minnesota

John J. Callaghan, MD
Professor
Department of Orthopaedic Surgery
The University of Iowa
Iowa City, Iowa

William N. Capello, MD
Professor
Department of Orthopaedic Surgery
Indiana University School of
　Medicine
Indianapolis, Indiana

Michael J. Christie, MD
Director
Southern Joint Replacement Institute
Nashville, Tennessee

Dennis K. Collis, MD
Orthopedic Health Care Northwest
Eugene, Oregon

Clifford W. Colwell, Jr., MD
Director, Musculoskeletal Center
Director, Scripps Center for
　Orthopaedic Research and
　Education
Division of Orthopaedics
Scripps Clinic
La Jolla, California

David K. DeBoer, MD
Director
Southern Joint Replacement Institute
Nashville, Tennessee

Craig J. Della Valle, MD
Assistant Professor
Department of Orthopaedic Surgery
Rush-Presbyterian–St. Luke's
　Medical Center
Chicago, Illinois

Clive P. Duncan, MD, MSc, FRCSC
Professor and Chairman
Department of Orthopaedics
University of British Columbia
Vancouver, British Columbia, Canada

Roger H. Emerson, Jr., MD
Texas Center for Joint Replacement
Plano, Texas

C. Anderson Engh, Jr., MD
Anderson Orthopaedic Research
    Institute
Alexandria, Virginia

Charles A. Engh, MD
Medical Director
Anderson Orthopaedic Research
    Institute
Alexandria, Virginia

Gracia Etienne, MD, PhD
Attending Physician
Department of Orthopaedics
Sinai Hospital of Baltimore
Baltimore, Maryland

Andrew A. Freiberg, MD
Chief, Arthroplasty Service
Department of Orthopaedic Surgery
Massachusetts General Hospital
Boston, Massachusetts

Reinhold Ganz, MD
Professor and Chairman Emeritus
Department of Orthopaedic Surgery
Inselspital-University of Bern
Bern, Switzerland

Donald S. Garbuz, MD, MHSC,
FRCSC
Assistant Professor
Department of Orthopaedics
University of British Columbia
Vancouver, British Columbia, Canada

Jean W.M. Gardeniers, MD
Orthopedic Surgeon
Department of Orthopedics
University Medical Center Nymegen
Nymegen, The Netherlands

Kevin L. Garvin, MD
L. Thomas Hood Professor and
    Chairman
Department of Orthopaedic Surgery
University of Nebraska Medical
    Center
Omaha, Nebraska

Graham A. Gie, FRCS Ed (Orth)
Princess Elizabeth Orthopaedic
    Centre
Royal Devon and Exeter N.H.S.
    Healthcare Trust
Exeter, Devon, England

Stuart B. Goodman, MD, PhD,
    FRCSC, FBSE
Professor of Orthopaedic Surgery
Stanford University
Stanford, California

Richard E. Grant, MD
Associate Professor
Department of Orthopaedics
Howard University
Washington, DC

Allan Gross, MD, FRCSC
Bernard Sherl Family Foundation
Chair in Reconstructive Surgery
Mt. Sinai Hospital
Professor of Surgery
Division of Orthopaedic Surgery
University of Toronto
Toronto, Ontario, Canada

Arlen D. Hanssen, MD
Professor of Orthopedics
Mayo College of Medicine
Mayo Clinic
Rochester, Minnesota

William L. Healy, MD
Chairman, Orthopaedic Surgery
Lahey Clinic
Professor, Orthopaedic Surgery
Boston University School of
    Medicine
Department of Orthopaedic Surgery
Lahey Clinic
Burlington, Massachusetts

Jonathan R. Howell, MB, BS, FRCS
(Tr & Orth)
Clinical and Research Fellow
Division of Reconstructive
    Orthopaedics
Department of Orthopaedics
University of British Columbia
Vancouver, British Columbia, Canada

William James Hozack, MD
Professor of Orthopedic Surgery
Director, Hip and Knee Replacement
    Service
Rothman Institute Orthopedics
Thomas Jefferson University Medical
    School
Philadelphia, Pennsylvania

Michael H. Huo, MD
Associate Professor
Department of Orthopedic Surgery
University of Texas Southwestern
    Medical School
Dallas, Texas

Richard Iorio, MD
Senior Attending Orthopaedic
    Surgeon
Associate Professor of Orthopaedic
    Surgery
Boston University School of
    Medicine
Department of Orthopaedic Surgery
Lahey Clinic
Burlington, Massachusetts

Joshua J. Jacobs, MD
Crown Family Professor of
    Orthopaedic Surgery
Rush-Presbyterian–St. Luke's
    Medical Center
Chicago, Illinois

Victor T. Jando, MD, FRCSC
Former Fellow of Reconstructive
    Orthopaedics
Department of Orthopaedics
University of British Columbia
Vancouver, British Columbia, Canada

Brian A. Jewett, MD
Orthopedic Healthcare Northwest
Eugene, Oregon

William A. Jiranek, MD
Associate Professor
Department of Orthopaedics
Medical College of Virginia
Virginia Commonwealth University
Richmond, Virginia

Scott S. Kelley, MD
Clinical Professor
North Carolina Orthopaedic Clinic
Duke University Medical Center
Durham, North Carolina

Paul F. Lachiewicz, MD
Professor
Department of Orthopaedics
University of North Carolina
Chapel Hill, North Carolina

Tony D. Lamberton, MB, ChB,
   FRACS (Orth)
Orthopaedic Surgeon
Department of Orthopaedic Surgery
Tauranga Hospital
Tauranga, New Zealand

Jo-ann Lee, MS
New England Baptist Hospital
Boston, Massachusetts

David G. Lewallen, MD
Professor of Orthopedic Surgery
Department of Orthopedic Surgery
Mayo Clinic College of Medicine
Rochester, Minnesota

Steve S. Liu, MD
Research Assistant
Orthopaedic Surgery
University of Iowa
Iowa City, Iowa

Adolph V. Lombardi, Jr., MD, FACS
Clinical Assistant Professor
Department of Orthopaedics
Clinical Assistant Professor
Department of Biomedical
   Engineering
The Ohio State University
Columbus, Ohio

Steven J. MacDonald, MD, FRCSC
Associate Professor
Division of Orthopaedic Surgery
The University of Western Ontario
Chief of Orthopaedics
London Health Sciences Centre
London, Ontario, Canada

Thomas H. Mallory, MD, FACS
Clinical Professor
Department of Orthopaedics
The Ohio State University
Columbus, Ohio

William J. Maloney, MD
Professor of Orthopaedic Surgery
Chief of Service
Department of Orthopaedic Surgery
Washington University School of
   Medicine
St. Louis, Missouri

David Manning, MD
Assistant Professor
Division of Orthopaedic Surgery
Department of Surgery
University of Chicago
Chicago, Illinois

Bassam A. Masri, MD, FRCSC
Associate Professor and Head
Division of Lower Limb
   Reconstruction and Oncology
Department of Orthopaedics
University of British Columbia
Vancouver, British Columbia, Canada

Joel M. Matta, MD
Los Angeles, California

David A. Mattingly, MD
Associate Clinical Professor of
   Orthopaedic Surgery
Tufts University School of Medicine
Department of Orthopaedic Surgery
New England Baptist Hospital
Boston, Massachusetts

James P. McAuley, MD, FRCSC
Anderson Orthopaedic Research
   Institute
Alexandria, Virginia

Joseph C. McCarthy, MD
Clinical Professor of Orthopedic
   Surgery
Tufts University School of Medicine
Department of Orthopedic Surgery
New England Baptist Hospital
Boston, Massachusetts

Ramin Mehin, MD, FRCSC
London Health Sciences Centre
London, Ontario, Canada

Michael A. Mont, MD
Director, Center for Joint
   Preservation and Reconstruction
Department of Orthopaedics
Sinai Hospital of Baltimore
Baltimore, Maryland

J. Craig Morrison, MD
Southern Joint Replacement Institute
Nashville, Tennessee

Stephen B. Murphy, MD
Center for Computer Assisted and
   Reconstructive Surgery
New England Baptist Hospital
Boston, Massachusetts

Charles L. Nelson, MD
Assistant Professor of Orthopaedic
   Surgery
Department of Orthopaedic Surgery
University of Pennsylvania
Philadelphia, Pennsylvania

Mary I. O'Connor, MD
Chair, Department of Orthopaedic
   Surgery
Mayo Clinic, Jacksonville
Jacksonville, Florida

Matthew Olin, MD
Attending Surgeon
Greensboro Orthopaedic Center
Greensboro, North Carolina

Michael R. O'Rourke, MD
Assistant Professor
Department of Orthopaedic Surgery
University of Iowa
Iowa City, Iowa

Wayne G. Paprosky, MD, FACS
Associate Professor
Rush Medical College
Rush-Presbyterian–St. Luke's
    Medical Center
Chicago, Illinois

Vincent D. Pellegrini, Jr., MD
James L. Kernan Professor and Chair
Department of Orthopaedics
University of Maryland School of
    Medicine
University of Maryland Medical
    Center
Baltimore, Maryland

Paul M. Pellicci, MD
Associate Director of the Joint
    Replacement Service
Chief of the Hip Service
Department of Orthopaedic Surgery
Hospital for Special Surgery
New York, New York

Brent A. Ponce, MD
Department of Orthopaedics
Massachusetts General Hospital
Boston, Massachusetts

Philip S. Ragland, MD
Physician
Department of Orthopaedics
Sinai Hospital of Baltimore
Baltimore, Maryland

Chitranjan S. Ranawat, MD
Chairman, Department of
    Orthopedic Surgery
Lenox Hill Hospital
New York, New York

Amar S. Ranawat, MD
Department of Orthopedic Surgery
Lenox Hill Hospital
New York, New York

Mark Cameron Reilly, MD
Assistant Professor, Department of
    Orthopaedics
Co-Chief Orthopaedic Trauma
    Service
New Jersey Medical School
Newark, New Jersey

Cecil H. Rorabeck, MD, FRCSC
Professor of Surgery
Division of Orthopedic Surgery
The University of Western Ontario
The London Health Sciences Center
London, Ontario, Canada

Aaron G. Rosenberg, MD, FACS
Professor of Surgery
Department of Orthopaedic Surgery
Rush-Presbyterian–St. Luke's
    Medical Center
Chicago, Illinois

Harry E. Rubash, MD
Chief of Orthopaedic Surgery
Massachusetts General Hospital
Edith M. Ashley Professor
Harvard Medical School
Boston, Massachusetts

Richard F. Santore, MD
Clinical Professor
Department of Orthopaedic Surgery
University of California, San Diego
San Diego, California

Thomas P. Schmalzried, MD
Associate Director Joint Replacement
    Institute
Orthopaedic Hospital
Los Angeles, California

B. William Schreurs, MD, PhD
Orthopedic Surgeon
Department of Orthopedics
University Medical Center Nymegen
Nymegen, The Netherlands

Khemarin Seng, MD
Resident
Department of Orthopaedics
Massachusetts General Hospital
Boston, Massachusetts

Peter F. Sharkey, MD
Associate Professor
Department of Orthopaedic Surgery
Rothman Institute Orthopaedics
Thomas Jefferson University Medical
    School
Philadelphia, Pennsylvania

Werner E. Siebert, MD, MBA
Professor, Doctor of Medicine
Chairman, Orthopedic Center Kassel
Adult Hip and Knee Reconstruction
Orthopaedic Center Kassel
Kassel, Germany

Bonnie M. Simpson, MD
Clinical Professor
Department of Orthopaedic Surgery
Howard University Hospital
Washington, DC

Tom J. J. H. Slooff, MD
Emeritus Professor of Orthopedics
Department of Orthopedics
University Medical Center Nymegen
Nymegan, The Netherlands

Mark J. Spangehl, MD
Assistant Professor of Orthopaedics
Mayo Medical School, Mayo
    Foundation
Department of Orthopaedics
Mayo Clinic Arizona
Scottsdale, Arizona

Andrew I. Spitzer, MD
Medical Director
Joint Replacement Program of
    Century City Hospital
Kerlan–Jobe Orthopaedic Clinic
Los Angeles, California

Scott M. Sporer, MD, MS
Assistant Professor
Rush Medical College
Rush Presbyterian–St. Luke's Medical
    Center
Chicago, Illinois

Bernard N. Stulberg, MD
Director
Center for Joint Reconstruction
Cleveland Orthopaedic and Spine
    Hospital
Cleveland Clinic Health System
Cleveland, Ohio

Edwin Su, MD
Adult Reconstruction Fellow
Hospital for Special Surgery
New York, New York

A.J. Timperley, FRCS Ed.
Consultant, Orthopaedic Surgery
Princess Elizabeth Orthopaedic
    Centre
Exeter, Devon, England

Robert T. Trousdale, MD
Associate Professor
Mayo Graduate School of Medicine
Department of Orthopaedics
Mayo Clinic
Rochester, Minnesota

Joseph P. Turk, MD
Resident, Orthopaedic Surgery
Department of Orthopaedic Surgery
Hospital of the University of
    Pennsylvania
Philadelphia, Pennsylvania

Thomas Parker Vail, MD
Associate Professor of Orthopaedic
    Surgery
Director of Adult Reconstructive
    Surgery
Duke University Medical Center
Durham, North Carolina

Frank R. Voss, MD
AAHKS Representative to AAOS
    Coding Committee
University Specialty Clinics
University of South Carolina
Columbia, South Carolina

Stuart L. Weinstein, MD
Ignacio V. Ponseti Chair and
    Professor of Orthopaedic Surgery
Department of Orthopaedic Surgery
The University of Iowa
Iowa City, Iowa

Richard E. White, Jr., MD
Medical Director
New Mexico Center for Joint
    Replacement Surgery
New Mexico Orthopaedics
Albuquerque, New Mexico

Preface

Many textbooks have been written on the adult hip. The obvious question follows: Is another textbook necessary? We believe that this text on the adult hip is unique because it is not just another reference; rather, it is a surgical guide. When developing *Advanced Reconstruction Hip* in conjunction with the American Academy of Orthopaedic Surgeons and the Hip Society, we envisioned that surgeons would use this text to help plan and carry out a specific surgical technique or manage a difficult clinical problem.

The book has been divided into five sections: primary total hip arthroplasty; complex total hip arthroplasty; complications after total hip arthroplasty; revision total hip arthroplasty; and alternative reconstructive procedures. The section on primary total hip arthroplasty reviews both standard and minimal incision approaches. Chapters are organized to allow the surgeon to prepare quickly for a particular surgical procedure. Therefore, the book is not heavily referenced. Each chapter contains photographs, illustrations, diagrams, and radiographs to highlight specific surgical techniques and management strategies.

The authors of the 66 chapters in this book were invited to contribute because of their special expertise related to a particular topic. They describe their indications, contraindications, and the techniques they use when confronted with a particular hip problem or when using particular implants. In addition, each chapter also reviews al-ternative management options and potential pitfalls. This format is conducive for a rapid review of a surgical technique and allows for more detailed study of a specific problem related to adult hip disease.

We thank the authors for dedicating their time and expertise in creating this text, particularly for the outstanding photographs, illustrations, and radiographs, all of which required extra effort to research and supply. We also thank Lynne Shindoll, Managing Editor, and Joan Abern, Senior Editor, for their hard work and editorial expertise. This book would never have been published without their efforts. Finally, we thank the American Academy of Orthopaedic Surgeons and The Hip Society for their support of this endeavor. Our hope is that you find this book to be a valuable tool and that you use it frequently when dealing with problems of the adult hip.

Jay R. Lieberman, MD
Professor of Orthopaedic Surgery
David Geffin School of Medicine at UCLA

Daniel J. Berry, MD
Professor and Chairman
Department of Orthopedic Surgery, Mayo Clinic
Rochester, Minnesota

Table of Contents

SECTION 1
Primary Total Hip Arthroplasty

Chapter 1

Primary Total Hip Arthroplasty: Posterolateral Approach

Paul M. Pellicci, MD
Edwin Philip Su, MD

 Indications

The posterolateral approach is suited to any procedure about the hip that requires excellent exposure of the proximal femur and acetabulum. It may be used for the treatment of osteoarthritis of the hip, osteonecrosis of the femoral head, failed total hip arthroplasty (THA), hip joint infections, and other forms of intra-articular pathology. The posterolateral approach can be used for THA or partial hip arthroplasty, surface replacement, revision THA, resection arthroplasty, osteochondral grafting, and removal of loose bodies.

 Contraindications

Because the principal blood supply to the femoral head can be compromised with this approach, the viability of the femoral head may be affected. Thus, if preservation of the femoral head is a goal, a more limited posterolateral approach, with preservation of the obturator externus and quadratus femoris muscles, or another approach to the hip is preferred.

Aside from this relative contraindication, there are few reasons to avoid the posterolateral approach to the hip. Body habitus and preexisting deformity do not prevent the wide exposure provided by this approach. In rare situations, a posterolateral approach will need to be converted to a transtrochanteric or an extended trochanteric osteotomy for additional exposure of the acetabulum.

 Alternative Treatments

Alternative approaches that provide good exposure of the acetabulum include the anterior (Smith-Peterson), anterolateral (Watson-Jones), direct lateral (Hardinge), and transtrochanteric approaches. Reported benefits of these alternatives include decreased risk of postoperative dislocation, but the higher risks for heterotopic ossification, abductor mechanism weakness, postoperative limp, and trochanteric nonunion make them less appealing to some surgeons.

 Results

The posterolateral approach for THA is most commonly used in the United States today because of its ease of use, excellent exposure of the femur and acetabulum, and low incidence of heterotopic ossification. It was developed as an alternative to the transtrochanteric approach and has been in use since the 1970s. Proponents of this approach have cited benefits such as decreased surgical time, reduced blood loss, and faster recovery. Although this approach offers unobstructed access to the proximal femur and acetabulum, detractors have cited the higher rate of postoperative dislocation.

Earlier reports of postoperative dislocation of THA using the posterolateral approach range from 4% to 10%. Better understanding of the importance of the integrity of the posterior structures as a soft-tissue restraint to dislocation led to repair of the external rotators and capsule. Recent reports from several authors using this method cite dramatically reduced dislocation rates (less than 1%). **Table 1** provides a summary of results.

 Technique

The patient must be positioned securely in the lateral decubitus position, with the pelvis level (**Figure 1**). If the pelvis is tilted, rotated, or the patient is not adequately secured, the position of the acetabular component will be affected. The dependent leg also must be properly cushioned and

Table 1 Dislocation Rate Following THA Using the Posterior Approach

Author(s) (Year)	Number of Hips	Implant Type	Type of Repair	Mean Patient Age (Range)	Mean Follow-up (Range)	Results
Robinson, et al (1980)	160	Cemented	None	63 years (29–85)	7.6 months (1–23)	7.5% dislocation
Woo and Morrey (1982)	735*	Varied	Piriformis	62.1 years (13–95)	3.1 years (1–10.4)	5.8% dislocation
Pellicci, et al (1998)	395* 395*	Hybrid Hybrid	SER SER, capsule, QF, GM	NS NS	1 year (NS) 1 year (NS)	4% dislocation 0% dislocation
White, et al (2001)	1,078 437*	Varied Varied	None SER, capsule	NS NS	6 months (NS) 6 months (NS)	4.8% dislocation 0.7% dislocation
Weeden, et al (2003)	945*	Uncemented	SER, capsule, GM	62.3 years (36–86)	6.4 years (2–9.3)	0.85% dislocation
Suh, et al (2004)	250 96*	Varied Varied	None SER, capsule	53.5 years (SD 10.4) 53.3 years (SD 10.8)	1 year (NS) 1 year (NS)	6.4% dislocation 1% dislocation

*Some form of posterior repair was performed. SER = short external rotators, QF = quadratus femoris muscle, GM = gluteus maximus tendon. NS = not specified, SD = standard deviation

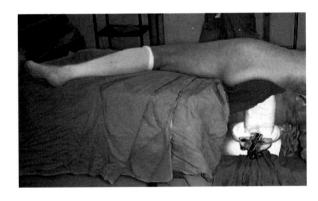

Figure 1 The patient is positioned on the hip table with the pelvis stabilized between the pubic and ischial posts. The dependent leg is well padded, and an axillary roll is present.

an axillary roll inserted under the torso to relieve pressure from the down shoulder.

Exposure

SKIN INCISION

Exposure of the hip begins with identification of the bony landmarks. First, the posterolateral corner of the greater trochanter and the anterior/posterior borders of the proximal femoral shaft are marked. Next, the osseous insertion of the gluteus maximus tendon is palpated onto the posterior femur; the midpoint of the femur is marked at this level. The incision then begins at

this point, extending obliquely over the posterolateral corner of the greater trochanter, continuing proximally so that the acetabulum is centered in the incision. The usual length of the incision is 20 cm, though this will vary depending on the patient's body habitus, and a minimal incision can be easily used (chapter 3).

Once the subcutaneous tissue is divided, the fascia lata is identified and incised in line with the incision. The fibers of the gluteus maximus muscle belly are bluntly separated to the proximal extent of the incision. Care is taken to avoid splitting the fas-

cia too posteriorly, or the gluteus maximus may obscure the exposure. A Charnley self-retaining retractor is placed to retract the gluteus maximus and fascia. We no longer routinely take down the osseous insertion of the gluteus maximus tendon and have had no problems with exposure in the primary arthroplasty setting.

ARTHROTOMY

The hip is internally rotated, which offers an excellent exposure of the posterior structures. The piriformis tendon is identified by palpation, and a curved retractor is placed deep to the abductors, just superior to the piriformis. An Aufranc, or cobra, retractor (George Tiemann, Hauppauge, NY) is then placed inferior to the femoral neck (**Figure 2**). The piriformis and conjoined tendons are divided as close to their insertions as possible and tagged with nonabsorbable suture for later repair.

Following reflection of the short external rotators, the capsule is isolated by repositioning the superior and inferior retractors. The curved su-

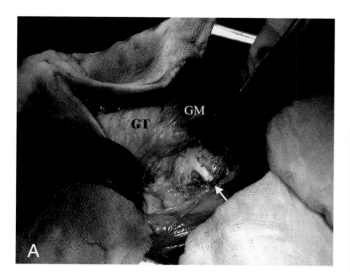
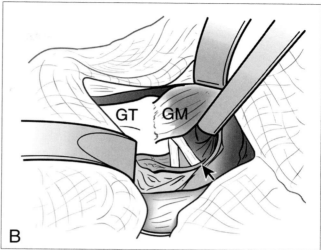

Figure 2   A, The short external rotators of the hip are exposed. The arrow points to the piriformis tendon; GM = gluteus medius; GT = greater trochanter. **B,** An anatomic drawing of same.

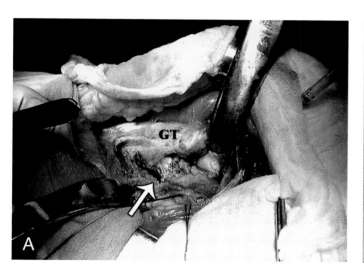
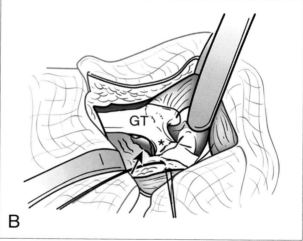

Figure 3   A, The posterior capsule is taken down in a continuous sleeve to the level of the lesser trochanter. The arrow points to the hip capsule; the asterisk represents the femoral neck; GT = greater trochanter. **B,** An anatomic drawing of same.

perior retractor is placed deep to the gluteus minimus, just over the superior femoral neck and capsule. A portion of the obturator externus muscle is divided at the level of the femoral neck, and the Aufranc retractor is placed just inferior to the femoral neck. A capsulotomy is then performed from the posterosuperior acetabulum and continued to the tip of the trochanter in line with the posterior border of the abductors. Care is taken to preserve the length of the capsule to facilitate later closure. The capsulotomy is continued inferiorly along the femoral neck. Instead of making an oblique posterior limb of the capsulotomy, we now favor reflecting the capsule as a continuous sleeve to the level of the lesser trochanter (**Figure 3**). The quadratus femoris is taken down along with the capsule, leaving a small muscular cuff for later reattachment. This provides a thick capsular layer that heals well, providing a soft-tissue restraint to posterior dislocation. The capsule is not tagged at this point; we prefer instead to set the tension of the capsular repair after prosthesis implantation.

ACETABULAR EXPOSURE

The hip is then gently dislocated, using a combination of flexion, internal rotation, and adduction. The leg is held in 90° of internal rotation so that

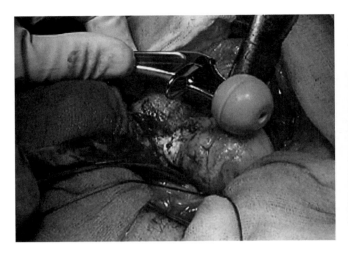

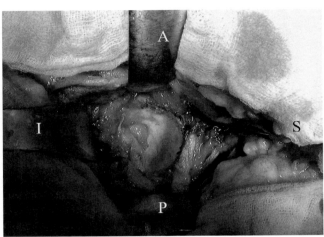

Figure 4 A trial prosthesis is placed along the exposed femoral head and neck to determine the level of neck osteotomy.

Figure 5 The exposed acetabulum is shown. S = superior; I = inferior; A = anterior; P = posterior.

the femoral neck is parallel to the ground. After confirming the level of resection with a trial prosthesis (**Figure 4**), the neck osteotomy is made using an oscillating saw, which allows for unobstructed access to the acetabulum.

Initially, a curved C-retractor is placed anteriorly, retracting the proximal femur out of the view of the acetabulum. Placing the operated extremity in a slightly flexed position will aid in exposure; occasionally, the reflected head of the rectus femoris will need to be released from the supra-acetabular region to allow for more excursion of the femur. A Steinmann pin is placed in the ilium to reflect the abductors, and a small capsulotomy is made inferiorly to allow placement of an Aufranc retractor deep to the transverse acetabular ligament. Finally, a bent Hohmann retractor is placed posteriorly, taking care first to palpate the sciatic nerve to ensure it is out of harm's way. The acetabulum is now ready for bony preparation (**Figure 5**).

Bone Preparation

With this excellent exposure, the acetabulum is easily prepared using hemispherical reamers. Depending on the surgeon's preference, the acetabular component may be cemented or press-fit into place. The complete visualization of the acetabulum facilitates the assessment of the anteversion and inclination of the component (**Figure 6**).

After implantation of the acetabular component, the leg is flexed and internally rotated to expose the proximal femur. The leg is held in approximately 90° of internal rotation and 70° of flexion, bringing the osteotomized neck into the surgeon's view (**Figure 7**). A modified Aufranc retractor with teeth is placed under the anterior aspect of the femoral neck, lifting it out of the wound. This allows for unencumbered preparation of the femoral canal. As the femoral canal is prepared, it is important to limit the spread of marrow contents into the surrounding soft tissue because we believe that this is a significant source of heterotopic ossification.

Prosthesis Implantation

As the femoral component is inserted, its anteversion should be noted because it may play a role in impingement and stability. Again, the wide exposure afforded by the posterolateral approach allows for assessment of the component position (**Figure 8**).

Before hip relocation, we make two drill holes in the posterior aspect of the greater trochanter for repair of the capsule and short external rotators.

Wound Closure

This is the area in which most of the improvements in the posterolateral approach have been made in recent years. Once the hip has been relocated, two nonabsorbable sutures are placed in the capsular flap. By waiting until the prosthesis has been implanted, the suture position can be adjusted to achieve adequate tensioning (**Figure 9**). The capsular and external rotator tagging sutures are brought through the drill holes in the greater trochanter and tied in layers. By extending and abducting the hip, excellent tension of these posterior structures can be obtained.

The enhanced posterior repair consists of repairing the quadratus femoris muscle (**Figure 10**) and the gluteus maximus osseous insertion, if it had been taken down. The quadratus femoris is reapproximated to its cuff and sutured with figure-of-eight bioabsorbable suture. The posterior fascia of the vastus lateralis muscle may be incorporated to prevent the stitch from pulling out. Multiple stitches are placed in the muscle belly,

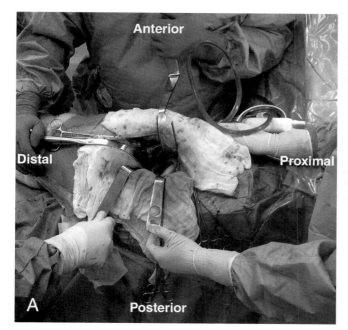

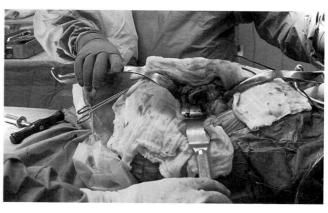

Figure 7 The operated limb is positioned with the aid of an assistant in approximately 70° of flexion and 90° of internal rotation.

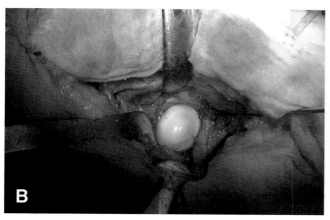

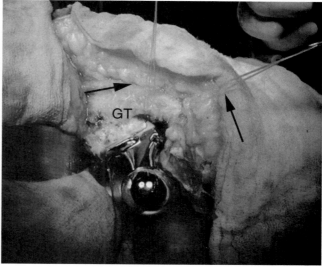

Figure 6 **A,** Posterior approach to the hip with retractors in place. **B,** An implanted acetabular component is shown. The excellent exposure facilitates assessment of component position.

Figure 8 Tagging sutures are shown (arrows) in the drill holes made in the greater trochanter for reattachment of the posterior structures. The component position is easily assessed with this excellent exposure. GT = greater trochanter.

leading to closure of the entire posterior soft-tissue sleeve of the hip (**Figure 11**).

Postoperative Regimen

The postoperative regimen consists of prompt physical therapy and mobilization. The operated hip is placed in an abducted position while the patient is at rest. Hip dislocation precautions include limiting hip flexion to 90° and avoiding internal rotation or adduction. In addition, the patient is in-structed to sit only in high-backed chairs, to use raised toilet seats, and to sleep with a pillow between the legs. The amount of weight bearing depends on the particular prosthesis used.

At the 6-week follow-up visit, barring any complications, the hip precautions will gradually be relaxed. Eventually, the patient can return to all previous activity except flexion and internal rotation.

Avoiding Pitfalls and Complications

Some of the complications reported with but not exclusive to the postero-lateral approach to the hip include sciatic and femoral nerve injury, early postoperative dislocation, and hetero-topic ossification.

Because of its proximity to the acetabulum, the sciatic nerve may be injured during any approach for hip

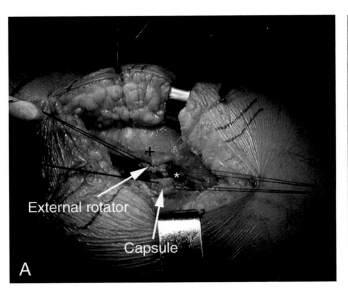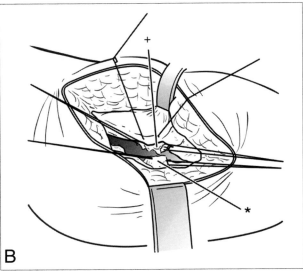

Figure 9   A, The hip capsule (+) and short external rotators (*) are tagged separately with nonabsorbable suture. **B,** An anatomic drawing of same.

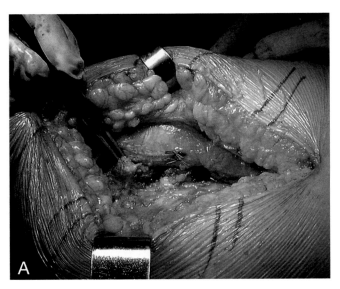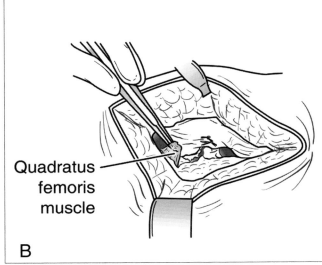

Figure 10   A, The quadratus femoris muscle is reapproximated to its muscular cuff. The forceps are shown grasping the muscle belly. **B,** An anatomic drawing of same.

arthroplasty. Several times during the posterolateral approach we pay particular attention to the location of the sciatic nerve to avoid injuring it. First, the incision should be long enough to avoid undue tension on the nerve with posterior retraction during acetabular and femoral exposure. The position of the leg during exposure of the proximal femur is also important. Intraop-

erative monitoring has demonstrated increased tension on the sciatic nerve with flexion, internal rotation, and adduction. Therefore, we place a soft roll under the thigh to avoid adduction during femoral preparation. Finally, during the repair of the quadratus femoris, the sciatic nerve should be palpated to ensure it is safely protected.

The femoral nerve may be injured during placement of the anterior acetabular retractor. This retractor must hug the anterior acetabular wall to avoid inadvertent positioning near the femoral nerve.

The incidence of heterotopic ossification has been reported to be less with the posterolateral approach compared with other surgical exposures of

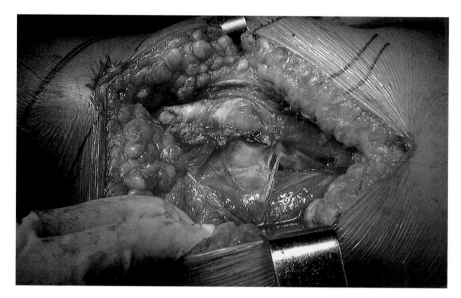

Figure 11 The completed enhanced posterior repair is shown.

the hip. We believe expulsion of the marrow contents during femoral canal preparation is a significant potential source of heterotopic ossification.

Thus, we carefully suction these contents and irrigate the soft tissues copiously. Excessive trauma to the soft tissues is also avoided to limit heterotopic ossification.

The incidence of early postoperative dislocation following the posterolateral approach has been shown to be decreased with an enhanced posterior repair. We believe the repair of the posterior soft tissues creates a check-rein to posterior dislocation in the postoperative period. Furthermore, it provides a scaffolding for the pseudocapsule to form. It is our opinion that the difference in dislocation rates between the posterolateral and other approaches can be minimized with this meticulous reapproximation of the posterior soft tissues.

References

Patiala H, Lehto K, Rokkanen P, Paavolainen P: Posterior approach for total hip arthroplasty. *Arch Orthop Trauma Surg* 1984;102:225-229.

Pellicci PM, Bostrom M, Poss R: Posterior approach to total hip replacement using enhanced posterior soft tissue repair. *Clin Orthop* 1998;355:224-228.

Robinson RP, Robinson HJ, Salvati EA: Comparison of the transtrochanteric and posterior approaches for total hip replacement. *Clin Orthop* 1980;147:143-147.

Suh KT, Park BG, Choi YJ: A posterior approach to primary total hip arthroplasty with soft tissue repair. *Clin Orthop* 2004;418:162-167.

Weeden SH, Paprosky WG, Bowling JW: The early dislocation rate in primary total hip arthroplasty following the posterior approach with posterior soft-tissue repair. *J Arthroplasty* 2003;18:709-713.

White RE Jr, Forness TJ, Allman JK, Junick DW: Effect of posterior capsular repair on early dislocation in primary total hip replacement. *Clin Orthop* 2001;393:163-167.

Woo R, Morrey BF: Dislocations after total hip arthroplasty. *J Bone Joint Surg Am* 1982;64:1295-1306.

Coding

CPT Codes		Corresponding ICD-9 Codes		
26990	Incision and drainage, pelvis or hip joint area; deep abscess or hematoma	682.5 711.45 730.05 998.1	682.6 711.95 924.01 998.5	711.15 726.5 958.3
26992	Incision, bone cortex, pelvis and/or hip joint (eg, osteomyelitis or bone abscess)	711.15 730.05 996.67	711.45 730.15 996.78	711.95 958.3 998.5
27030	Arthrotomy, hip, with drainage (eg, infection)	711.05 998.5	730.25	958.3
27033	Arthrotomy, hip, including exploration or removal of loose or foreign body	716.15 890.0	729.6 890.1	732.7
27036	Capsulectomy or capsulotomy, hip, with or without excision of heterotopic bone, with release of hip flexor muscles (ie, gluteus medius, gluteus minimus, tensor fascia latae, rectus femoris, sartorius, iliopsoas)	343.0 343.3 728.13	343.1 343.9 781.2	343.2 718.45 905.1
27052	Arthrotomy, with biopsy; hip joint	682.5		
27054	Arthrotomy, with synovectomy; hip joint	714.0	719.25	
27087	Removal of foreign body, pelvis or hip; deep (subfascial or intramuscular)	729.6 996.67	890.0 996.78	890.1 998.4
27090	Removal of hip prosthesis; (separate procedure)	996.4	996.66	996.77
27091	Removal of hip prosthesis, complicated, including total hip prosthesis, methylmethacrylate with or without insertion of spacer	996.4	996.66	996.77
27125	Hemiarthroplasty, hip, partial (eg, femoral stem prosthesis, bipolar arthroplasty)	715.15 716.15 733.42	715.25 718.6 905.6	715.35 733.14
27130	Arthroplasty, acetabular and proximal femoral prosthetic replacement (total hip arthroplasty), with or without autograft or allograft	711.45 714.30 715.35 718.6 733.42	711.95 715.15 716.15 720.0 808.0	714.0 715.25 718.5 733.14 905.6
27132	Conversion of previous hip surgery to total hip arthroplasty, with or without autograft or allograft	715.15 718.2 733.14 996.4	715.25 718.5 733.42 996.66	715.35 718.6 905.6 996.77
27134	Revision of total hip arthroplasty; both components, with or without autograft or allograft	996.4	996.66	996.77
27137	Revision of total hip arthroplasty, acetabular component only, with or without autograft or allograft	996.4	996.66	996.77
27138	Revision of total hip arthroplasty, femoral component only, with or without allograft	996.4	996.66	996.77
27236	Open treatment of femoral fracture, proximal end, neck, internal fixation or prosthetic replacement	733.14 820.03 820.13	820.00 820.10 820.8	820.02 820.12 820.9

CPT copyright © 2004 by the American Medical Association. All Rights Reserved.

Chapter 2

Primary Total Hip Arthroplasty: Anterolateral and Direct Lateral Approaches

David G. Lewallen, MD

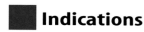 ## Indications

Anterolateral and direct lateral approaches with anterior arthrotomy of the hip joint are useful in both primary and revision total hip arthroplasty (THA). In most patients, these approaches also can be used selectively as adjuncts to the posterior approach. Anterior arthrotomy and an anterolateral or lateral approach to the hip is especially useful in management of patients at risk for dislocation or instability.

A variety of anterior and anterolateral approaches to the hip have been described for primary THA. The main indications for these approaches consist of the following: (1) routine primary THA, depending on surgeon preference and (2) primary THA in patients at increased risk for dislocation, specifically those who have Parkinson's disease, spasticity, or dementia, or those undergoing primary THA for femoral neck fracture.

The main advantages of an anterior hip arthrotomy and use of these approaches to the hip include reduced risk of dislocation related to preservation of the posterior capsule and external rotators, avoiding direct exposure of the sciatic nerve, excellent acetabular exposure, and the opportunity to visualize any defects, prepare the bone, and implant a prosthesis while viewing the acetabulum directly from the abdominal side of the patient.

Contraindications

Contraindications to these approaches include exposure of the posterior aspect of the acetabulum to remove plates, screws, or heterotopic ossifications or to bone graft a deficient posterior wall. In general, reconstructions of the hip that are associated with high hip centers, such as the more severe forms of degenerative dysplasia of the hip, and revision procedures that require extensive superior exposure of the acetabulum should not use a direct lateral approach. When performing a direct lateral approach to the hip, the proximal extent of the exposure is via direct muscle splitting of the gluteus medius and is limited by potential injury to the superior gluteal nerve. The superior gluteal nerve innervates the gluteus medius, gluteus minimus, and the tenor fascia latae. There is a so-called safe zone that extends 5 cm superior to the tip of the greater trochanter where the dissection can be extended without injury to the nerve. However, the distribution of the nerve is variable and may be found only 3 or 4 cm proximal to the tip of the greater trochanter in some patients. Therefore, excessive retraction on the gluteus medius flap should be avoided.

Alternative Treatments

The posterolateral and transtrochanteric approaches are alternatives that provide excellent exposure to the acetabulum and the femur. The benefits of the posterolateral approach are enhanced exposure and decreased risk of a postoperative limp, but there is a higher risk of dislocation. The transtrochanteric approaches also provide excellent exposure, but there is a risk of trochanteric nonunion and trochanteric bursitis secondary to hardware.

Results

Although both anterolateral and direct lateral approaches are commonly used, few studies evaluate their efficacy. Woo and Morrey reported a significantly lower dislocation rate compared with the posterior approach. In a more recent study, no dislocations were reported with the direct lateral approach. **Table 1** summarizes results of these studies.

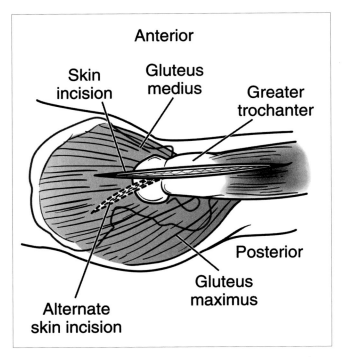

Figure 1 The skin incision may either be straight and centered over the femoral shaft or have a gentle proximal posterior curve to facilitate exposure of the femoral canal.

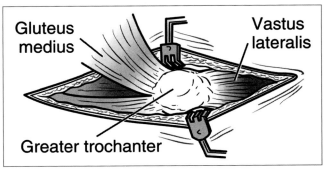

Figure 2 The skin, subcutaneous tissue, and fascia are retracted with the Charnley self-retaining retractor. The anterior portion of the gluteus medius is released from the anterior portion of the greater trochanter. The split is extended proximally through the substance of the muscle. The split should not extend more than 5 cm proximal to the tip of the trochanter to protect the superior gluteal nerve.

Technique

Anterolateral Approach

EXPOSURE

With the patient in the lateral decubitus position, the hip is prepared and the leg is draped free. This allows the leg to be positioned over the side of the table into a sterile pocket on the abdominal side of the patient. The incision is centered over the trochanter and extends in line with the femur distally. Proximally, the incision continues in line with the femur or curves slightly posteriorly, which can facilitate access to the femoral canal in larger or obese patients (**Figure 1**).

The fascia is divided in line with the skin, and the inferior margin of the anterior portion of the gluteus medius is identified.

The most anterior portion of the gluteus medius inserts obliquely into the trochanter, and the central and more posterior portions are oriented vertically in line with the femur. A curving, J-shaped incision is made (either sharply or with cautery) to detach the anterior portion of the gluteus medius directly off of the trochanter, allowing proximal and anterior retraction of the anterior-most portion of the gluteus medius (**Figure 2**). In primary THA, approximately 40% of the muscle is mobilized, leaving the central and more dense tendinous portion posteriorly intact and attached to the trochanter. Splitting of the gluteus medius must not extend beyond 5 cm above the tip of the greater trochanter to avoid injury to the superior gluteal nerve. The gluteus minimus is identified and divided from its attachment to the trochanter and tagged for later repair. Anterior capsulotomy is then performed with either complete capsulectomy or T-shaped capsular flaps, depending on surgeon preference (**Figure 3**).

BONE PREPARATION

The hip is dislocated anteriorly by external rotation of the adducted and flexed hip. Capsular attachments around the base of the neck are divided to mobilize the femur, and osteotomy of the femoral neck is performed during primary THA. Mobilization and posterior retraction of the femur allows access to the acetabular cavity.

Excellent acetabular exposure is achieved with the surgeon on the abdominal side of the patient, allowing easy reference for component insertion, particularly when the entire acetabular rim is exposed. Following the acetabular procedure, the femur can be accessed with the leg dislocated and the foot and leg held in the sterile

Table 1 Dislocation Rates Associated With Direct Lateral Approach for Primary THA

Author(s) (Year)	Number of Hips	Dislocation (%)
Woo and Morrey (1982)	8,944	2.3%
Moskal and Mann (1996)	306	0%

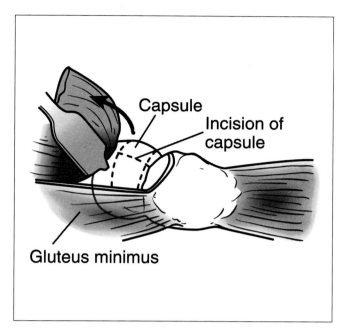

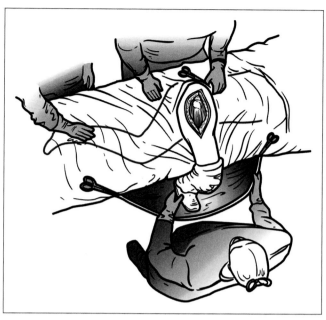

Figure 3 The gluteal muscles are retracted superiorly and held with acetabular pin retractors or a broad, spiked (Bickel) retractor driven into the supracetabular region of the ilium. The anterior and lateral portions of the capsule are incised or excised.

Figure 4 After dislocation of the hip by adduction, external rotation, and longitudinal traction, the foot and leg can be placed into the sterile pocket. When the leg is perpendicular to the floor, the surgeon can assess the version of the femoral prosthesis in a clinically reproducible manner.

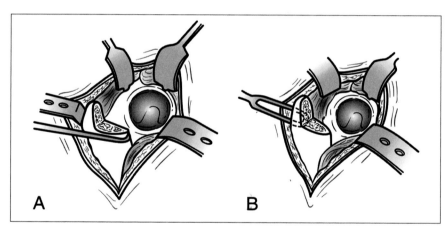

Figure 5 **A**, A large bone hook placed around the femoral neck assists the posterior retraction of the femur during acetabular exposure and preparation. **B**, A large, spoon-shaped retractor placed beneath the greater trochanter elevates the proximal femur during preparation of the femoral canal and insertion of the femoral prosthesis.

pocket at the side of the bed (**Figure 4**). A blunt retractor placed beneath the posterior aspect of the greater trochanter helps elevate the proximal femur out of the wound (**Figure 5**).

The anterolateral approach and this type of patient positioning are especially helpful in large or obese patients because the assistant does not need to support or hold an extremely large limb after dislocation, as is required with the posterior approach. The overhanging trochanter and intact, attached portions of the gluteus medius must be protected during femoral access and preparation to avoid damaging the intact portion of the tendon and muscle or creating a greater trochanteric fracture. The greater trochanter and the intact posterior portion of the gluteus medius may force femoral preparation instruments into a position of flexion and/or varus unless care is taken to prevent this problem.

Direct Lateral Approach
With the direct lateral approach, the anterior portion of the gluteus medius is elevated, along with the anterior portion of the vastus lateralis distal to the trochanter. This continuous soft-tissue sleeve is raised subperiosteally off of the trochanter by sharp dissection or cautery.

Variations of the direct lateral approach involve changes in the amount of vastus lateralis or gluteus medius included in the flap. In the 1980s, Hardinge popularized a version that curved posteriorly into the gluteus medius; this approach releases most of the gluteus medius tendon from the tro-

construction is possible with no adverse effect on abductor strength.

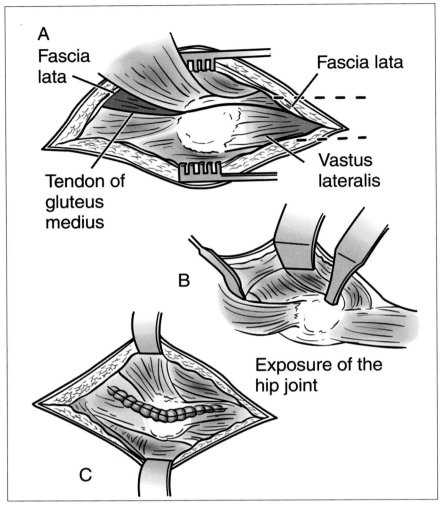

Extensile Variations of the Direct Lateral Approach
When more extensile exposure of the femur is required distal to the trochanter to remove laterally positioned femoral plates, access cortical defects, or create cortical windows, the vastus slide is used. This approach involves release of the entire vastus lateralis from posterior to anterior, beginning just below the trochanter and extending distally (**Figure 7**). Proximally, the release extends around the trochanter to the anterior portion of the gluteus medius. After elevation of the vastus lateralis, both femoral exposure and subsequent access to the acetabulum through an anterior arthrotomy are excellent.

Another more extensile exposure that begins to overlap with formal trochanteric osteotomy approaches is the trochanteric slide. With this approach, the entire vastus lateralis distally is elevated and then followed by trochanteric osteotomy, which allows elevation of the gluteus medius proximally (**Figure 8**). This digastric flap allows retraction of the gluteus medius and vastus lateralis in continuity and provides excellent exposure of the femur.

The acetabulum is prepared in the interval between the osteotomy fragment, which can be reflected anteriorly, and the femur, which can be translated posteriorly with the external rotators intact and with arthrotomy and dislocation of the hip anteriorly. The osteotomy provides secure repair of the vastus lateralis and gluteus medius back to the proximal femur and reduces the risk of dislocation when the external rotators are left intact.

Wound Closure
Following arthroplasty and relocation of the hip, capsular repair may be performed if the capsular flaps have been preserved. The gluteus minimus and the anterior portion of the gluteus me-

Figure 6 The direct lateral approach of Hardinge. **A**, The insertion of the gluteus medius is removed from the anterior portion of the greater trochanter and extended proximally into the substance of the gluteus medius and minimus muscles. The vastus lateralis is split distally. Care is taken to remove the abductors anteriorly so as to leave a tendinous cuff on the trochanter. **B**, The vastus lateralis is subperiosteally elevated, and the entire myofascial unit is retracted anteriorly to expose the hip capsule. **C**, The myofascial unit is repaired in a side-to-side fashion with multiple interrupted sutures that provide a secure reattachment. Care is taken to divide the abductors anteriorly to leave a tendinous cuff on the trochanter. The split in the abductor muscle should not extend more than 5 cm proximal to the tip of the greater trochanter to protect the superior gluteal nerve.

chanter (**Figure 6**). Other more recent versions involve releasing less of the gluteus medius proximally to reduce the risk of residual abductor weakness. Variations on this approach include elevation of a wafer of bone from the anterior portion of the trochanter along with the anterior portion of the gluteus medius and vastus lateralis, to facilitate secure repair and healing of that flap.

Regardless of the technique used, excessive splitting or proximal dissection into the gluteus medius must be avoided to avoid injuring the superior gluteal nerve as it courses within the medius muscle. If the supra-acetabular soft tissues are lifted rather than split, and with adequate distal exposure to relax the sides of the incision, safe yet extensive acetabular re-

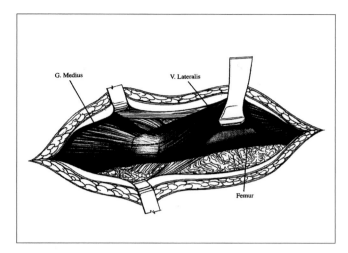

Figure 7 Extensile modification of the direct lateral approach. The gluteus medius and minimus are reflected anteriorly as is the vastus lateralis. (Reproduced with permission from McGann WA: Surgical approaches in Callaghan JJ, Rosenberg AG, Rubash HE (eds): *The Adult Hip*. Philadelphia, PA, Lippincott-Raven, 1998, pp 678-681.)

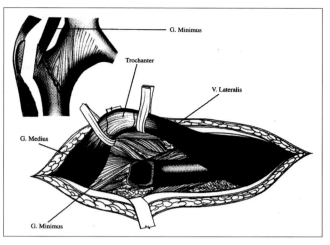

Figure 8 The trochanteric slide. The soft tissue is retracted anteriorly and may be held with retractors. The anterior capsule can then be dissected for exposure of the hip joint. (Reproduced with permission from McGann WA: Surgical approaches in Callaghan JJ, Rosenberg AG, Rubash HE (eds): *The Adult Hip*. Philadelphia, PA, Lippincott-Raven, 1998, pp 678-681.)

dius are repaired separately using nonabsorbable sutures through bone in the trochanter. Meticulous repair is important to prevent detachment and potential for pain, weakness, or a limp.

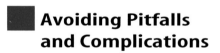

Avoiding Pitfalls and Complications

The main disadvantages of the anterolateral approaches include the following: (1) the potential for a limp due to abductor weakness resulting from injury to the superior gluteal nerve (which can occur with excessive splitting of the gluteus medius) or failure of the muscle-tendon repair to the greater trochanter; (2) slower recovery of abductor power (compared with the posterior approach); and (3) lack of visualization or access to the femoral shaft distally. Additional disadvantages include the potential for femoral stem malposition or trochanteric fracture as a result of trochanteric impingement during prosthesis insertion. To minimize these risks, careful attention is essential during reaming and insertion of femoral components using anterior arthrotomy. With careful attention to technique, anterior arthrotomy and the family of anterolateral and direct lateral approaches can greatly facilitate complex reconstructions of the acetabulum and femur and provide safe, reproducible, excellent exposure for these reconstructive efforts.

References

Moskal JT, Mann JW III: A modified direct lateral approach for primary and revision and total hip arthroplasty: A prospective analysis of 453 cases. *J Arthroplasty* 1996;11:255-266.

Woo RY, Morrey BF: Dislocations after total hip arthroplasty. *J Bone Joint Surg Am* 1982;64:1295-1306.

Coding

CPT Codes		Corresponding ICD-9 Codes		
27087	Removal of foreign body, pelvis or hip; subcutaneous tissue, deep (subfascial or intramuscular)	714.0 716.15 729.6 890.0 996.4 996.77	714.30 718.X5 733.14 890.1 996.66 996.78	715.X5 720.0 733.42 905.6 996.67 998.4
27090	Removal of hip prosthesis (separate procedure)	714.0 716.15 733.14 890.1 996.66	714.30 718.X5 733.42 905.6 996.77	715.X5 720.0 890.0 996.4
27125	Hemiarthroplasty, hip, partial (eg, femoral stem prosthesis, bipolar arthroplasty)	714.0 715.25 718.X5 733.14 890.1 996.66	714.30 715.35 718.6 733.42 905.6 996.77	715.15 716.15 720.0 890.0 996.4
27130	Arthroplasty, acetabular and proximal femoral prosthetic replacement (total hip arthroplasty), with or without autograft or allograft	711.45 714.30 720.20 733.14 905.6 996.77	711.95 715.X5 718.X5 733.42 996.4	714.0 716.15 718.6 808.0 996.66
27132	Conversion of previous hip surgery to total hip arthroplasty, with or without autograft or allograft	714.0 716.15 718.6 733.42 996.4	714.30 718.2 720.0 808.0 996.66	715.X5 718.X5 733.14 905.6 996.77
27134	Revision of total hip arthroplasty; both components, with or without autograft or allograft	714.0 716.15 733.14 996.4	714.30 718.X5 733.42 996.66	715.X5 720.0 905.6 996.77
27137	Revision of total hip arthroplasty; acetabular component only, with or without autograft or allograft	714.0 716.15 733.14 996.4	714.30 718.X5 733.42 996.66	715.X5 720.0 905.6 996.77
27138	Revision of total hip arthroplasty; femoral component only, with or without allograft	714.0 716.15 733.14 996.4	714.30 718.X5 733.42 996.66	715.X5 720.0 905.6 996.77
27236	Open treatment of femoral fracture, proximal end, neck, internal fixation or prosthetic replacement	714.0 716.15 733.14 820.02 820.12 820.9 996.66	714.30 718.X5 733.42 820.03 820.13 905.6 996.77	715.X5 720.0 820.00 820.10 820.8 996.4

Mini-Incision Total Hip Arthroplasty: Posterior Approach

Thomas Parker Vail, MD

Indications

The posterior approach to the hip joint is favored by many surgeons because it avoids damage to the gluteus medius muscle and yields excellent functional results. The "mini" posterior approach evolved from the standard posterior approach and eliminates all but the most essential parts of the posterior exposure required to accomplish a successful total hip arthroplasty (THA). Development of the mini posterior approach was facilitated by increased knowledge of the anatomy, careful placement of the incision, and the availability of lower profile instruments and retractors.

The goal of the mini-incision approach is not simply to make the incision small but to perform a successful THA with the smallest possible incision. In the ideal patient, incision length can be as small as 6 to 8 cm. However, the exact length of the incision depends on the surgeon's experience and the patient's body habitus. The length of the mini-incision required to access both the femur and the acetabulum depends on the distance between the surface of the skin and the lowest depth of the wound.

Minimal tissue trauma and mobilization of bone and soft tissue used in the posterior incision approach are applicable to all patient types and all levels of surgical experience.

Once a surgeon understands the basic surgical skills required for this approach, incisions can be made progressively smaller in all patients as the surgeon gains experience in the technique. The mini posterior incision is thus indicated for any primary THA. However, there is no evidence-based data available to prove superiority of the mini-incision over standard approaches.

The universal indication for the mini posterior incision derives from the fact that it can be extended into a standard approach or lengthened to a degree less than a standard approach to accommodate patient size, joint stiffness, or other impediments to successful use of a small incision. The ultimate goals of the mini posterior approach are to facilitate quicker recovery, produce a more cosmetically pleasing incision, reduce pain, and decrease the rate of transfusion. The approach is used for patients meeting appropriate criteria when it furthers the overall goals of a highly functional hip replacement and a low rate of revision.

Contraindications

The mini posterior incision may be contraindicated in obese or very muscular patients or those with stiff joints, acetabular protrusio, or retained hardware. Mini-incision hip arthroplasty is not possible in most hip revision cases. A small posterior incision is not indicated if it might lead to excessive soft-tissue damage, improper bone preparation, such as eccentric reaming of the acetabulum, or improper implant positioning. The appropriate length of the incision is a surgeon's judgment call, and a successful outcome is clearly more important than the incision's length.

Alternative Treatments

There are many alternative approaches to the hip, the most common being the standard posterior approach. The decision to convert the mini-incision to a standard incision can be made at any time during the surgery.

The most common minimally invasive alternatives to the mini posterior incision are the mini anterolateral or direct lateral incision. Surgeons choosing these approaches often cite the low dislocation rate as the main advantage. The two-incision open technique or the fluoroscopically guided technique are also alternative mini-incision approaches that can be used with selected patients. No accepted algorithm exists for selecting

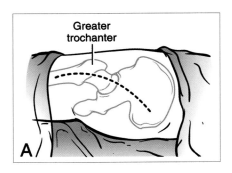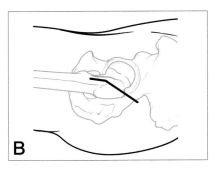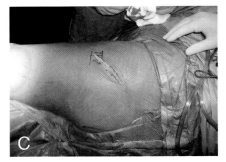

Figure 1 The standard (**A**) and mini-incision (**B** and **C**) posterior approaches to THA. Note that the skin incision for the mini posterior approach is centered over the acetabulum or slightly posterior to it and requires approximately only the middle third of the standard posterior approach. (Figure 1, A is reproduced with permission from Vail TP: Posterior mini-incision. *Semin Arthroplasty* 2004;15:83-86.)

an approach because indications for each approach overlap. The choice of alternative exposures may be influenced by the surgeon's training or the patient's specific needs and expressed desires.

Results

The current results of mini posterior total hip procedures are preliminary and conflicting. In a recent report that randomly compared mini-incision to standard length incision THA, higher rates of soft-tissue complications and component malposition were reported with the mini approach. Other short-term cohort studies report a higher rate of patient satisfaction and a lower rate of transfusion with the smaller posterior incision. The length of the incision reportedly increases with higher patient body mass index. Early indications from the reported series suggest that wound and implant positioning problems can arise when the primary goal is limiting the length of the skin incision. However, when the mini posterior approach is applied with careful attention to soft-tissue protection and technique, and by lengthening the incision as required, results can be achieved in early follow-up that are at least equal to those obtained with the standard posterior approach. Long-term reports of im-

plant performance with the mini posterior incision are not currently available.

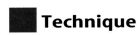

Technique

Exposure

To successfully perform the mini posterior approach, first visualize the standard posterior approach and then eliminate all parts of it that are not necessary to complete the THA. The smaller approach generally uses the middle third of the standard approach. Instrument modifications that can aid in exposure include using more slender and lower profile instruments, limiting the number of retractors used, and using lighted retractors, in-line broach handles, and offset reamers. Avoid excessive or prolonged pressure on soft tissues by retractors or instruments. Important technical points include using the skin incision as a window to the bone structures that move with the retractors, moving the limb as needed to facilitate visualization, and mobilizing the femur anterior to the acetabulum for acetabular exposure.

The skin incision for the mini posterior approach is a short, oblique incision centered over the acetabulum or slightly posterior to it (**Figure 1**). Some surgeons make the incision in

line with the posterior border of the femur, but an oblique incision facilitates acetabular reaming because the incision is more in line with the direction of acetabular reaming. Useful surface landmarks are the tip of the greater trochanter, the sciatic notch, and the anterior edge of the vastus lateralis ridge. The sciatic notch is a soft spot just dorsal to the posterior inferior iliac spine and posterior to the greater trochanter. I usually begin with a 4- to 5-cm skin incision that passes directly over the acetabulum by centering over the posterior two thirds of the greater trochanter in line with the sciatic notch and the anterior border of the femur at the vastus ridge.

Once the skin is incised, a small self-retaining retractor facilitates visualization of the fascia. The fascial incision is made within the thin investing fascia of the gluteus maximus muscle, stopping distally at the musculotendinous junction of the tensor fascia muscle. The goal is to make the fascial incision primarily transmuscular rather than through the iliotibial band (**Figure 2**). The incision in the tensor fascia can be extended below the skin distally, if needed for exposure. The gluteus maximus muscle is then divided in line with its fibers at a raphe between the middle and posterior thirds of its pennate structure. The muscle is separated proximally until the sciatic notch is palpable deep to the muscle (it is sometimes difficult to

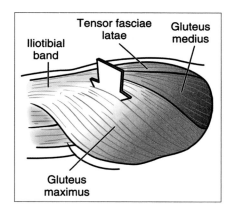

Figure 2 The transmuscular approach through the gluteus maximus muscle is the first part of the deep exposure. The goal of this approach is to make the fascial incision mostly transmuscular rather than through the iliotibial band.

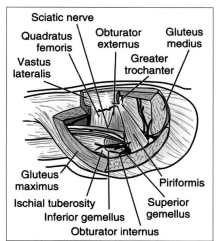

Figure 3 The sciatic nerve exits the greater sciatic notch below the piriformis muscle and proceeds distally over the short external rotator muscles and ischial tuberosity before exiting into the posterior compartment of the thigh.

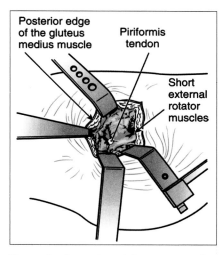

Figure 4 Retraction of the posterior edge of the gluteus medius muscle reveals the piriformis tendon, proceeding toward its insertion on the top of the femur, and the short external rotators below. The piriformis tendon is an important landmark for creating the upper limb of the L-shaped capsular incision. (Reproduced with permission from Vail TP: Posterior mini-incision. *Semin Arthroplasty* 2004; 15:83-86.)

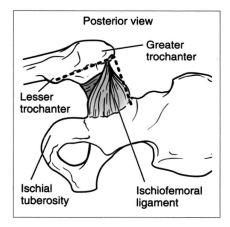

Figure 5 This posterior view of the hip capsule shows the capsular incision and the ischiofemoral ligament within the hip capsule from the surgeon's point of view. The L-shaped incision spares the ligament, allowing repair during closure of the incision.

palpate in a deep wound). Placement of a Charnley retractor deep to the gluteus maximus will hold the muscle apart and allow visualization of the trochanteric bursa, the posterior border of the gluteus medius muscle as it inserts into the greater trochanter, and the short external rotator muscles.

The next step is to expose the piriformis and the short external rotator muscles by excising or bluntly displacing the trochanteric bursa with a sponge. Hemostasis must be carefully maintained with cautery during this part of the exposure because the trochanteric bursa is well vascularized and there are often large veins lying over the piriformis tendon and the short rotator muscles. Palpate and protect the sciatic nerve as it exits the greater sciatic notch and proceeds distally over the ischial tuberosity (**Figure 3**) into the posterior compartment of the thigh. There is no need to expose the sciatic nerve.

A retractor placed under the posterior border of the gluteus medius muscle reveals the piriformis tendon as it courses toward its insertion in the piriformis fossa (**Figure 4**). The short external rotator muscles, consisting of the obturator externus, superior gemellus, obturator internus, inferior gemellus, and quadratus femoris, are also known as the conjoint tendon. The capsulotomy can be performed by creating a capsule-tendinous flap with the short rotator muscles and piriformis, or by dissecting the layers separately. Whether created in one layer with the overlying tendons or in two separate layers, the capsular flap should be tagged with a suture to facilitate anatomic repair at the time of wound closure.

The capsulotomy is an L-shaped incision that courses along the superior border of the piriformis tendon, starting at the acetabular rim and following the piriformis tendon down to its insertion in the piriformis fossa. The lower part of this L-shaped incision then extends distally along the intertrochanteric line of the femur and stops at the superior border of the quadratus femoris muscle. The reason for the L-shaped incision is to incorporate the strong ischiofemoral ligament of the posterior hip capsule (**Figure 5**).

Bone Preparation
With the capsular flap retracted posteriorly, the femoral head is exposed,

thus allowing posterior dislocation of the femoral head from the acetabulum. A femoral neck osteotomy can be performed with a sagittal saw. The surgeon must be careful not to notch the greater trochanter with the saw be-

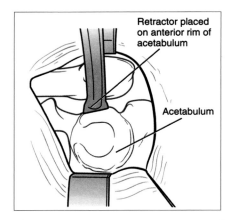

Figure 6 Elevation of the deep fibers of the anterior capsule from the anterior acetabular rim facilitates anterior translation of the femur to allow an unobstructed view of the acetabulum. (Reproduced with permission from Vail TP: Posterior mini-incision. *Semin Arthroplasty* 2004;15:83-86.)

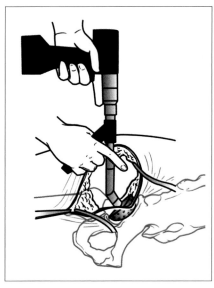

Figure 7 An angled reamer can be a useful adjunct to the posterior approach, allowing reaming without soft-tissue impingement.

cause a notch creates a stress riser that could lead to a fracture of the greater trochanter. Preoperative templating identifies the tip of the greater trochanter as an easily accessible reference point for making the neck cut. If femoral head dislocation is difficult, the femoral neck can be cut in situ before dislocation by resecting a segment of the femoral neck with two transverse cuts. Once this segment of the femoral neck is removed, the remaining femoral head bone can be pulled from the acetabulum by drilling into it with a threaded pin on a handle. With the femoral head removed, acetabular preparation can begin.

To successfully perform the mini posterior approach, the femur must be mobilized anteriorly to allow an unobstructed view of the acetabulum. Mobilization is facilitated by four critical steps: (1) elevation of the anterior hip capsule from the anterior rim of the acetabulum; (2) placement of a retractor under the femur and over the anterior rim of the acetabulum; (3) division of the inferior hip capsule, if tight; and (4) flexion/forward translation of the femur. The deep fibers of the anterior hip capsule can be seen

inserting into the anterior rim of the acetabulum when the femur is retracted forward. Elevating these fibers from the anterior rim with either a knife or cautery facilitates anterior translation of the femur and allows the anterior acetabular retractor to be placed onto the anterior rim under direct visualization. The anterior capsular fibers can be further elevated, if necessary, once the anterior retractor is in place (**Figure 6**).

The anterior acetabular retractor ideally has both a sharp tip and a light, thus allowing it to be securely placed into the anterior column and to illuminate the acetabulum. With the anterior retractor in place and the anterior capsular fibers elevated, the only remaining obstruction to adequate anterior femoral translation is the inferior capsule. It can be palpated and radially divided at the six o'clock position with electrocautery, provided that acetabular exposure is limited. Electrocautery is preferred because branches of the obturator artery can sometimes be encountered when dividing the inferior capsule. The transverse acetabular ligament does not at-

tach to the femur and does not need to be excised or divided unless it obstructs a clear view of osteophytes at the inferior border of the acetabulum.

The final step in acetabular exposure is flexion of the femur. Flexion, combined with adduction of the femur, helps move the femur anterior to the acetabulum and encourages the skin incision to move anteriorly and distally. Movement of the skin incision with the limb and retractors allows acetabular reaming without excessive skin tension.

With the femur retracted anteriorly, the degenerative acetabular labrum can be excised, marginal osteophytes on the acetabular rim can be removed, and acetabular reaming can begin. It may be helpful to remove the Charnley retractor at this point. A limited number of retractors in the incision make it easier to place the acetabular reamers without stretching the skin. Visualization requires only the anterior acetabular retractor and a Hibbs or Hohmann retractor, carefully placed posteriorly, without putting traction or applying pressure on the sciatic nerve. The posterior retractor needs to be placed in a different position for exposure and removed for reaming if its position interferes with the reamer.

Successful acetabular reaming requires creating a spherical socket shape and avoiding asymmetric or misdirected reaming. It is particularly important to ensure that the femur does not push the reamer into the posterior column and that the skin and soft tissue at the inferior aspect of the wound do not raise the reamer into the lateral rim of the acetabulum. Angled reamers and cup inserters can be valuable tools for navigating a small wound and avoiding soft-tissue impingement (**Figure 7**). A curette can be used to uncover the fovea to allow visualization of its floor, which is the landmark for the end point of medial reaming. Straight reamer handles allow more direct pressure and therefore more aggressive bone removal than angled reamer handles. Thus, it may be useful to start reaming with the straight handles and finish with the angled reamers once medialization is complete.

Femoral preparation is generally performed after placement of the acetabular component to minimize bleeding from the femoral canal. Limb positioning is important for femoral exposure. The hip should be flexed so that the femoral shaft aligns with the skin incision, and the proximal femur is pushed cephalad up into the wound as much as possible. The limb is internally rotated to 90° or more, and a narrow proximal femoral elevator is placed under the resected femoral neck. A second retractor, such as a sharp Hohmann retractor, can be placed medial to the calcar femorale, if necessary. The combination of limb positioning and retractor placement will allow exposure of the proximal femur, visualization of the calcar, and standard preparation with reamers and broaches. As with any approach, trial reduction should be performed to ensure implant fit, limb length, joint stability, and motion without impingement. An intraoperative radiograph is often useful to assess implant position, size, limb length, and offset restoration.

Prosthesis Implantation

Implanting the prosthesis requires carefully passing the components through the wound to avoid contamination by the skin edges or obstruction of the implant's porous surface by soft tissue. It is sometimes possible to protect the implant with a plastic wrapper before placing it into the wound, removing the plastic once the implant is in the wound but before its final seating. The principles of soft-tissue management reviewed above in the section on bone preparation are also relevant to prosthesis implantation, including movement of the limb

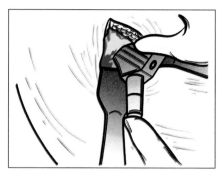

Figure 8 Once the femoral component is placed into the femoral canal, extension of the hip brings the trunion of the implant in line with the incision so that the implant can be fully seated.

and retractors to avoid excess skin tension.

For acetabular component placement, it is important to have the femur retracted forward to avoid risk of retroversion or vertical socket placement by bone or soft-tissue obstruction. Placing the final femoral component requires exposure of the proximal femur by limb positioning and retractor placement. A very small wound requires placing the femoral component partly into the femur with the hip flexed. The component neck or trunion may overhang the posterior edge of the wound (**Figure 8**), requiring movement of the hip into a more extended position to fully seat the femoral component. The femoral component can be implanted with direct visualization of the femoral neck osteotomy site to ensure full seating of the component without overimpaction that might result in femoral fracture.

Wound Closure

Wound closure should be preceded by thorough wound cleansing using a mechanical lavage system. Devitalized tissue should be sharply débrided. Skin edges should be carefully inspected, and any edges that appear macerated or damaged should be débrided. Removal of any damaged tissue will minimize the chance of wound dehiscence, infection, or hematoma. Hemostasis

should be ensured before closure. Particular attention should be directed to the inferior capsular branches of the obturator vessels and the branches of the medial femoral circumflex vessels running in the quadratus femoris muscle on the posterior aspect of the femoral neck. Suction drains can be placed, if necessary.

Repair of the hip capsule is the first step in wound closure. An intact hip capsule contributes to hip stability and increases the torque required to dislocate the hip joint. Several clinical studies support repair of the hip capsule, and link capsule repair to a lower dislocation rate.

The apex of the triangular capsular flap and piriformis tendon are pulled beneath the posterior border of the gluteus medius tendon toward the piriformis fossa. The suture is then passed through the gluteus medius tendon or trochanteric drill holes and tied over the top of the tendon. Passing the suture through the tendon maintains some compliance in the repair. The upper limb of the capsular repair can be strengthened by placing sutures directly into the hip capsule. The remainder of the wound is closed in layers, starting with the gluteus fascia and tensor fascia, proceeding to the subcutaneous layer, and finishing with nylon skin sutures or skin adhesive. A small, moisture-proof dressing is then applied.

Postoperative Regimen

The postoperative regimen focuses more on the implant than the approach used. Some surgeons using uncemented implants prefer to restrict weight bearing in the early postoperative period, citing concerns about bone ingrowth. However, there are protocols showing equally reliable bone ingrowth with early weight bearing in both tapered titanium and cylindrical cobalt chrome porous stems. Weight-bearing issues aside, most surgeons use a mini-incision in combination with accelerated rehabilitation for patients motivated to early discharge and quicker return to function than had previously been reported with standard incisions.

Preoperative protocols include thorough patient education and the use of nonsteroidal anti-inflammatory drugs. Other protocols include administering regional anesthetics, using long-acting oral narcotic agents postoperatively, and limiting use of intravenous narcotic agents. Patients on a "fast track" are typically mobilized the day of surgery and targeted for discharge in 48 to 72 hours if medically stable.

The pain management protocol includes a preoperative dose of a nonsteroidal anti-inflammatory drug the day before surgery and continuing during hospitalization. However, this protocol is modified based on patient comorbidities.

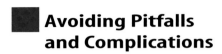

Avoiding Pitfalls and Complications

Some pitfalls in performing the mini posterior incision are related to poor visualization that can result in soft-tissue injury, inaccurate reaming, and suboptimal component placement. These pitfalls are avoided by lengthening the incision when the procedure becomes uncomfortable for the surgeon, or if excess pressure on soft tissue is required to place instruments into the appropriate position in the wound.

Mobilization of the femur anterior to the acetabulum is the most important step for accurate acetabular component placement.

An intraoperative radiograph with trial components in place is an extremely valuable preventive measure. The intraoperative radiograph provides real-time feedback regarding component position and hip mechanics while the surgeon can still make corrections before closing the wound. Gradual adoption of the mini posterior approach will ensure success without unexpected complications.

References

Berry DJ, Berger RA, Callaghan JJ, et al: Minimally invasive total hip arthroplasty: Development, early results, and critical analysis. *J Bone Joint Surg Am* 2003;85:2235-2246.

Chimento G, Sculco TP: Minimally invasive total hip arthroplasty. *Oper Tech Orthop* 2001;11:270-273.

DiGioia AM, Blendea S, Jaramaz B, Levison TJ: Less invasive total hip arthroplasty using navigational tools. *Instr Course Lect* 2004;53:157-164.

Waldman BJ: Advancements in minimally invasive total hip arthroplasty. *Orthopedics* 2003;26:S833-S836.

Weeden SH, Paprosky WG, Bowling JW: The early dislocation rate in primary total hip arthroplasty following the posterior approach with posterior soft-tissue repair. *J Arthroplasty* 2003;18:709-713.

Wenz JF, Gurkan I, Jibodh SR: Mini-incision total hip arthroplasty: A comparative assessment of perioperative outcomes. *J Orthopedics* 2002;25:1031-1043.

Coding

CPT Codes		Corresponding ICD-9 Codes		
27130	Arthroplasty, acetabular and proximal femoral prosthetic replacement (total hip arthroplasty), with or without autograft or allograft	711.45 711.95 714.0 714.30 715.15	715.25 715.35 716.15 718.5 718.6	720.0 733.14 733.42 808.0 905.6
27132	Conversion of previous hip surgery to total hip arthroplasty, with or without autograft or allograft	715.15 715.25 715.35 718.2	718.5 718.6 733.14 733.42	905.6 996.4 996.66 996.77

Chapter 4

Mini-Incision Total Hip Arthroplasty: Anterolateral Approach

William J. Hozack, MD
Matthew Austin, MD

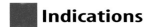 Indications

The indications for mini-incision total hip arthroplasty (THA) are the same as for traditional THA, with some additional criteria regarding patient selection and surgeon experience. The patient should have relatively uncomplicated degenerative joint disease and a body mass index (BMI) no higher than 30 kg/m^2. A thorough discussion with the patient about the risks and benefits of small incision surgery is critical, as is emphasizing realistic expectations regarding outcomes. The surgeon must have realistic expectations regarding incision size relative to the patient's body habitus and must be able to obtain adequate visualization for safe and proper component insertion. As with traditional THA, adequate exposure, minimal blood loss, and respect for the soft tissues apply to mini-incision techniques as well.

Contraindications

Mini-incision THA is not conducive to complicated primary THA, such as that associated with moderate to severe dysplasia or revision surgery, or for patients with a BMI that greatly exceeds 30 kg/m^2. One of the most important contraindications to using this approach is surgeon inexperience. Mini-incision THA should be approached gradually; surgeons should observe others who are facile with the technique before attempting the approach themselves. The surgeon should try to gradually minimize the size of the incision using the most familiar approach. A radical change from a traditional hip exposure to a minimal incision approach is fraught with potential complications and is a disservice to the patient.

Alternative Treatments

The alternative to the mini-incision approach is traditional THA through anterior, anterolateral, or posterior approaches.

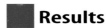 Results

The results of mini-incision THA are controversial. Some surgeons report excellent short-term results, whereas others report an increased incidence of complications. Current literature is insufficient to draw any definitive conclusions.

Technique

Acetabulum
The patient is placed in the supine position, which provides several advantages. Limb length is easily and accurately measured by simply palpating the malleoli without the use of external devices. The acetabular component can be positioned without concern for pelvic shift, as is common with the lateral decubitus position. Finally, the anatomic landmarks of the pelvis are easily palpated to assist in component orientation.

EXPOSURE
The anterolateral approach allows direct visualization of the muscle

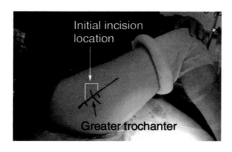

Figure 1 The incision is generally centered over the anterior third of the greater trochanter (arrow).

planes, acetabulum, and femur. Unlike the two-incision approach, the mini-incision approach does not require two-dimensional fluoroscopic imaging to appreciate three-dimensional surgical anatomy.

The length of the incision, which can range from 8 to 12 cm, depends on surgical skill, patient weight, local adipose thickness, muscle mass, stiffness, and anatomy. The incision should extend from the anterior third of the tip of the greater trochanter to a point several centimeters distal along the femoral shaft (**Figure 1**). This incision should be centered so that it can be extended proximally for femoral exposure or distally for acetabular exposure. In heavier patients, the greater trochanter cannot be precisely located until the incision extends into the fascial layer. In these patients, making a smaller initial incision into the fascia to help locate the greater trochanter is

advised before committing to a longer incision.

The initial incision extends down to the level of the fascia. The fat is then dissected from the fascia, creating a "mobile window" (**Figure 2**, *A*) that can be shifted to maximize visualization of the acetabulum and allow for adequate exposure of the proximal femur (**Figure 2**, *B*). The incision must be of sufficient length to extract the femoral head (**Figure 2**, *C*).

At this point, the most lateral aspect of the greater trochanter can be palpated. The fascial incision should be just anterior to this landmark. The anterior soft tissues are retracted, and the anterior and posterior borders of the gluteus medius are identified. The anterior third of the gluteus medius, the entire gluteus minimus, and the anterior half of the hip capsule are elevated as one flap. The vastus lateralis should be protected to minimize bleeding, swelling, and pain. This flap is analogous to a "curtain" that can be elevated to expose the acetabulum and femur (**Figure 3**), and it can be repaired anatomically. This flap can be accomplished with minimal trauma to the abductor muscles. The hip capsule is then incised in two locations: superiorly along the posterior border of the gluteus minimus tendon, and inferomedially just superior to the iliopsoas tendon. This technique of capsular incision rather than excision maximizes exposure yet maintains the integrity of

the hip capsule for improved stability and allows for full, unrestricted activity immediately after surgery.

Acetabular retractors specially designed to facilitate the mini-incision approach are placed in the following order: anterior, superior, inferior, and posterior (**Figure 4**). A cobra retractor is used anteriorly, placed with the hip flexed to relax the anterior neurovascular structures. The superior retractor is placed at the 10 o'clock position (right hip) or the 2 o'clock position (left hip). This retractor has been modified to accommodate a small incision approach and is now smaller and has a fiberoptic light. The initial inferior retractor is a double-angle device placed onto the ischium, which puts the pubofemoral ligament on stretch. The ligament is then incised, taking care not to violate the iliopsoas tendon. A double-footed retractor can replace the double-angle retractor if acetabular visualization is suboptimal. The incision also can be extended distally to improve exposure. The labrum and contents of the cotyloid fossa are resected. At this point, the entire periphery of the acetabulum should be visualized.

Before reaming, the anterior and posterior walls and columns, medial wall, and acetabular notch should be identified. The pelvis must be level to the floor. Proper placement of the acetabular retractors protects the skin

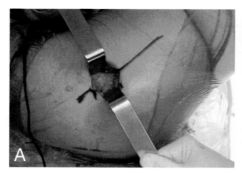
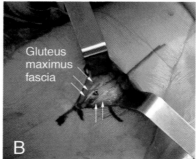
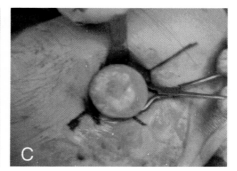

Figure 2 **A,** The "mobile window" allows soft tissues to be shifted for optimal visualization. **B,** Gluteus maximus and fascia lata are split. Note the anterior position of the split. **C,** The lower limit of incision size is limited by the size of the femoral head to be extracted.

from damage from the reamers, regardless of incision size.

BONE PREPARATION

Reaming should progress sequentially to form a hemisphere that is fully medialized with the inferior edge of the shell at the level of the teardrop. The anterior and posterior walls and columns should not be reamed away. The reamer heads may be disconnected from the reamer shaft while in the acetabulum to facilitate extraction (**Figure 5**).

PROSTHESIS IMPLANTATION

The cup is generally underreamed by 1 mm to obtain a press-fit. The component is then inserted under direct visualization. The pelvis is parallel to the floor, making component positioning easier. Excellent visualization of the acetabulum facilitates proper cup orientation. A curved cup insertion device is available for component insertion. Screws are generally not needed but may be used to improve initial fixation. At this point the liner is inserted.

Femur

EXPOSURE

The acetabular retractors are removed, and the limb is adducted and externally rotated. A double-footed retractor is placed posterior to the femur, and a second double-footed retractor is placed lateral to the femur (**Figure 6**). The retractors, if properly placed, will protect the soft tissues from injury during reaming, broaching, and insertion. Exposure can be improved by releasing the posterior capsule from the posterior femur to allow the limb greater adduction and to enhance visualization of the proximal femur (**Figure 7**). If exposure is still suboptimal, the incision can be extended proximally. The entire circumference of the proximal femur must be seen to assess version, axial stability, and rotational stability and to allow early de-

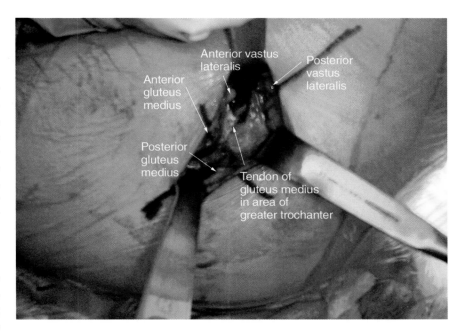

Figure 3 The soft-tissue curtain consisting of the anterior third of the gluteus medius, the entirety of the gluteus minimus, and the anterior half of the hip capsule.

tection of fracture during femoral preparation and component insertion.

BONE PREPARATION

The starter reamer is used to open the canal, and the femur is sequentially broached. The use of a single reamer to open the canal limits potential damage to the abductors.

PROSTHESIS IMPLANTATION

The broach serves as a trial component. A special head-neck insertion device is available to make trial reduction easier (**Figure 8**). The hip is then tested for stability, impingement, and limb length, and the final component is inserted.

Wound Closure

The incision is closed in layers, with careful attention directed to repair of the gluteus medius tendon (**Figure 9**). The hip can be internally rotated to facilitate repair. The gluteus maximus fascia and fascia lata are repaired with the hip in external rotation. The skin is closed with bioabsorbable suture and staples.

Postoperative Regimen

Bracing, hip precautions, or protected weight bearing typically are not required. Patients generally are encouraged to walk with a walker on the day of the procedure and with the aid of a physical therapist. The urinary catheter and all intravenous medications and fluids are discontinued, and the patient is encouraged to be out of bed as much as possible. While hospitalized, patients work with physical therapists twice daily.

No intravenous pain medication is used. Oral pain management consists of standardized, twice daily oxycodone during the inpatient stay and a COX-2 inhibitor unless the patient has a history of cardiac disease.

The patient is discharged 2 or 3 days postoperatively with crutches, depending on physical therapy goals. Patients generally progress to a cane by 2 weeks after discharge.

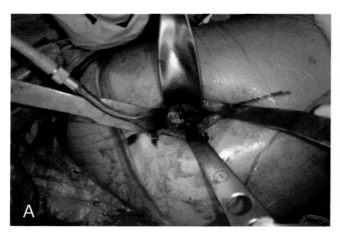

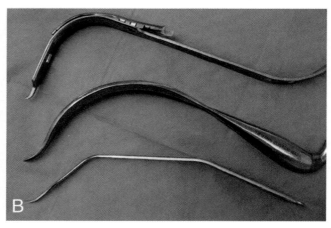

Figure 4 Acetabular exposure. **A,** The anterior retractor is placed through the anterior hip capsule just over the edge of the anterior acetabular rim. The superior lighted retractor is placed through the superior hip capsule and anchored into the ilium. The inferior retractor is placed into the ischium just inferior to the acetabular rim. The modified retractors and addition of a fiberoptic light result in excellent visualization of the acetabulum. **B,** The retractors used.

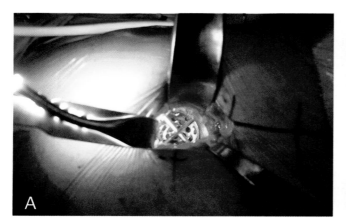

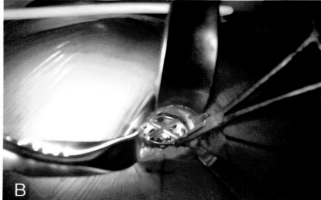

Figure 5 **A,** At times, it may be difficult to remove the reamer from the acetabulum because of soft-tissue impingement. **B,** In this situation, the reamer head is released from the reamer and removed separately from the acetabulum.

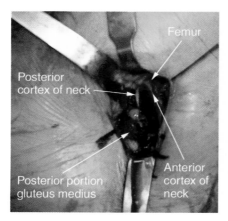

Femur

Posterior
cortex of neck

Posterior portion
gluteus medius

Anterior
cortex of
neck

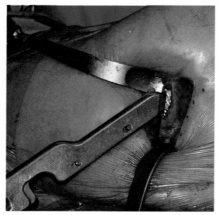

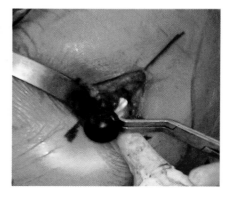

Figure 8 A special head-neck insertion device aids intraoperative assembly and trialing.

Figure 6 Femoral exposure. Note that the soft tissues are protected. The leg is adducted and externally rotated across the opposite limb (figure 4 position).

Figure 7 Release of the posterior capsule improves femoral exposure.

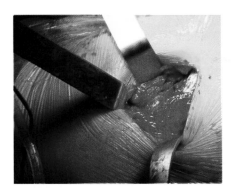

Figure 9 The gluteus medius prior to closure. Note the atraumatic technique. Closure is accomplished using bioabsorbable suture in which the anterior flap is sutured directly to the posterior flap.

Avoiding Pitfalls and Complications

The anterolateral mini-incision technique for THA balances the desire for less invasive surgery with the need for optimal visualization. Surgeons should not attempt an immediate radical change in surgical technique but should progress through a series of gradual steps aimed at reducing the size of the incision while maintaining a high priority on adequate exposure. The initial incision may be extended as needed to improve exposure and spatial orientation, thus ensuring accurate component positioning.

The incidence of serious complications, such as nerve injury, limb-length discrepancy, dislocation, and intraoperative fracture should not be greater than complication rates associated with the traditional approaches. Reaming away the medial wall or the acetabular supportive rim should be avoided because of direct visualization of the bony anatomy of the acetabulum. Fluoroscopic imaging is not required.

———————■

References

Ahrengart L: Periarticular heterotopic ossification after total hip arthroplasty: Risk factors and consequences. *Clin Orthop* 1991;263:49-58.

Barber TC, Roger DJ, Goodman SB, Schurman DJ: Early outcome of total hip arthroplasty using the direct lateral vs the posterior surgical approach. *Orthopedics* 1996;19:873-875.

Downing ND, Clark DI, Hutchinson JW, Colclough K, Howard PW: Hip abductor strength following total hip arthroplasty: A prospective comparison of the posterior and lateral approach in 100 patients. *Acta Orthop Scand* 2001;72:215-220.

Hardinge K: The direct lateral approach to the hip. *J Bone Joint Surg Br* 1982;64:17-19.

Masonis JL, Bourne RB: Surgical approach, abductor function, and total hip arthroplasty dislocation. *Clin Orthop* 2002;405:46-53.

Coding

CPT Codes		Corresponding ICD-9 Codes		
27125	Hemiarthroplasty, hip, partial (eg, femoral stem prosthesis, bipolar arthroplasty)	715.15 716.15 733.42	715.25 718.6 905.6	715.35 733.14
27130	Arthroplasty, acetabular and proximal femoral prosthetic replacement (total hip arthroplasty), with or without autograft or allograft	711.45 714.30 715.35 718.6 733.42	711.95 715.15 716.15 720.0 808.0	714.0 715.25 718.5 733.14 905.6
27132	Conversion of previous hip surgery to total hip arthroplasty, with or without autograft or allograft	715.15 718.2 733.14 996.4	715.25 718.5 733.42 996.66	715.35 718.6 905.6 996.77
27137	Revision of total hip arthroplasty; acetabular component only, with or without autograft or allograft	996.4	996.66	996.77
27236	Open treatment of femoral fracture, proximal end, neck, internal fixation or prosthetic replacement	733.14 820.10 820.8	820.00 820.12 820.9	820.03 820.13

CPT copyright © 2004 by the American Medical Association. All Rights Reserved.

Mini-Incision Total Hip Arthroplasty: Two-Incision Approach

Bassam A. Masri, MD, FRCSC
Victor T. Jando, MD, CM, FRCSC
Clive P. Duncan, MD, MSc, FRCSC

Indications

Several techniques of the so-called minimal incision total hip arthroplasty (MIS THA) have been described, despite the lack of consensus regarding its exact definition. Two categories of MIS THA have emerged: modified single-incision approaches and a two-incision approach. The single-incision approaches are modifications of the standard posterolateral, anterolateral, or anterior approaches commonly used for THA and are performed through 3- to 4-inch incisions. The two-incision technique, developed by Mears and refined by Berger, constitutes a radically different approach for THA and has been the subject of much controversy. The goal of this approach is to use strategically located incisions to insert the prosthesis components into specific intermuscular and internervous planes in an effort to minimize disruption of muscles and tendons and ultimately allow rapid rehabilitation. Note, however, that cemented components cannot be inserted using this technique. In addition to the change in surgical technique, changes in patient care pathways and rehabilitation are required to ensure maximum patient benefit. The indications for a two-incision THA are essentially the same as those for a standard uncemented THA, specifically the presence of disabling pain associated with advanced joint degeneration. The underlying causes may include osteoarthritis, rheumatoid arthritis, osteonecrosis, or mild acetabular dysplasia.

Contraindications

Although the indications seem to be broad, the complexity of the technique requires that the contraindications be carefully considered. As with any THA, adequate access to the acetabulum and proximal femur is essential, as is accurate component implantation without compromising soft-tissue and neurovascular structures. Along with the general contraindications to standard THA, a number of contraindications specific to the two-incision technique apply.

The most important contraindication is lack of appropriate surgeon training. This operation should not be attempted after simply reviewing a surgical technique manual, watching a videotape, or after reading a publication. Cadaveric training, mentoring, and proctoring are necessary to avoid potential serious complications.

Second, patient selection is key to avoid difficulties in exposure that may compromise the safety of the procedure. Obese patients are not candidates for two-incision MIS THA, particularly those who are significantly obese around the buttock and proximal thigh. Patients who are moderately obese around the center of the body but have slim lower limbs can be offered this procedure without much difficulty, provided that they are capable of rapid rehabilitation to achieve maximum benefit from the technique. Nevertheless, slim patients (body mass index of less than 25) should be selected for the first few cases; thereafter and in most cases, patients' body mass index should be less than 30. Very muscular male patients, even if they are not obese, similarly are not good candidates because they may pose difficulties with exposure, retraction, manipulation of the limb, and reduction of the hip. Finally, patients with significant contractures pose difficulties with this approach and in the soft-tissue balancing of the hip; thus, they are best treated with other surgical techniques.

Patients also may be excluded after thorough inspection of their radiographs. Those with severe hypertrophic changes, ankylosis, near ankylosis, heterotopic ossification, or moderate to severe protrusio acetabuli should be excluded. Patients with severe dysplasia (Crowe III or IV) also should be excluded. Patients with posttraumatic deformities, previous osteotomies, or retained hardware also are not candidates because of the difficulty in reconstructing the femur. The femur should be templated carefully in the lateral view to ensure that

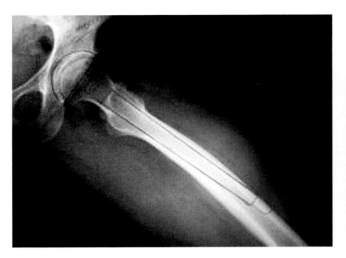

Figure 1 Lateral radiograph of the femur shows that the stem cannot fit because of the excessive bowing of the femur. Attempting a two-incision MIS THA may result in an intraoperative fracture. (Courtesy of Dr. Paul Duwelius).

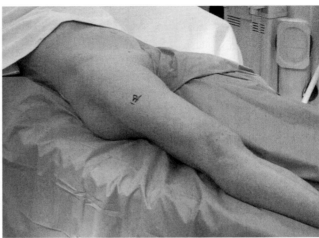

Figure 2 Proper placement in the supine position with adequate exposure.

the bow of the femur allows the use of a straight tapered or extensively coated stem. If there is an implant-bone conflict (**Figure 1**), a fracture may occur, and other techniques should be used. Finally, patients with significant osteoporosis or very small or very large femoral canals should be excluded because of the risk of fracture or undersizing of the stem.

We acknowledge that these contraindications seem strict and that they clearly encompass a spectrum of severity. However, with surgeon experience and improved competence with the technique, some of these contraindications may be relaxed. We want to stress that two-incision MIS THA is technically demanding, and patients with characteristics that may pose additional difficulty should be excluded by most surgeons.

Alternative Treatments

The patient's body habitus and radiographic appearance of the bony anatomy are used to determine whether a two-incision approach can be used. If a two-incision approach is contraindi-

cated, then one of the standard incisions can be used. One advantage of the anterolateral and posterolateral approaches is that a small incision can easily be converted to a more extensile approach.

Results

The only published results of this technique to date are the combined experience of four surgeons who reported on 375 patients with short-term follow-up. This work, however, has not been peer reviewed. The most common significant complication was intraoperative fracture of the proximal femur, usually in the calcar region, which occurred in six patients. All fractures requiring treatment were fixed with cerclage wire and healed without loosening of the femoral component. Neurologic injuries consisted of two partial femoral nerve palsies, both of which resolved, and neurapraxias of the lateral cutaneous nerve to the thigh that resolved in 9 of 16 patients. Other reported complications included dislocation (two patients; both posterior), mild heterotopic ossification (two patients), deep vein thrombosis (one patient), and

late infection (one patient at 9 months postoperatively). Stem subsidence of 5 mm was also noted in one patient, but the patient was asymptomatic. Long-term results are not available at this time, and the durability of prostheses inserted using the two-incision technique is unknown.

Technique

Patient Positioning

The patient should be placed in a supine position on a radiolucent table or a standard operating table that may be adapted by the addition of a radiolucent extension to allow intraoperative fluoroscopy (**Figure 2**). Next, an inflatable bolster is placed under the ipsilateral buttock. This bolster serves two purposes: it allows the appropriate surgical preparation and draping of the buttock; and it elevates the buttock off of the table to simplify femoral preparation. With experience, however, we now use a noninflatable bolster for draping and subsequently remove it before the acetabular component is inserted. The operative limb is then free draped with as much proximal, medial, and posterior exposure

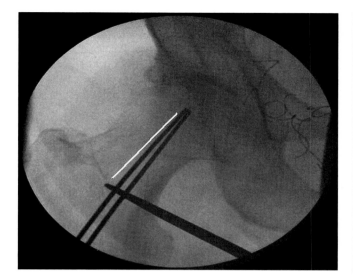

Figure 3 Fluoroscopic view of the hip joint. The tip of the proximal forceps points to the posterior acetabular margin, and the tip of the distal forceps points to the intertrochanteric line. The white line represents the anterior incision.

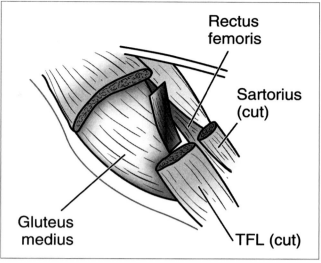

Figure 4 The superficial plane of dissection for the anterior incision is between the tensor fascia lata (TFL) and the sartorius muscles, which are shown as detached in this illustration. This allows access to the deep plane of dissection between the rectus femoris and the gluteus medius.

as possible. The drapes are typically placed at the abdominal midline, above the iliac crest, and as posteriorly and superiorly to the greater trochanter as possible. The use of towel clips or drape tape may facilitate holding the drapes in place prior to application of an adhesive surgical sheet.

The Acetabulum
EXPOSURE

Skin Incision   The surface landmark is a line that joins the anterosuperior iliac spine and the tip of the greater trochanter. The incision is typically located three to four fingerbreadths distal, medial, and parallel to this line and is confirmed with fluoroscopy by drawing a line that connects the posterior margin of the acetabulum to the intertrochanteric line (**Figure 3**). Typically, the incision is 1.5 to 2 inches in length, but its exact length is of little relevance to the technique; therefore, the surgeon should not hesitate to extend it somewhat if there is excessive skin tension or potential skin compromise. A longer incision does not necessarily help with exposure unless a large acetabular component is to be

inserted. In that case, a larger incision prevents contact between the component and the edge of the skin. The area of dissection is typically quite thin in most patients. Sharp dissection should be reserved for the skin incision only. Subsequent deeper dissection can be done bluntly.

Deep Dissection   The remainder of the exposure follows a modified Smith-Peterson approach to the hip in which the plane of dissection is initially between the sartorius and the tensor fascia lata muscles. This is not only an intermuscular plane but also an internervous plane between the femoral and superior gluteal nerves, respectively. This plane is easier to palpate distally within the incision. The fascia is then incised in that location, or slightly more laterally, to avoid injuring the lateral cutaneous nerve, and the dissection is extended proximally. Blunt dissection is used to develop this interval.

Deep within the distal end of this interval lies a leash of vessels that constitutes the anterior ascending branches of the lateral femoral circumflex vessels. These vessels are im-

portant not only because of their propensity to bleed if cut but also because they confirm that the interval dissected is the correct one. A more medial interval, just medial to the sartorius muscle, will place the femoral nerve at risk. If these vessels are not visualized, the surgeon should reexamine the landmarks and reestablish the correct interval. If in doubt, the dissecting finger may be extended proximally until the anterosuperior iliac spine is located. The dissection planes should be lateral to the origin of the sartorius muscle. Once the vessels are located, the tensor fascia lata and the sartorius muscles are retracted using right-angle retractors or "Army-Navy" retractors, and the vessels are carefully and completely ligated or coagulated. Significant bleeding may result if this step is neglected.

The deep plane is next identified between the rectus femoris medially and the gluteus medius laterally (**Figure 4**). Ligation of the anterior branches of the lateral femoral circumflex allows safe retraction of the rectus femoris muscle medially. A Cobb elevator is then used to develop

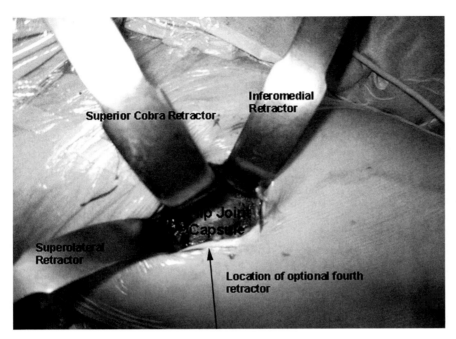

Figure 5 Proper positioning of the cobra retractors, which allows an excellent, unimpeded view of the hip joint capsule.

the interval between the capsule and overlying rectus femoris muscle. Palpation of the femoral head during hip rotation will confirm that the surgeon has reached the capsule. The hip joint capsule is then exposed by placing a narrow cobra retractor superiorly at the junction between the superior pubic ramus and the anterior acetabular wall, typically in the region of the reflected head of the rectus femoris muscle. A second, narrow cobra retractor is then placed over the superolateral aspect of the hip joint capsule, perpendicular to the long axis of the femoral neck, and a third narrow cobra retractor is placed over the inferomedial aspect of the hip joint capsule perpendicular to the long axis of the femoral neck (**Figure 5**). The precise placement of these retractors is critical for exposure, and even slight deviation may significantly compromise the exposure. If the visualization is not satisfactory, subtle repositioning of the retractors significantly improves exposure, which is learned with experience. Care is needed when placing the inferomedial retractor to prevent

injury to the femoral nerve. This retractor should be lateral to the iliacus muscle at all times. If the retractor is placed medial to the muscle, the femoral nerve may be compromised. Although this next step is optional, we find that the placement of a fourth cobra retractor (**Figure 5**) over the tip of the greater trochanter is quite helpful not only to help retract the anterior border of the abductors but also to allow the direct visualization and palpation of the greater trochanter, which will facilitate the femoral neck osteotomy later in the procedure.

This retractor arrangement gives excellent exposure of the anterior aspect of the hip joint capsule in preparation for the hip joint capsulotomy. A linear, T-shaped, inverted T-shaped, or an H-shaped capsulotomy may be performed at this time. We prefer using an H-shaped capsulotomy from the edge of the acetabulum to the intertrochanteric line. Gentle flexion of the hip joint at this stage will allow easy palpation of the vastus tubercle, which helps locate the intertrochanteric line without the need for fluoros-

copy. We typically move the image intensifier away from the surgical field after the incision is made because it is not required for any of the above dissection. The superolateral and inferomedial cobra retractors are then reinserted in an intracapsular location but in a similar arrangement. The capsular flaps should be retained for repair at the end of the procedure.

BONE PREPARATION

Osteotomy of the Femoral Neck It is nearly impossible to dislocate the hip using the two-incision approach without first performing an in situ osteotomy of the femoral neck. The distal level of the osteotomy must be precisely referenced. First, the distance between (1) the vertical limb and the tip of the greater trochanter and (2) the neck osteotomy and the superolateral aspect of the femoral neck is measured on preoperative radiographs. Intraoperatively, the neck cut is marked on the surface of the bone using electrocautery with reference to these two landmarks. Finally, the image intensifier is used to confirm the distance from the top of the greater trochanter to the neck cut. Because the magnification of the image intensifier is not known, measurements are not exact; however, we correlate that distance as a proportion of the length of the lesser trochanter.

Once the location is confirmed, the neck cut is made initially using a reciprocating saw for the vertical limb of the osteotomy (**Figure 6**, *A*, line 1) and an oscillating saw for the horizontal limb (**Figure 6**, *A*, line 2), taking great care to avoid extending the cut through the greater trochanter. Use of a fourth cobra retractor over the tip of the greater trochanter is helpful in this regard. Once the neck cut is completed, traction is applied to the leg, and an osteotome is placed within the cut and gently rotated to ensure that the neck osteotomy is complete. A third cut is made with the oscillating saw, beginning at the femoral head-

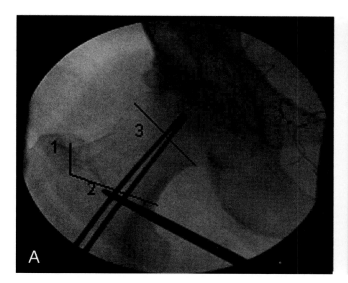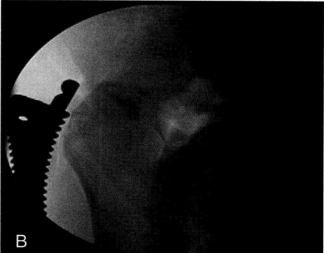

Figure 6 **A,** The sequence of femoral neck cuts is shown by the numbers in ascending order. **B,** After the femoral neck cuts are completed, a broach may be placed next to the femur at the level of the bone to help the surgeon estimate the distance between the neck cut and the lesser trochanter. The surgeon can count the teeth on the broach and then measure the broach to determine the exact distance between the femoral neck cut and the lesser trochanter. This is an alternate method to what is described in the text.

neck junction (**Figure 6**, *A*, line 3). The saw should be parallel or slightly convergent posteriorly to the horizontal neck cut to create a wedge of bone that can be easily removed. In this orientation, the saw will avoid inadvertent osteotomy of the posterior wall of the acetabulum. An osteotome is placed in the second neck cut to ensure that it is free. The interposed neck segment is then removed using a threaded Steinmann pin or a Schanz screw. Finally, the femoral head is removed using a threaded Steinmann pin or corkscrew in combination with a spoon elevator or by morcellization in situ. Some traction distally on the limb will create additional space to aid in removal of the femoral head.

Acetabular Preparation To achieve adequate exposure of the acetabulum, at least three narrow cobra retractors are used: one is positioned directly superiorly over the rim of the acetabulum; the second and third retractors are placed opposite each other over the anteroinferior and posteroinferior rims of the acetabulum. These retractors may be angled or repositioned slightly to create a "mobile window" that allows complete visualiza-

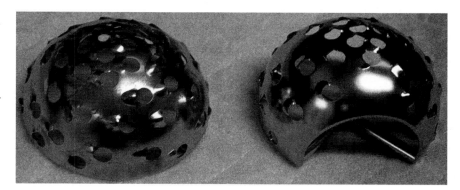

Figure 7 Standard hemispheric reamer (right) next to the modified cut-off reamer (left).

tion of the acetabulum. Any remaining labrum is excised, and the cotyloid notch medially is exposed by removing any remaining synovial tissue or remnant of the ligamentum teres. The inferior acetabular ligament is exposed to identify the inferior acetabular margin.

At this time, the bolster either has been or should be deflated or removed from beneath the buttock so that the reaming can be directed toward the plane of the table with the patient supine. The acetabulum is then reamed in a fashion similar to a standard THA. Modified cut-off reamers can be used because they are easier to insert into the acetabulum, but we prefer standard

reamers because they work well in our hands (**Figure 7**). Note that the direction of reaming is not familiar to most surgeons because of the patient's position. The angle between the reamer shaft and the sagittal plane bisecting the patient is the so-called abduction angle, which should be about 40°. The angle between the reamer handle and the plane of the operating table surface is the anteversion angle, which should be about 20°. Because of the patient's supine position and the presence of the thigh, overanteversion is a common error. This problem can be avoided by keeping the hand pushed down toward the table as much as possible. Fluoros-

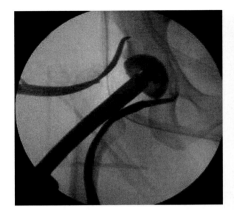

Figure 8 The accuracy of acetabular reaming may be verified radiographically.

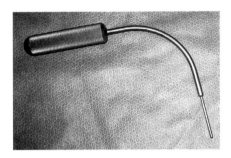

Figure 10 A curved awl is used to help locate the posterior incision.

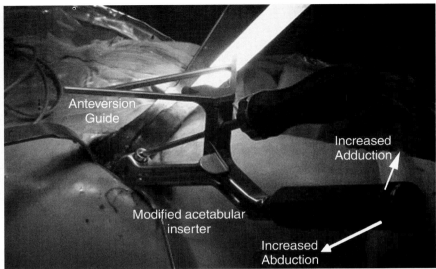

Figure 9 Intraoperative photograph shows use of a modified curved acetabular inserter. The anteversion guide must be parallel to the floor to ensure anteversion of 20°. In this photograph, the position of the socket is too anteverted but can be corrected if the surgeon brings his or her hand toward the floor. To control for abduction and adduction of the socket, the handle of the insertion device is moved either in the direction of the solid arrow to increase abduction or in the direction of the dashed arrow to reduce abduction.

copy may be used to verify the alignment and medialization of the reamers until the surgeon gains adequate experience with this approach (**Figure 8**). Placing the limb in slight flexion may facilitate introduction of the reamers into the wound. Minimizing the number of times the reamers are inserted and extracted avoids unnecessary trauma to the surrounding soft tissues.

PROSTHESIS IMPLANTATION
Once the acetabulum has been prepared, cobra retractors are kept in the same position and care is taken to prevent the soft tissues from invaginating between the component and the prepared acetabular bed. The definitive prosthesis is impacted into 40° of abduction and 20° of anteversion using a specially designed curved inserter (**Figure 9**), with an alignment guide that is especially designed for the supine position. This curved inserter al-

lows the proximal femur to be cleared, minimizing the risk of malpositioning the socket in excessive anteversion or abduction. Proper cup alignment is confirmed with fluoroscopy during impaction and once it is fully seated. For final confirmation, the retractors may need to be removed to avoid obscuring the image. If augmentation of the initial press-fit fixation is necessary, one or two screws may be inserted in the postero-superior quadrant using a flexible drill and an articulated screw driver. Finally, acetabular rim osteophytes are removed with an osteotome or rongeur, and the definitive liner can be inserted.

At this stage, the lesser trochanter may be brought into view by flexion, adduction, and external rotation of the lower limb. This way, the level of the femoral neck cut can be confirmed one final time before moving to the femoral preparation (**Figure 6**, *B*).

The Femur
EXPOSURE
Skin Incision The inflatable bolster, if used, is reinflated at this stage. The lo-

cation of the posterior skin incision should allow straight reamer and rasp access to the femoral canal. Because of the bow in the proximal femur, the incision tends to be more posterior and more proximal than anticipated. A more anteriorly placed incision results in an oblique pathway into the femur, resulting in reaming of the anterior cortex and an increased risk of proximal femoral fracture. One method to identify the correct location of the posterior skin incision is to use the intersection of colinear lines drawn along the long axes of the femur over both the anterior and the lateral thigh. The leg should be positioned in about 15° to 20° of adduction, neutral rotation, and slight flexion. The proper location of the posterior incision is then confirmed by passing a curved awl (**Figure 10**) through the anterior incision and behind the edge of the short rotators and the posterior margin of the gluteus medius and minimus complex through the posterior capsule. The curved awl is then palpated through the skin of the buttock, and a 0.25-inch oblique incision is made over it. This incision is

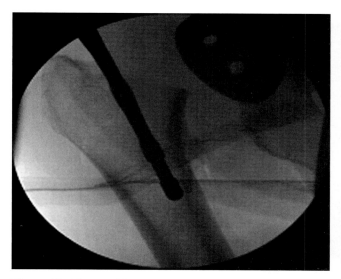

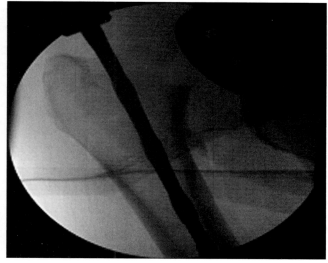

Figure 11   The tip of the lateralizing reamers should be just distal to the trochanter (left), not well distal to it (right).

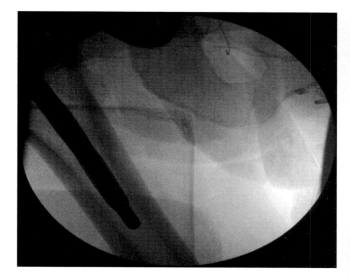

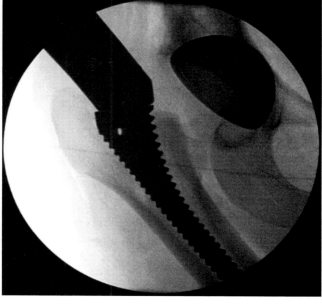

Figure 12   Fluoroscopy is used to ensure central reaming of the medullary canal to the correct depth. This is one of the first few reamers; further reaming is needed in this example.

Figure 13   Fluoroscopy is used to guide broaching of the femur.

subsequently extended into a 1- to 1.5-inch incision once the accurate location of the incision is confirmed.

Dissection   The fascia over the gluteus maximus is divided with electrocautery, and the fibers of the muscle are spread with scissors. This is the only intramuscular plane of dissection in this procedure. Long scissors are then passed through this rent in the gluteus maximus and behind the glu-

teus medius-minimus complex and short external rotators, which are not detached from their insertion into the piriformis fossa. The scissors are then guided by the surgeon's other hand, which has been placed through the anterior incision, until the tips pass into the medullary canal of the femur. Once intraosseous placement of the scissors is confirmed, the scissors are withdrawn slowly, as the jaws of the

scissors are opened to enlarge the entry point within the posterior capsule.

BONE PREPARATION

The leg must be kept in adduction, neutral rotation, and slight flexion to maintain the coaxial relationship between the femoral canal and the soft-tissue interval that extends to the posterior wound. With a soft-tissue protector in place, a Charnley awl is in-

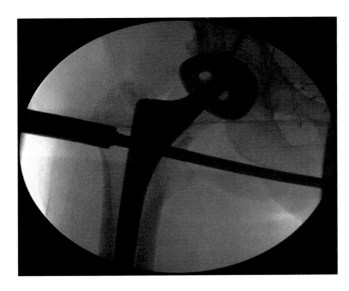

Figure 14 Fluoroscopy is used to ensure proper seating of the stem. The straight rod shown in this example references the lesser trochanter to the ischial tuberosities in both hips to ensure equalization of limb length.

serted from the posterior wound and directed into the piriformis fossa to gain access into the intramedullary canal. Fluoroscopy is used to confirm the position of the awl within the canal.

Because a box osteotome cannot be used to lateralize the entry point into the femur and thus ensure central placement of the stem within the intramedullary canal, side-cutting reamers are used to remove the remaining bone off of the medial aspect of the greater trochanter and to achieve proper lateralization. These lateralizing reamers have a blunt tip and should be inserted just distal to the lesser trochanter (**Figure 11**) and centrally in the anteroposterior plane. They are then sequentially increased in size up to the anticipated size of the femoral stem. They are inserted with a power reamer but not advanced distally; rather, they remove bone by moving laterally, pivoting against the blunt distal tip, which is placed just distal to the lesser trochanter. A channel is created within the lateral-most portion of the calcar during lateralization. Digital palpation ensures that this channel is central in the anteroposterior plane. Errors are easily corrected by moving the power reamer anteriorly or posteriorly as required. Fluoroscopy is used intermittently to ensure that reaming is

performed in neutral alignment and to the correct depth.

Next, distal reaming is done with flexible and/or straight reamers (**Figure 12**), followed by sequential broaching (**Figure 13**) until the broach is stable according to the surgical technique for the desired stem. It is useful to look through the anterior incision as the broach is torqued, as is done in an open THA, to ensure broach stability. Digital palpation alone can be quite misleading, and it is easy to undersize the stem unless visual confirmation is made through the anterior incision. Intermittent fluoroscopic images are used to ensure proper insertion of the reamers and broaches.

The limb must be kept in the same position (with the patella pointing up) during broaching to maintain the same degree of anteversion and to match the definitive stem anteversion with the broach anteversion. Capsular entrapment between the broach and the calcar may impede further broach advancement. If this happens, a partial posterior capsular release using electrocautery along the broach is necessary to allow proper seating of the broach and to facilitate transfer of the neck of the prosthesis from the posterior incision into the anterior incision to allow definitive reduction of the arthroplasty. This release is done under

direct visualization through the anterior incision with proper retraction and protection of any structures that may be at risk.

It is almost impossible to reattach the broach handle to the broach if the broach is detached. For this reason, it is necessary to use a locking broach handle, and the surgeon should check the locking mechanism before each successive broaching. Also, it is not possible to perform a trial reduction with the broach. The only trial reduction is performed after definitive implantation of the stem. This is why preoperative planning is of utmost importance with this technique.

PROSTHESIS IMPLANTATION

With the leg in the same position as during broaching, the femoral prosthesis is inserted through the posterior wound and advanced into the femoral canal. Initially, the prosthesis is malrotated by 180°, but once the femoral neck clears the skin incision, it is rotated into correct alignment and is advanced by hitting it with the stem inserter, which typically has an anteversion guide to maintain correct anteversion during stem advancement. We typically use the 7.5° of anteversion setting. Alignment and depth of insertion are guided by fluoroscopy (**Figure 14**) and confirmed by direct visualization through the anterior wound. These assessments must be made before the femoral component is fully seated to avoid fracture of the proximal femur. Through the anterior wound, the surgeon should ensure that no soft tissues are caught between the stem and prepared femur. It may be necessary to release more of the posterior capsule to allow delivery of the femoral neck into the joint. Before attempting a trial reduction, the surgeon should communicate to the anesthesiologist the need for full neuromuscular relaxation, particularly if the procedure is being done under general anesthesia.

A trial reduction is performed after the neck of the prosthesis is delivered into the anterior incision. This is done with one assistant applying traction to the leg while the surgeon maneuvers the neck into the anterior incision using a large bone hook and applies gentle flexion, abduction, and external rotation. The collar and the neck of the prosthesis occasionally cannot be delivered into the anterior incision unless a linear cut is made along the neck of the implant using electrocautery to release any tethered capsule. Once the neck is delivered into the anterior incision, side-mounting trial femoral heads are inserted onto the trunnion. We recommend placing a suture through the holes of the trial head so that it may be easily retrieved should it inadvertently disengage. Because of the small incision, the head may be lost in the buttock if this is not done. After the trial head component is inserted, the hip is reduced with gentle traction and internal rotation. Hip stability is then checked using standard maneuvers, and limb-length is checked by approximating the ankles and ensuring that the medial malleoli are at the same level, provided that the pelvis is level on the table. Limb length also may be verified fluoroscopically by comparing the level of the lesser trochanters to the obturator foramina or ischial tuberosities (**Figure 14**).

Once the correct neck length has been determined, the trial component is removed and the definitive head is impacted onto the Morse taper of the stem using a side-hitting femoral head impactor (**Figure 15**). The definitive components are then reduced, and the wounds copiously irrigated with normal saline solution.

Wound Closure

Suture repair of the anterior capsule should be attempted to increase postoperative stability. The use of local anesthetic may assist in postoperative pain control. We inject a local anesthetic mixture of 200 to 300 mg of ropivicaine (depending on patient size),

5 mg of morphine, and 1 mL of 1:1,000 epinephrine, diluted with normal saline solution for a total volume of 100 mL. The mixture is infiltrated into the capsule and surrounding soft tissues (avoiding the femoral neurovascular bundle medially), as well as the subcutaneous tissues and skin for both anterior and posterior wounds. Posteriorly, the fascia over the gluteus maximus is repaired. Anteriorly, the fascia between the sartorius and tensor fascia lata is repaired with care to avoid entrapment of the lateral femoral cutaneous nerve. The subcutaneous tissues are then reapproximated, and the skin is closed with bioabsorbable subcuticular suture. The use of a suction drain in the anterior incision for a few hours postoperatively is optional but may reduce the risk of hematoma formation or excessive drainage. The wounds are covered with small occlusive dressings just long enough to cover the length of each incision.

Postoperative Regimen

All patients are mobilized on the day of surgery, with weight bearing as tolerated and the assistance of a physical therapist. Patients are taught safe ambulation skills with walking aids in preparation for their discharge the next day. To this end, all patients receive intensive preoperative education to ensure that the appropriate supports are in place and that the home environment is safe.

Preemptive analgesia with 1,000 mg of acetaminophen and 20 mg of sustained-release oxycodone and an anti-inflammatory are used preoperatively. Celecoxib is held in patients with a cardiac history, and oxycodone is held if the anesthesiologist has used intrathecal morphine. Regional anesthesia is our preferred method of anesthesia. Acetaminophen and celecoxib are continued, along with regular oxycodone, for the first few postoperative days. Oxycodone is given for breakthrough pain. Thromboembolic prophylaxis is achieved using low molec-

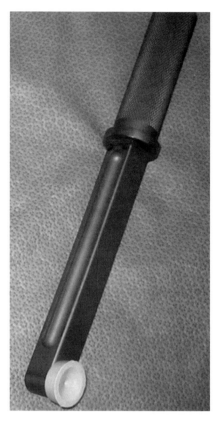

Figure 15 The side-hitting femoral head impactor is useful for the final impaction of the femoral head on the Morse taper through a limited incision.

ular weight heparin for 10 days for low-risk patients and up to 35 days for high-risk patients. All patients receive prophylactic antibiotics preoperatively and for 24 hours postoperatively.

Physical therapy is started in the hospital and is continued by a home care physical therapist or at an outpatient facility, depending on the patient's individual needs.

Avoiding Pitfalls and Complications

The potential advantages of this technique are lower dislocation rates and more rapid rehabilitation and discharge from hospital, typically 1 to 2 days after the procedure. Same-day discharge also is possible with this technique. The main disadvantage, however, is the higher risk of intraoperative fracture, particularly if the surgeon has little experience with the technique. Fractures of the proximal femur are most common, but distal fractures also have been reported. The reasons for these fractures are numerous but may be related to some pitfalls that may be easy to avoid.

Improper lateralization may lead to varus placement of the stem, with a potential for perforation or fracture. Proper lateralization will avoid this problem. Insertion of the lateralizing reamers too far distally initially also may cause fracture as a result of either excessive leverage on the lateral femur or reaming away of medial bone. With the latter, the cutting teeth of the reamer may come in contact with the medial bone stock as the reamer is levered laterally. This also should be avoided. Entering the femur from an anterior direction allows reaming of the anterior cortex, which also increases the risk of fracture. For this reason, proper placement of the posterior incision is critical. Similarly, avoiding excessive valgus or varus placement of reamers or broaches reduces the risk of fracture.

Reaming to the correct depth is important when using an extensively porous-coated stem; otherwise, the risk of fracture is increased. Reaming too distal in the canal may compromise the anterior cortex, and insufficient distal reaming may lead to reamer-stem mismatch, which increases the hoop stresses within the femur and can lead to fracture.

Failure to maintain the same rotational alignment between the broaches and the stem leads to proximal femoral fracture. Thus, proper position of the leg in space is essential while the stem is being inserted. Attempting to insert the stem deeper than the broach also may result in a fracture. If the neck cut is too long and then subsequently revised, reaming and broaching to the new correct depth should be repeated before stem insertion.

Soft-tissue complications also have been reported. Attempting to use an incision that is simply too small to easily insert the components requires vigorous retraction, which can compromise the wound edges, increase the risk of wound-edge necrosis, and potentially increase the risk of infection. The soft tissue should be handled as gently as possible to avoid these problems. Use of the anterior approach puts the lateral femoral nerve at inherent risk; therefore, all patients should be advised about this risk preoperatively. Straying too far medially during the anterior portion of the procedure will compromise the femoral nerve and possibly the femoral vessels.

References

Berger RA: The technique of minimally invasive total hip arthroplasty using the two-incision approach. *Instr Course Lect* 2004;53:149-155.

Berger RA, Duwelius PJ: The two-incision minimally invasive total hip arthroplasty: Technique and results. *Orthop Clin North Am* 2004;35:163-172.

Berry DJ, Berger RA, Callaghan JJ, et al: Minimally invasive total hip arthroplasty: Development, early results, and a critical analysis. *J Bone Joint Surg Am* 2003;85:2235-2246.

Irving JF: Direct two-incision total hip replacement without fluoroscopy. *Orthop Clin North Am* 2004;35:173-181.

Mears DC: Development of a two-incision minimally invasive total hip replacement. *J Bone Joint Surg Am* 2003;85:2238-2240.

Coding				
CPT Code		**Corresponding ICD-9 Codes**		
27130	Arthroplasty, acetabular and proximal femoral prosthetic replacement (total hip arthroplasty), with or without autograft or allograft	711.45 711.95 714.0 714.30 715.15	715.25 715.35 716.15 718.5 718.6	720.0 733.14 733.42 808.0 905.6

CPT copyright © 2004 by the American Medical Association. All Rights Reserved.

Chapter 6

Primary Total Hip Arthroplasty: Preoperative Planning and Templating

Kevin L. Garvin, MD

Introduction

The primary goals for total hip arthroplasty (THA), pain relief and improvement of function, are affected by the precision of the surgical procedure. Templating improves the surgeon's ability to restore limb length and offset precisely, place the components accurately, and ensure proper implant selection based on the patient's anatomy. This chapter provides guidelines for templating and surgical reconstruction of the hip based on preoperative planning.

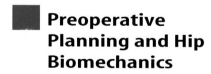

Preoperative Planning and Hip Biomechanics

Comprehensive preoperative planning is critically important for a successful outcome in THA. A comprehensive history and physical examination, including radiographs of the affected limb, are essential because they may reveal medical diagnoses that dictate further evaluation by the patient's internist or other specialists. These specialists also are frequently asked to assist with the perioperative management of the patient.

Once the patient's health is determined to be acceptable for anesthesia and surgery, the next step is templating of the hip. Restoration of hip biomechanics (including limb length and offset) can be considered a critical secondary goal and is a major factor in obtaining excellent results.

Better postoperative function is increasingly important as younger patients undergo THA. With the advent of new materials, longevity of the implant system will gradually be taken for granted. Any appreciable limb-length discrepancy and failure to obtain adequate offset can compromise the patient's function and biomechanics after THA. Malalignment and the imbalance of resulting forces can affect more than function; by causing increased micromotion and loosening, they also influence the long-term success of THA.

In one study, lengthening of the operated leg was determined to be an important factor in explaining aseptic loosening of the prosthesis. Data from other studies indicate that a limb-length inequality of 10 mm leads to an asymmetric increase in muscle group activity and lateral imbalance in the erect posture. The lumbar spine is subjected to sagittal and rotational stresses. The hip on the side of the longer leg is subjected to greater stresses at the articulating surfaces, and these stresses are believed to pro-mote chondral damage and unilateral arthrosis. Limb-length discrepancy is one of the easiest parameters by which the quality of a THA can be quantified; therefore, it is bound to be of increased interest. Of the 14,979 orthopaedic malpractice claims in the United States from 1985 to 1998, 29% involved joint procedures (ranked as number one). Patient dissatisfaction because of unequal limb length is the type of imperfection after surgery that can lead to claims of "improper performance of surgery" and can result in legal action. Patients ranked unequal limb length similarly to nighttime pain, difficulty with standing, difficulty with toileting, and difficulty with sexual activity.

The interest in research focusing on the measurement and assurance of quality in performing THA has attracted much recent attention, especially with the increased use of navigation and other computer-assisted surgery tools.

Measurements in hip replacement, limb length, and offset have clear definitions and can be quantified accurately. True limb-length discrepancy is an absolute difference in the length of the limbs as measured by scanography or, more typically, from the anterior spine to the medial malleolus. Placing standing blocks under the foot is another measurement technique. Functional (ie, apparent) limb-length discrepancy is caused by tightness of the soft tissues, primarily the adductors, or a fixed obliquity of the lumbosacral spine. Five degrees of such deformity causes a 1.6-cm limb-length discrepancy.

Femoral offset is the distance (along the mediolateral direction) from the center of the femoral head to a line bisecting the long axis of the femur (**Figure 1**, *A*). Femoral compo-nent (stem) offset is the distance (along the mediolateral direction) from the center of rotation of the pros-thetic femoral head to a line bisecting the long axis of the stem (**Figure 1**, *B*). Larger offset results in less impinge-ment of components and reduces the need for skirted heads, which may im-pinge on the acetabular component. Increased offset also enhances soft-tis-sue tension, resulting in increased hip stability or less risk of dislocation. Be-cause increased offset improves lever-age, it reduces the abductor muscle force needed, thereby improving effi-ciency and gait. The reduced abductor muscle force, in turn, results in a smaller compressive force across the hip joint and decreased stresses in the articulating surfaces with understand-able improvement in prosthesis wear. Strain of the proximal femur, cement, and femoral prosthesis is not signifi-cantly altered by an increase in offset in vivo. However, there is some concern about a relationship between large off-set femoral stems and failure of fixa-tion if the geometry of the stem makes it difficult to achieve an adequate ce-ment mantle.

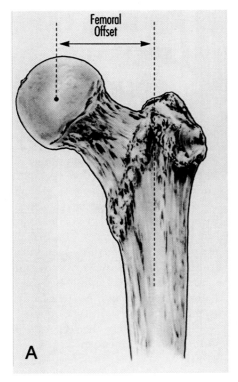
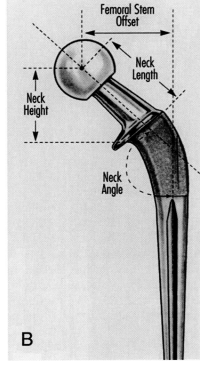

Figure 1   **A,** Femoral offset. **B,** Femoral component offset.

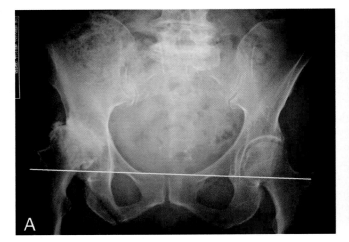
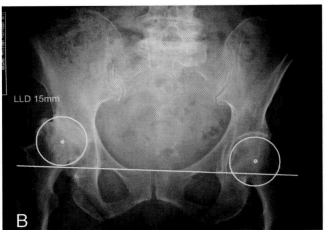

Figure 2   **A,** AP view of the pelvis with a horizontal line drawn using the teardrops as a reference. **B,** The horizontal line is used as a reference for component position. The circles identify the center of rotation of each hip. LLD = limb-length discrepancy.

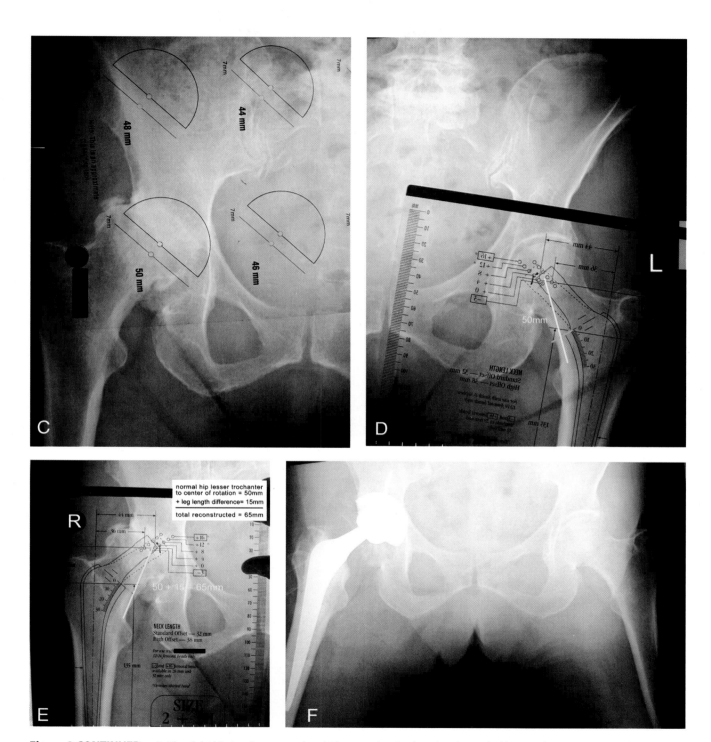

Figure 2 CONTINUED **C,** The right hip has been templated. The template is placed at the probable site of reconstruction. Although the component is cephalad based on the patient's disease, it was believed to be the best site for cup placement. **D,** The femur of the normal, unaffected hip is templated as a reference for the reconstructed hip. **E,** The affected hip is then templated. The sum of measurements (65 mm = 15 mm for the cephalad cup and 50 mm for the normal anatomic length from the lesser trochanter to the center of the femoral head) is used to determine placement of the femoral component. **F,** The postoperative radiograph shows the position of the prosthesis.

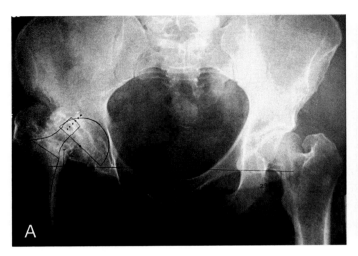
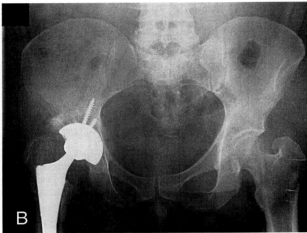

Figure 3 A, AP radiograph of the right hip of a 38-year-old man who had a femoral neck fracture at age 12 years after which posttraumatic osteoarthritis of the right hip developed. The measurement shows a 45-mm limb-length discrepancy on the right side. **B,** Postoperative AP radiograph showing anatomic placement of the cup and restoration of most of the limb-length discrepancy.

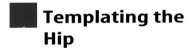

Templating the Hip

Templating is one of the final steps necessary in preparing for surgical management of patients with hip disease. Templating for THA has several purposes: First, it helps facilitate the appropriate selection of implants; the implant selected for a large-boned elderly patient with osteopenia may differ from that selected for a young patient with congenital or developmental dysplasia of the hip. Second, it enables the surgeon to determine placement of the acetabular and femoral components to restore limb length and offset. Finally, it helps the surgeon prepare for both expected and unexpected problems. A patient with a varus femoral neck angle requires a femoral component that restores offset. The selection of a femoral component with inadequate offset for a patient with this condition can lead to a limb-length discrepancy. Intraoperatively, the surgeon may find that the only way to achieve adequate soft-tissue tension is by increasing the limb length to compensate for the lack of offset in the femoral component. Templating for the acetabular component may reveal that a dysplastic hip

requires an autogenous femoral head graft to provide adequate stability for the acetabulum.

Imaging

The essential tools for templating include appropriate radiographs of the hip, a full range of templates, and radiograph-marking pencils. The hip should be templated with adequate time remaining before surgery to obtain the necessary components and instruments required for surgical reconstruction.

Both an AP view of the entire pelvis and a lateral view of the femur should be obtained. If the hip cannot be internally rotated, then the patient should be prone with slight external rotation of the limb to mimic an anatomic position. In this position, the limb is in 15° to 20° of external rotation. The preferred lateral radiograph is a modification of the frog lateral or the table down (Lowenstein lateral) view. It also is useful to template the contralateral hip. Templates are normally magnified 20% to match the radiographic magnification, and the surgeon must know the amount of magnification before using templates. If the radiographs are digitized the surgeon should confirm the amount of

magnification with the radiology technician.

Technique

Preoperative templating is performed to reconstruct the hip to its anatomic length. Data from the physical examination and radiographs should be used to determine limb length.

Before the template is placed on the radiographs, several landmarks must be identified. The acetabular teardrop, which is the landmark of the inferomedial acetabulum, is one of the most reliable (**Figure 2**, *A*). A line connecting the teardrops serves as the reference from which the center of rotation can be measured. This line is also helpful for the acetabular and femoral measurements. The acetabular component is normally placed at the lateral edge of the teardrop, with abduction inclination of 45°, as drawn on **Figure 2**, *B*. In the ideal situation, the lateral aspect of the template will extend to the lateral rim of the acetabulum. Component placement may vary from this anatomic position, depending on the requirements for reconstruction. The components also should be placed to maximize bony containment and the surface area of contact. In this patient's hip, the ac-

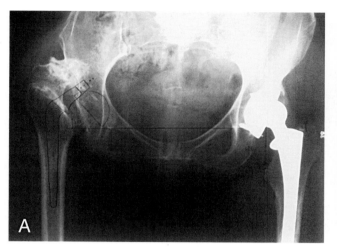
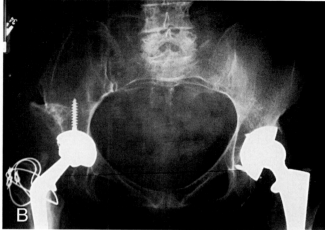

Figure 4 **A,** AP radiograph of a 70-year-old woman with a high iliac hip dislocation secondary to a congenital hip. **B,** Postoperative AP radiograph shows that the hip has been reconstructed to the anatomic acetabulum.

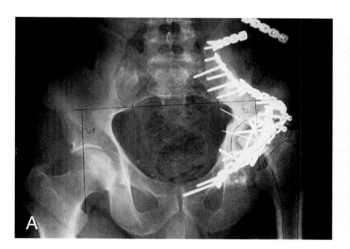
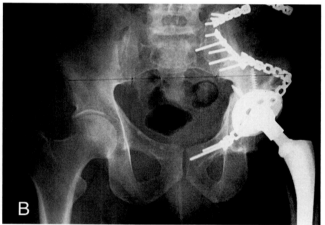

Figure 5 **A,** AP radiograph of a 39-year-old man who had an acetabular fracture 8 years ago, resulting in posttraumatic osteoarthritis and a 36-mm limb-length discrepancy. The sacroiliac joint was used for referencing because of alteration of the patient's anatomy. **B,** Postoperative AP radiograph shows near restoration of the patient's limb length and offset.

etabular template is placed superior and medial to the center of rotation and has affected limb length (**Figure 2**, *C*). The acetabular component is placed 15 mm proximal to the measured center of rotation.

Templating of the femur occurs next. It is helpful to first template the normal, unaffected side, which is then used as a reference for the affected hip (**Figure 2**, *D*). Both limb length and offset are measured to restore the appropriate anatomy. Offset is defined as the horizontal difference from the center of the femoral component to its

center of rotation. The offset of the femoral component should include the anatomic offset of the patient's proximal femur plus any difference that might be measured from the medially placed acetabular component. For example, in this patient, the cup is medialized; therefore, increased offset is required to restore offset in the hip. The femoral anatomic markings for limb length include the center of the femoral head and the lesser trochanter.

The next step is to select the femoral component that will restore limb length and offset. Most components

currently have dual offset (standard and high) options to accommodate the anatomic variability (**Figure 2**, *E*). The distance from the lesser trochanter to the center of the femoral head on the normal left hip is templated to be 50 mm. The acetabular component on the right hip is placed 15 mm higher than the center of the femoral head on the normal left hip. Making the distance from the lesser trochanter to the femoral head 65 mm on the right hip will compensate for the 15-mm difference and result in equal limb lengths. The postoperative

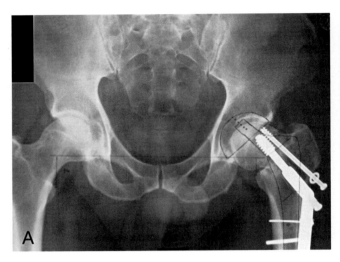
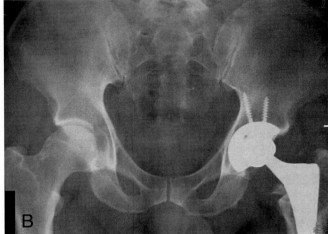

Figure 6　**A,** AP radiograph of a 52-year-old man with a history of femoral neck and shaft fractures sustained during a fall while snow skiing. The femoral neck fracture failed to heal, and he had a 15-mm limb-length discrepancy on the left side. **B,** Postoperative AP radiograph showing full restoration of limb length.

radiograph shows the reconstructed hip (**Figure 2**, F). The acetabular component is cephalad because of bone deficiency. The femoral component has been placed to reconstruct the hip and restore length and offset.

Case Examples

The anatomy of the hip in a patient with dysplasia may differ, depending on the severity of the disease. Patients with very mild dysplasia have nearly normal anatomy, and anatomic reconstruction of the acetabulum is possible. Patients with moderate involvement or a high-riding hip may require cephalad replacement of the acetabu-

lar component or augmentation of the bone and/or component so it can be placed in an anatomic position (**Figure 3**). Finally, patients with severe dysplasia frequently require small-sized components that can be placed in the anatomic position (**Figure 4**). The femur is shortened to compensate for the acetabular component's anatomic position.

Patients with posttraumatic osteoarthritis also require special attention during preoperative planning and templating (**Figures 5** and **6**). First, it is necessary to remove the retained hardware if it interferes with component placement. Several questions

also arise during this preoperative planning: Is it necessary to augment the bone during placement of the component? Has the acetabular fracture been anatomically reconstructed? If not, can it be augmented? Is the femur anatomically reconstructed? How will removal of the retained hardware affect the integrity of the bone? In a patient with minimal trauma to the acetabulum, the templated acetabular component should have a center of rotation equal to that of the anatomic hip.

References

Austin MS, Hozack WJ, Sharkey PF, Rothman RH: Stability and leg length equality in total hip arthroplasty. *J Arthroplasty* 2003;18:88-90.

AAOS Committee on Professional Liability: *Managing Orthopaedic Malpractice Risk*, ed 2. Rosemont, IL, American Academy of Orthopaedic Surgeons, 2000.

Maloney WJ, Keeney JA: Leg length discrepancy after total hip arthroplasty. *J Arthroplasty* 2004;9(suppl 1):108-110.

Ranawat CS, Rao RR, Rodriguez JA, Bhende HS: Correction of limb-length inequality during total hip arthroplasty. *J Arthroplasty* 2001;16:715-720.

Wright JG, Young NL: The patient-specific index: Asking patients what they want. *J Bone Joint Surg Am* 1997;79:974-983.

Chapter 7

Primary Total Hip Arthroplasty: Cemented Acetabulum

Chitranjan S. Ranawat, MD
Amar S. Ranawat, MD

Indications

Cemented fixation is a durable, reproducible, and cost-effective technique that has stood the test of time, in part because wear rates with cemented all-polyethylene acetabular components are considerably lower than uncemented fixation.

For a variety of reasons, however, cemented all-polyethylene acetabular components are rarely used in the United States, despite the fact that cemented fixation remains the most commonly used acetabular fixation technique in the world. As a result, an entire generation of orthopaedic surgeons in the United States has not been exposed to the technique. Nonetheless, it remains a valuable technique if only to practice the skills necessary to cement a new liner into a well-fixed, metal-backed acetabular shell.

Our indications for cemented total hip arthroplasty (THA) with a highly cross-linked, all-polyethylene acetabular socket include all patients older than age 60 years who have hip osteoarthritis with adequate acetabular bone stock.

Contraindications

Cemented fixation is contraindicated in patients with excessive acetabular bleeding after reaming, extensive cyst formation, and/or weak cancellous bone such as in inflammatory arthropathies, dysplasia, or protusio deformities. The use of cement is also generally contraindicated in patients with significant cardiopulmonary disease to minimize embolization secondary to cement pressurization.

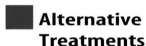 Alternative Treatments

In younger patients and patients with the aforementioned contraindications to cemented acetabular fixation, press-fit, porous-coated, hemispheric titanium acetabular shells, with and without supplemental screw fixation, have been used with excellent results. These shells have the added benefit of accepting multiple, alternative bearing surfaces.

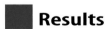

Results

The long-term results of cemented all-polyethylene sockets are excellent, especially within a defined indication. Revision rates at 10 to 20 years vary between 2% and 14% for osteoarthritis.

Similarly, radiographic loosening over the same time period ranges from 6% to 23% (**Table 1**). Nonetheless, confusion about their durability has arisen given the results of many studies focusing on the long-term survivorship of cemented cups have been confounded with differing designs, diagnoses, and definitions of failure. Using the historical literature, if 32-mm heads, metal-backed sockets, rheumatoid arthritis, dysplasia, and revisions were eliminated from consideration, the long-term results of cemented all-polyethylene cups are impressive. In fact, our data demonstrate an 88% survivorship of 236 hips with cemented all-polyethylene cups at 15-year follow-up for all diagnoses, which increases to 98% survivorship of 160 hips at 20 years for osteoarthritis alone.

Using direct compression-molded polyethylene, wear rates have been documented as low as 0.075 mm/year. As a result, 10-year follow-up data in 235 consecutive hips using this material have yielded no clinical failures.

Technique

Exposure

Exposure occurs through the posterior approach under hypotensive epidural anesthesia (defined as mean arterial

Table 1 Failure Rate With Cemented Cups

Author(s) (Year)	Number of Hips	Implant Type	Minimum Follow-up (Years)	Revision Rate (%)
DeLee and Charnley (1976)	141	Charnley	10	No revision
Stauffer (1982)	231	Charnley	10	3%
Brick and Poss (1988)	267	Mixed	11	3.1%
Ritter, et al (1992)	238	Charnley	10	4.6%
Wroblewski and Siney (1993)	193	Charnley	18	3%
Kavanagh, et al (1994)	112	Charnley	20	16%
Ranawat, et al (1995)	236	Mixed	5	0.8%
Mulroy, et al (1995)	105	CAD, HD-2	10	5%
Callaghan, et al (2004)	27	Charnley	30	12%
Della Valle, et al (2004)	40	Charnley	20	23%

CAD = computer assisted design; HD-2 = Harris-II (Stryker Howmedica Osteonics, Allendale, NJ)

pressure ≤ 50 mm Hg) to help achieve a dry cancellous acetabular bed to allow for cement intrusion during pressurization. After trapezoidal capsulotomy, release of the short external rotators and release of the quadratus femoris, an Aufranc retractor is placed just inferior to the transverse ligament at the level of the obturator foramen. Anterior femoral mobilization is enhanced by partial release of the insertion of the gluteus maximus tendon, release of the reflected head of the rectus femoris, and excision of the labrum. Attention is given to the identification and preservation of the transverse ligament, which helps in containment and pressurization of cement. A curved C-retractor is placed anteriorly, bringing the femur forward and out of the field of view. A Steinmann pin is placed superiorly to retract the gluteus medius muscle. The exposure is completed with a narrow, 90°-bent Hohmann retractor placed in the ischium in the interval between the capsule and labral remnant.

Bone Preparation

Circumferential reaming commences in a stepwise fashion until the blush of cancellous bleeding bone is noted in both anterior and posterior columns where the pubis and ischial tuberosity meet the pelvis. Medialization to the inner mantle is avoided to preserve medial cancellous bone (**Figure 1**). Trial fitting using a hemispherical device allows for optimization of orientation (40° lateral opening and 15° anteversion) and assessment of the cement mantle (the trial component should spin easily between two fingers

to accommodate for adequate thickness of the cement mantle) (**Figure 2**).

Multiple fixation holes are burred into the superior dome in the area of the cancellous bone of the posterior column (**Figure 3**), and two larger cavities are created in the pubis and ischium to facilitate macrointerlock. Pulsatile lavage is used to remove blood and fat debris, and the bed is dried with sponges and pressure (**Figure 4**). Heated cement is allowed to cure to a doughy consistency during the setting phase (**Figure 5**). Cement is then introduced into the bony cancellous bed and pressurized using a special bulb syringe device (Bard, Murray Hill, NJ) to enhance microinterlock via cement intrusion. Care is taken to remove excess cement from the inferior teardrop area prior to insertion of the all-polyethylene cup.

Prosthesis Implantation

Current design parameters allow for a high-walled, highly cross-linked polyethylene acetabular component with a 28-mm inner diameter to mate with a chromium-cobalt femoral head (**Figure 6**). The cup is inserted with a cup holder engaging inferiorly first, and then in a medial-superior direction (**Figure 7**, *A*). Cement is reinforced over the superior edge with the finger, and final positioning is achieved with the cup holder. Removal of the cup holder allows for circumferential inspection, final adjustments of orientation, and removal of excess cement. The cup is held in place with medial pressure, and the cement is allowed to polymerize (**Figure 7**, *B*).

Attention can now be turned to the femur for preparation of femoral component.

Wound Closure

Prior to closure, the wound is irrigated. The insertion of the tendon of the gluteus maximus and the quadratus femoris are repaired with nonabsorbable sutures. The superior capsule is closed with another nonabsorbable suture.

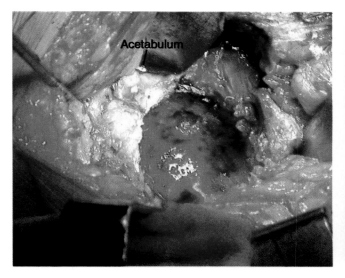

Figure 1 Acetabular exposure with the Steinmann pin superiorly, the Aufranc retractor inferiorly, the C-retractor anteriorly, and the 90°-bent Hohmann retractor posteriorly. The medial wall should not be reamed.

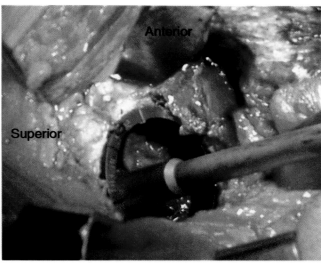

Figure 2 The acetabular trial component should spin easily between two fingers.

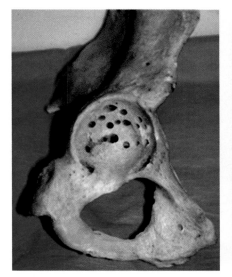

Figure 3 Multiple fixation holes located in the ilium, ischium, and pubis.

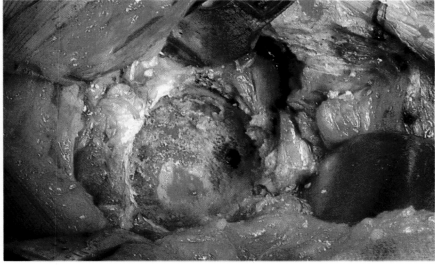

Figure 4 The dry cancellous bed after preparation.

The posterior capsule and short external rotators are repaired with two nonabsorbable sutures passed through drill holes in the greater trochanter. A drain is pulled through the anteroinferior aspect of the incision and placed in the posterior gutter. The fascia is approximated with interrupted bioabsorbable sutures superimposed with a continuous running baseball stitch.

Care must be taken to avoid sewing in the drain. The subcutaneous tissue is closed with bioabsorbable suture, and nylon is used for the skin.

Postoperative Regimen

Our postoperative THA protocol consists of a pain management program with multiple modalities combined with immediate weight bearing as tolerated. Deep venous thrombosis prophylaxis relies on operative time of less than 1 hour, early ambulation, mechanical compression, and warfarin. All patients undergo Doppler ultrasound on postoperative day 3. Patients with negative results are placed on aspirin; otherwise, they are treated appropriately. The average hospital stay is less than 4 days. With this protocol,

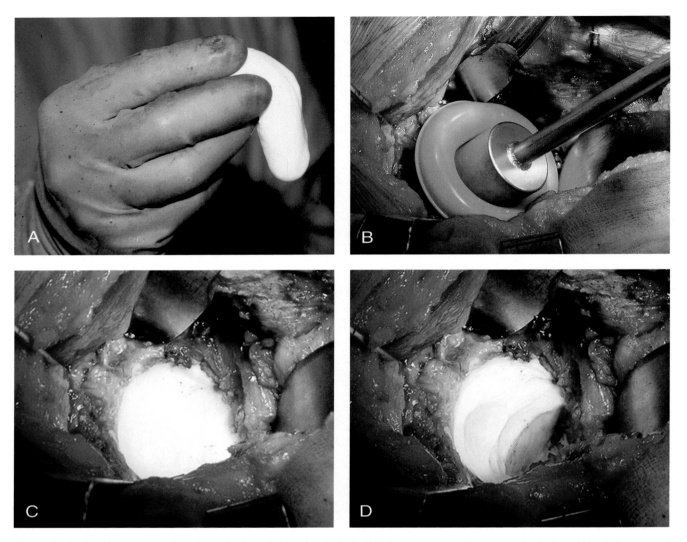

Figure 5 **A,** Doughy cement prior to insertion into the dry acetabular bed. **B,** Pressurization of cement with a bulb syringe. **C,** Pressurized cement prior to component insertion. **D,** Elevation of cement out of the teardrop.

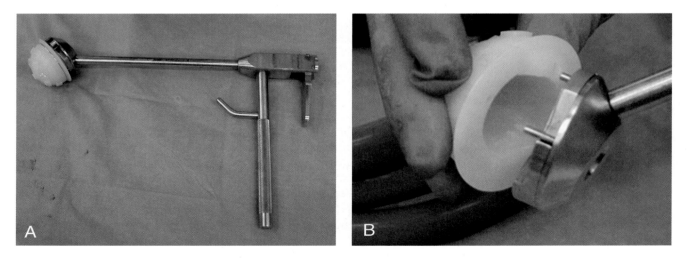

Figure 6 Highly cross-linked polyethylene component **(A)** and cup holder device **(B)**.

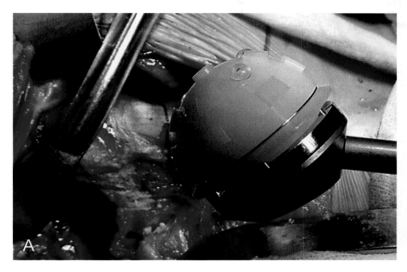
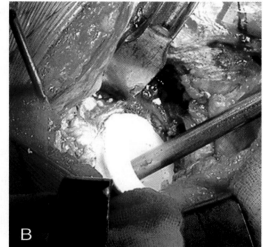

Figure 7　**A,** Insertion of cup with holder. **B,** Awaiting polymerization of cement.

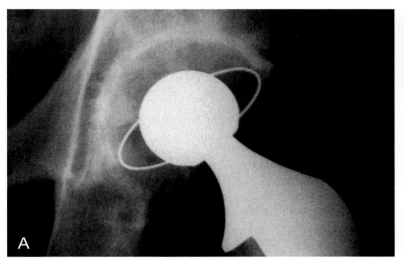
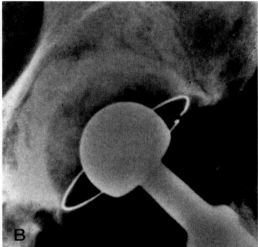

Figure 8　**A,** AP radiograph showing excellent cement interdigitation in all three zones. **B,** AP radiograph showing early demarcation in all three zones.

most patients are walking unassisted and without a limp by 6 weeks.

■ Avoiding Pitfalls and Complications

Although cementing in an all-polyethylene cup is a demanding surgical technique, it can be learned and its results are reproducible. Fixation and durability have been excellent between 10 and 20 years, with survivorship approaching 99% for patients with osteoarthritis. Wear rates of the cemented all-polyethylene cup have been superior compared with those of metal-backed cups (less than 0.1 mm/ year). The primary cause of early failure (less than 10 years) of cemented acetabular fixation is directly related to failure to achieve satisfactory initial cement-bone macro- and microinterlock. This is technique dependent and can be predicted based on early postoperative radiographs, which would show evidence of demarcation at the cement-bone interface (**Figure 8**).

References

Brick GW, Poss R: Long-term follow-up of cemented total hip replacement for osteoarthritis. *Rheum Dis Clin North Am* 1988;14:565-577.

Callaghan JJ, Templeton JE, Liu SS, et al: Results of Charnley total hip arthroplasty at a minimum of thirty years: A concise follow-up of a previous report. *J Bone Joint Surg Am* 2004;86:690-695.

Della Valle CJ, Kaplan K, Jazrawi A, Ahmed S, Jaffe WL: Primary total hip arthroplasty with a flanged, cemented all-polyethylene acetabular component: Evaluation at a minimum of 20 years. *J Arthroplasty* 2004;19:23-26.

DeLee JG, Charnley J: Radiological demarcation of cemented sockets in total hip replacement. *Clin Orthop* 1976;121:20-32.

Kavanagh BF, Wallrichs S, Dewitz M, et al: Charnley low-friction arthroplasty of the hip: Twenty-year results with cement. *J Arthroplasty* 1994;9:229-234.

McCombe P, Williams SA: A comparison of polyethylene wear rates between cemented and cementless cups: A prospective, randomized trial. *J Bone Joint Surg Br* 2004;86:344-349.

Mulroy WF, Estok DM, Harris WH: Total hip arthroplasty with use of so-called second generation cementing techniques: A fifteen-year-average follow-up study. *J Bone Joint Surg Am* 1995;77:1845-1852.

Ranawat CS, Deshmukh RG, Peters LE, Umlas ME: Prediction of the long-term durability of all-polyethylene cemented sockets. *Clin Orthop* 1995;317:89-105.

Ranawat CS, Peters LE, Umlas ME: Fixation of the acetabular component: The case for cement. *Clin Orthop* 1997;344:207-215.

Ritter MA, Faris PM, Keating EM, Brugo G: Influential factors in cemented acetabular cup loosening. *J Arthroplasty* 1992;7(suppl):365-367.

Schmalzried TP, Kwong LM, Jasty M, et al: The mechanism of loosening of cemented acetabular components in total hip arthroplasty: Analysis of specimens retrieved at autopsy. *Clin Orthop* 1992;274:60-78.

Stauffer RN: Ten-year follow-up study of tot al hip replacement. *J Bone Joint Surg Am* 1982;64:983-990.

Wroblewski BM, Siney PD: Charnley low-friction arthroplasty of the hip: Long-term results. *Clin Orthop* 1993;292:191-201.

Coding

CPT Codes		Corresponding ICD-9 Codes		
27130	Arthroplasty, acetabular and proximal femoral prosthetic replacement (total hip arthroplasty), with or without autograft or allograft	711.45 714.30 715.35 718.6 733.42	711.95 715.15 716.15 720.0 808.0	714.0 715.25 718.5 733.14 905.6
27132	Conversion of previous hip surgery to total hip arthroplasty, with or without autograft or allograft	715.15 718.2 733.14 996.4	715.25 718.5 733.42 996.66	715.35 718.6 905.6 996.77

CPT copyright ©2004 by the American Medical Association. All Rights Reserved.

Chapter 8

Primary Total Hip Arthroplasty: Uncemented Acetabulum

Robert L. Barrack, MD

 ## Indications

In the early years of total hip arthroplasty (THA), acetabular fixation was obtained with polymethylmethacrylate. Loosening of cemented sockets emerged as a major clinical problem 10 years postoperatively, particularly in younger, more active patients. Improvements in cement technique of the 1970s and 1980s seemed more applicable to the femoral than to the acetabular side, which lead to the popularity of uncemented fixation of the acetabular component. The advantages of uncemented fixation include (1) the need for less exposure, (2) the ability to change component position after initial insertion, and (3) the flexibility of combining a metal shell with a wide variety of modular liner options, including numerous inner diameters, elevated rim, lateralized, anteverted, and constrained liners. Uncemented components are also easier to insert through more limited approaches, which is an important advantage with the increasing interest in minimal incision THA.

Despite generally good clinical results, versatility, and the popularity of uncemented acetabular fixation, surgeons must recognize the proper indications and follow optimal technique to consistently obtain excellent long-term results and avoid numerous potential complications.

Uncemented acetabular fixation can be used for most patients undergoing primary THA. The basic requirements are the ability to obtain immediate mechanical stability and intimate contact with host bone, with biologic potential for bone ingrowth over at least 60% of the porous surface.

 ## Contraindications

Contraindications include severe osteopenia and bone loss in which case a press-fit acetabular component is associated with a high risk of fracture, and adjunctive fixation with screws, pegs, or spikes cannot ensure immediate mechanical stability. Micromotion of 50 to 100 μm or more is associated with failure of bone ingrowth. Other contraindications include radiation necrosis, primary or metastatic periacetabular tumor, and severe metabolic bone disease that precludes reliable bone ingrowth.

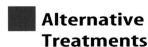 ## Alternative Treatments

The principal alternative to uncemented acetabular fixation is a cemented all-polyethylene component. In patients with severe osteopenia, bone loss, and/or protrusio, an all-polyethylene component alone may be suboptimal and is frequently combined with impaction grafting of cancellous bone and an antiprotrusio ring or cage. This approach is occasionally indicated, however, in patients with severe rheumatoid arthritis who require primary THA.

 ## Results

Ten-year results of the success of uncemented acetabular components are now emerging, particularly intermediate- and long-term results for the HG-I and HG-II (Zimmer, Warsaw, IN). These components were initially implanted with line-to-line reaming and screw fixation, and in the past 10 years, reports of loosening or the need for component revision have virtually disappeared. Of some concern, however, is the incidence of osteolysis, which has ranged from 5% to 23% and seems to be related to patient age and activity level (**Table 1**). The incidence of lysis after 10 years is of some concern, particularly with younger patients. These early-generation components had suboptimal locking mechanisms, liner conformity, and backside surface finishes. More recent

Table 1   Intermediate-Term Results of Uncemented Acetabular Components

Cup Type	Number of Hips	Average Follow-up (Years)	Lysis	Loose or Revised
HG-I	196	10.2	5%	0
HG-I	56	11	23%	0
HG-II	78 (age < 50 years)	10	16%	1.3%
Omnifit HA Threaded	124	7.9		1%
Dual-geometry HA Press-fit	156	7.9		11%
Dual-geometry HA porous	103	7.9		2%

HG = Harris-Galante (Zimmer, Warsaw, IN)
Omnifit (Stryker, Mahwah, NJ)

reports, with short and intermediate follow-up, have noted low revision rates in acetabular components implanted without adjunctive screw fixation. With improvements in polyethylene sterilization, processing, and optimization in modular uncemented component design characteristics, it is hoped that polyethylene wear and lysis will substantially diminish over the next 10 to 20 years.

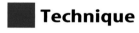

Technique

Exposure

The patient is placed in a lateral position in a positioning device with the torso and pelvis held as rigidly as possible perpendicular to the table. The hips and knees are flexed 30° and overlapped so that the knees and feet can be felt as references for relative limb length. The posterior and direct lateral approaches are most commonly used. For most patients, I prefer the posterior approach with capsular repair.

After the femoral neck cut is made, the anterior capsule is incised, when necessary, to allow retraction of the femur anteriorly and insertion of the acetabular component in 20° to 30° of anteversion. For large patients or those with stiff hips, it may be necessary to release the reflected head of the rectus tendon and part or all of the gluteal sling to allow adequate mobilization of the femur. After the femur has been levered forward, a self-retaining retractor is placed on the posterior capsular flap and the edge of the medius tendon to expose the anterior and posterior acetabular margins and to protect the sciatic nerve with soft tissue.

A retractor is also placed inferiorly into the obturator foramen to provide circumferential exposure to the acetabular rim. The labrum is completely excised, as is at least the superior half of the transverse acetabular ligament. Removing soft tissue from the entire acetabular rim allows for more accurate positioning of the acetabular component based on bony landmarks. The cotyloid notch is cleared of all soft tissue with a curette and rongeur. The base of the notch is clearly defined, which closely corresponds to the acetabular teardrop visualized on the AP radiograph during templating (**Figure 1**, *A*). In some cases a large medial osteophyte may be present rather than the soft tissue typically encountered. The osteophyte can be removed with an osteotome to locate the cotyloid notch. The base of the notch and the transverse acetabular ligament are consistent landmarks for the inflexor border of the true acetabulum (**Figure 1**, *B*). Before reaming, the templated radiographs should be checked for the anticipated component diameter and depth of reaming necessary to obtain adequate coverage and placement of the acetabular component at the anatomic position adjacent to the teardrop.

Bone Preparation

Reaming commences with a hemispheric reamer 8 to 10 mm smaller than the anticipated component diameter. Initial reaming is straight and medially centered over the cotyloid notch. Medial reaming normally progresses to within 2 to 4 mm of the base of the notch (**Figure 1**, *C*). If complete coverage can be obtained without reaming to the base of the notch, medial bone can be retained to preserve bone stock, particularly in young patients. If the thickness of the medial wall is in question and further medialization is necessary to obtain adequate coverage, a drill can be used through the medial wall without plunging, and the thickness measured with a depth gauge. After all of the cartilage has been removed and the reamer is near the base of the notch, reaming is directed at 45° inclination and 20° to 30° of anteversion. Sequentially larger reamers are used until the anterior and posterior walls are firmly engaged. Once this occurs, increasing reamer size should be done with caution because it is easy to ream away the anterior and posterior rims, which compromises the ability to obtain a press-fit. A circumferential bleeding bone surface is desirable (**Figure 1**, *C*). Once the periphery shows bleeding bone and rigidly engages the reamers (**Figure 1**, *D*), bone preparation is normally complete, and a trial shell can be used.

Prosthesis Implantation

Retractors are replaced to ensure complete circumferential exposure of the bony rim at the time of component insertion (**Figure 2**). A 1- to 2-mm press-fit is desirable depending on bone quality and cup diameter. For larger diameters of 60 mm or more, a 2-mm press-fit normally can be obtained. A trial component 1 to 2 mm larger than the last reamer size is introduced and should sit several millimeters proud to ensure obtaining a press-fit. The component is then impacted at 40° to 45° of abduction and 20° to 30° of anteversion.

Before impaction, the patient's position should be checked to ensure that the trunk and pelvis are perpendicular to the table. The templated radiograph is also checked for the anticipated position of the cup relative to the superior acetabular margin. If the acetabulum is dysplastic, up to 20% of the acetabular component is often uncovered despite medialization to the teardrop. Impacting a component to allow complete coverage in this situation will result in more vertical than optimal component position, which is a common technical error.

If the bone is very rigid and the component cannot be seated with firm blows, changing a 2-mm to a 1-mm press-fit shell is often advisable. Once the shell has been seated, the holes in the cup should be checked to ensure complete seating. The edge of the shell should be firmly grasped with an instrument to ensure mechanical stability. Finally, the edge of the cup should be inspected relative to the acetabular rim as a check for component position. If the anterior edge of the cup is recessed relative to the anterior wall of the acetabulum, excessive component anteversion may have occurred. Conversely, if the posterior edge of the component is recessed relative to the

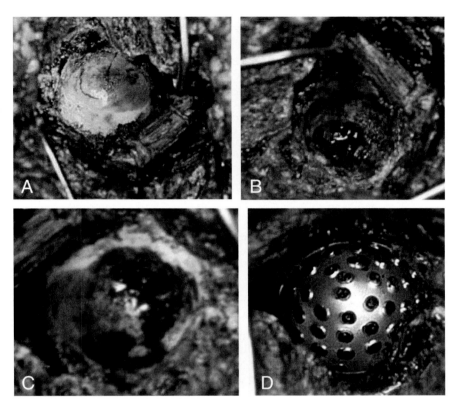

Figure 1 A, Circumferential exposure of the acetabular rim outlining the cotyloid notch. **B,** The base of the cotyloid notch is outlined in curetted and defined. Straight medial reaming is performed to the base of the notch **(C)** or until adequate coverage of the reamer is obtained **(D)**.

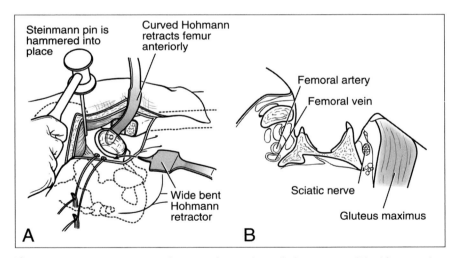

Figure 2 Retractor placement for circumferential acetabular exposure **(A)** with protection of neurovascular structures **(B)**. (Reproduced with permission from Pellici PM, Padgett DE: Acetabular exposure and reaming, in *Atlas of Total Hip Replacement*, New York, NY, Churchill Livingstone, 1995, pp 33-47.)

posterior wall, component retroversion may have occurred. Using the acetabular rim as a guide for cup placement may be dangerous if extensive

osteophytes are present. This should be judged on plain radiographs.

Once the acetabular metal shell has been fully seated, the necessity for

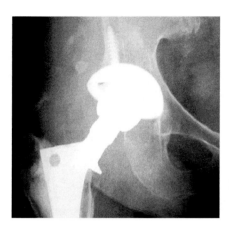

Figure 3 Reaming at a 45° angle prior to medialization resulted in proximal placement and partial uncovering of the acetabular component.

screw fixation must be determined. If the shell is completely covered by bone, completely seated, and rigidly fixed, the use of additional screws is optional. In a dysplastic acetabulum in which a portion of the rim is uncovered, additional screw fixation is probably advisable. One strategy to avoid wasting metal shells is to use a shell that has two or three holes for adjunctive screw fixation and to orient the screw holes inferiorly, out of the weight-bearing area, if it is anticipated that a press-fit without screw fixation should be obtainable. If the cup is not fully covered or the orientation needs to be changed after initial impaction, the screw holes can be reoriented superiorly or posteriorly after reimpaction of the component. If screw fixation is elected, screws should be secure and fully seated. The screw head should be felt to ensure that it is countersunk and will not impede seating of the polyethylene liner. In a patient undergoing routine primary THA, the actual liner may be impacted at this point. If the orientation of the component is in doubt or if any anatomic variations are present, it is probably prudent to insert a trial liner to preserve the options of using an elevated rim, lateralized or anteverted liner, or a larger femoral head size

based on the stability noted during trial reduction.

Wound Closure

Immediately before wound closure, hip stability must be tested in full extension and external rotation. This is one of the most important steps in inserting an uncemented acetabular component to prevent impingement of the neck of the stem and the liner, which can lead to anterior instability. The hip should then be checked in midposition with slight traction to ensure adequate tension on the reconstruction. The hip also should be tested at 90° of flexion with adduction, then at 90° of flexion with mild abduction, and internal rotation. The hip should easily internally rotate 50° to 70° without subluxation. If impingement or subluxation occurs, the position of the acetabular component should be reassessed to ensure that the shell does not need repositioning. One of the principal advantages of uncemented acetabular components is the ability to reorient the shell with much greater ease compared with a cemented component.

Postoperative Regimen

If an uncemented acetabular component is mechanically stable and well positioned, immediate weight bearing as tolerated is allowed. In the rare case when there is any doubt about mechanical stability, protected weight bearing for the first 6 to 8 weeks is advisable. This precaution should be exceedingly rare following primary THA, but it is possible in unusual cases of dysplasia in which more than 10% to 20% of the component is uncovered or there is severe protrusio in which medial bone grafting has been performed, and there is contact with allograft over a substantial portion of the prosthesis-bone interface.

———————■

 Avoiding Pitfalls and Complications

Despite the consistently good long-term results reported for uncemented acetabular components, several potential complications have been associated with their use. These pitfalls can occur during reaming, component seating, or screw insertion. In addition, a number of long-term complications, many of which are to some degree preventable, are associated with use of these components.

Failure to ream appropriately can result in at least three complications: (1) proximal placement of the acetabular component; (2) excessive reaming with loss of stability; and (3) lateral placement of the acetabular component, which also leads to suboptimal stability and the potential for cup dislodgement. These pitfalls can be avoided by exposing the entire acetabular rim, carefully removing soft tissue from the cotyloid notch, defining the base of the notch, and straight medial reaming close to the base of the notch before reaming in the orientation of cup insertion. Reaming at a 45° angle before medialization will result in proximal placement of the acetabular component, which could result in shortening, instability, and use of skirted heads to compensate for the proximal cup placement (**Figure 3**). Failure to medialize also increases the likelihood of excessive reaming because the reamers will contact less of the anterior and posterior rim, thus reaming away part or all of the acetabular rim and compromising component stability. Finally, lateral placement of the component can result from failure to adequately medialize, which alters hip mechanics and compromises component stability. Failure to use screws with a lateralized uncovered component can cause the shell to dislodge from the pelvis, particularly if a dislocation is reduced (**Figure 4**).

Seating of the uncemented shell is also associated with a number of pitfalls, including acetabular fracture, incomplete seating, and soft-tissue impingement. Avoiding excessive press-fit minimizes the risk of fracture. Press-fitting of more than 2 mm is rarely necessary or advisable in primary THA. Incomplete seating is an additional pitfall. Complete clearing of soft tissue from the rim helps ensure optimal seating and stability. If the mechanical stability of the shell is in doubt, additional screw fixation is advisable.

A unique complication of uncemented shells is symptomatic soft-tissue impingement that occurs when the metal shell extends beyond the bony margin anteriorly. This problem can lead to groin pain from psoas tendinitis and has been described as a cause for component revision (**Figure 5**). Once the shell is seated it should be checked circumferentially to determine whether metal is extending beyond the margin of the acetabulum.

Once the shell is seated, potentially catastrophic complications can occur if the screws are placed through the shell. The key to avoiding these complications is familiarity with the quadrant system. A line extending from the anterosuperior iliac spine through the polar hole of the component divides the acetabular shell into anterior and posterior quadrants (**Figure 6**). Screws should be used only in the posterior quadrants. Screws longer than 30 mm are only consistently appropriate for use in the posterosuperior quadrant. Bicortical fixation frequently is not necessary to obtain adequate mechanical strength, regardless of the quadrant. If bicortical fixation is used, the surgeon must be completely confident that the drill is encountering steady, firm resistance and that the screws do not plunge beyond the second cortex. A very firm end point also must be consistently obtained with a depth gauge

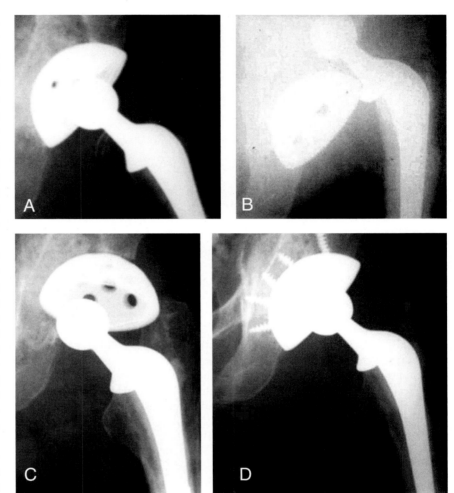

Figure 4   A, AP radiograph showing an uncemented acetabular component without screw fixation. **B,** AP radiograph demonstrating component dislocation. **C,** Attempt at closed reduction resulted in the shell becoming dislodged from the pelvis. **D,** Revision THA with replacement of the shell with screw fixation was required.

to ensure that excessively long screws that extend into the pelvis are not used. Finally, once seated, screws must obtain a good bite and be rigidly fixed to the bone. Loose screws should not be left in place because they increase the risk of fretting and wear debris. Screw heads should be countersunk to avoid impinging on the backside of the polyethylene liner, which can compromise the strength of the locking mechanism and increase the risk of wear between the screw head and the liner.

Long-term complications include failure of ingrowth and in-creased incidence of polyethylene wear and osteolysis. Both of these complications were much more common with early modular uncemented designs and can be largely avoided by selecting components with optimal design characteristics. Lack of ingrowth rarely occurs with uncemented components and is largely the result of suboptimal component design or surgical technique. Designs associated with inconsistent ingrowth include hydroxyapatite-coated components on either a smooth or plasma sprayed substrate. The use of fiber metal mesh, sintered beads, and can-

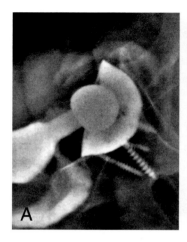
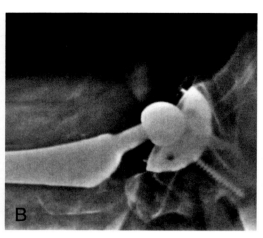
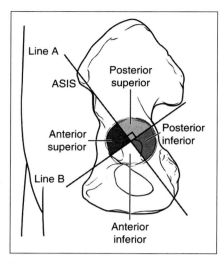

Figure 5 **A,** Lateral arthrogram shows anterior extension of the uncemented acetabular shell from less than optimal component anteversion with impingement on the psoas tendon. **B,** Revision surgery was required to reposition the shell. (Reproduced with permission from Trousdale RT, Cabanela ME: Uncemented acetabular components, in Morrey BF (ed): *Reconstructive Surgery of the Joints,* ed 2. New York, NY, Churchill Livingstone, 1996, pp 961-978.)

Figure 6 The quadrant system as described by Wasielewski. Screws should be placed in the posterior quadrants. (Reproduced with permission from Wasielewski RC, Cooperstein LA, Druger MP, Rubash HE: Acetabular anatomy and the transacetabular fixation of screws in total hip arthroplasty. *J Bone Joint Surg Am* 1990;72:501-508.)

cellous structured titanium has been a high percentage of patients.

Liner dislodgement is a unique complication associated with modular uncemented acetabular components but was much more common with early-generation liners. With current locking mechanisms, the incidence of dislodgement should be virtually eliminated, particularly if complete initial seating is confirmed. Once a liner is seated, it must be tested to make sure that it cannot be easily dislodged with an instrument. Accelerated wear and lysis were associated with suboptimal characteristics of early component designs. Use of components with improved locking mechanisms, backside conformity, a smooth shell backside, and appropriate polyethylene thickness should minimize the long-term complications associated with uncemented acetabular components.

————————■

■ References

Archibeck MJ, Berger RA, Jacobs JJ, et al: Second-generation cementless total hip arthroplasty: Eight- to eleven-year results. *J Bone Joint Surg Am* 2001;83:1666-1673.

Clohisy JC, Harris WH: The Harris-Galante porous-coated acetabular component with screw fixation: An average ten-year follow-up study. *J Bone Joint Surg Am* 1999;81:66-73.

Crowther JD, Lachiewicz PF: Survival and polyethylene wear of porous-coated acetabular components in patients less than fifty years old: Results at nine to fourteen years. *J Bone Joint Surg Am* 2002;84:729-735.

Maloney WJ, Galante JO, Anderson M, et al: Fixation, polyethylene wear, and pelvic osteolysis in primary total hip replacement. *Clin Orthop* 1999;369:157-164.

Manley MT, Capello WN, D'Antonio JA, Edidin AA, Geesink RG: Fixation of acetabular cups without cement in total hip arthroplasty: A comparison of three different implant surfaces at a minimum duration of follow-up of five years. *J Bone Joint Surg Am* 1998;80:1175-1185.

Sharkey PF, Hozack WJ, Callaghan JJ, et al: Acetabular fracture associated with cementless acetabular component insertion: A report of 13 cases. *J Arthroplasty* 1999;14:426-431.

.

Coding

CPT Codes		Corresponding ICD-9 Codes		
27130	Arthroplasty, acetabular and proximal femoral prosthetic replacement (total hip arthroplasty), with or without autograft or allograft	711.45 714.30 715.35 718.6 733.42	711.95 715.15 716.15 720.0 808.0	714.0 715.25 718.5 733.14 905.6
27132	Conversion of previous hip surgery to total hip arthroplasty, with or without autograft or allograft	715.15 718.2 733.14 996.4	715.25 718.5 733.42 996.66	715.35 718.6 905.6 996.77
27134	Revision of total hip arthroplasty; both components, with or without autograft or allograft	996.4	996.66	996.77
27137	Revision of total hip arthroplasty; acetabular component only, with or without autograft or allograft	996.4	996.66	996.77
Modifier 22	Unusual procedural services			

CPT copyright ©2004 by the American Medical Association. All Rights Reserved.

On rare occasions when more extensive procedures involving extensive grafting are necessary, such as use of a structural graft and/ or acetabular protrusio cage or ring, modifier 22 may be used to indicate a substantially greater degree of work, risk, and time involved in the occasional complex primary THA.

Chapter 9

Primary Total Hip Arthroplasty: Cemented Femur

William N. Capello, MD

 ## Indications

The reasons for cementing a femoral stem vary greatly from surgeon to surgeon and from institution to institution. I believe cemented femoral stems are indicated in patients with poor bone quality, such as those with Dorr type C and even some type B bone. Some of these patients can be difficult to manage with uncemented implants because they require either massive, canal-filling, uncemented implants that frequently produce significant stress shielding of the femur, or they have proximally filled implants that can make accurate adjustment of limb lengths very difficult. I believe cemented stems are indicated in patients with anomalies of the proximal femur that are unsuitable for uncemented fixation, and in elderly patients (70 years of age and older), because the literature clearly demonstrates that cemented femoral stems can routinely last 10 to 25 years.

Antibiotic-impregnated cement might be advisable for certain groups of patients, such as those undergoing certain revision arthroplasties and those with a history of sepsis who have no options other than the use of a cemented stem. Some patients, such as those on renal dialysis, may be more prone to sepsis, and it might be advisable to consider using antibiotic-impregnated cement for these patients. Cemented stems should also be con-

sidered for patients with defects in the proximal femur secondary to an intertrochanteric or low femoral neck fracture or from a tumor resection. For these patients, the use of cement with a bone-replacing prosthesis may be the preferred treatment, independent of age or bone quality.

———■

Contraindications

Cemented implants have few absolute contraindications. Because of the embolic load secondary to the pressurization of cement during total hip arthroplasty (THA), many surgeons avoid cementing components in patients with a history of cardiopulmonary disease. In addition, an increased incidence of infection in cemented THA has been reported in certain patient populations, eg, those with Gaucher's disease or those on long-term renal dialysis. Cementing is also contraindicated in those settings where aggressive reaming of the femoral canal is necessary to accommodate both the cement and the implant. I believe these patients would be better served with other means of implant fixation.

Many surgeons are reluctant to offer cemented implants to younger, more active patients, but this is more a reflection of surgeon preference than a contraindication. Regardless of the patient's age, no compelling data

prove that modern cemented stems implanted with careful third-generation techniques are less able to withstand activity than their uncemented counterparts.

Finally, both experimental and clinical data suggest an unacceptably high probability of failure when cementing into femoral canals that previously contained cemented implants. Femurs devoid of cancellous bone have been shown to have a much lower load-carrying capacity than those in which the cement interlocks with the cancellous bone. Therefore, options for revision of a failed cemented implant may be more limited than for a failed uncemented implant.

———■

Alternative Treatments

Nonsurgical treatments include ongoing activity modification, use of analgesics and/or anti-inflammatory medications, assistive devices for ambulation, and weight loss for the overweight patient. Surgical alternatives to THA may include femoral or pelvic osteotomies. A periacetabular osteotomy may provide excellent pain relief and improved short-term functionality (2 to 4 years later) in patients with hip dysplasia. However, these procedures have a definite learning

Table 1   Results of Cemented Femoral Components in Primary THA

Author(s) (Year)	Number of Hips	Implant Type	Mean Patient Age (Range)	Mean Follow-up (Range)	Results* %
Berger, et al (1996)	150	Harris Precoat (Zimmer, Warsaw, IN)	67 years (39–85)	7–10 years	1.6%
Madey, et al (1997)	142	Charnley (DePuy, Warsaw, IN)	62 years (24–88)	15+ years	5%
Bourne, et al (1998)	195	HD-2 (Howmedica, Rutherford, NJ)	68 years (31–89)	12 years (10–15)	5%
Smith, et al (1998)	161	117 CAD (Stanmore Implants, Middlesex, England) 44 HD-2 (Howmedica)	61 years (21–85)	15 years (2–20)	9%
Clohisy and Harris (1999)	100	Harris Precoat (Zimmer)	65 years (45–87)	10 years (7–13)	4%
Kale, et al (2000)	132	Spectron (Smith & Nephew, Memphis, TN)	68 years (17–85)	10 years (5–13)	6%
Sanchez-Sotelo, et al (2002)	256	HD-2 (Howmedica)	66 years (16–89)	15 years (10–20)	10%
Williams, et al (2002)	325	Exeter Universal (Stryker Orthopaedics, Mahwah, NJ)	68 years (24–87)	8–12 years	0%
Meneghini, et al (2003)	102	Omnifit (Stryker Orthopaedics, Rutherford, NJ)	68 years (46–84)	9 years (5–14)	2%

* Results = Femoral Mechanical Failure Rate =

$$\frac{\text{Number of stems revised for aseptic loosening} + \text{Number of radiographically loose stems}}{\text{Total number of stems in study}}$$

curve and not all surgeons may be comfortable in performing periacetabular osteotomies. Surface replacement, a procedure popular in the early 1970s but largely abandoned because of component loosening secondary to excessive polyethylene wear, is now reemerging as a bone-conserving alternative to THA because of the advent of improved bearing surfaces. In certain difficult posttrauma or postinfection cases, hip fusion remains a viable alternative. Current techniques provide acceptable fusion rates with

acceptable functional outcomes. Finally, using an uncemented femoral component is a viable alternative to using a cemented femoral component.

I consider many factors in deciding on the fixation of a femoral component, including the patient's cardiopulmonary status, the etiology of the hip arthritis, and the patient's age and functional demands. In my opinion, uncemented implants may be more durable and therefore a better alternative in younger, more active patients. Alternative bearing surfaces

such as alumina ceramic on alumina ceramic can be used only with titanium stems, and therefore options for use of a cemented stem are extremely limited.

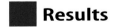

Results

Table 1 shows the femoral mechanical failure rates with a variety of cemented implants, all inserted with either second- or third-generation cementing techniques. Follow-up at about 10 years indicated failure rates ranging from 0% to 10%.

■ Technique

Exposure

A cemented stem can be implanted through a number of surgical exposures, including anterolateral, posterolateral, or direct lateral approaches as well as transtrochanteric osteotomy. I am most familiar and comfortable with the posterolateral approach, and this approach is described below.

The patient is placed in a lateral decubitus position with the affected side facing up. The entire extremity is prepared from the rib cage to the toes and draped in sterile fashion. A modest posterolateral skin incision is created, centered over the greater trochanter, and extended distally about 3 to 4 cm and proximally about 7 to 8 cm, with the dissection carried out through the subcutaneous tissues to the underlying fascia. The fascia of the gluteus maximus is then split, as is the muscle in line with its fibers. The tensor fascia lata is split for a short distance, and a self-retaining retractor is placed to hold the fascia and gluteus maximus apart, thus exposing the external rotators of the hip.

I prefer elevating the posterior margin of the gluteus medius with a retractor because this permits easy visualization of the external rotators. I isolate four tendons (piriformis, superior gemellus, obturator internus, and inferior gemellus) and tag them with a heavy nonbioabsorbable No. 5 suture. Using electrocautery, I release those tendons from the posterior side of the trochanter. The gluteus medius muscle is then lifted off the posterior capsule of the hip to protect it while I incise the posterior capsule, retaining as much capsule as possible for subse-quent repair. The capsule is tagged with the same suture (nonbioabsorbable No. 5) proximally and distally, allowing a large flap to be repositioned at the conclusion of the operation. The quadratus femoris is then taken down, permitting identification of the lesser trochanter. An atraumatic posterior dislocation of the hip is performed.

The femoral neck is resected in accordance with the specific implant system being used. I prefer referencing off the lesser trochanter and following a preoperative plan that dictates the level of resection. I then release the anterior capsule, permitting easy translation of the femur anteriorly for acetabular preparation and, just as importantly, allowing the femur to be elevated from the wound, thus providing excellent access into the femoral canal. This step is particularly important in larger patients. Occasionally, a small portion of the gluteus maximus tendon is released at the point where it inserts onto the femur, enhancing femoral exposure by allowing more internal rotation while augmenting acetabular exposure.

Bone Preparation

Femoral preparation begins once the acetabular component is implanted. A retractor is placed beneath the anterior surface of the remaining femoral neck to facilitate elevation of the femur out of the wound. A small rake retractor is used to hold the posterior margin of the gluteus medius away from the trochanter. I routinely identify and clean the trochanteric fossa and make a pilot hole in it. A blunt-tipped T-handled reamer is inserted through this pilot hole to seek the long axis of the femoral canal. The residual femoral neck is cleared with a box chisel to ensure direct access into the femoral canal and minimize the possibility of varus implantation of the prosthesis (**Figure 1**). Sometimes a lateralizing reamer is used to facilitate this step.

Reaming of the femoral canal is not a part of the usual preparation for cementing. In fact, all preparation is done with a toothed broach or rasp (**Figure 2**). Instruments are frequently sized according to the size of the implant. I start about two sizes smaller than the intended prosthesis size selected in preoperative planning. Broaches are frequently oversized relative to the final implant size, thereby ensuring a minimum cement mantle around the implant. With that assumption in mind, the final broach is determined when it adequately fills the proximal femur. The final broach thus also serves as a trial component, and trial reduction is then performed. When I am satisfied with stability, limb length, and offset, femoral cementing can proceed.

Prosthesis Implantation

The broach is removed, and the canal gently curetted to remove any incompetent cancellous bone, especially medially and posteriorly (**Figure 3**, *A*). The canal is then brushed. I prefer brushing it well below the level of the intended placement of the plug (**Figure 3**, *B*) so that the cement remains in contact with the femoral canal prepared for it in case the plug translates distally during the pressurization process. After brushing, the canal is irrigated with a long, pulsating irrigating tip (**Figure 3**, *C*). This is also done well below the intended level of the plug placement. High-quality cancellous bone should remain in the femoral canal following this preparation (**Figure 3**, *D*). The canal is then sounded to identify the appropriate diameter of a distal centralizer on the prosthesis. I believe that centralizing the prosthesis is important to ensure an uninterrupted cement mantle around the implant.

A plug is placed after irrigation of the canal (**Figure 4**). Many types of plugs are available. I try to allow for 1 to 2 cm of cement below the tip of the implant and place the plug at that

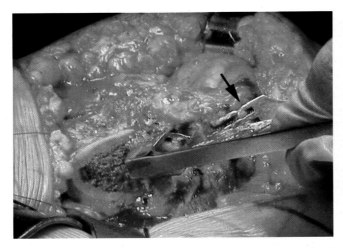

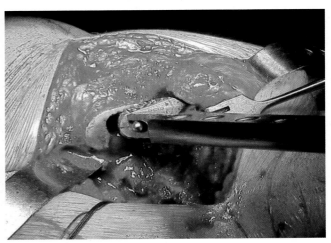

Figure 1 Use of a box chisel to remove the residual femoral neck. Note the placement of the retractors. There is a self-retaining fascia retractor, a retractor under the anterior neck to elevate the femur out of the wound, and a rake retractor to hold the posterior margin of the gluteus medius away from the trochanter.

Figure 2 Broaching of the femoral canal.

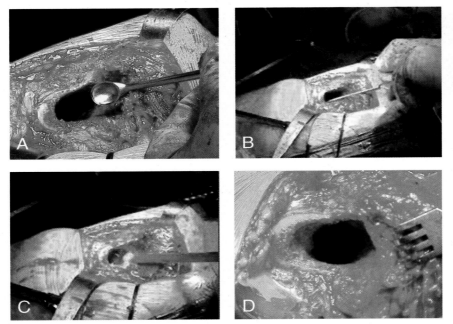

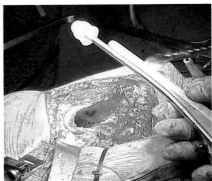

Figure 4 Plugging of the femoral canal.

Figure 3 **A**, Curetting of the femoral canal. **B**, Brushing of the femoral canal. **C**, Irrigation of the femoral canal. **D**, Femoral canal with residual high-quality cancellous bone following canal preparation.

level. It must be secure enough to withstand pressurization.

The cement is then mixed. I prefer a vacuum mixing system and usually mix three packs of cement, each containing 40 g of powder. While the cement is being mixed the canal is irrigated again and dried with a sponge. After about 2.5 minutes of cement mixing, the sponge in the canal is removed, and the canal is irrigated again and then dried with a different sponge. The proximal part of the canal is sprayed with thrombin, and the canal is packed with a thrombin-saturated sponge. It is important to keep the canal dry during cementing. Other drying agents, such as hydrogen peroxide, can be used, and some surgeons use continuous suction to keep the canal dry.

The viscosity of the cement is an important consideration in the cementing technique. I believe a cement with too much liquid is not only difficult to manage but also makes it quite difficult to obtain a blood-free interface between bone and cement. I prefer a somewhat doughy cement delivered with a cement gun. To determine the appropriate viscosity, I watch the cement flow from the tip of the gun. Cement that is somewhat resistant to gravity is nearing what I think is the appropriate consistency. It should have lost its sheen, and the surgeon should be able to break off small pieces and roll them between the fingers without having them stick to the surgical gloves. In my experience, this consistency occurs between 5.5 to 6.5 minutes of setting time, assuming a complete setting time of 11 to 12 minutes. I use Simplex cement (Stryker Orthopaedics, Mahwah, NJ).

Once the cement reaches the appropriate viscosity, packing is removed and the canal suctioned. The cement is delivered retrograde into the canal. Once the canal is filled with cement, a pressurizing unit is placed over the proximal femur and more cement is injected into the femur, thereby pressurizing the column of cement within (**Figure 5**).

The prosthesis is then inserted into the doughy mass of cement with the centralizer attached to the tip. Several prostheses have some form of proximal centralizing that is helpful in maintaining the prosthesis in a neutral attitude during insertion and the final curing process. I tend to occlude the proximal medial part of the canal as the stem is being inserted, thereby allowing further pressurization. If the cement is of the proper viscosity, fairly vigorous pushing and occasionally a few taps with the mallet should be required to fully seat the implant the last few centimeters within the cement mantle. The stem is held steady while the cement cures. Excessive cement is removed from the proximal femur and surrounding areas. The femoral head is attached, the hip is reduced, and closure begun.

Wound Closure

My preferred closure starts by drilling two holes through the posterior trochanter. A suture passer is then pushed through the gluteus medius tendon at the tip of the greater tro-

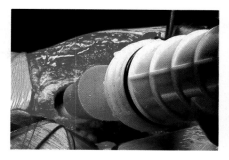

Figure 5 Pressurization of the cement in the femoral canal.

chanter, and two suture ends are pulled up through the tendon, one suture tag from the superior capsule and one from the external rotators. Then the suture passer is pushed through the most proximal drill hole, pulling up the remaining suture tags from the superior capsule and external rotators and one tag from the inferior capsule. Finally, the suture passer is pushed through the distal drill hole and the remaining suture tag of the inferior capsule is pulled through.

With the extremity held in neutral abduction and adduction and slight external rotation, these suture tags are tied upon themselves, resulting in three knots in the final capsule repair. This repositions the capsule and the external rotators in their anatomic position. I then close the quadratus femoris in a continuous fashion, including the gluteus maximus tendon if it has been released. I then reposition and close the bursa over this deeper suture line to tighten up this space. I think covering the ends of the nonbioabsorbable sutures may minimize the likelihood of a postoperative trochanteric bursitis. After this is accomplished, the fascia over the gluteus maximus is closed in a running fashion, and the fascia lata is closed with a few interrupted sutures. Finally, the subcutaneous tissue and skin are closed. Use of a wound drainage system is optional; I use such a system most often with patients who

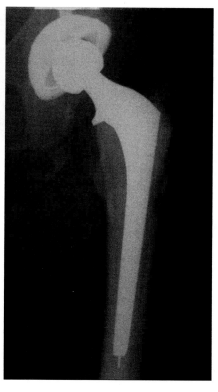

Figure 6 AP radiograph of a cemented femoral component showing excellent cement technique.

have 5 cm or more of subcutaneous fat around the hip.

Postoperative Regimen

The day after surgery the patient is encouraged to bear weight as tolerated with the use of crutches or a walker. Average length of hospitalization is 2 to 4 days, and the patient has physical therapy twice daily during that time. Patients should be able to climb a flight of stairs and move in and out of bed with minimal assistance at discharge. TED hose (Kendall-Futuro, Cincinnati, OH) should be worn for 2 weeks after surgery. Patients are asked to use crutches or a walker for 3 or 4 weeks and then progress to a cane or single crutch. They are instructed to use an elevated toilet seat, to place a pillow between their legs for sleeping at night, to avoid sitting on low or soft surfaces, and to avoid crossing the leg or flexing the hip beyond 90° for 6 weeks after surgery. I place patients on a multivitamin regimen and an iron supplement as well as appropriate pain medication. I encourage patients to be as active as they wish, and allow them to drive within 2 weeks of surgery if they feel comfortable doing so.

The skin staples are removed 7 to 10 days after the procedure, and patients return for follow-up about 6 to 7 weeks after surgery, when I ask them to initiate a program of progressive resistive exercises with weights to strengthen both the abductors and hip flexors. At that time the patient is allowed to walk unassisted for short distances and to continue using a cane for longer walks for about another 4 to 6 weeks.

Avoiding Pitfalls and Complications

Careful preoperative planning and accurate templating to determine offset and limb-length equalization are important first steps in ensuring the long-term success of a cemented stem. Other critical factors in implant longevity are a cement mantle thickness of 2 to 5 mm proximally and medially with neutral orientation of a stem that fills more than half of the distal part of the medullary canal (**Figure 6**). It is also important to avoid an incomplete cement mantle. This is done by appropriately sizing the implant relative to the canal and by choosing an implant system that provides instruments that allow this to be accomplished routinely.

Varus or valgus placement of the prosthesis should be avoided, and centralizers are useful in this regard. It is important to avoid jostling or moving the implant during the setting process, as this could lead to premature loosening. Cement that is too liquid in consistency might compromise the bone-cement interface. I believe the critical tasks in cementing a stem are interdigitating the cement with the existing high-quality cancellous bone, creating an uninterrupted but not necessarily uniform cement mantle, and centralizing the implant within the femoral canal.

References

Berger RA, Kull LR, Rosenberg AG, Galante JO: Hybrid total hip arthroplasty: 7- to 10-year results. *Clin Orthop* 1996;333:124-146.

Berger RA, Seel MJ, Wood K, et al: Effect of a centralizing device on cement mantle deficiencies and initial prosthetic alignment in total hip arthroplasty. *J Arthroplasty* 1997;12:434-443.

Bourne RB, Rorabeck CH, Skutek M, et al: The Harris Design-2 total hip replacement fixed with so-called second-generation cementing techniques: A ten to fifteen-year follow-up. *J Bone Joint Surg Am* 1998;80:1775-1780.

Callaghan JJ, Albright JC, Goetz DD, Olejniczak JP, Johnston RC: Charnley total hip arthroplasty with cement: Minimum twenty-five year follow-up. *J Bone Joint Surg Am* 2000;82:487-497.

Clohisy JC, Harris WH: Primary total hip replacement, performed with insertion of the acetabular component without cement and a precoat femoral component with cement: An average ten-year follow-up study. *J Bone Joint Surg Am* 1999;81:247-255.

DiGiovanni CW, Garvin KL, Pellicci PM: Femoral preparation in cemented total hip arthroplasty: Reaming or broaching? *J Am Acad Orthop Surg* 1999;7:349-357.

Dohmae Y, Bechtold JE, Sherman RE, Puno RM, Gustilo RB: Reduction in cement-bone interface shear strength between primary and revision arthroplasty. *Clin Orthop* 1988;236:214-220.

Ebramzadeh E, Sarmiento A, McKellop HA, Llinas A, Gogan W: The cement mantle in total hip arthroplasty. *J Bone Joint Surg Am* 1994;76:77-87.

Harris WH: Options for primary femoral fixation in total hip arthroplasty: Cemented stems for all. *Clin Orthop* 1997;344:118-123.

Kale AA, Frankel VH, Stuchin SA, Zuckerman JD, diCesare PE: Hip arthroplasty with a collared straight cobalt-chrome femoral stem using second-generation cementing technique: A 10-year average follow-up study. *J Arthroplasty* 2000;15:187-193.

Madey SM, Callaghan JJ, Olejniczak JP, Goetz DD, Johnston RC: Charnley total hip arthroplasty with use of improved techniques of cementing: The results after a minimum of fifteen years of follow-up. *J Bone Joint Surg Am* 1997;79:53-64.

Meneghini RM, Feinberg JR, Capello WN: Primary total hip arthroplasty with a roughened femoral stem: Integrity of the stem-cement interface. *J Arthroplasty* 2003;18:299-307.

Noble PC, Collier MB, Maltry JA, Kamaric E, Tullos JS: Pressurization and centralization enhance the quality and reproducibility of cement mantles. *Clin Orthop* 1998;355:77-89.

Patterson BM, Healey JH, Cornell CN, Sharrock NE: Cardiac arrest during hip arthroplasty with a cemented long-stem component. *J Bone Joint Surg Am* 1991;73:271-277.

Pitto RP, Koessler M, Draenert K: Prophylaxis of fat and bone marrow metabolism in cemented total hip arthroplasty. *Clin Orthop* 1998;355:23-34.

Sanchez-Sotelo J, Berry DJ, Harmsen S: Long-term results of use of a collared matte-finished femoral component fixed with second-generation cementing technique: A fifteen-year median follow-up study. *J Bone Joint Surg Am* 2002;84-A:1636-1641.

Shepard MF, Kabo JM, Lieberman JR: The Frank Stinchfield Award: Influence of cement technique on the interface strength of femoral components. *Clin Orthop* 2000;381:26-35.

Smith SW, Estok DM, Harris WH: Total hip arthroplasty with use of second-generation cementing techniques: An eighteen-year average follow-up study. *J Bone Joint Surg Am* 1998;80:1632-1640.

Star MJ, Colwell CW, Kelman GL, Ballock RT, Walker RH: Suboptimal (thin) distal cement mantle thickness as a contributory factor in total hip arthroplasty femoral component failure: A retrospective radiographic analysis favoring distal stem centralization. *J Arthroplasty* 1994;9:143-149.

Trumble SJ, Mayo MA, Mast JW: The periacetabular osteotomy: Minimum 2 year followup in more than 100 hips. *Clin Orthop* 1999;363:54-63.

Williams HD, Browne G, Gie GA, Ling RS, Timperley AJ, Wendover NA: The Exeter universal cemented femoral component at 8 to 12 years: A study of the first 325 hips. *J Bone Joint Surg Br* 2002;84:324-334.

Coding

CPT Codes		Corresponding ICD-9 Codes		
27125	Hemiarthroplasty, hip, partial (eg, femoral stem prosthesis, bipolar arthroplasty)	715.25 715.35	716.15 718.6	733.14 733.42 905.6
27130	Arthroplasty, acetabular and proximal femoral prosthetic replacement (total hip arthroplasty), with or without autograft or allograft	711.45 711.95 714.0 714.30 715.15	7715.25 715.35 716.15 718.5 718.6	720.0 733.14 733.42 808.0 905.6
27132	Conversion of previous hip surgery to total hip arthroplasty, with or without autograft or allograft	715.15 715.25 715.35 718.2	718.5 718.6 733.14 733.42	905.6 996.4 996.66 996.77
27134	Revision of total hip arthroplasty; both components, with or without autograft or allograft	996.4	996.66	996.77
27138	Revision of total hip arthroplasty; femoral component only, with or without allograft	996.4	996.66	996.77

CPT copyright © 2004 by the American Medical Association. All Rights Reserved.

Chapter 10

Primary Total Hip Arthroscopy: Extensively Porous-Coated Femoral Components

C. Anderson Engh, Jr, MD

Indications

The Anatomic Medullary Locking (AML) femoral component (DePuy, Warsaw, IN), the first extensively porous-coated femoral component approved for use without cement, was released in 1983. Many implants available today have a similar amount of porous coating.

The hallmarks of these porous-coated implants are a cylindrical shape distally and a triangular metaphyseal shape. They are also known as parallel-sided, extensively porous-coated devices because the anterior, posterior, and lateral sides are parallel. Only the medial aspect flares to create a proximal triangle to fill the metaphysis. The proximal triangle generally comes in two or three sizes for each diaphyseal diameter. The porous coating is usu-

ally three-dimensional, with a mean pore size of 200 µm. Because heat is required to apply the porous coating, the stem is cast cobalt chromium rather than titanium. The stems are 6 inches long so that the cylindrical distal portion of the stem can contact 2 to 3 inches of femoral diaphysis length.

These design characteristics match the philosophy of distal fixation, which is to make the femur fit the stem. Extensively porous-coated components attain their initial stability in the femoral diaphysis. This is accomplished by preparing the femur with straight reamers until the femoral cortex is engaged and then inserting a slightly larger straight femoral component. Two to three inches of cortical bone will always be available for fixation of a straight 6-inch stem, regardless of femur shape or degree of patient osteoporosis.

The indications for the use of extensively porous-coated femoral components are the same as those for total hip arthroplasty (THA). Patients must have clinical and radiographic evidence of arthritis, and nonsurgical treatment has failed.

Contraindications

The only contraindication is active infection.

Alternative Treatments

Alternative treatments for use of extensively porous-coated femoral components are the same as those for THA. I use extensively porous-coated femoral implants in all of my THA patients.

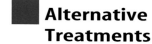

Results

Since 1983 my associates and I have used extensively porous-coated femoral components in all patients (**Table 1**). Our earliest series of patients is a consecutive, nonselected group of 204

Table 1 Recent Published Femoral Results From Anderson Orthopaedic Research Institute

Diagnosis	Number of Hips	Mean Follow-up (Years)	Loose or revised (%)
All diagnoses	211	13.9	3.4%
Rheumatoid arthritis	71	11.4	7%
Osteonecrosis	48	9.7	0%
Elderly	196	8.2	2%

Table 2 Published Femoral Results From Other Centers

Author(s) (Year)	Number of Hips	Mean Follow-up (Years)	Loose or Revised Components (%)
Nercessian, et al (2001)	52	10.5	4%
Woolson and Adler (2002)	50	4.4	0%
Chiu, et al (2001)	27	7.6	0%
Kronick, et al (1997)	174	8.3	1%

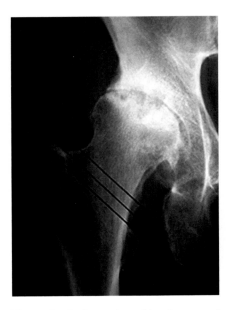

Figure 1 Radiograph marking the general location of high, standard, or low neck resection levels corresponding to my starting point. The levels depicted correspond to intraoperative anatomic measurements that reference the greater and lesser trochanters.

patients (211 hips) that have been followed for a mean of 14 years. The combined (loose and revised) femoral failure rate for this group was only 3%. In addition, we have studied patients with disease processes not originally thought to work well with uncemented techniques. In our series of patients with rheumatoid arthritis, 36 of 64 patients were taking steroids at the time of surgery. At a mean 11-year follow-up, only one femoral component needed revision. In 203 patients 65 years of age or older (212 hips), there was only one failure. We reviewed series of patients younger than age 50 years and patients with developmental dysplasia, but our youngest series is a group of 45 patients (55 hips) with osteonecrosis and a mean age of 31 years. There were no femoral failures in this series at a mean of 10 years.

Other authors and institutions have reported results obtained with the extensively porous-coated AML femoral component (**Table 2**). Kronick and associates reported the largest series (174 hips in 154 patients younger than 50 years of age). Chiu and associates studied young patients, comparing the results of 27 AML femoral components to 34 proximally coated anatomic-shaped femoral components. Nercessian and associates reported the longest follow-up, with a

mean of 10 years (range, 9 to 12 years). Woolson and Adler compared 25 patients allowed full weight bearing with 24 patients (25 hips) limited to partial weight bearing. At 2-year follow-up, none of Woolson and Adler's patients experienced loosening.

These excellent mid- to long-term results were achieved because of the extensive porous coating on the implants, the strong diaphyseal bone ingrowth, and a simple, reproducible surgical technique.

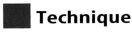

Technique

Exposure

Preoperative templating information, including planned limb-length correction, anticipated stem diameter and triangular segment size, and the level of the femoral neck osteotomy must be available to the surgeon before the procedure begins. Patient positioning during surgery is based on surgeon preference and training. My colleagues and I prefer a lateral decubitus position and use either a posterior or modified Hardinge approach. The nonoperative knee must be palpable through the drapes so that limb lengths can be checked throughout the procedure.

Bone Preparation

Femoral lengths are measured at the knee and a pin is placed in the ilium to measure hip joint length and offset. The level of the femoral neck osteotomy is determined from preoperative templating. The initial cut is a high, standard, or low neck cut that is fine-tuned during the trial reductions (**Figure 1**). The tip of the greater trochanter and the top of the lesser trochanter are the references for the three neck cut levels.

Assuming a 45° angle for the femoral neck cut, a high neck cut is more than one fingerbreadth above the lesser trochanter and exits superiorly in the femoral neck. A standard neck cut is one fingerbreadth above the lesser trochanter medially, exiting superiorly at the junction of the greater trochanter and the anterior femoral neck. A low neck cut is less than one fingerbreadth above the lesser trochanter and below the level of the superior femoral neck. Although an initial high neck cut can always be lowered, a neck cut higher than needed makes acetabular exposure more difficult. The neck osteotomy controls the height of the neck cut and the initial femoral anteversion. Except in patients with excessive femoral anteversion (developmental dysplasia of the hip) or retroversion (old slipped capital femoral epiphysis), the neck cut is made perpendicular to the patient's existing anteversion.

The goal of femoral reaming is to prepare 5 to 7 cm of the proximal diaphysis to match the cylindrical portion of the femoral component. To accomplish this, the direction of the reamer must be controlled by the diaphysis, not by the greater trochanter or femoral neck. A posterolateral pilot hole near the insertion of the piriformis tendon is necessary to prevent deflection of the femoral reamer. Reaming progresses with 1-mm increases in reamer diameter until cortical contact is encountered, after which the reamers progress in 0.5-mm increments. If the reamer is binding or contacting either the greater trochanter or the posterior femoral neck, the pilot hole must be enlarged with a high-speed burr or a side-cutting drill to prevent undersizing the femoral component (**Figure 2**).

Reaming depth is determined by preoperative templating. Reference marks on the reamer refer to either the level of the neck cut or the distance from the tip of the greater trochanter, which itself is not influenced by the neck cut. Reaming too far distally can notch the femur, and not reaming far enough can prevent full seating of the prosthesis. I prefer to use the greater trochanter reference because the reamer is closer to the greater trochanter than the medial femoral neck, making the reference marks easier to see. If the neck cut is used as a reference for the reaming depth, a poor neck cut will lead to the wrong depth of reaming. The last reamer used should be 0.5 mm smaller in diameter

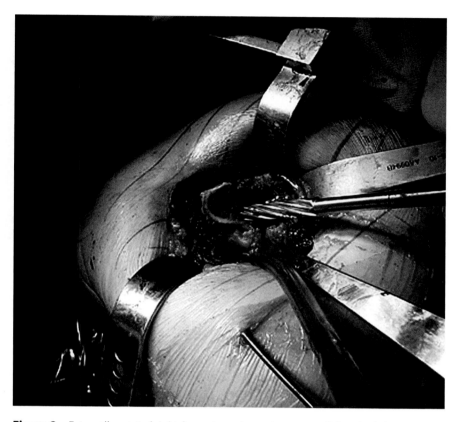

Figure 2 Externally rotated right femur (anterior at the top, medial to the left). The initial pilot hole (medial and anterior) was enlarged posterolaterally to allow correct reamer alignment.

than the actual component and should have a minimum of 6 cm cortical contact when the reamer is at the appropriate depth. This can be checked by hand inserting a reamer that is the same size as the prosthesis until it contacts cortical bone, and then measuring how proud the reamer remains (**Figure 3**, A).

Femoral broaching follows canal reaming. Broaching determines which of the two metaphyseal sizes is used. The larger triangular segment provides greater rotational control. More importantly, it allows greater offset options. Broaching begins at a diameter two to three sizes smaller than the final implant diameter using the small triangle broach. When the appropriately sized small triangle broach is seated to the templated level, a trial reduction is performed to check limb

lengths. If the limb length is correct, the surgeon chooses between the small and large triangular implants. In general, the large triangle is preferable if there is enough metaphyseal bone to accommodate it. The greater femoral offset will improve hip joint stability and increase the abductor moment arm, strengthening the abductors and decreasing the joint reaction forces. If more offset is needed but the metaphysis is not large enough to take a large triangle, the surgeon has three options. The first is to use a longer ball, thereby increasing offset and lengthening the limb. The second is to lower the small triangle stem in the femur and use a longer ball, thus maintaining the same limb length while increasing offset. The third option is to remove metaphyseal cortical bone so that a large triangle implant

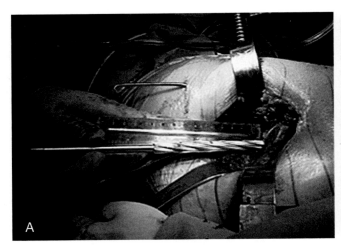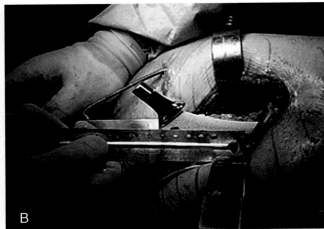

Figure 3 **A,** At the top, a reamer 0.5 mm larger than the last reamer used and the same size as the femoral component is inserted until it comes into contact with the femoral diaphysis. **B,** This measures 7 cm, which corresponds to the amount of scratch fit measured with the actual femoral component prior to impaction.

fits. This requires a high-speed burr, a side-cutting reamer, or a milling device. Although it requires additional instruments and increases the risk of a metaphyseal fracture, I prefer this option if the amount of calcar removed is small.

I always perform the final trial reduction with a middle-length ball. This allows the option of using either a longer or shorter femoral head length after the final implants are inserted. The purpose of the trial reduction is to confirm hip joint stability and check limb length. Hip joint stability is more a function of acetabular position and femoral offset, whereas limb length is principally influenced by the seating level of the femoral component.

Prosthesis Implantation

The insertion of the final femoral implant should take 30 to 80 mallet blows. Typically, the final implant is inserted by hand until it engages cortical bone. This is typically 5 to 10 cm above the final seating level corresponding to the amount of cortical bone that was in contact with the final reamer (**Figure 3**, *B*). The initial impaction blows will advance the stem 5 mm at a time. As the stem advances,

the same blows will move the stem 0.5 to 1 mm at a time over the final 2 to 3 cm. In patients with hard bone, the stem may advance only every other blow for the last centimeter. Usually the impaction force needs to be slightly increased over the final 2 cm. Knowing how hard to hit the femoral stem is a matter of both surgeon experience and patient bone quality. As a rough guide, inserting a straight, fully porous-coated stem takes slightly more force than inserting a femoral intramedullary nail for a fracture.

Postoperative Regimen

Postoperative rehabilitation depends on how tightly the stem is inserted and on the postoperative radiograph. If the stem is tight and the radiograph is good, the patient is allowed full weight bearing. If the stem was easy to insert or the radiograph demonstrates varus and/or undersizing, the patient is permitted 25% to 50% full weight bearing for 4 to 6 weeks. The decision is essentially the surgeon's choice. The radiograph is used to confirm proper alignment, a tight fit, and the absence of fracture.

■ Avoiding Pitfalls and Complications

The most common complication after THA is hip dislocation. Postoperative dislocations are always related to soft-tissue tension and component orientation. The surgeon has very little control over orientation on the femoral side of the hip joint, but tremendous control over soft-tissue tension. Preoperative templating and reductions with trial implants are the primary mechanisms surgeons have to confirm soft-tissue tension, component orientation, and hip joint stability. I prefer to address soft-tissue laxity with increased femoral offset. Whenever possible, I use the femoral component with the greater offset because hip joint stability is thereby increased without lengthening the patient's limb. One advantage of extensively coated parallel-sided femoral components is that soft-tissue tension can be adjusted by changing the seating level of the implant. Changing femoral head length can also result in small changes in offset and tissue tension. However, I avoid skirted femoral heads because the skirt can impinge on the polyethylene and cause dislocation. The final available option on the femoral side of the hip joint is to decrease the amount of instability by increasing the head diameter. These femoral options are combined with the standard acetabular options, including reorienting the shell, offset, face changing, and lipped polyethylene liners.

Failure of ingrowth is often related to undersizing the femoral component. Placing the pilot hole in the wrong position or failing to enlarge it when the reamer impinges proximally are the main causes of an undersized femoral component. If a reamer smaller than the templated size seems to be tight, the surgeon should access the pilot hole, making sure it is lateral enough and that the femoral diaphysis, not the proximal pilot hole, determines the femoral orientation. If the reamer is still tighter than expected, intraoperative AP and lateral radiographs with the reamer in place will confirm its appropriate size and orientation.

Insertional femoral fractures are either proximal or distal, displaced or nondisplaced (**Figure 4**). All fractures are protected by limiting the patient to 10% to 25% weight bearing for 6 weeks. Nondisplaced fractures do not need additional fixation. Displaced proximal fractures need only a cable. Displaced distal fractures need a cable and a plate device to stabilize the fracture. Patients should always be informed of this complication and assured that it has been treated.

Proximal fractures occur when the triangular portion of the component does not fit into the femoral metaphysis. They occur most commonly in female patients, in patients of small stature, in those with coxa vara, or when a low neck cut is needed. Identifying these patients during the templating process permits

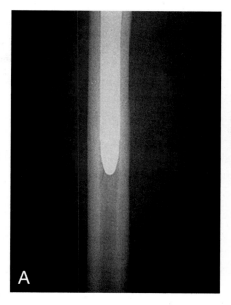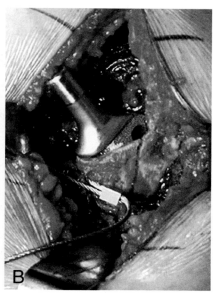

Figure 4   **A**, Nondisplaced distal fracture as seen on postoperative radiograph. Protected weight bearing without additional fixation is the appropriate treatment. **B**, A displaced proximal fracture treated with a cable and 6 weeks of protected weight bearing.

use of an implant with a lower neck-shaft angle that allows the stem to sit higher in the femur, decreasing the chance of a proximal fracture. If the broach is still limited by the proximal medial calcar, the bone must be removed with a side-cutting reamer or a high-speed burr.

Distal fractures are rarely displaced and almost always occur when the implant is inserted. If fracture is suspected because the stem suddenly advances 2 mm during impacting when it was previously advancing only 0.5 mm, an intraoperative radiograph will confirm nondisplacement. However, it is more common to identify a nondisplaced diaphyseal fracture on immediate postoperative radiograph. In either situation, if the fracture is seen on only one view, no additional fixation is needed and the patient is treated with protected weight bearing.

Extensively porous-coated femoral components have the longest

track record of any uncemented devices in the United States and have been available for more than 20 years. Concerns about thigh pain and stress shielding leading to reoperations have not been validated. The medical literature confirms that osseointegration with these components reliably occurs. In addition, clinical studies, some with more than 10 years of follow-up, consistently show a femoral failure rate of less than 7%. The consistently good results achieved with these components, in combination with a simple and reproducible surgical technique that can be used in patients regardless of diagnosis and bone quality, make these implants the benchmark for uncemented femoral fixation. My colleagues and I use extensively porous-coated femoral components for all primary and revision THA.

References

Chiu KY, Tang WM, Ng TP, et al: Cementless total hip arthroplasty in young Chinese patients: A comparison of 2 different prostheses. *J Arthroplasty* 2001;16:863-870.

Engh CA Jr, Claus AM, Hopper RH Jr, Engh CA: Long-term results using the anatomic medullary locking hip prosthesis. *Clin Orthop* 2001;393:137-146.

Hartley WT, McAuley JP, Culpepper WJ, Engh CA Jr, Engh CA Sr: Osteonecrosis of the femoral head treated with cementless total hip arthroplasty. *J Bone Joint Surg Am* 2000;82:1408-1413.

Jana AK, Engh CA Jr, Lewandowski PJ, Hopper RH Jr, Engh CA Sr: Total hip arthroplasty using porous-coated femoral components in patients with rheumatoid arthritis. *J Bone Joint Surg Br* 2001;83:686-690.

Kronick JL, Barba ML, Paprosky WG: Extensively coated femoral components in young patients. *Clin Orthop* 1997;344:263-274.

McAuley JP, Moore KD, Culpepper WJ II, Engh CA: Total hip arthroplasty with porous-coated prostheses fixed without cement in patients who are sixty-five years of age or older. *J Bone Joint Surg Am* 1998;80:1648-1655.

Nercessian OA, Wu WH, Sarkissian H: Clinical and radiographic results of cementless AML total hip arthroplasty in young patients. *J Arthroplasty* 2001;16:312-316.

Woolson ST, Adler NS: The effect of partial or full weight bearing ambulation after cementless total hip arthroplasty. *J Arthroplasty* 2002;17:820-825.

Coding

CPT Codes		Corresponding ICD-9 Codes		
27125	Hemiarthroplasty, hip, partial (eg, femoral stem prosthesis, bipolar arthroplasty)	715.25 715.35	716.15 718.6	733.14 733.42 905.6
27130	Arthroplasty, acetabular and proximal femoral prosthetic replacement (total hip arthroplasty), with or without autograft or allograft	711.45 711.95 714.0 714.30 715.15	7715.25 715.35 716.15 718.5 718.6	720.0 733.14 733.42 808.0 905.6
27132	Conversion of previous hip surgery to total hip arthroplasty, with or without autograft or allograft	715.15 715.25 715.35 718.2	718.5 718.6 733.14 733.42	905.6 996.4 996.66 996.77
27134	Revision of total hip arthroplasty; both components, with or without autograft or allograft	996.4	996.66	996.77
27138	Revision of total hip arthroplasty; femoral component only, with or without allograft	996.4	996.66	996.77
27236	Open treatment of femoral fracture, proximal end, neck, internal fixation or prosthetic replacement	733.14 820.00 820.02	820.03 820.10 820.12	820.13 820.8 820.9

Chapter 11

Primary Total Hip Arthroplasty: Tapered Stems

Robert B. Bourne, MD, FRCSC

Indications

Total hip arthroplasty (THA) has revolutionized the care of patients with end-stage hip disorders. Surgeons may choose from a variety of surgical procedures, including cemented fixation, hybrid fixation (cementing the femoral stem and inserting an uncemented acetabular component), reverse hybrid fixation (uncemented femoral stem and cemented socket), or uncemented implants.

Uncemented femoral stems can be categorized as tapered, anatomic, or distal fixation implants. All have proven durability, but each has disadvantages of varying degrees, specifically, associated thigh pain and frequent stress shielding. The prevalence of thigh pain varies across implant types, occurring in 3% of patients with uncemented tapered stems, in 8% to 15% with uncemented distal fixation stems, and in more than 20% of patients with anatomic stems. Some degree of stress shielding occurs with all endosteally fixed stems, less with uncemented tapered and anatomic stems, and more with distal fixation stems. Engh has described significant stress shielding with extensively coated distal fixation stems in 23% of patients.

More than 85% of patients have Dorr type A or B femurs with funnel-shaped medullary canals. These patients, regardless of age, are ideal candidates for uncemented tapered femoral stems. Secondary factors in the selection of a femoral stem type include patient age, the underlying arthritic condition, and patient activity level. Hence, patients younger than age 70 years with osteoarthritis or osteonecrosis and a high activity level are particularly well suited to uncemented tapered stems.

I prefer uncemented tapered femoral stems. Since 1987, my associates and I have implanted a total of 1,958 uncemented tapered stems, including 30 Cementless Locking Stems (CLS, Centerpulse, Winterthur, Switzerland), 1,147 Mallory Head stems (Biomet, Warsaw, IN), and 781 Synergy stems (Smith & Nephew, Memphis, TN). The recommendations in this chapter reflect our experience with these uncemented tapered femoral stems.

Contraindications

The only absolute contraindication to use of an uncemented tapered femoral stem is active sepsis, although there are several relative contraindications. Dorr type C femurs require very large stems and carry the risks of stress shielding and thigh pain; I prefer to use cemented femoral stems in these patients. Many patients with developmental dysplasia of the hip are better treated with a modular THA that allows correction of excessive femoral neck anteversion. If an uncemented tapered femoral stem is used in a severely dysplastic hip, I recommend a low femoral neck cut to prevent excessive anteversion of the uncemented tapered femoral component. Uncemented tapered stems should not be used in high-riding developmental dysplasia of the hip where a shortening subtrochanteric osteotomy is needed because these stems do not allow ample fixation of the distal femoral fragment.

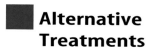

Alternative Treatments

Nonsurgical treatment (ie, analgesics, anti-inflammatory agents, walking aids, physical therapy, or hip injections) must be considered when patients have end-stage arthritic hip conditions. Femoral or periacetabular osteotomy might be considered in selected patients younger than age 50 years, and hip arthrodesis is a possibility for treating unilateral hip disease in young male laborers. Options for patients who require THA include the following: cemented femoral stems; tapered, anatomic, or distal fixation uncemented femoral implants; or surface replacement THA.

Table 1 Results of Uncemented Tapered Femoral Stems at 10 or More Years Follow-up

Author(s) (Year)	Number of Hips	Implant Type	Mean Patient Age (Range)	Mean Follow-up (Range)	Results (%)		
					Thigh Pain	Revisions	Fibrous Ingrowth
Bourne, et al (2001)	307	Mallory Head	NA	NA	3%	0.5%	0%
Hellman, et al (1999)	76	Omnifit	NA	NA	3%	2.6%	NA
Mallory, et al (2001)	120	Mallory Head	NA	NA	0%	2.5%	0%
Sakalkale, et al (1999)	61	Taperloc	NA	NA	1.4%	0%	5%

NA = Not Available

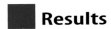

Results

Tapered femoral stems have proven extremely durable, with more than 99% in place at 10 or more years' follow-up. Uncemented tapered femoral components produce only a 3% prevalence of thigh pain, similar to the rate for cemented femoral stems and much lower than the rates for other types of uncemented femoral stem designs. Stress shielding is confined to Gruen zones 1 and 7, with hypertrophy of cortical bone in Gruen zones 3 and 5 in more than 50% of patients. A summary of results appears in **Table 1**.

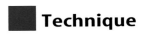

Technique

Exposure
Uncemented tapered femoral stems may be inserted through various surgical approaches, including anterolateral, direct lateral, posterolateral, or mini-incision techniques. I prefer a direct lateral approach because it gives wide exposure of both the acetabulum and femur and minimizes the risk of postoperative dislocation (< 0.3%).

The skin incision is centered on the greater trochanter and extends proximally one handbreadth and distally one half handbreadth to the tip of the greater trochanter (**Figure 1**). The incision is carried through the subcutaneous tissue and iliotibial band. The iliotibial band is first incised distally, and the incision is carried proximally in the interval between the tensor and gluteus maximus muscles. The trochanteric bursa is then incised and the skin and iliotibial band retracted with a Charnley self-retaining retractor. Using capsular scissors, a muscle split is made in the interval between the anterior and posterior portions of the gluteus medius muscle. Right angle retractors are used to gently open this interval.

Electrocautery is used to carry the incision along the anterior aspect of the greater trochanter, past the vastus tubercle and into the posterior aspect of the vastus lateralis (**Figure 2, A**). The fat overlying the gluteus minimus is swept proximally and retracted to protect the terminal branch of the superior gluteal nerve, which courses 9 cm proximal to the posterior tip of the greater trochanter. A vertical cut is then made through the gluteus mini-

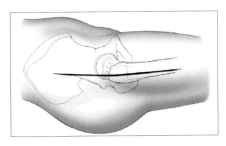

Figure 1 Skin incision for a direct lateral approach to the hip.

mus muscle and capsule using an electric knife, and this incision is carried distally, reflecting the anterior attachment of the gluteus medius, gluteus minimus, and capsule from the anterior aspect of the greater trochanter. The incision continues distally, releasing the vastus lateralis from the proximal femur (**Figure 2, B**). A pin is placed in the iliac crest and a mark placed on the greater trochanter. With the operated limb resting on the nonoperated limb under the sheets, limb length and offset are measured (**Figure 3**). The hip is then dislocated and the femoral neck osteotomized. The acetabulum is exposed and reamed, and an uncemented acetabular component is inserted in the usual fashion.

Bone Preparation
The femur is adducted and placed in a sterile bag opposite the surgeon (**Figure 4**). The femur is opened with a box osteotome and awl and then reamed by hand or power reamer, progressing from small to large size reamers (**Figure 5**). It is important to protect the abductor muscles during this process. Reaming stops when the templated size is reached and good cortical chatter is encountered. Difficulty reaming to the templated size usually means that the stem is in varus. Once this is corrected, the femur is broached, beginning with a broach at least three sizes smaller than that of the final reamer and progressing to the same sized broach used in the last reaming. It is important to keep working laterally and posteriorly with these broaches.

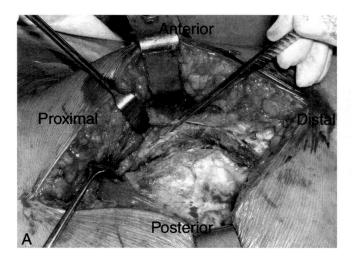
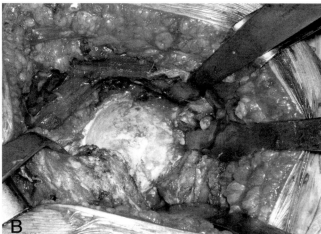

Figure 2 **A,** Vertical split incision through the gluteus medius, gluteus minimus, capsule, and vastus lateralis used in direct lateral approach to the hip. **B,** Wide exposure provided by the direct lateral approach to the hip.

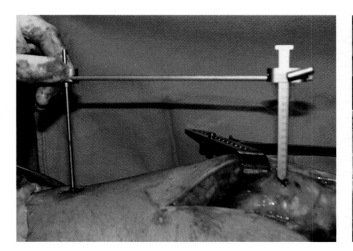
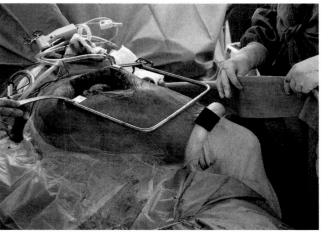

Figure 3 Intraoperative limb length and offset measurements made before the hip is dislocated.

Figure 4 Ipsilateral leg positioning for femoral stem preparation using the direct lateral approach to the hip.

Once the final broach is in place and the implant is both axially and rotationally stable, the impaction tool is removed from the broach and a trial neck placed on the broach. The hip is then reduced and limb length and offset measured. Fine tuning of limb length and offset can be achieved by using standard or high offset femoral necks, different femoral head neck lengths, or a lateralized acetabular insert (**Figure 6**). Once limb length and offset have been restored, the hip is dislocated and the trial components removed.

When performing an uncemented tapered THA, templating is an important first step not only to select the proper stem size and femoral offset but also to determine the level of the femoral neck osteotomy and plan for correction of any limb-length discrepancy. Templating may be performed on standard radiographs or digital images. The magnification of most templates has been determined for a low-centered, AP radiograph of the pelvis. Imaging both hips helps assess limb-length problems and femoral head off-

set. I template both the ipsilateral and contralateral hips.

To assess limb-length discrepancies, it is important to ask the patient whether he or she perceives a limb-length problem. When assessing radiographs for limb-length inequality, the most accurate way is to draw a horizontal line connecting both teardrops and then measure the perpendicular distance from this line to the center of the femoral heads. This technique minimizes the effect of a hip flexion contracture that might be a problem if

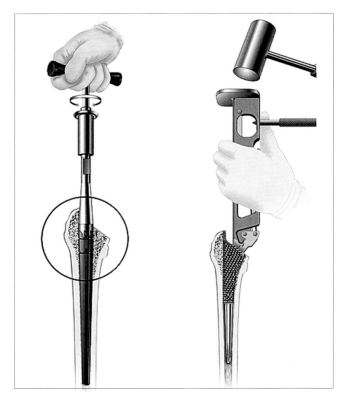

Figure 5 Reaming (top) and broaching (bottom) of the proximal femoral medullary canal with a tapered reamer.

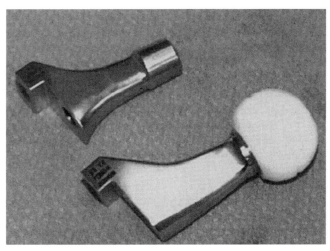

Figure 6 Options that the surgeon has to soft-tissue balance the hip, restoring both limb length and femoral head offset, while using the broach as a trial implant.

the surgeon assesses limb lengths by drawing a horizontal line connecting the ischial tuberosities and noting the relationship of this line to both lesser trochanters (**Figure 7**).

After templating the acetabulum for socket implant size and hip center, the proximal femurs are templated for the neck cut level, femoral component size, and the required femoral head offset (**Figure 8**). I use the junction of the greater trochanter and the lateral femoral neck as a radiographic landmark to identify the location of the proximal and lateral shoulder of the femoral implant. Femoral stem size is then determined using the series of templates. The best-fitting femoral head offset is determined by templating both hips. The surgeon must be aware that arthritic hips usually have an external rotation contracture, which tends to result in underestimation of the required femoral head offset. Therefore, tem-

plating the unaffected hip in unilateral disease can be useful.

Prosthesis Implantation

The uncemented tapered femoral stem corresponding to the femoral stem size, as determined by reaming and broaching, and the femoral neck offset, as determined by limb-length and offset measurements, are selected at this time. The uncemented tapered femoral stem should be toggled to within 1 cm of its final resting position and then the femoral stem gently tapped into place. This tapping should stop once the stem stops advancing. It does not matter if 1 to 2 mm of the porous coating is left exposed. However, if limb length is an issue and the femoral stem will not fully seat, removing the femoral component is advisable. Deeper reaming and broaching should then be performed, and the same femoral stem should be rein-

serted. The femoral head is applied to the Morse taper of the femoral stem and the hip relocated. Once again, limb length and offset should be measured (**Figure 9**). The Ranawat test, useful in assessing proper acetabular and femoral implant positioning, is performed by flexing the hip 30°. If the femoral head sits concentrically in the acetabular polyethylene insert, component positioning is correct.

Next, the hip should be assessed for stability. The key maneuvers are extension, maximal external rotation, and hip flexion in the plane of the body to 90°, with at least 45° of internal rotation. I also test for hip abduction, stretching the shortened adductors to at least 45°. Open adductor tenotomy is rarely needed.

Wound Closure

The wound should be thoroughly irrigated, and the conjoint gluteus minimus and capsule then closed with a running suture. I prefer to use No. 0 polydioxone surgical (PDS) sutures. The conjoint gluteus medius, gluteus minimus, and capsule are then closed using an interrupted No. 1-0 PDS suture, reapproximating the anterior sleeve of the gluteus medius, gluteus

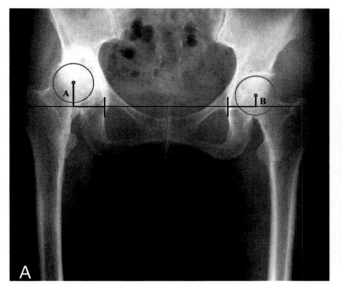
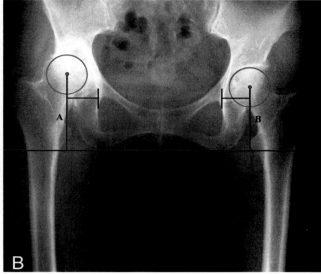

Figure 7 Two methods to determine limb length from preoperative radiographs. Use of the "teardrops" (**A**) is preferred to a line joining the ischial spine (**B**).

minimus, and capsule to the soft-tissue cuff left on the anterior aspect of the greater trochanter (**Figure 10**). All layers of the conjoint tendon must be captured anteriorly. The iliotibial band is then closed with interrupted No.1-0 PDS sutures. The subcutaneous tissue is closed in layers with interrupted No. 2-0 Vicryl (Ethicon, Somerville, NJ) sutures, and the skin is closed with staples.

Postoperative Regimen

Postoperatively, I allow weight bearing as tolerated (**Figure 11**). Patients usually prefer an assistive walking aid (crutches) for the first 3 to 4 weeks, and then progress to use of a single contralateral crutch or cane before beginning independent ambulation. I discourage crossing the leg or flexing the hip more than 90° during the first 6 weeks after surgery.

At 6 weeks postoperatively, resisted abductor strengthening exercises and full weight bearing are encouraged, range of motion precautions are removed, and most patients are allowed to resume driving an automobile.

Avoiding Pitfalls and Complications

Vertical cracks in the anterior femoral cortex occur in approximately 2% of patients at the time of femoral stem insertion. Two important criteria in preventing these cracks are patient selection and surgical technique. Uncemented tapered femoral stems should not be used for elderly, osteoporotic patients with type C femurs.

It is important that the femoral stem be tapped into place and not struck heavily with a mallet during surgery. Once the femoral stem stops advancing, the surgeon must stop hitting it. An uncemented tapered femoral stem is a wedge that will split the femur if continued force is applied.

Anterior femoral cracks are easily repaired. The femoral stem is backed out, and one or two cerclage wires are placed around the proximal femur (**Figure 12**). Care should be taken to remain on bone and to pass the wires posterior-to-anterior to avoid a potential neuromuscular injury. The same femoral stem is then tapped back into place. Patients with

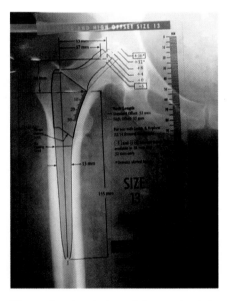

Figure 8 Templating of the proximal femur for stem size, femoral head offset, and the level of the neck osteotomies.

an anterior femoral split fracture should be restricted to toe-touch weight bearing for 6 weeks rather than weight bearing as tolerated. After following patients for at least 10 years postoperatively, my colleagues and I reported no difference in clinical out-

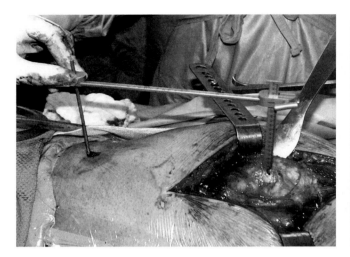

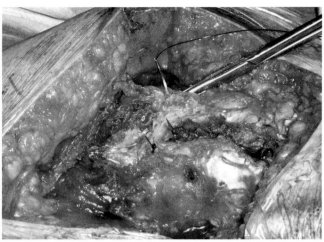

Figure 9 Final limb-length and offset measurements using the intraoperative guide.

Figure 10 Closure of the conjoint gluteus medius, gluteus minimus, and capsule.

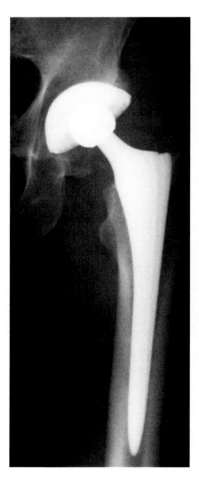

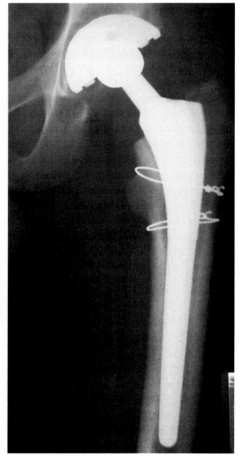

Figure 11 Postoperative radiograph of a well-balanced uncemented tapered total hip replacement.

Figure 12 Patient who sustained an intraoperative anterior split fracture of the proximal femur at 9-year follow-up. The femoral stem was backed out, the proximal femur encircled with a cerclage wire, and the uncemented tapered stem reinserted.

come for these patients compared with patients in whom no crack occurred.

Careful preoperative templating of both the affected hip and the contralateral hip permits appropriate preoperative planning and helps guide implant placement, offset selection, and femoral neck length. Use of an intraoperative limb-length and offset guide identifies what corrections have been made in limb length and offset during surgery (**Figure 5**). I use high-offset femoral stems in about 50% of my patients undergoing THA surgeries. Failure to control offset or limb length can result in soft-tissue laxity and impingement, factors that contribute to postoperative dislocation. Proper restoration of offset is important in maximizing abductor muscle function, thereby improving abductor strength and reducing the need for walking aids.

References

Bourne RB, Rorabeck CH, Patterson J, Guerin J: Tapered titanium cementless total hip replacements: A 10- to 13-year followup study. *Clin Orthop* 2001;393:112-120.

Hellman EJ, Capello NN, Feinberg JR: Omnifit cementless total hip arthroplasty: A 10-year average follow-up. *Clin Orthop* 1999;364:164-174.

Mallory TH, Lombardi AV, Leith JR, et al: Minimal 10-year results of a tapered cementless femoral component in total hip arthroplasty. *J Arthroplasty* 2001;16:49-54.

Mulliken BD, Bourne RB, Rorabeck CH, Nayak NN: A tapered titanium femoral stem inserted without cement in a total hip arthroplasty: Radiographic evaluation and stability. *J Bone Joint Surg Am* 1996;78:1214-1225.

Sakalkale DP, Engh K, Hozack WJ, Rothman RH: Minimum 10 year results of a tapered cementless hip replacement. *Clin Orthop* 1999;362:138-144.

Coding

CPT Codes		Corresponding ICD-9 Codes		
27125	Hemiarthroplasty, hip, partial (eg, femoral stem prosthesis, bipolar arthroplasty)	715.25 718.6 905.6	715.35 733.14	716.15 733.42
27130	Arthroplasty, acetabular and proximal femoral prosthetic replacement (total hip arthroplasty), with or without autograft or allograft	711.45 714.30 715.35 718.6 733.42	711.95 715.15 716.15 720.0 808.0	714.0 715.25 718.5 733.14 905.6
27132	Conversion of previous hip surgery to total hip arthroplasty, with or without autograft or allograft	715.15 718.2 733.14 996.4	715.25 718.5 733.42 996.66	715.35 718.6 905.6 996.77
27134	Revision of total hip arthroplasty; both components, with or without autograft or allograft	996.4	996.66	996.77
27138	Revision of total hip arthroplasty; femoral component only, with or without allograft	996.4	996.66	996.77
27236	Open treatment of femoral fracture, proximal end, neck, internal fixation or prosthetic replacement	733.14 820.03 820.13	820.0 820.10 820.8	820.02 820.12 820.9

Chapter 12

Primary Total Hip Arthroplasty: Modular Stems

William P. Barrett, MD

▮ Indications

Femoral head and neck modularity of total hip arthroplasty (THA) components was introduced in the early 1980s. This design feature offers several advantages, including adjustable limb length and offset once the femoral component is in place, a wide variety of acceptable materials for the head and stem, decreased stem inventory, simplifying exposure to facilitate isolated acetabular revisions, and adjustable head size and neck length to address instability. The disadvantages of these junctions include fretting and corrosion wear, third-body generation, mechanical failure of the junction, head dissociation, and decreased range of motion associated with use of skirted heads.

Fretting and corrosion wear depend on a variety of factors, including

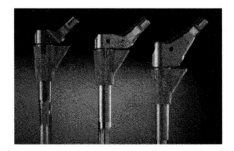

Figure 1 Proximal modular implant. The fluted stem attaches to metaphyseal sleeve via a Morse taper. Multiple sizes of sleeves can fit with any given stem.

load, number of loading cycles, contact stress distribution, and surface finish. Although some wear is inevitable at these modular junctions, 6- to 10-year follow-up studies report success rates similar to monoblock stems without evidence of the catastrophic wear associated with modular junctions or a significant increase in the rate of osteolysis.

The S-ROM (DePuy, Warsaw, IN) was introduced in the mid 1980s in an attempt to achieve a consistently tight fit both proximally and distally. The S-ROM stem is a proximal modular system. The diaphyseal stem obtains distal stability via flutes and bony ingrowth proximally into metaphyseal sleeves, both of which are necessary to obtain metaphyseal fill and attach to the stem via a Morse taper (**Figure 1**). The stem is undersized proximally; therefore, it can be inserted into the metaphyseal sleeve in any degree of anteversion. Straight or bowed stems of varying lengths can be used with any metaphyseal component. The stability of modular stems and the modular head-neck junction relies on the use of Morse tapers. These tapers are truncated cones that attach via an interference fit to a similar socket. The wedge shape of the tapered cone results in a mechanical interlock. All nonwelded junctions have some degree of micromotion under load.

This chapter focuses on the S-ROM stem because I have extensive

experience with this stem, and at present I am not aware of any other modular femoral prosthesis with midterm results from multiple centers. The principles discussed in this chapter can be applied to any modular stem, but specific techniques may need to be modified according to the recommendations of the manufacturer.

Modular uncemented stems can be used in any situation in which an uncemented stem is indicated based on surgeon preference and experience. Typically, young, active patients with type A or B bone are good candidates. A modular stem is particularly indicated in patients with (1) developmental dysplasia of the hip (DDH), (2) juvenile rheumatoid arthritis, (3) previous trauma or surgery, or (4) metabolic bone disease.

DDH, with its associated excessive femoral neck anteversion, altered femoral head and neck anatomy, and proximal location of the femoral head, is well suited to reconstruction with a modular implant. The modular stem allows placement of the proximal metaphyseal sleeve in the best available bone. The stem can be placed in the diaphysis independent of the metaphyseal anatomy, which allows correction of excessive anteversion. In patients with congenital high hip dislocation, in which anatomic placement of the acetabular component is desired, a subtrochanteric shortening osteotomy can be performed to avoid

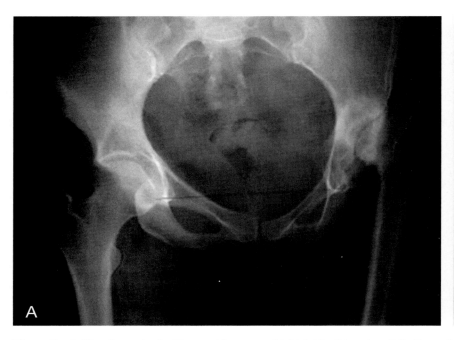

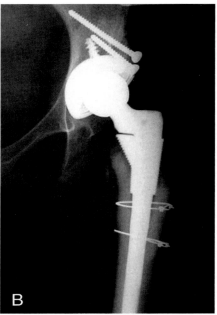

Figure 2   **A,** AP radiograph of a 42-year-old woman with high hip dislocation. **B,** Radiograph obtained 5 years following uncemented THA using a modular stem, subtrochanteric, shortening osteotomy shows that the osteotomy has healed. The proximal portion of the osteotomy has ingrowth into the metaphyseal sleeve, and the distal portion is stabilized by five flutes on the modular stem.

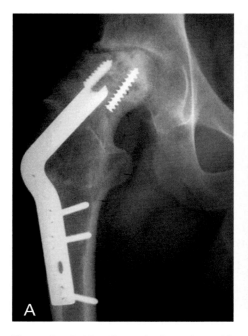

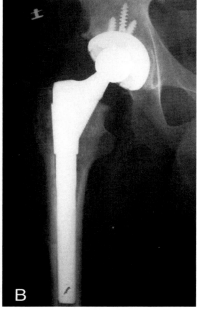

Figure 3   **A,** AP radiograph of a patient with posttraumatic osteoarthritis secondary to a femoral neck fracture. Nonunion developed, and a valgus osteotomy was required. Osteonecrosis of the femoral head developed postoperatively. **B,** AP radiograph obtained 3 years after THA with a modular stem.

excess stretch on soft tissue and neurovascular structures (**Figure 2**). In this situation, the fluted distal stem allows independent fixation of the distal fragment of the osteotomy, whereas the proximal metaphyseal sleeve allows fixation to the portion above the osteotomy. Stability is provided by the modular junction, which has adequate strength to resist the torsional loads during healing of the osteotomy.

Juvenile rheumatoid arthritis can affect proximal and distal femoral anatomy, as well as overall bone quality. A proximal modular system allows independent sizing of the distal and proximal femur, as well as correction of excess anteversion that is often associated with this condition.

In patients who have had previous trauma or surgery, the anatomy of the proximal femur is often distorted. The presence of previous hardware creates defects that must be bypassed, and malrotation is often present (**Figure 3**). These challenges can be addressed by using a modular implant. Varying stem lengths allow the lowest screw hole to be bypassed by at least two canal diameters. Proximal and distal fixation allows correction of angular or rotational malalignment with a corrective osteotomy.

Metabolic bone disease is often associated with bowing of the femur, which precludes use of a monoblock stem. In this situation, corrective osteotomy, realignment, and rotational correction of the femur can be obtained with use of a modular stem.

Contraindications

Contraindications for modular uncemented stems are generally similar to those for uncemented stems in THA. Inability to obtain either proximal or distal fixation as a result of a patulous femur precludes the use of an uncemented device. When a modular stem is fixed, both proximally and distally, it has been reported to have a load to failure, similar to a cemented stem inserted with third-generation cementing techniques. However, when the stem is fixed only proximally or only distally, the load to failure is only half of that obtained with both proximal and distal fixation.

Alternative Treatments

In most patients with excellent bone and typical endosteal anatomy, the monoblock stems currently available will achieve rigid fixation, which prevents micromotion and allows contact of the roughened femoral surface with endosteal bone. The advantages of a modular system are not required in these patients, and the theoretical concern of fretting, corrosion, and third-body wear can be avoided by use of a monoblock stem. The decision to use proximal or distal fixation of the stem is based on surgeon preference and experience.

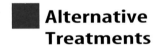

Table 1   Results of Modular Stems for THA

Author(s) (Year)	Number of Hips	Implant Type	Mean Patient Age (Range)	Mean Follow-up (Range)	Results
Christie, et al (1999)	175	S-ROM	59 years (22–93)	5.3 years (4–7.8)	98% bone ingrowth 7% osteolysis 7% thigh pain 2 revisions of acetabular component
Tanzer, et al (2001)	59	S-ROM	56 years (14–76)	8.5 years (6–12.9)	100% bone ingrowth 42% osteolysis No revision for aseptic loosening
Sporer, et al (2004)	135	S-ROM	77.2 years (70–90)	5 years (2–8.5)	100% bone ingrowth 7% osteolysis 1.5% thigh pain No revisions

Results

Results with the S-ROM prosthesis are summarized in **Table 1**.

Technique

Exposure
A standard posterolateral or direct lateral approach can be used, depending on surgeon preference. The details of these approaches were described previously. In general, care must be taken to protect the abductor muscles during reaming to avoid damage while lateralizing the reamers in the greater trochanter.

Bone Preparation
After a trial component or a real component with a trial liner is placed in the acetabulum, attention is turned to the femur. The technique for the S-ROM prosthesis is described here because no generic modular technique is currently in use. The femoral osteotomy for an S-ROM stem is transverse to the longitudinal axis of the femur (**Figure 4**). A definitive cut based on preoperative templating, or a provisional cut that is revised once the bone is prepared, can be performed with a saw.

The femur is prepared in a three-step reaming process, beginning distally, then proximally after sizing the diaphysis, and finally in the calcar area. Patients with type A bone often have a very narrow diaphyseal canal; thus, to avoid a potential step-off from a straight rigid reamer, the diaphyseal canal is initially reamed with flexible reamers. A bulb-tipped guide rod is inserted, and flexible reamers are used up to the minor diameter of the stem (stem diameter minus the flutes). Circumferential reaming should be obtained at the desired stem size. Next, straight rigid reamers (ie, 1-mm smaller than the last flexible reamer) are used to prepare the diaphysis and progress to the minor diameter of the stem or 0.5 mm over the minor diameter, depending on bone quality. During this reaming process, it is important to remain lateral at the starting point and to avoid varus placement of the stem as the reaming progresses distally (**Figure 5**). Use of a bent Hohmann retractor over the tip of the greater trochanter to protect the abductors aids the reaming process and protects

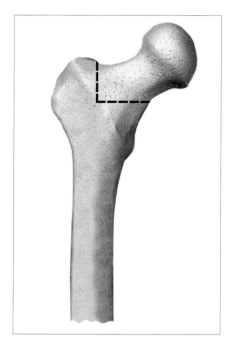

Figure 4 The femoral neck osteotomy for a modular stem is made transverse to the longitudinal axis of the femur.

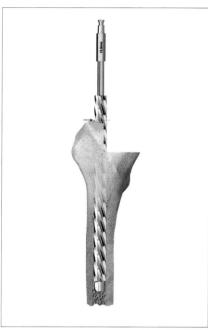

Figure 5 Distal reaming with a rigid reamer. Note the lateral starting point and that varus position was avoided.

cone reamer into the medial side of the greater trochanter is important to avoid varus placement of the stem. This requires retraction of the abductors using a rake or bent Hohmann retractor. Progressively larger cone reamers are then used until cortical contact is achieved. This occurs first in the subtrochanteric region anteriorly. The depth of proximal reaming is determined by advancing the cone reamer until the reference line for the desired neck length is level with the tip of the greater trochanter. The triangular portion of the proximal sleeve is prepared with the appropriate milling reamer until cortical contact is obtained in the medial proximal femur. However, because placement of the proximal sleeve does not determine stem anteversion, the triangle can be placed anywhere in the proximal femur to obtain the best bone (**Figure 6**, *B*)

Prosthesis Implantation

A trial proximal sleeve is placed on the sleeve introducer, the triangular portion is rotated to the appropriate position, and then the sleeve is impacted into the metaphysis. Overzealous impaction should be avoided because this can act as a splitting wedge in the proximal femur. A trial stem with appropriate neck length is inserted in the desired anteversion (**Figure 7**). Trial reduction of the reconstruction occurs next. Stability in flexion and internal rotation and in extension and external rotation is checked. If stability is not adequate, then cup placement or stem version is adjusted (**Figure 8**).

Once stability is judged to be adequate, the real components are placed. After seating the proximal sleeve, the Morse taper junction is cleaned and dried, and then the real stem is placed in the appropriate version and driven into the sleeve until the Morse taper is engaged. Appropriate engagement is confirmed by an audible change in the pitch of impaction and visually by a gap of 1 to 3 mm between the sleeve and neck of the

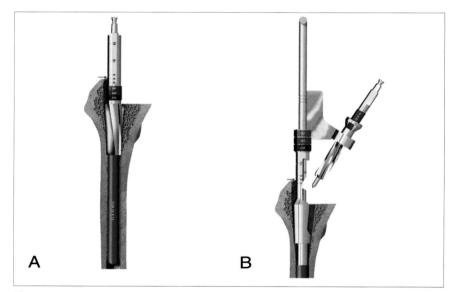

Figure 6 **A,** Proximal reaming with cone reamers. **B,** Milling of the proximal stem.

the gluteus medius. The depth of distal reaming is determined by progressing until the reference line on the reamer reaches the tip of the greater trochanter.

Next, proximal reaming of the metaphysis is performed with cone

reamers that are 5-mm larger than the corresponding distal stem size selected. The smallest cone reamer for a given size is attached to a pilot shaft, which is equal to the selected distal stem size, and then reaming is initiated (**Figure 6**, *A*). Lateralization of the

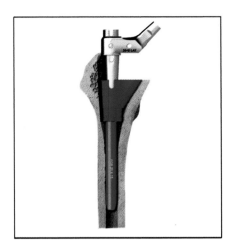

Figure 7 Trial stem inserting into a trial metaphyseal sleeve. Stem version is independent of sleeve placement.

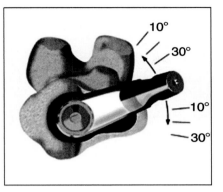

Figure 8 With trial components, stem version can be changed to enhance stability or correct excess anteversion. The position of the trial implants is recorded so that the real implants are placed in proper orientation.

prosthesis. The stem has sharp flutes that engage the endosteal bone early; thus, version cannot be changed once the flutes have engaged the bone. The appropriate neck length and head size are chosen to restore limb length and offset.

The advantage of the modular prosthesis is that version of the femoral stem can be altered to compensate for femoral anatomy. For example, patients with DDH usually have increased femoral anteversion. If a standard stem is implanted in this type of femur, there may be excessive anteversion of the femoral component, which can lead to anterior instability. A modular stem allows placement of the stem in "relative retroversion" to compensate for the excessive femoral anteversion.

These modular stems allow the surgeon to select the appropriate version to compensate for the patient's anatomy, which may be quite variable, particularly in those with a history of a

proximal femoral fracture or femoral osteotomy.

Wound Closure

If a posterior approach was used, the posterior capsule and short external rotators are reattached to the posterior trochanter or tendon of the gluteus medius using No. 5 nonabsorbable sutures. The quadratus femoris is loosely tacked down to its stump with No. 1 bioabsorbable suture. The fascia lata is closed with No. 1 bioabsorbable suture, the subcutaneous tissue is closed with No. 2 bioabsorbable sutures, and the skin closed with staples.

Postoperative Regimen

Physical therapy is initiated the day of surgery with the patient standing at the bedside and walking, if tolerated. Weight bearing with a walker or crutches is allowed as tolerated for 4 weeks, followed by progression to a cane, if postoperative radiographs are satisfactory. Home strengthening exercises are prescribed before the patient leaves the hospital. Total hip pre-

cautions are followed for 8 weeks after surgery.

Avoiding Pitfalls and Complications

Varus placement of the stem is the most common technical error with this system and can lead to undersizing of the stem and ultimately compromised fixation. This problem can be avoided by stressing a lateral starting point for the reaming process and maintaining lateralization during distal and proximal reaming. If the position of the stem is in question, an intraoperative radiograph can be obtained with the trial components in place. Overly aggressive reaming of the proximal bone with cone reamers can thin the anterior cortical bone, increasing the risk of fracture. Forceful seating of the proximal sleeve (given its triangular shape) can split the proximal femur, much like a wedge in wood. Malrotation of the stem within the modular sleeve during seating can affect the stability of the hip construct. This problem can be avoided by assessing the proper version of the stem for maximum stability of the hip construct with trial components and noting that amount of version so it can be repeated during stem impaction. Failure to engage the Morse taper of the sleeve can occur without adequate overreaming of the distal bone or when seating a long bowed stem, which can achieve early three-point fixation and cause the stem to become stuck before fully seating.

References

Cameron HU: Modularity in primary total hip replacement. *J Arthroplasty* 1996;11:332-334.

Christie MJ, DeBoer DK, Trick LW, et al: Primary total hip arthroplasty with use of the modular S-ROM prosthesis. *J Bone Joint Surg Am* 1999;81:1707-1716.

Sporer SM, Obar RJ, Bernini PM: Primary total hip arthroplasty using modular proximally coated prosthesis in patients older than 70. *J Arthroplasty* 2004;19:197-203.

Tanzer M, Chan S, Brooks CE, Bobyn JD: Primary cementless total hip arthroplasty using a modular femoral component. *J Arthroplasty* 2001;16(suppl 1):64-70.

Coding

CPT Codes		Corresponding ICD-9 Codes		
27130	Arthroplasty, acetabular and proximal femoral prosthetic replacement (total hip arthroplasty), with or without autograft or allograft	711.45 714.30 715.35 718.6 733.42	711.95 715.15 716.15 720.0 808.0	714.0 715.25 718.5 733.14 905.6

CPT copyright © 2004 by the American Medical Association. All Rights Reserved

Chapter 13
Surface Replacement
Thomas Parker Vail, MD

Indications

Surface replacement is an appropriate treatment for active patients with advanced hip degeneration. The ideal candidate has good bone quality and activity demands that would benefit from bone conservation and joint stability. Surface replacement is indicated for degenerative conditions that irretrievably destroy the articular surface of the hip, resulting in pain and disability. Common conditions include osteoarthritis, posttraumatic arthritis, femoral head osteonecrosis, and degenerative sequelae of childhood hip diseases such as slipped capital femoral epiphysis with chondrolysis or developmental dysplasia. Because nonsurgical treatments have not resulted in improvement, candidates for surface replacement present at an advanced stage of degeneration not treatable with procedures that spare the femoral head, such as intertrochanteric osteotomy or grafting. Hemiresurfacing is appropriate when the articular surface of the acetabulum is relatively free from degenerative changes (no full-thickness chondral loss).

Hip joint surface replacement is either a hemiresurfacing (**Figure 1**, *A*) of the femoral head or a total surface replacement of both the femoral head and the acetabular surface (**Figure 1**, *B*). Total articular surface replacement of the hip with a metal-on-metal bearing (class III, category B) is not currently approved by the US Food and Drug Administration (FDA) but is used extensively in other countries (**Figure 2**). This procedure is appropriate when acetabular degenerative changes accompany femoral head degenerative changes. Appropriate diagnoses for consideration of total articular hip replacement, in addition to the diagnoses above, include later stages of osteonecrosis associated with secondary degenerative changes of the acetabulum (**Figure 3**). Total surface replacement can also be used to treat degenerative sequelae arising from less severe cases of developmental dysplasia of the hip.

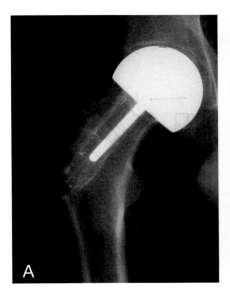
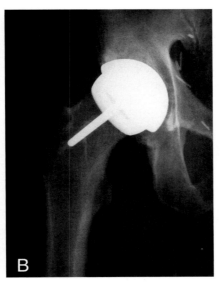

Figure 1 **A**, Radiograph showing a femoral head hemiresurfacing. **B**, AP radiograph of metal-on-metal total articular resurfacing. (Note: This device [class III, category B] is not approved by the FDA for clinical use.)

Contraindications

Femoral head surface replacement is contraindicated in patients without enough femoral head and neck bone to achieve fixation of the resurfacing component, such as those with femoral neck osteoporosis (more than one standard deviation below the norm), large cysts of the femoral head or neck, primary or metastatic neoplasms, posttraumatic arthrosis with

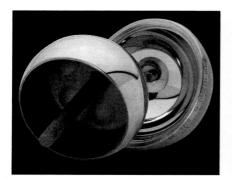

Figure 2 Total hip resurfacing component. (Note: This device is not approved by the FDA for clinical use.) (Courtesy of DePuy, Warsaw, IN.)

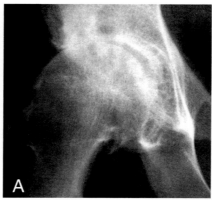

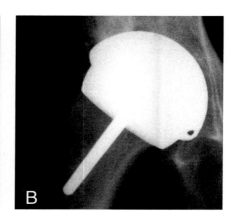

Figure 3 **A,** Preoperative AP radiograph of a patient with degenerative joint disease in the hip. **B,** Postoperative AP radiograph demonstrating total articular resurfacing of the hip.

extensive femoral neck bone loss, large segments of osteonecrosis of the femoral head with collapse of the head into the neck, and proximal femoral deficiencies. Anatomic variations leading to a short, wide femoral neck, as seen in some patients with Legg-Calvé-Perthes disease, are also relative contraindications. Achieving reliable femoral side fixation and restoration of offset and length by resurfacing is quite difficult in such patients. Hemisurface replacement (femoral head only) is not indicated in patients with developmental dysplasia with subluxation of the femoral head.

Additional contraindications to total resurfacing include any condition unfavorable to a metal-on-metal articulation, such as metal allergy or hypersensitivity and renal insufficiency (see chapter 14 on bearing surfaces). Active infection is also a contraindication to any type of surface replacement.

Alternative Treatments

The diagnoses for which surface replacement is commonly considered affect many patients, and treatment alternatives depend on the particular condition of the hip to be treated. Treatment alternatives include restor-

ative and bone-sparing procedures such as bone grafting of the femoral head, osteotomy of the proximal femur and acetabulum, and cartilage repair strategies. Within the context of arthroplasty, alternatives to femoral head resurfacing include hemiarthroplasty with fixed or bipolar bearing. Unlike femoral head resurfacing, these options require removal of the femoral head and placement of a femoral stem with a modular or nonmodular femoral head replacement. Hemiresurfacing implant systems are generally available in increments of 1 to 2 mm in diameter to accommodate the inner diameter of the native acetabulum.

Alternatives to total resurfacing include total hip arthroplasty (THA) with standard or jumbo bearing surfaces. Many widely available total hip systems include the option of using heads larger than 32 mm that articulate with a polyethylene, metal, or ceramic counterface on the acetabular side. The advantages of a larger femoral head can thus be realized if sparing the femoral head bone is technically impossible or the procedure for total resurfacing is not FDA approved.

Results

Hemiresurfacing of the hip provides pain relief and improved function for

most patients. However, most studies indicate that these benefits are not as predictable or long-lasting as those obtained with THA. Some reports suggest declining survivorship with hemiresurfacing because of recurrent pain at relatively short follow-up (**Table 1**).

Results of total articular surface replacement are difficult to analyze because follow-up periods were generally short, and the designs in these studies were abandoned because of rapid advances in metal-on-metal bearing technology (**Table 2**). The FDA has sanctioned ongoing clinical trials for several metal-on-metal total resurfacing systems through its Investigational Device trials.

Technique

Optimal outcomes in hip resurfacing depend on appropriate indications, preoperative assessment of the femoral neck bone, and surgical technique, including optimization of implant geometry and size and achievement of durable fixation of the implant to the bone.

Exposure

The anterolateral approach to the hip is the preferred exposure for hemiresurfacing because it takes advantage of

Table 1   Results of Hemiresurfacing

Author(s) (Year)	Number of Hips	Implant Type	Mean Patient Age (Range)	Mean Follow-up (Range)	Results
Scott, et al (1987)	25	TARA*	38 years (22–55)	3 years (2–5)	88% Good/Excellent
Hungerford, et al (1998)	33	TARA*	41 years (25–65)	10.4 years (4–14)	61% Good/Excellent
Beaulé, et al (2001)	37	Various	34 years (18–51)	15 years	Survivorship 79% (5 years) 59% (10 years) 45% (15 years)

*Total Articular Replacement Arthroplasty head (BioPro, Port Huron, MI)

Table 2   Results of Metal-on-Metal Total Hip Resurfacing

Author(s) (Year)	Number of Hips	Implant Type	Mean Patient Age (Range)	Mean Follow-up (Range)	Results (Survival)
Daniel, et al (2004)	439	McMinn, Birmingham	48 years (27–55)	3.3 years (1.1–8.2)	99% (1996 patients excluded)
Amstutz, et al (2004)	400	Wright Medical	48 years	3.5 years	94.4%
Wagner and Wagner (1996)	35	Wagner	36 years (15–64)	20 months (6–54)	86%

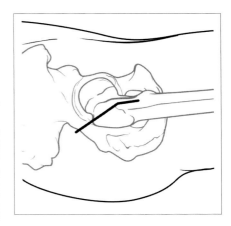

Figure 4   Diagram demonstrates correct placement of the skin incision over the greater trochanter.

the femoral neck's natural anteversion, which conveniently brings the femoral head into view when the hip is flexed and externally rotated, dislocating the femoral head anteriorly. The skin incision (**Figure 4**) is placed obliquely over the greater trochanter from a point 2 to 3 cm distal to the tip of the trochanter, anterior to the femoral shaft, and extends proximally over the trochanter toward the sciatic notch. The tensor fascia and gluteus medius are divided in line with the muscle fibers.

Once the gluteus medius muscle is exposed beneath the fascial layer, the hip capsule can be approached through either a direct lateral exposure or a modified Hardinge approach. The latter is performed by incising the fibers of the gluteus medius at the anterior third of the greater trochanter. The gluteus medius tendon is elevated from the trochanter, creating a continuous soft-tissue sleeve, extending no more than 4 cm into the medius muscle proximally, and 4 cm into the vastus lateralis muscle distally. Once this soft-tissue sleeve is reflected forward, the hip capsule is exposed and incised in an L-shape, extending from the acetabular rim at the 11 o'clock position toward the piriformis fossa, and extended distally along the intertrochanteric line. The capsule is reflected forward, bringing the femoral head into view. The femoral head can then be dislocated anteriorly by flexing and externally rotating the hip joint. Further flexion and external rotation of the hip bring the femoral head up into the wound, allowing preparation of the femoral head for the resurfacing prosthesis.

The alternative to the modified Hardinge approach is the direct lateral approach for femoral head resurfacing. Direct lateral exposure is achieved by elevating a small wafer of bone from the greater trochanter. This bone wafer is 8- to 12-mm thick and includes the attachment of the gluteus medius and minimus. When the combination of the trochanteric bone and abductors is reflected forward, the hip joint capsule and reflected head of the rectus femoris are visualized. The remainder of the approach is the same as that of the modified Hardinge approach.

The posterior approach to the hip is the preferred approach for total hip resurfacing. This approach begins with an oblique skin incision similar to the one described for the anterolateral approach. The incision is placed over the greater trochanter and is followed by splitting of the gluteus maximus, proceeding posterior to the gluteus medius muscle insertion on the greater trochanter. With the hip inter-

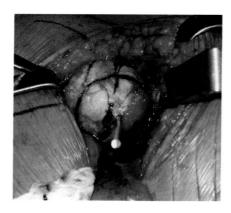

Figure 5 Osteophytes obscure the approach to the femoral neck. The circle drawn on the femoral head outlines the position of the femoral neck relative to the femoral head. Note the correct placement of the guide pin down the center of the femoral neck.

nally rotated and the posterior edge of the gluteus medius retracted anteriorly, the piriformis and short external rotators down to the quadratus femoris are visualized. Gentle traction of the gluteus medius is required so that undue traction is not placed on the neurovascular pedicle to the gluteus muscle tracking out of the greater sciatic notch. The short external rotators are tagged with a heavy suture and incised along with the posterior capsule. The capsular incision proceeds along the superior border of the piriformis, moving toward the piriformis fossa from a position anterior to the sciatic notch. The distal limb of the capsular incision proceeds down the intertrochanteric line to the lesser trochanter. With the capsule and short external rotators reflected posteriorly, the femoral head can be dislocated posteriorly by flexion and internal rotation of the hip joint, and then prepared for the femoral resurfacing device.

The femoral head and neck must be mobilized anteriorly to allow acetabular exposure. The key step in this mobilization is elevating the anterior capsule from the acetabulum's anterior lip to allow translation of the femoral head and neck into a recess anterior and superior to the acetabulum.

With the hip flexed and the femoral head translated forward, the acetabulum comes into clear view for reaming and acetabular component preparation.

Bone Preparation

Unlike THAs, femoral resurfacing prostheses must follow strict sizing requirements to properly link with the acetabulum during both hemiresurfacing and total articular resurfacing. The resurfaced femoral head must be prepared so that it creates an exact fit with the native acetabular inner diameter (for hemiresurfacing) or the inner diameter of the acetabular prosthesis (for total articular resurfacing). The femoral head must not be overreamed, making the outer diameter too small for the hip socket. Similarly, an excessively large femoral head will not articulate properly within the acetabulum. Careful templating and trialing of the acetabular diameter will help prevent such errors. In total articular resurfacing, the size of the acetabular component is linked to the size of the femoral head component, with a large femoral head component requiring a correspondingly large acetabular component that matches the diameter of the templated native acetabulum.

The linked size requirements between the femur and acetabulum make it clear that templating and size determination are key points to success in a resurfacing operation. The first step in both hemiresurfacing and total articular resurfacing is to measure the acetabular diameter, because this measurement dictates the femoral component sizes. When hemiresurfacing the femur, the size of the femoral component and the appropriate amount of bone resection in the femoral neck are determined by placing trial components in the acetabulum to gauge the best fit within the native acetabulum. With total articular resurfacing, templating the femoral head after the acetabular size is determined ensures that the femoral head size

matching the templated acetabular component will safely fit the proximal femur. If the appropriate resurfacing component for the acetabulum appears to require a femoral component that is too small for the femoral neck, the size of the acetabular component will need to be increased. Newer resurfacing components are designed with the smallest component wall thickness to minimize both the total volume of bone excised during the procedure and the need to increase the size of the acetabular component to accommodate the femoral neck.

Femoral head bone preparation requires four key steps: placing a guide pin down the center of the femoral neck, cylindrical reaming of the femoral neck over the guide pin, creating a proximal head resection, and chamfer reaming of the top of the head. Depending on instrumentation, these steps can be performed sequentially or simultaneously.

Most instrumentation systems begin by centering a guide pin on the femoral neck axis rather than on the center of the femoral head. Accurate placement is critical to avoid inadvertent notching of the femoral neck during cylindrical reaming. Most femoral heads being resurfaced have some degree of eccentricity relative to the femoral neck. In end-stage degenerative hip conditions, the femoral head is flattened superiorly, resulting in an acquired varus anomaly accentuated by an osteophyte in the inferior recess of the joint. Osteophytes at the osteoarticular border of the femoral head dramatically distort the perception of the actual location of the femoral head relative to the neck (**Figure 5**). Therefore, the entry point of the guide pin is often located in what appears to be a superior valgus (**Figure 6**, *A*) and anterior (**Figure 6**, *B*) position on the flattened femoral head to allow centering of the guide pin in the femoral neck.

Accurate placement of the guide pin can be accomplished by using pin alignment guides and repositioning

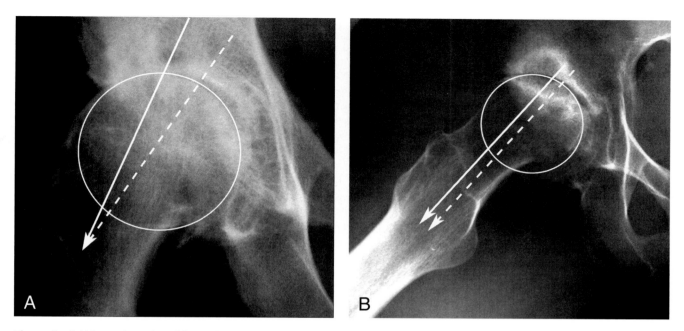

Figure 6 **A**, Valgus orientation of the guide pin. The guide pin should be placed down the center of the femoral neck at approximately 140° relative to the femoral shaft. The dotted line, although in the center of the femoral head, is incorrectly positioned, producing a varus orientation of the femoral neck preparation. The smooth line is correctly positioned down the center of the femoral neck. Note the entry point is well above the equator of the femoral head. **B**, Center position of the femoral neck on lateral view. The guide pin often appears high on the femoral head to achieve a pin position centered in the femoral neck. The dotted line is centered on the femoral head but is incorrectly positioned because it is posterior to the center of the femoral neck.

devices to control angulation and translation of the pin entry point on the femoral head. The starting point for the guide pin can be estimated by drawing two lines up the center of the femoral neck, one each on the superior and anterior quadrants. The intersection of these two lines provides a reasonable estimate of the point where the guide pin should enter the femoral head. Ideal preparation of the femoral head bone places the femoral component in slight valgus alignment, with a neck-shaft angle near 140°. Whether placed manually or with a pin driver, the final pin position should be checked with a stylus to reference the femoral neck. If placed centrally within the neck, the guide pin should pass unimpeded to the lateral cortex of the femur. If the guide pin stops short while being driven down the femoral neck, it has probably impinged on the anterior femoral neck cortex.

Femoral head reaming is performed in most systems by cannulated reamers that pass over the central guide pin. A series of reaming or milling devices turns the femoral neck into a cylindrical shape with a chamfered proximal edge (**Figure 7**). Centering of the cylindrical head reamers ensures proper positioning of the femoral component and minimizes the risk of notching the superior and anterior surfaces of the femoral neck. These are the tension surfaces of the femoral neck, and notching them could place the patient at a higher risk of femoral neck fracture. Centering the femoral head component also ensures adequate clearance of the femoral neck from the acetabular rim when the hip is flexed. Posterior or inferior translations of the resurfacing will decrease the femoral neck clearance in flexion, abduction, and external rotation.

To ensure that the femoral and acetabular component sizes match the patient's anatomy, the preferred technique is to stop reaming the femoral neck when it is at least one size larger

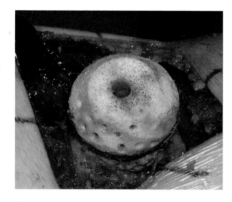

Figure 7 Final preparation of the femoral head and neck.

than the templated size, and then begin acetabular preparation. Once this is completed, and the size of the acetabular component is correct, final preparation of the femur can be safely performed. It is not necessary to remove all of the osteophytes from the femoral neck distal to the area that will be covered by the resurfacing prosthesis. Aggressive removal of osteophytes can lead to weakening of the femoral neck. Similarly, the femoral neck is more vulnerable to fracture if there is exposed cancellous bone surface distal to the area of the femoral neck covered by the resurfacing device. However, it is appropriate to remove large osteophytes that could lead to impingement or restricted range of motion of the hip joint.

A femoral head resurfacing device affords limited ability to alter the length or offset of the femoral neck. The proximal neck cut employs a measured resection technique that removes bone thickness equal to the size of the prosthetic device. Fixation of the femoral head resurfacing component depends on contact with the femoral neck. Therefore, placing the prosthesis above the resected surface diminishes the bone-prosthesis contact area and creates an excessively thick cement mantle.

Chamfer reaming of the proximal neck follows the proximal resection, creating a uniform surface beneath the femoral resurfacing prosthesis and providing a larger surface area for fixation. Once the bone cuts are completed, final preparation of the femoral head bone to maximize the cement interface is performed, including curettage of cysts, drilling of sclerotic bone, and removal of loose or mechanically inferior bone.

Acetabular bone preparation for the total resurfacing procedure is the same as standard reaming for uncemented sockets during THA. The most important features are creation of a spherical cavity with uniform bone-implant contact, adequate press-fit for initial stability, and placement of the prosthesis at the anatomic center of hip joint rotation whenever technically possible. Dome holes for screw fixation will disrupt bearing lubrication in the acetabular component. Therefore, adequate initial stability without dome screws is required to withstand frictional torque and resist

micromotion that could lead to a fibrous interface.

Prosthesis Implantation

Implantation of the femoral resurfacing prosthesis requires creation of an optimal prosthesis-bone interface. Proper preparation of the femoral head and fixation of the implant are critical to success. Most femoral head resurfacing implants are designed for use with cement, and most acetabular components are designed for uncemented application. On the femoral side, cement interdigitation is accomplished by using cement pressurization during implant insertion or by suctioning cement into the femoral head. Liquid cement is poured into the top quarter of the femoral component, and the prepared femoral head is coated with cement. Cannulating the lesser trochanter with a metal suction device prior to implantation draws cement into the bone. Spilling cement into the wound or pouring cement out of the femoral component during implantation should be avoided. A uniform cement mantle with up to 3 mm of cement penetration is desirable.

Implantation of the acetabular component is the same as acetabular insertion in primary THA. The acetabular bone is generally underreamed by 1 to 2 mm to ensure press-fit of the component without excessive force. It is critical that the acetabular component be designed to withstand insertion without deformation so that the diametral clearance between the femoral head and acetabular components is not altered during implantation.

Wound Closure

A standard layered wound closure is performed, and the capsule and short external rotators are repaired. Using monofilament bioabsorbable suture in layers on the fascia and subcutaneous layers is preferred. The skin is closed with a running subcuticular suture and adhesive strips.

Postoperative Regimen

Patients are restricted to partial (50%) weight bearing on crutches or with a walker for approximately 2 to 4 weeks. Partial weight bearing is suggested in the initial postoperative period to permit acetabular bone ingrowth and optimal patient comfort. Full weight bearing can be initiated 4 weeks after surgery. Sporting activities or aggressive physical activity are delayed for 12 weeks postoperatively to allow some degree of femoral neck bone remodeling to be achieved. Some surgeons advocate immediate full weight bearing, and there is great variability in weight-bearing protocols. All patients are mobilized on the first postoperative day and receive prophylaxis for deep venous thrombosis.

———————————■

Avoiding Pitfalls and Complications

Complications causing early failure are related to patient selection and technical errors but can be avoided by selecting patients carefully and adhering to important surgical principles. Femoral neck fracture after resurfacing seems to occur within the first 3 months after surgery, before the femoral neck has remodeled sufficiently to resist fatigue and bending stresses. Protecting the affected hip by using a cane, crutches, or a walker during the first weeks after surgery should be considered, especially for patients with known risk factors such as insufficient bone density in the femoral neck or the presence of stress risers in the femoral neck after bone preparation. Therefore, patient selection should focus on those candidates with femoral neck bone densities that fall within the normal, age-adjusted range. The exact point at which the degree of osteoporosis changes from acceptable to high risk is not known.

Stress risers in the femoral neck created during bone preparation may increase the risk of femoral neck fracture. Stress risers are caused by notching of the femoral neck during reaming, aggressive removal of osteophytes at the junction of the femoral head and neck, and excessive reaming of the femoral neck below the distal rim of the femoral head resurfacing prosthesis. All exposed cancellous bone created by reaming should ideally be covered by the implant. Reaming should not continue distal to the covered area on the femoral neck. The superior and anterior surfaces of the femoral neck are the tension sides of the bone, and avoiding notching in these locations is particularly important. Notching can be minimized by avoiding excessive valgus positioning of the femoral reamers and by centering the reamers on the femoral neck. Templating of the femoral component, choosing the appropriate starting point for the reamers, and repeated use of a stylus can keep the reamers on the appropriate trajectory.

Patients with a very wide or foreshortened femoral neck, as sometimes occurs in Legg-Calvé-Perthes disease, may not be good candidates for resurfacing. The width of the femoral neck may be broader than the appropriate femoral resurfacing component, making notching of the femoral neck more likely. The lack of available neck length also makes it very difficult to restore normal offset and mechanics.

Uncommon potential pitfalls of resurfacing include early femoral loosening and femoral component failure. Risk factors for femoral loosening include varus component position, an excessively thick cement mantle, and poor cement interdigitation with the femoral neck bone. The cement mantle can be optimized by cyst débridement, drilling of excessively sclerotic bone surfaces, cancellous bone lavage, and pressurization of cement into the femoral head. Additionally, the femoral component must be fully seated on the prepared bone surface. The small stem present on most femoral resurfacing components is meant for implant centering, not load sharing, and it is not advisable to try to regain femoral neck length by leaving the prosthesis above the resected bone surface. Incomplete seating of the component could lead to failure of the cement interface or fracture of the stem because of cantilever bending stress.

Potential pitfalls on the acetabular side include incomplete seating of the acetabular component or component malposition. Soft-tissue or bone impingement, excessive socket medialization, and socket malposition are risk factors for dislocation. Achieving a concentric, spherically reamed acetabulum facilitates prosthesis seating. Avoiding overly aggressive press-fit also facilitates seating of the acetabular component within the acetabulum. Most implant systems recommend no more than 2 mm underreaming of the acetabular component as ideal.

Late failures of total resurfacing components relate to component wear and are particularly problematic with large-diameter metal-on-polyethylene bearings. The newer components are metal-on-metal bearings, which generate smaller volumes of wear particles. The particle counts and metal ion levels generated by these bearings are greater than those of metal-on-polyethylene bearings. The long-term effects of metal ion dissemination in the body are not fully understood. However, improved metal surface finishes, closer tolerances between femoral and acetabular components, sphericity of components, and the potential for fluid film lubrication with larger bearings suggest great potential for durability and low wear rates with these bearings.

———■

References

Amstutz HC, Beaulé PE, Dorey Frederick FJ, et al: Metal-on-metal hybrid surface arthroplasty: Two to six-year follow-up study. *J Bone Joint Surg Am* 2004;86:28-39.

Beaulé PE, Schmalzried TP, Campbell P, Dorey F, Amstutz HC: Duration of symptoms and outcome of hemiresurfacing for hip osteonecrosis. *Clin Orthop* 2001;385:104-117.

Campbell P, Mirra J, Amstutz HC: Viability of femoral heads treated with resurfacing arthroplasty. *J Arthroplasty* 2000;15:120-122.

Daniel J, Pynsent PB, McMinn DJW: Metal on metal resurfacing of the hip in patients under the age of 55 years with osteoarthritis. *J Bone Joint Surg Br* 2004;86:177-184.

Hungerford MW, Mont MA, Scott R, et al: A surface replacement hemiarthroplasty for the treatment of osteonecrosis of the femoral head. *J Bone Joint Surg Am* 1998;80:1656-1664.

Mont MA, Rajadhyaksha AD, Hungerford DS: Outcomes of limited femoral resurfacing arthroplasty compared with total hip arthroplasty for osteonecrosis of the femoral head. *J Arthroplasty* 2001;16:134-139.

Scott RD, Urse JS, Schmidt R, Bierbaum BE: Use of TARA hemiarthroplasty in advanced osteonecrosis. *J Arthroplasty* 1987;2:225-232.

Wagner M, Wagner H: Preliminary results of uncemented metal on metal stemmed and resurfacing hip replacement arthroplasty. *Clin Orthop* 1996;329:S78-S88.

Coding

CPT Codes		Corresponding ICD-9 Codes		
27130	Arthroplasty, acetabular and proximal femoral prosthetic replacement (total hip arthroplasty), with or without autograft or allograft	711.45 711.95 714.0 714.30 715.15	715.25 715.35 716.15 718.5 718.6	720.0 733.14 733.42 808.0 905.6
27132	Conversion of previous hip surgery to total hip arthroplasty, with or without autograft or allograft	715.15 715.25 715.35 718.2	718.5 718.6 733.14 733.42	905.6 996.4 996.66 996.77
27299	Total articular resurfacing (unlisted procedure, pelvis or hip joint)	N/A	N/A	N/A

CPT copyright © 2004 by the American Medical Association. All Rights Reserved.

Chapter 14
Bearing Surfaces
Joshua J. Jacobs, MD

 Introduction

Total hip arthroplasty (THA) represents one of the greatest success stories in modern orthopaedic surgery. It has revolutionized the treatment of end-stage congenital, traumatic, neoplastic, and degenerative conditions of the hip. Furthermore, considerable data amassed over the last 2 decades demonstrate excellent long-term survival of well-designed and well-implanted THA components. Although THA has had excellent results, in some clinical settings and patient populations results can be further improved. In particular, the high-demand patient with a long life expectancy continues to represent a challenge, given the higher prevalence of osteolysis and aseptic loosening in these patients. In response to this challenge, there has been a tremendous effort over the last 15 years to understand the pathogenesis of osteolysis and to develop strategies to minimize its impact and prevalence.

Numerous investigators have made it clear that the cellular reaction to particulate degradation products plays a major role in the onset and progression of aseptic loosening and osteolysis. Two principal strategies have emerged to address this problem: (1) using materials in joint replacement applications that are more resistant to in vivo degradation, and (2) modifying the host response to deg-

radation products from these implants. This chapter describes the use of so-called alternative bearing surfaces in THA. Historically, the most popular bearing couple has been a cobalt-chromium-molybdenum (CoCrMo) alloy femoral head that articulates with an ultrahigh molecular weight polyethylene (UHMWPE) acetabular component. Alternatives to this traditional bearing couple discussed in this chapter include contemporary highly cross-linked UHMWPE-on-CoCrMo alloy, ceramic-on-ceramic, and metal-on-metal bearing couples.

━━━━━▪

Polyethylene Wear

There is increasing evidence that the biologic reaction to particulate wear debris, particularly UHMWPE debris, is a major factor limiting the longevity of contemporary THA components. The study of wear is quite complex, and discussion of the basic science of wear is beyond the scope of this chapter. However, some background in this area is important to provide a framework for understanding the rationale for the introduction of alternative bearing surfaces. The use of the CoCrMo/conventional UHMWPE bearing couple results in wear that can be measured radiographically as linear

penetration of the metallic head into the radiolucent UHMWPE component. Linear wear rates of UHMWPE have been reported to vary from 0.04 to 0.25 mm/year, with a typical value in the range of 0.1 mm/year. The corresponding volumetric wear rate, which is the volume of UHMWPE that is lost through wear, ranges from 27 to 172 mm^3/year, with a typical value of approximately 100 mm^3/year. Based on a mean UHMWPE particle diameter of 0.5 µm, this amount of volumetric wear translates into 5×10^{11} particles/year or roughly 50,000 particles per step. Clearly, a very large particulate burden is introduced into the periprosthetic tissues. The cellular reaction to this large burden of debris ultimately leads to periprosthetic bone loss and aseptic loosening.

Numerous factors contribute to UHMWPE wear. Factors intrinsic to the material properties of the UHMWPE itself that have been shown to affect the wear performance of UHMWPE include the following: (1) the presence of fusion defects or inclusions; (2) the use of ionizing radiation, which is associated with residual free radicals in the matrix; (3) the stiffness of the polyethylene; (4) the nature of the base resin; (5) the molecular weight; (6) the method of fabrication (machined versus molded); and (7) the degree of cross-linkage. The degree of cross-linkage is particularly germane in that it serves as the basis for a new generation of UHMWPE materials introduced in THA applications. Other factors unrelated to the material properties of the UHMWPE (extrinsic factors) include femoral head size, the counterface material, counterface roughness, the presence and stability of modular connections, the thickness of the UHMWPE, the presence or absence of metal backing, and the presence of any third bodies.

Data from preclinical studies and retrieval analyses have revealed much about how these factors influence UHMWPE wear performance. The orthopaedic implant industry has responded by improving the quality of UHMWPE. Most manufacturers have also modified sterilization and packaging procedures to minimize the oxidation that may lead to deleterious effects on the mechanical properties and wear performance of UHMWPE. These improvements in the fabrication of conventional UHMWPE will likely reduce the intermediate and long-term failures related to its wear. Additional approaches have been sought, however, to further reduce the wear debris burden in an attempt to extend the long-term survival of THA components, particularly in high-demand patient populations. Manufacturers have responded to this challenge by enhancing the wear resistance of UHMWPE through the production of a highly cross-linked molecular structure and by removing UHMWPE from the bearing system entirely in favor of the so-called hard-on-hard bearing surfaces: ceramic-on-ceramic and metal-on-metal.

Highly Cross-linked UHMWPE

The use of ionizing radiation to sterilize UHMWPE components transiently produces free radicals that are highly reactive intermediates. If there is oxygen in the environment, these free radicals may combine with oxygen, resulting in chain scission and degradation in the mechanical and wear performance of the polyethylene. However, if ionizing radiation is introduced in an oxygen-free environment, the free radicals that are formed are more likely to combine with free radicals on adjacent polymer chains, forming a cross-linked molecular structure that has proved to be more resistant to wear. Results of many hip simulation studies indicate an inverse correlation between the dose of radiation and the rate of UHMWPE wear. This reduction in wear is accompanied by a decrease in the tensile strength and fracture toughness of the polyethylene. Therefore, the dose of radiation must be optimized to leverage the beneficial effects of cross-linking (reduction of wear) without substantially compromising other mechanical properties. Although the dose of gamma radiation used for sterilization of conventional polyethylenes ranges from 2.5 to 4.0 megarads (Mrad), the dose of radiation used in the highly cross-linked materials currently on the market ranges from 5 to 10 Mrad.

Highly cross-linked UHMWPE materials have been studied more extensively in clinically validated hip simulation studies under a variety of conditions than other "improved" polyethylenes introduced over the last 15 years. In nearly all of these studies, the highly cross-linked UHMWPEs outperformed their conventional counterparts, providing the rationale for their use in the clinical environment, particularly in high-demand populations at the greatest risk for osteolysis and aseptic loosening. Highly cross-linked UHMWPE was approved by the US Food and Drug Administration (FDA) for use in THA in 1997. Nonetheless, until quite recently no clinical data confirmed the in vivo superiority of contemporary highly cross-linked polyethy-lenes, although scattered clinical data exist for other highly cross-linked polyethylenes that have been available since the 1960s. Using both Roentgen stereophotogrammetry and computer-based methods of radiographic wear measurements, investigators report that in the short term (2 to 3 years) the steady-state wear rate of highly cross-linked UHMWPE materials is significantly less than that seen in conventional polyethylenes (**Figure 1**). Given that these are short-term results, additional follow-up is clearly required. Close surveillance of patient populations with highly cross-linked UHMWPE implants is recommended to ensure that other failure modalities, such as polyethylene fracture, are not more prevalent and that the decreased wear rates translate into improved implant survivorship.

Ceramic-on-Ceramic Bearings

The use of ceramic materials as a bearing surface in THA was introduced in 1970. Both zirconium oxide and aluminum oxide have been used in THA applications and are inert, stable, dense, and hard ceramics. These materials are highly wettable secondary to their hydrophilic nature. In addition, a surface protein monolayer develops in vivo, which helps decrease adhesive and abrasive implant wear. Alumina ceramics are reported to resist abrasive forces 30 to 40 times greater than those causing comparable damage to titanium-aluminum-vanadium and cobalt-chrome alloys. Ceramics are also stiffer than the metal alloys currently in use in total joint arthroplasties. Because of this increased stiffness, ceramic components are better able to maintain congruence, which allows for distribution of forces over a larger area and, ultimately, decreased wear. Laboratory wear testing of ce-

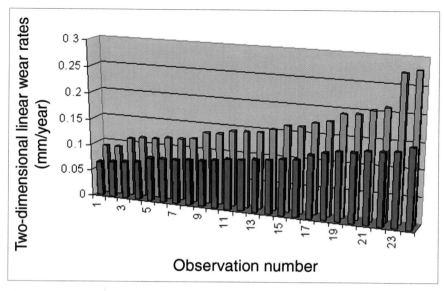

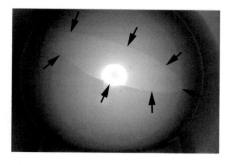

Figure 2 Photograph of a retrieved ceramic head with evidence of stripe wear. This wear pattern has been postulated to result from edge loading in deep flexion activities.

Figure 1 Two-dimensional linear wear rates at latest follow-up (between 18 and 42 months) in 24 patients with highly cross-linked polyethylene (10 Mrad gamma irradiated in inert atmosphere, red columns) and 24 patients with conventional polyethylene (2.5 Mrad gamma irradiated in inert atmosphere, blue columns). Although there is variability within each group, the mean wear rate for the highly cross-linked material is significantly lower. (Courtesy of John Martell, MD.)

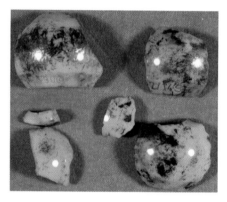

Figure 3 Photograph of a fractured ceramic head that was retrieved 5 years after implantation. Note the discoloration due to smearing of metal on the ceramic surface.

ramics shows dramatic improvements in wear performance over metal-on-polyethylene bearings. Wear of ceramic-on-ceramic bearings has been reported between 0.025 and 10 μm/year. This is, at worst, an order of magnitude better than the accepted average rate for metal-on-conventional UHMWPE. In certain circumstances, however, ceramic bearing surfaces have demonstrated a pattern of "stripe" wear, most likely due to localized edge loading in deep flexion (**Figure 2**).

Ceramic components are more brittle than other materials in current use. This increased brittleness decreases the component's resistance to fracture, which is a catastrophic problem when it occurs in vivo (**Figure 3**). Factors implicated in ceramic component fracture include poor material quality, large grain size, small head size, residual internal stress, and poor taper design. Intraoperative component positioning also has been shown to be very important. Incorrect positioning of the femoral or acetabular components can lead to impingement,

edge loading, subsequent fracture, and accelerated wear. Ceramic component fracture is widely reported in the literature, with frequency ranging from a low of 1 in 1,763 hips to a high of 9 in 130 hips. Revision in this situation is mandatory, with problems arising from the difficulty in removing all retained ceramic material. Any ceramic left behind can cause severe and rapid third-body wear of both polyethylene and metal alloy components. Revision of nonmodular acetabular components is recommended to remove any ceramic material embedded in the acetabular bearing surface that can lead to accelerated wear of the newly revised head. A failed ceramic head should be replaced with a metallic head because imperfections in the trunion may lead to stress risers, predisposing to recurrent fracture of a newly implanted ceramic head.

The manufacturing of ceramics has improved to address the problem of fracture. The design of the taper has also improved, minimizing unacceptable stresses in the head. Quality con-

trol has improved as well as a result of International Organization for Standardization standards first adopted in 1979 and revised in 1994. Furthermore, the use of finer-grained microstructures and individual component proof testing prior to distribution should incrementally decrease the propensity for fracture. Since receiving FDA approval in 2003, contemporary ceramic-on-ceramic bearings have been generally available in the US marketplace.

Historically, osteolysis and aseptic loosening have been reported in association with the early designs of ceramic-on-ceramic bearings. In some series, the prevalence of these complications was comparable to that observed with metal-on-polyethylene

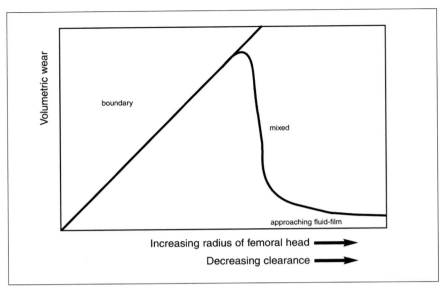

Figure 4 Theoretical relationship between volumetric wear, head size, and clearance. Within a certain range, as head size increases and clearance decreases, boundary lubrication transitions to mixed and then fluid-film regimes, which are associated with reduced wear rates. (Reproduced with permission from Dowson D: New joints for the millenium: Wear control in total replacement hip joints. *I Mech E J Engng Med* 2001;215:335-358.)

bearings. Histologic analysis has revealed ceramic particulate debris within the periprosthetic tissues; the mean ceramic particle size of 0.7 μm was comparable with the size of polyethylene debris observed in association with failed polyethylene bearings. Thus, patients with ceramic bearing couples are not necessarily immune to the complications of osteolysis and aseptic loosening.

Other studies evaluating ceramic-on-ceramic designs have reported more favorable results, with survival at 10 years of more than 95%. A multicenter prospective analysis of a contemporary alumina-on-alumina THA using a modular acetabular component with a metal backing reported clinical results comparable with conventional bearings at short-term (3-year) follow-up. It remains to be seen if contemporary ceramic-on-ceramic THA components will demonstrate improved survival compared with CoCrMo/UHMWPE bearings in the long term.

Metal-on-Metal Bearing Surfaces

Metal-on-metal bearing surfaces were available for general use in the 1960s but because of their inferior clinical performance compared with those used in Charnley low-friction arthroplasty, these bearing surfaces fell out of favor. With the emergence of the concept of "particle disease," (ie, particulate wear debris as the proximate cause of osteolysis and aseptic loosening), metal-on-metal bearing surfaces for THA components were reintroduced in the late 1980s with improved manufacturing and material properties. Currently, the metal-on-metal bearing surfaces available for use in THA components are fabricated from CoCrMo alloy. Metal-on-metal bearing surfaces have been marketed and generally available in the United States since 1999 when certain devices received FDA approval.

Retrieval studies of the new-generation metal-on-metal implants have reported initial (first year) wear rates

ranging from 15 to 20 μm per component per year. The wear rate significantly decreases to 2 to 5 μm per component per year after the second or third year. Thus, the steady-state linear wear rate of these bearing surfaces is approximately two orders of magnitude less than that of conventional metal-on-polyethylene bearing surfaces. In theory, within a certain range, the wear rate of metal-on-metal bearing surfaces decreases as head size increases and clearance (the difference between the inner diameter of the acetabular bearing surface and the diameter of the femoral head) decreases as a result of more efficient entrainment of lubricant (**Figure 4**).

However, the size of the metallic wear particles produced from metal-on-metal THA components is considerably smaller (most particles are smaller than 50 nm) than those of polyethylene wear particles generated from CoCrMo/UHMWPE THA components. Therefore, for a given volume of wear, many more metal particles will be released from metal-on-metal bearing surfaces than polyethylene particles from CoCrMo-on-conventional UHMWPE bearing surfaces. This large number of nanoscale particulate debris is associated with a very large specific surface area available for corrosion and the subsequent transport of metal ions into the system.

Corrosion and wear of metal-on-metal bearing surfaces and their particulate degradation products lead to increases in cobalt and chromium levels in the serum and urine of patients with well-functioning metal-on-metal bearing surfaces compared with patients who have well-functioning CoCrMo-on-UHMWPE bearing surfaces (**Figure 5**). Metal levels have been reported to remain elevated even after the initial wear-in period, usually defined as the first year of service (approximately 1 million cycles). From previous studies of patients with long-term metal-on-metal McKee-Farrar

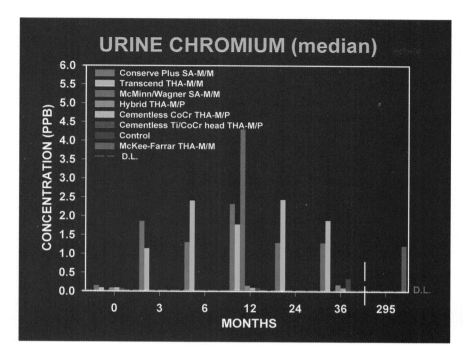

Figure 5 Graph summarizing several longitudinal and cross-sectional cohort studies on urine chromium levels in patients undergoing THA with either metal-on-metal (M/M) resurfacing arthroplasty (Conserve Plus, Wright Medical Technology, Arlington, TN; McMinn/Wagner), metal-on-metal THA (Transcend, Wright Medical Technology, Arlington, TN; McKee-Farrar, Howmedica International, Limerick, Ireland), or metal-on-polyethylene (M/P) THA (Hybrid, Cementless CoCr, Cementless Ti/CoCr head). All of these studies used identical analytic techniques. Metal-on-metal bearings were associated with substantial elevations in urine chromium with respect to metal-on-polyethylene bearings, even in patients with clinically successful long-term (>20 years) McKee-Farrar implants. Urine chromium levels in patients with contemporary metal-on-metal surface replacements were similar to those in patients with contemporary metal-on-metal THAs.

tions of these persistent elevated metal concentrations.

Clinically, the intermediate-term (4- to 7-year) results with new-generation metal-on-metal bearing surfaces in the United States are similar to those of THA components with conventional bearing surfaces at comparable time periods in terms of patient-derived outcome scores, the prevalence of osteolysis and aseptic loosening, and the failure rate. Further follow-up will establish whether long-term outcomes and survival have improved with these low-wear bearings.

Summary

The use of new bearing surfaces in THA components is attractive given the improved wear performance of these components compared with that of conventional metal-on-UHMWPE articulations. However, each of the newer low-wear bearing couples has potential drawbacks, including diminished fracture toughness (highly cross-linked UHMWPE and ceramic-on-ceramic bearing surfaces) and elevated systemic metal levels (metal-on-metal bearing surfaces). These concerns, in concert with the lack of clinical evidence demonstrating improved function or survival, temper the enthusiasm for widespread use of these couples. Therefore, these couples should be recommended for patients at high risk for osteolysis and aseptic loosening. The role of these bearing couples in the armamentarium of the adult reconstruction surgeon will be established only through long-term high-quality clinical trials.

(Howmedica International, Limerick, Ireland) implants, these elevated levels appear to persist for the life of the implant. However, no toxic effects have been directly attributed to these elevated levels. Elevated metal ion levels are of particular concern to younger, more active patients and their surgeons because the patient's life expectancy after implantation may exceed 30 years.

Epidemiologic studies of populations with orthopaedic implants conducted to date have predominantly shown that the overall cancer risk is slightly less than that observed in the general population. Some studies, however, have also reported an increased incidence of lymphoma and leukemia when individual cancers are examined. At this time, no cause-and-effect relationship between cancer and metal-on-metal implants has been established. However, there is growing evidence suggesting that metal hypersensitivity plays a role in implant failure in a small proportion of patients with metal-on-metal bearing surfaces. Further study is needed to fully understand the local and systemic implica-

■ References

D'Antonio J, Capello W, Manley M, Bierbaum B: New experience with alumina-on-alumina ceramic bearings for total hip arthroplasty. *J Arthroplasty* 2002;17:390-397.

Dorr LD, Wan Z, Longjohn DB, Dubois B, Murken R: Total hip arthroplasty with use of the Metasul metal-on-metal articulation: Four to seven-year results. *J Bone Joint Surg Am* 2000;82:789-798.

Greenwald AS, Garino JP: Alternative bearing surfaces: The good, the bad, and the ugly. *J Bone Joint Surg Am* 2001;83(suppl):68-72.

Jacobs JJ, Hallab NJ, Skipor AK, Urban RM: Metal degradation products: A cause for concern in metal-metal bearings? *Clin Orthop* 2003;417:139-147.

McKellop H, Shen FW, Lu B, Campbell P, Salovey R: Effect of sterilization method and other modifications on the wear resistance of acetabular cups made of ultra-high molecular weight polyethylene: A hip-simulator study. *J Bone Joint Surg Am* 2000;82:1708-1725.

Chapter 15

Optimizing Stability and Limb Length
Charles A. Engh, Sr, MD

 ## Introduction

Patient satisfaction with total hip arthroplasty (THA) depends in part on the surgeon's ability to equalize the patient's limb length and to produce a stable hip that will not dislocate. Experienced surgeons learn how to identify patients who are at high risk for postoperative dislocation and in whom it will be difficult to achieve equal limb lengths. To provide these patients with the best outcome, the surgical approach may need to be altered, different surgical implants used, or in some cases postoperative bracing may be required. Patients must understand that producing a stable hip takes precedence over equalizing limb length and that it is always easier to lengthen the leg by THA than to shorten it. Most importantly, patients must be advised about realistic expectations. For example, patients needing limb-length correction may not be good candidates for hip resurfacing procedures or for the currently popular minimally invasive surgical techniques. Understanding and discussing expectations with patients can minimize postoperative dissatisfaction.

This chapter is divided into five sections: (1) identifying the high-risk patient, (2) physical examination of the patient with limb-length inequality, (3) radiographic examination of the THA patient, (4) templating for limb length, and (5) the intraoperative

measures that I use to minimize the risk of postoperative dislocation.

 ## Identifying High-Risk Patients

Patients who are particularly susceptible to limb overlengthening are those with naturally short stature and those with coxa vara. Treating these patients with an uncemented femoral stem sometimes requires a special prosthesis. Promising to equalize limb length in patients who have shortening of more than 2 cm is unwise. Patients whose limb-length discrepancy is caused by pelvic obliquity also present a challenge, and planning their limb-length correction is complicated.

Identifying patients who are at high risk for postoperative dislocation is also important. In general, elderly female patients are at greater risk for dislocation than young male patients. Patients with joint hypermobility are also more prone to dislocate. Another high-risk group consists of patients who are likely to have poor muscle control of the hip postoperatively. This group includes (1) patients who have been treated for an intertrochanteric fracture by hip replacement, (2) those who have high-riding dislocations, (3) those undergoing a fusion takedown, and (4) patients who have

been previously treated by a resection arthroplasty. High-risk patients may require postoperative bracing until adequate hip muscle function returns. Performing THA on noncompliant patients and patients with hip muscle imbalance caused by neuromuscular disorders requires caution because these patients are prone to dislocation.

 ## Physical Examination of the Patient With Limb-Length Inequality

To equalize limb length by THA, the apparent cause of the discrepancy must first be determined. I refer to "apparent difference" as the difference perceived by the patient when he or she is examined in the standing position. Limb length is measured with a measuring tape from the anterosuperior iliac spine to the medial malleoli. Limb-length difference is measured by placing blocks under the foot of the shorter leg until the patient feels comfortable. This apparent limb-length difference can be an actual shortening of the extremity (**Figure 1**), or it can be caused in part by the abnormal position in which the patient is forced to hold his or her hip. A fixed abduction

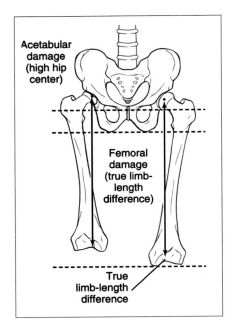

Figure 1 Diagram illustrates a true limb-length difference caused by arthritic damage. The shortening of the right leg is caused by the high acetabular center and the flattened femoral head.

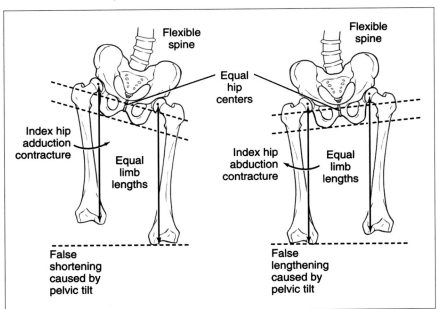

Figure 2 Diagram illustrates how pelvic obliquity can produce false limb lengthening (right) or false shortening (left) of the arthritic hip. Once this problem has been identified, the surgeon must determine whether it is correctable by THA.

contracture of the hip causes false lengthening, and a fixed adduction posture causes false shortening (**Figure 2**). On physical examination, I suspect that at least a portion of the limb-length difference is false if the pelvis is not level after the apparent difference has been corrected using blocks to the patient's satisfaction. It is also helpful to compare the standing and supine limb-length measurements. The supine measurement more accurately shows a true limb-length difference.

Pelvic obliquity caused by conditions such as ankylosis of the contralateral hip or a fixed scoliosis is not correctable by THA. However, if the obliquity is caused by the ankylosed position in which the patient is forced to hold his or her hip, and if the surgeon believes that normal range of motion in that hip can be restored, the obliquity is probably correctable. My planning of the limb-length correction differs for these two situations.

To determine the cause of the pelvic obliquity, range of motion in

both hips and spine flexibility must be checked. The latter is checked with the patient seated and then asked to bend laterally in both directions. If the spine is not flexible, the pelvic obliquity probably is not correctable by THA. In these patients, I lengthen the shortened limb the distance that feels most comfortable, which was determined by placing blocks under the patient's foot on standing examination. If the spine is flexible and I think the pelvic obliquity will be corrected by the THA, I plan differently. In this situation, I make the limbs equal in length and presume that when motion returns to the involved hip the pelvis will become level, resulting in limbs that are equal in length. If I fail to anticipate that restoring hip motion will level the pelvis, the pelvis will not be level and the operative limb will be longer than the normal limb.

One word of caution, subtle abduction and adduction contractures of the hip sometimes can be difficult to detect on physical examination. In some cases hip contractures are more

easily detected on an AP radiograph of the pelvis.

———■

Radiographic Examination of the THA Patient

The most important radiograph for planning limb-length correction is an AP view of the pelvis. This view is not the usual flat plate of the abdomen. Rather, the x-ray beam is centered about 2 inches below the pubic symphysis. This view should include both femurs to a level below the ends of the proposed femoral implants and the pelvis to only about 2 inches above the acetabuli. The technician should position the patient so that the legs are parallel with toes turned in. In addition, the legs should be perpendicular to an imaginary line through the iliac crest (**Figure 3**). When I am confident that the patient is in the proper position, I can sometimes detect abduc-

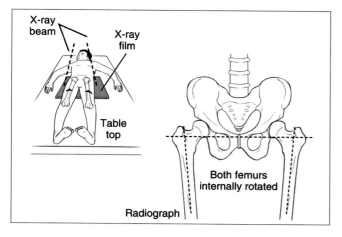

Figure 3 Diagram illustrates the way in which to obtain an AP radiograph of the pelvis. Both legs are maximally internally rotated with the toes touching, and the legs are placed in a position that is perpendicular to an imaginary line through the iliac crests. Note that the x-ray beam is centered below the pelvis (inset).

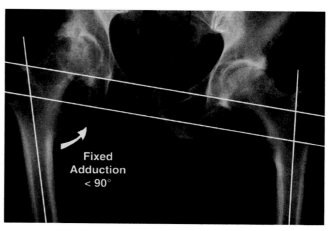

Figure 4 AP radiograph of the pelvis demonstrates the importance of the previously described method to obtain a radiograph for detecting pelvic obliquity.

tion and adduction contractures that I missed on physical examination (**Figure 4**). The severity of this fixed adduction contracture might have been missed if an AP view of the femur had not included the pelvis.

Templating for Limb Length

Most modern implant systems have a large inventory of stem and cup sizes. Therefore, in preoperative planning, I do not concentrate so much on exact stem or cup size but on optimizing limb length and hip stability. Most importantly, I want to ensure with my templates that when I seat an uncemented stem at the desired level inside the femur, the shortest ball will not overlengthen the leg.

I also consider postoperative hip stability. Postoperative hip dislocation can be minimized by maintaining good postoperative hip muscle tension without excessive limb lengthening. When possible, it is usually better to eliminate joint laxity by increasing femoral offset (ie, the distance the fe-

mur is displaced laterally away from the pelvis) than by overlengthening the leg. Optimizing the correct balance between femoral offset and limb length may require altering the shape of the femoral neck of the prosthesis (a standard versus a high offset stem). It also may involve altering the cup position, the seating level of the stem, and the position of the ball on the taper neck of the femoral prosthesis. All of these factors can be planned preoperatively with templates.

Obtaining the Correct Radiographs

The correct radiographs can be properly obtained only on a view in which the femur has been rotated to the plane in which the femoral prosthesis will be inserted into the femur. This is the plane shown on the stem template. The AP view of the pelvis must therefore be obtained with the femurs internally rotated approximately 15°. One of the most common errors in templating is placing the overlay on a radiograph of an externally rotated femur. As shown in **Figure 5**, the inside shape of the proximal femur and the femoral head offset of the externally rotated femur differ dramatically

when a radiograph is obtained with the femur internally rotated to the plane in which the femoral prosthesis will be inserted. It is useless to put a manufacturer's template on an improperly rotated femur.

Planning Bilateral Cases

Because it is sometimes impossible to obtain an internally rotated view of the femur and because hip abduction and adduction contractures can falsely exaggerate limb-length discrepancies, templating is not always a simple task. Surgical planning for patients with bilateral osteoarthritis of the hip is not a problem as long as the patient has been advised that he or she will have a temporary limb-length difference until after surgery is performed on the second hip. In these bilateral cases, hip stability usually can be easily obtained by lengthening the leg to achieve the desired muscle tension.

Templating From the Contralateral Hip

Patients with unilateral hip disease and major limb-length differences present more difficult challenges. In these cases, more extensive planning is necessary. In some patients, I use the

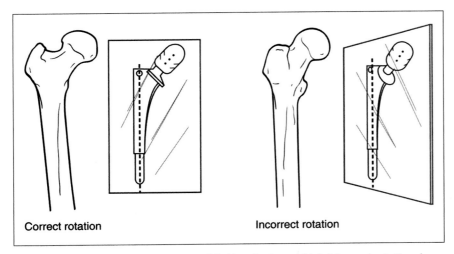

Figure 5 Diagram of femurs in internal (left) and external (right) femoral rotation shows different views of the proximal femur and the femoral head offset.

template overlays on the involved hip, whereas in others I use the contralateral, normal side for templating. In these cases, the normal side is used as the model for the limb length desired on the affected side. However, when I template the normal side, I also consider the possibility that the cup on the affected side might need to be seated slightly higher or more medial than normal, and I compensate for this possibility when I template the femoral component.

Decisions Affecting How to Template
The decision as to how to template depends on three factors: (1) whether the patient has a false limb-length discrepancy, (2) whether this discrepancy is correctable by THA, and (3) whether the affected hip can be internally rotated on the AP view of the pelvis. I always use the contralateral, normal hip as the basis for templating if the affected hip cannot be properly internally rotated. I also use the normal hip if the patient has pelvic obliquity that is correctable by hip surgery. If the patient has pelvic obliquity that cannot be corrected by THA, I prefer to plan the procedure using the affected side, lengthening the leg by the amount measured with the standing

blocks. The ways in which I alter the templating process based on these variables are illustrated below.

Templating With No Limb-length Difference
Figure 6 shows an AP view of a patient with no pelvic obliquity, both femurs properly internally rotated, and no limb-length difference. This is the simplest of cases. I place the components so that the distance separating the femur from the pelvis will not be changed by the THA. The acetabular cup template is placed in the desired position, and the biomechanical center is marked. The stem template is then placed over the center line of the femur and then lowered to a seating level in which one of the different neck length options allows a femoral head to be placed directly over the new acetabular biomechanical center (**Figure 7**).

Templating With Limb-length Difference Resulting From True Shortening
Figure 8 shows AP radiographs of a patient with no pelvic obliquity but who has an apparent standing limb-length difference of 1 cm. The discrepancy appears to be a true shortening

caused by a higher-than-normal acetabular socket center and a damaged femoral head. The radiograph also shows that the femur has been properly internally rotated for templating. The goal in this patient is to lengthen the leg the amount measured with blocks beneath the foot. Because the leg is properly internally rotated and the pelvis is level, I use the affected side for templating, placing the acetabular cup template first and then placing the femoral stem template over the center line of the femur. I then adjust the seating level of the stem to ensure that the femoral offset has been maintained and the limb length has been increased by the desired 1 cm. In this situation, the center of the proposed femoral head will be 1 cm directly above the socket center. If the components are placed in this position at surgery, the leg will be lengthened the desired 1 cm when the ball is placed in the socket.

Templating Complex Cases
Figure 9 shows an AP radiograph of a patient with both a true limb-length difference resulting from acetabular damage and a false limb-length difference caused by an adduction contracture. In this situation, I prefer to plan this surgery using templates on both sides. **Figure 10** shows an AP radiograph of a patient with a true limb-length difference, along with a fixed external rotation contracture, which makes it impossible to template the femur on the affected side. In this situation, I also prefer to do part of the templating on the contralateral, normal side.

The way in which I templated the patients shown in **Figures 9** and **10** is illustrated in **Figure 11**. In **Figure 11**, *A*, note the damage to the acetabular socket, which makes it impossible to place the acetabular cup in a normal position. This is similar to the acetabular socket damage shown in **Figures 9** and **10**. Because of the socket damage, the position of the ac-

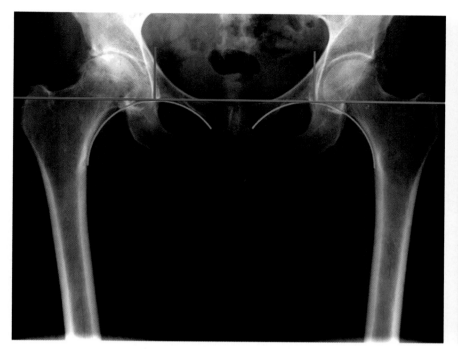

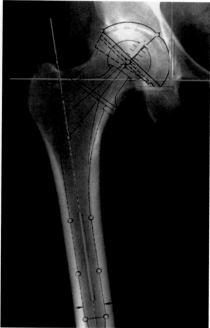

Figure 6 AP radiograph of the pelvis shows an arthritic hip with no limb-length difference, no pelvic obliquity, and internally rotated femurs. This radiograph resembles Figure 3 and is the easiest type of case to template. The goal is to maintain equal space between the femur and pelvis.

Figure 7 AP radiograph shows an example of templating with correct femoral rotation. In this case, there is no limb-length difference; therefore, the femoral template is adjusted within the femur until one of the femoral head options is centered in the cup.

etabular socket must be planned on the affected side and then transposed to the contralateral, normal side (**Figure 11**, *B*). Next, I decide whether this position is similar to the one in which I would place an acetabular cup on the normal side. In this situation, it is not. The acetabular damage on the affected side would result in a cup position that is a little higher than normal. Thus, the abnormal cup center position is marked on the normal side. The femoral component seating level and head position are planned on the normal side as well because this is the side in which the limb length is to be matched (**Figure 11**, *C*). I adjust the position of the femoral template so that one of the potential positions for the femoral head lies directly over the higher-than-normal acetabular center. If the cup is placed in the planned position on the affected side, the neck seating level and the head and neck

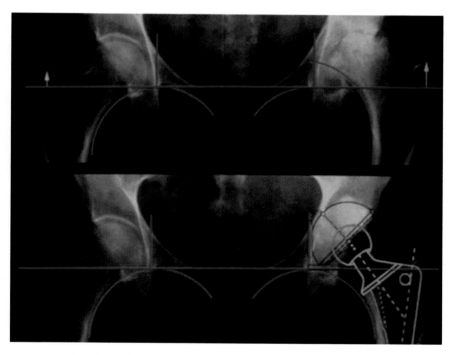

Figure 8 AP radiographs show a patient with a true limb-length difference (top). In this case, the limb-length correction can be planned on the affected side because the involved femur has been properly internally rotated (bottom).

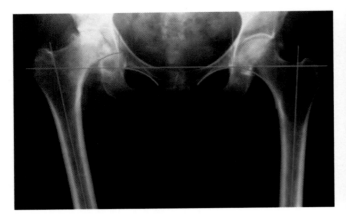

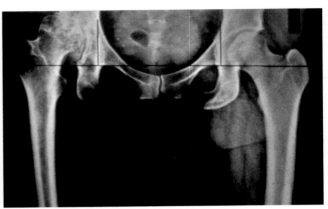

Figure 9 AP radiograph of the pelvis demonstrating true limb-length difference resulting from acetabular damage and a false limb-length difference caused by adduction contracture. Because this patient's radiograph shows a femoral adduction contracture, both-side templating is needed.

Figure 10 AP radiograph of the pelvis demonstrating a true limb-length difference resulting from acetabular dysplasia and a fixed external rotation contracture. Because this hip is ankylosed in an externally rotated position, a portion of the preoperative planning must be done on the contralateral, normal side.

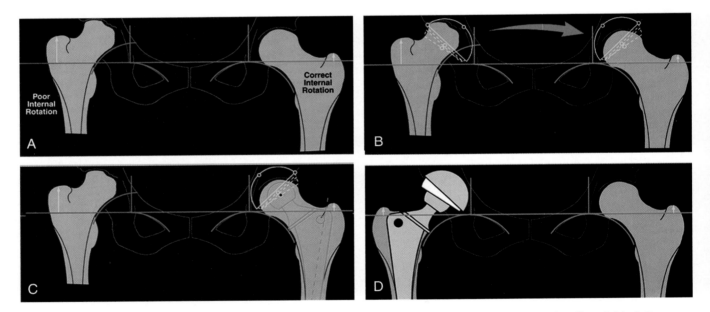

Figure 11 Templating method for a damaged acetabular socket. **A,** Template the acetabular socket position on the affected side. **B,** Determine the socket position on the damaged side, "flip" to the contralateral side, and mark the cup center. **C,** Select the stem seating level and head position on the contralateral side, with the head in the marked cup center. **D,** Reproduce the plan intraoperatively on the index hip.

segment position are placed as shown on the normal side, and surgery is performed as planned. The postoperative radiograph should demonstrate that the space separating the femurs from the pelvis should be nearly identical, Shenton's line should be restored, and limb length should be nearly equal (**Figure 11**, *D*).

I recognize that both-side templating can be a little confusing and that with difficult cases like this, templating cannot always be precise. However, I believe it is the best method for solving these more complex limb-length problems.

Minimizing Dislocation Risk

I follow two rules for minimizing the risk of hip dislocation. The first is to identify patients at high risk preoperatively and treat them with a different surgical approach and a different postoperative protocol. The second rule, which applies to all patients, is to perform the entire surgery using trial components; I do not insert final components until I am certain that the hip is stable. For patients at high risk of hip dislocation, I use an anterolateral rather than a posterior surgical approach. I detach the anterior third of the gluteus medius and the gluteus minimus from the femur and then reattach it through drill holes in the bone using strong nonabsorbable suture. The hip capsule is preserved beneath the gluteus minimus, opened with a vertical incision, and then closed with at least two bioabsorbable sutures. I use the largest femoral head size possible and count on the intact posterior capsule and the large head size to prevent posterior dislocations. The anterior capsular closure is protected postoperatively with bracing, which prevents full hip extension and external rotation.

Trial components should be checked before final components are inserted in all patients, not just those at high risk for dislocation. The hip should be put through a full range of motion and assessed for bone and soft-tissue impingement. Component impingement and joint laxity should be checked at the extremes of range of motion. Next, the orientation of the trial acetabular component is compared to the rim of the acetabulum. When I use a posterior approach, I leave a small portion of the trial component exposed directly posteriorly. The anterior rim of the acetabular trial component should be countersunk beneath the anterior acetabular rim by a corresponding amount. As a result, the cup is flexed forward and anteverted about 15° more than the normal acetabulum.

When using an anterolateral surgical approach, I rely on the posterior capsule to prevent posterior dislocations, and I do not antevert the trial component to the same degree. With both approaches, I usually attempt to insert the cup at an inclination angle of 45° horizontal. However, when using a posterior approach, I worry about posterior dislocations with the hip in maximum flexion. In this situation, if the cup is placed slightly more vertical, the combination of increased anteversion and increased verticality provides the most protection against posterior dislocation with the hip in hyperflexion. This increased verticality is not necessary with the anterolateral approach so the cup can be placed slightly more horizontal.

I find it much easier to measure femoral stem anteversion than cup anteversion. I also find it easier to measure the combined anteversion of both components than to measure cup anteversion alone. Combined anteversion should be measured with the hip in approximately 30° of flexion. The femur should then be internally rotated until the collar of the femoral prosthesis is parallel to the face of the acetabular cup and the cup appears to provide equal coverage of the head in all directions. Ideally, with these components parallel, the femur should be internally rotated about 45° to the coronal plane of the patient, making the combined anteversion of the two components 45°. I check the combined anteversion with the knee flexed to 90°. With the lower leg in this position, the angle between the plane of the lower leg and the coronal plane of the patient should be about 45°.

Soft-tissue and bone impingement at the extremes of hip motion can cause the femoral head to be levered out of the socket, which is another common cause of dislocation. In flexion and adduction, a thickened anterior hip capsule, anterior osteophytes on the femur or acetabulum, or anterior heterotopic bone can produce anterior impingement, which can result in posterior dislocation. The incidence of posterior dislocation can be minimized by removing this bone and its corresponding soft tissue. It also can sometimes be minimized by displacing the femur farther away from the pelvis so that the bony prominences no longer come in contact. The latter can be done by altering the trial components. Most implant systems have both standard and high offset femoral trial components. Most also have increased offset polyethylene liners for acetabular trial components, which can be used to decrease bone and soft-tissue impingement problems by increasing the distance the femur is separated from the pelvis so that these bony or soft-tissue prominences no longer come into contact when the hip is flexed.

Component-to-component impingement at the extremes of range of motion is another potential cause of dislocation. When this type of impingement occurs, the orientation of the femoral and acetabular trial components should be checked. This type of impingement often can be decreased by changing the anteversion of the cup. Cup anteversion also can be changed by using polyethylene liners that change the orientation of the face of the cup and by increasing the femoral head size to increase the difference in size between the diameter of the femoral head and that of the neck. This alteration will increase the range of motion before neck impingement occurs. In general, I prefer to use the largest head size possible. When the outside diameter of the acetabular component is 52 mm or more, I generally use either a 28- or 32-mm head and when the outside diameter is 54 mm or more, I consider using a femoral head that is 36-mm or larger in patients at high risk for dislocation.

Soft-tissue laxity also can be diminished by displacing the femur farther away from the pelvis. In general, it is preferable to increase soft-tissue tension by displacing the femur laterally away from the pelvis rather than by lengthening the leg. This is done by using lateralized femoral components. Balancing offset and limb length to achieve optimum soft-tissue tension also may involve dropping the stem lower to decrease limb length and using a longer head on the femoral stem to improve lateralization. All of this can be checked with trial components prior to inserting final components.

Summary

Templating and preoperative use of femoral and acetabular trial components are important ways to decrease the likelihood of limb-length and dislocation complications. However, templating is valuable only if the surgeon can consistently position the components in the operating room in the planned position. This usually is not difficult with the femoral stem. It is fairly easy to determine intraoperatively whether the stem has been placed in neutral, valgus, or varus. The seating level can be easily measured from the lateral shoulder of the stem to the top of the greater trochanter. The amount of femoral anteversion also can be easily measured by comparing the anteversion of the neck of the prosthesis to the position of the lower leg with the knee bent. Intraoperatively, calculating acetabular component orientation and position is more difficult. It is for this reason that I depend more on the method for measuring combined anteversion described in this chapter. Only with time does the experienced surgeon learn to place the acetabular cup consistently in the preoperatively planned position. In the future, intraoperative radiographs and surgical navigation tools will be relied upon more often to check and improve cup positioning intraoperatively.

References

Austin MS, Hozack WJ, Sharkey PF, Rothman RH: Stability and leg length equality in total hip arthroplasty. *J Arthroplasty* 2003;18(suppl 1):88-90.

Bourne RB, Rorabeck CH: Soft tissue balancing: The hip. *J Arthroplasty* 2002;17(suppl 1):17-22.

Eggli S, Pisan M, Muller ME: The value of preoperative planning for total hip arthroplasty. *J Bone Joint Surg Br* 1998;80:382-390.

Jasty M, Webster W, Harris W: Management of limb length inequality during total hip replacement. *Clin Orthop* 1996;333:165-171.

Ranawat CS, Rao RR, Rodriguez JA, Bhende HS: Correction of limb-length inequality during total hip arthroplasty. *J Arthroplasty* 2001;16:715-720.

White TO, Dougall TW: Arthroplasty of the hip: Leg length is not important. *J Bone Joint Surg Br* 2002;84:335-338.

SECTION 2
Complex Total Hip Arthroplasty

Chapter 16

Total Hip Arthroplasty: Degenerative Dysplasia of the Hip

Miguel E. Cabanela, MD

 ## Indications

The indications for total hip arthroplasty (THA) in patients with degenerative dysplasia of the hip (DDH) and subluxation without dislocation are the same as for any other form of hip disease. Clinical symptoms must be sufficient to warrant surgical intervention, and radiologic changes must be of enough magnitude to make alternative solutions impossible. Pain is usually the most important factor in surgical decision making. At times, limb-length inequality can be of importance to the patient, but it should not be the principal reason for THA.

Degenerative disease secondary to hip dysplasia occurs at an early age. Most patients who require THA usually undergo this surgery before age 50 years. THA in this population often demands special technique and is associated with a higher failure rate than arthroplasty that is done for other conditions. This is undoubtedly related to the altered anatomy associated with this condition.

 ## Contraindications

Radiologically, joint deformity per se is not enough to justify THA in patients with adequate cartilage space remaining. In these cases, conservative alternatives must be considered and ruled out.

 ## Alternative Treatments

In patients who have pain with activity but not at rest, reasonably well-preserved joint space, and reasonable range of motion, alternative joint-sparing procedures should be considered. Redirection pelvic (acetabular) osteotomies are indicated in patients with DDH that principally affects the acetabulum and is characterized by lack of coverage of the femoral head, subluxation, lateralization of the joint hip center, and a well-preserved cartilage space. Conversely, in patients with coxa valga luxans (ie, excess proximal femoral valgus but adequate articular cartilage), a varus femoral osteotomy (at times combined with medial derotation in the presence of excess femoral anteversion) is the procedure of choice. These alternative treatments should not be considered in patients with advanced joint destruction. Thus, THA should be reserved for patients in whom alternative joint-preserving procedures are not possible or reasonable.

 ## Results

The reported results of acetabular reconstruction using cemented components indicate a high rate of failure (16% to 52%) at more than 10 years' follow-up. This high failure rate results in part from younger patient age and possibly from the nonanatomic placement of the acetabular component. Uncemented components have fared somewhat better, but the reported follow-up is not quite as long, and thus the mode of failure might be different. **Table 1** summarizes published results of acetabular reconstruction with uncemented components, with and without acetabular augmentation. With follow-up that extends into the second decade, the incidence of loosening and mechanical failure (ie, revision for loosening plus revision for other causes) remains moderate. It is important to note, however, that the causes of failure appear to differ somewhat from those that occur with cemented components in that wear and osteolysis have been responsible for most of the revisions in the uncemented series. This difference is undoubtedly related in part to the fact that the component diameter often is small and thus has a thinner polyethylene that may wear at a higher rate.

With medialization of the acetabular reconstruction (cotiloplasty), very few results have been reported, but the failure rates reported after 7 years' follow-up are very low. There is some concern, however, with the difficulty of revision surgery after medialization.

Results of cemented femoral reconstruction for dysplasia generally

Table 1 Results of Acetabular Reconstruction

Author(s) (Year)	Number of Hips	Implant Type	Mean Patient Age (Range)	Mean Follow-up (Range)	Revision Loosening (%)	Mechanical Failure Rate (%)
Anderson and Harris (1999)	20	Uncemented	52 years (25–87)	6.9 years (5.3–8.5)	0	0
Silber and Engh (1990)	19	Uncemented with acetabular augmentation	45 years	3 years (2–6.3)	5	26
Morsi, et al (1996)	17	Uncemented with acetabular augmentation	50.3 years (36–65)	6.6 years (5.1–9.8)	0	0
Spangehl, et al (2001)	44	Uncemented with acetabular augmentation	39 years (12–67)	7.5 years (5–12.3)	4.5	9

have been better than acetabular results. With follow-up of 20 years and longer, the failure rate remains between 10% and 20%. There are no long-term reports of uncemented femoral reconstruction. In a series with one of the longest periods of follow-up reported (7.5 years), the failure rate was 7%.

Technique

Exposure

Hips with mild to moderate dysplasia can be approached through either a conventional anterolateral or posterolateral approach, depending on surgeon preference. Occasionally a transtrochanteric approach is necessary in the very stiff hip or in patients who have had previous surgery, such as a previous varus-producing osteotomy. When this approach is necessary, the surgeon must ensure that enough bone is available laterally on the femur after the prosthesis is implanted so that the trochanter can be reattached onto a bony base. A flat osteotomy of the trochanter usually is preferred to a more complex geometric osteotomy because the former facilitates anterior translation of a posteriorly displaced trochanter. In mild to moderate dysplasia, subtrochanteric shortening femoral osteotomies (described in chapter 17) are never necessary.

General Principles of Hip Reconstruction

Different methods of classifying the bony anatomic abnormalities of DDH have been described. Most focus on the amount of femoral subluxation or dislocation relative to the normal anatomic hip center. My preference is the Hartofilakidis system, which consists of three distinct types of congenital DDH in adults based on the relationship between the femoral head and the acetabulum. In dysplasia, the femoral head is in contact with the true acetabulum. In low dislocation, the femoral head is in contact, at least in part, with the true acetabulum but also in part with the false acetabulum; the deformity in this instance is the most severe. In high dislocation, the femoral head and the true acetabulum make no contact, and the head has migrated superiorly and posteriorly. Often in this deformity, the true acetabulum is reasonably well preserved although underdeveloped and osteoporotic.

Changes in the bony anatomy are associated with changes in the soft tissues; the more severe the bony abnormality, the more severe the changes in the soft tissues. Some element of capsular thickening is always present, as is hypertrophy of the psoas tendon. Shorten-

ing of the hamstrings, adductors, and rectus femoris is common. The abductors are oriented transversely as a result of the upward position of the femoral head and the proximal femur, but they are less foreshortened than might be predicted. The femoral and sciatic nerves might be shortened and, therefore, more vulnerable to injury at the time of arthroplasty.

Acetabular Reconstruction

Uncemented acetabular fixation is the method of choice of most surgeons in North America, particularly in younger patients with DDH. In most cases, the acetabular prosthetic component should be placed as close to the anatomic hip center as possible. However, in patients with moderate DDH, moving the center of rotation slightly proximal is permissible. It has been suggested that a proximal and medial location is better than a proximal and lateral position.

BONE PREPARATION

If the acetabular bone stock is insufficient (ie, if anterolateral coverage of the component is deficient), several alternative methods of management are available (**Figure 1**). Mild lack of anterolateral cup support is acceptable (**Figure 2**) if the construct is stable. If superior coverage is more severely deficient, one of three alternative solu-

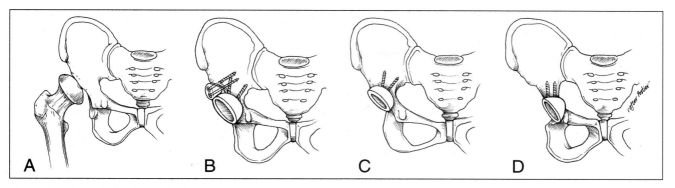

Figure 1 Three alternative methods to reconstruct **(A)** Crowe type II and III dysplastic acetabuli: **(B)** augmentation with bone grafting, **(C)** high hip center, and **(D)** medialization of the cup. (Reproduced with permission from the Mayo Foundation)

tions is advisable. (1) Further medialization of the socket beyond Köhler's line—producing a mild, deliberate perforation of the medial pelvic wall. The medial wall can be cracked (cotiloplasty) or reamed and the component translated slightly medially in a deliberate protrusio position. This approach is relatively simple and provides good coverage of the cup on host bone. However, it sacrifices some bone stock for the future, and if revision becomes necessary, less bone will be present. It also carries some risk of weakening the acetabulum sufficiently that failure by early protrusion of the cup into the pelvis can occur. (2) A small, uncemented component can be placed in a high hip center location. In this position, the component is completely covered by host bone, which facilitates osseointegration and avoids the need for grafting. This approach also has disadvantages, including decreased polyethylene thickness associated with the small acetabular component, limb equalization problems, altered hip mechanics, and hip instability related to femoral-pelvis impingement either in flexion or in extension. (3) The lack of superior coverage can be supplemented with augmentation bone graft. The graft usually comes from the patient's own femoral head and is fixed to the lateral pelvic wall with cancellous screws (**Figure 3**). I prefer to use augmentation bone graft using the patient's femoral head if there is lack of socket coverage beyond

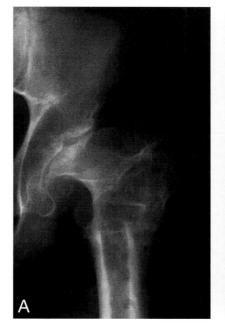
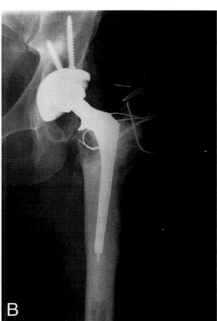

Figure 2 **A,** AP radiograph of the left hip of a 42-year-old man 15 years after undergoing a varus femoral osteotomy. Note the poor coverage of the deformed femoral head. **B,** Medializing to Köhler's line, but without perforating the medial wall, provided satisfactory coverage of an uncemented acetabular component. The femoral deformity was corrected with a cemented component in a slight valgus position, slightly "cheating" the anatomy. A trochanteric osteotomy was used for the approach and then fixed with wires.

15% to 20% of the superior-lateral cup. This approach restores hip mechanics by allowing the center of rotation to be placed in a more anatomic position. Furthermore, grafts may increase bone stock, which in turn facilitates future revision surgery should it become necessary. However, bone grafting increases the technical complexity of the procedure, and bone graft resorption leading

to late failure has been reported. In my experience, however, graft resorption typically has been minimal and limited to the nonstressed zones of the graft.

GRAFT PLACEMENT
Reaming is performed with the goal of preserving the anterior wall and should extend into the ischium and the posterior column because bone is typ-

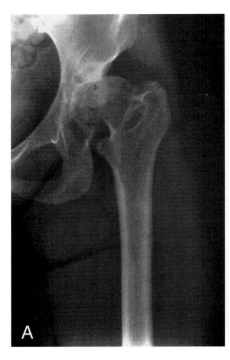 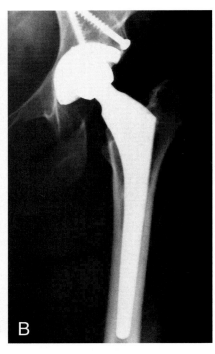

Figure 3 **A,** AP radiograph of a 27-year-old woman with osteoarthritis secondary to DDH. Her dysplasia would be classified as Hartofilakidis and Crowe type II following the Crowe system. **B,** AP radiograph of the hip obtained 2 years postoperatively. Note that a femoral head autograft was used for acetabular coverage and a standard press-fit metaphyseal-filling femoral component also was used given the minimal deformity of the femoral anatomy.

ically thicker in these patients. Reamer coverage is then assessed to determine if augmentation grafting is necessary. If it is, the femoral head is prepared by dividing it along the weight-bearing trabeculae and fashioned so that it can be grafted onto the prepared lateral pelvic wall. This step typically augments superior and anterior coverage, where the most common deficiencies are located. The head is temporarily fixed to the pelvic wall with either two 3.2-mm drills or two small Steinmann pins, taking care to leave enough grafted bone overhanging inferiorly for later reaming. At this point, one of the pins or drills is changed to a 6.5-mm cancellous screw of the proper length. The smooth portion of the screw should traverse the bone graft, and the threaded portion should engage the pelvis. No threads should be present in the grafted bone if possible. After the first screw is in place, additional reaming is necessary to complete acetabular preparation.

Typically, a congruous graft-native acetabulum junction can be obtained. The acetabular component is impacted, press-fit fixation is augmented with two or three screws, and a second 6.5-mm cancellous screw is placed through the graft. There is no advantage to having graft overhanging the socket component because it will not be mechanically stressed and will tend to resorb.

Femoral Reconstruction

The femoral anatomy often is distorted with excessive anteversion and coxa valga, and a small medullary canal, which may have a peculiar shape (typically narrow with smaller mediolateral than anteroposterior diameter). The greater trochanter may be located posteriorly.

BONE PREPARATION

The degree of anteversion must be carefully assessed. If there is increased acetabular anteversion, there is a tendency for over anteversion of the implants, which can make the reconstructed hip unstable anteriorly. Additionally, anteversion of the femoral components can lead to an internal rotation contracture of the hip.

PROSTHESIS IMPLANTATION

Either cemented or uncemented components can be used for patients with DDH or a low dislocation. Cemented components allow the surgeon to address femoral deformities, especially the above-mentioned increased anteversion. Many component systems have cemented stems specially designed for patients with DDH; these implants characteristically are smaller in size, straighter, and have minimal metaphyseal flare, thus accommodating the distorted anatomy of these femora. Alternatively, by downsizing the component, the surgeon can "cheat" the anatomy by placing the component in less anteversion than the femur.

Uncemented components can be used as well. Proximally (metaphyseally) fitted components may not allow freedom to correct anteversion and, in extreme situations, may require a simultaneous femoral derotation osteotomy to correct the abnormal femoral anteversion. A distally fixed extensively coated component would, in some cases, allow correction of the abnormal anteversion by ignoring the proximal femur and obtaining fixation in the diaphysis. Some modular components allow the surgeon to fit the proximal and distal femur separately, which simultaneously accommodates and corrects the femoral deformity. Modular implants allow anteversion of the femoral component, independent of the anatomy, and can be very useful in this specific situation (**Figure 4**).

Avoiding Pitfalls and Complications

Most of these patients are young; therefore, it is critically important to provide them with as good a reconstruction as possible so that a long-lasting satisfactory result may ensue. As deformity of the acetabular and femoral anatomy increases, so does the technical difficulty of the reconstruction.

In the acetabulum, following the abnormal anatomy too closely (ie, to overantevert the acetabular component) might lead to anterior instability. It is also important to recognize that a substantial degree of acetabular deformity can be present with a relatively normal-looking AP radiograph. The surgeon must be aware of this possibility and plan the procedure accordingly. Scrutinizing the AP radiograph of the pelvis usually suffices; following the outline of the anterior and posterior acetabular walls on this view typically provides a good indication of the amount of anteversion present. If in doubt, a false profile view obtained preoperatively will yield the best estimate of the amount of acetabular anteversion.

It is equally important to recognize that femoral anteversion might be difficult to assess. Even in a normal-appearing AP radiograph, considerable levels of femoral antetorsion can be present. Use of a cemented or a modular stem, as discussed above, can help avoid the unwanted proximal femoral fractures that can occur when attempting to fit a proximally coated uncemented stem in a deformed proximal femur.

Nerve injury is a risk in these patients and avoiding excessive lengthening may reduce this risk. Optimizing hip biomechanics and implant stability improves the postoperative potential to restore normal gait and reduce the significant potential long-term problem of implant loosening in these young patients.

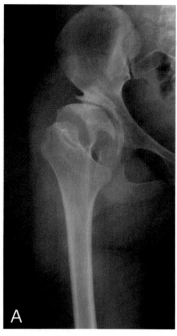
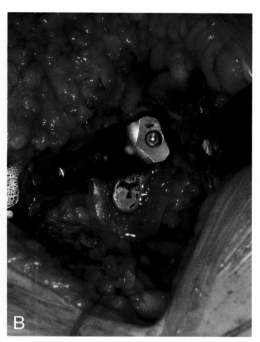
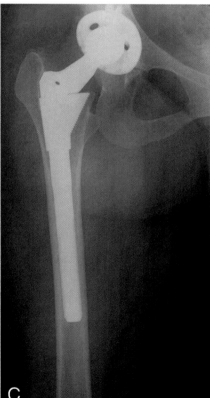
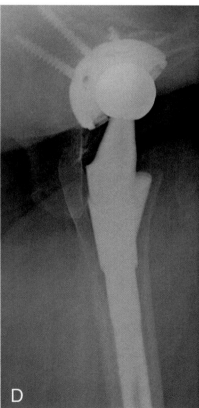

Figure 4 **A,** AP radiograph of the hip of a 34-year-old woman with significant anteversion of the proximal femur. **B,** Intraoperative photograph of the proximal femur shows the modular femoral component and the marked mismatch between the femoral anteversion and the anteversion of the prosthesis. The modular sleeve is oriented to the anatomy of the patient, and the prosthesis is derotated to produce normal femoral anteversion. AP **(C)** and lateral **(D)** postoperative radiographs show the modular prosthesis and the mismatch between the bony and the prosthetic anteversion.

█ References

Anderson MJ, Harris WH: Total hip arthroplasty with insertion of the acetabular component without cement in patients with congenital dislocation or marked congenital dysplasia. *J Bone Joint Surg Am* 1999;81:347-354.

Crowe FJ, Mani VJ, Ranawat CS: Total hip replacement in congenital dislocation and dysplasia of the hip. *J Bone Joint Surg Am* 1979;61:15-23.

Dorr LD, Tawakkol S, Moorthy M, Long W, Wan Z: Medial protrusion technique for placement of a porous-coated, hemispherical acetabular component without cement in a total hip arthroplasty in patients who have acetabular dysplasia. *J Bone Joint Surg Am* 1999;81:83-92.

Hartofilakidis G, Stamos K, Karachalios T, Ioannidis TT, Zacharakis N: Congenital hip disease in adults: Classification of acetabular deficiencies and operative treatment with acetabuloplasty combined with total hip arthroplasty. *J Bone Joint Surg Am* 1996;78:682-692.

Morsi E, Garbuz D, Gross AE: Total hip arthroplasty with shelf grafts using uncemented cups: A long-term follow-up study. *J Arthroplasty* 1996;11:81-85.

Numair J, Joshi AB, Murphy JC, Porter ML, Hardinge K: Total hip arthroplasty for congenital dysplasia or dislocation of the hip: Survivorship analysis and long-term results. *J Bone Joint Surg Am* 1997;79:1352-1360.

Silber DA, Engh CA: Cementless total hip arthroplasty with femoral bone grafting for hip dysplasia. *J Arthroplasty* 1990;5:231-240.

Sochart DH, Porter ML: The long-term results of Charnley low-friction arthroplasty in young patients who have congenital dislocation, degenerative osteoarthritis, or rheumatoid arthritis. *J Bone Joint Surg Am* 1997;79:1599-1617.

Spangehl MJ, Berry DJ, Trousdale RT, Cabanela ME: Uncemented acetabular components with bulk femoral head autograft for acetabular reconstruction in developmental dysplasia of the hip. *J Bone Joint Surg Am* 2001;83:1484-1489.

Coding

CPT Codes		Corresponding ICD-9 Codes		
27130	Arthroplasty, acetabular and proximal femoral prosthetic replacement (total hip arthroplasty), with or without autograft or allograft	711.45 714.30 715.35 718.6 733.42	711.95 715.15 716.15 720.0 808.0	714.0 715.25 718.5 733.14 905.6
27132	Conversion of previous hip surgery to total hip arthroplasty, with or without autograft or allograft	715.15 718.2 733.14 996.4	715.25 718.5 733.42 996.66	715.35 718.6 905.6 996.77
27165	Osteotomy, intertrochanteric or subtrochanteric including internal or external fixation and/or cast	715.15 731.0 736.1 754.31 754.35	715.25 732.1 736.32 754.32 755.61	715.35 733.81 754.30 754.33 755.62 755.63
Modifier 22	Unusual procedural services			

CPT copyright © 2004 by the American Medical Association. All Rights Reserved.

Chapter 17
Total Hip Arthroplasty: High Hip Dislocation

Cecil H. Rorabeck, MD, FRCSC
R. Stephen J. Burnett, MD, FRCSC

Indications

Reconstruction of the degenerative and severely dysplastic hip is one of the most challenging procedures for surgeons performing total hip arthroplasty (THA). Indications for surgery are (1) the symptomatic degenerative hip, including progressive pain and dysfunction, and (2) failure of nonsurgical management, including activity modifications, analgesics, anti-inflammatories, and the use of assistive aids for walking. Often the severely dysplastic, high-riding hip occurs bilaterally and, because of the articulation in a false high acetabulum, may become symptomatic later in life (40s to 50s) compared with the lower dysplastic hip (20s to 30s). Patients are frequently women of child-bearing age with active occupations and lifestyles, and after they have had previous treatment, including femoral or acetabular osteotomy, in childhood or later. The need for future revision is a reality in this patient population. The anatomic abnormalities increase the technical difficulty of hip surgery in the severely dysplastic hip (**Figure 1**); thus, familiarity and experience with advanced reconstruction techniques are necessary to manage the severely dysplastic hip. A femoral shortening procedure is often necessary to restore the hip to its anatomic center and to avoid overlengthening of the leg, which may result in neurologic compromise.

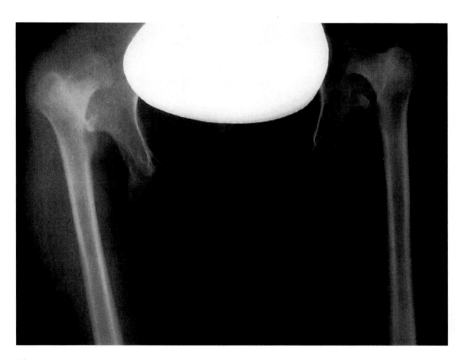

Figure 1 AP radiograph of high-riding Crowe IV degenerative dysplasia of the hip, which may occur bilaterally. Acetabular abnormalities include high dislocation with articulation in a false, small, shallow, and anteverted acetabulum. Femoral changes of coxa breva and coxa valga, often with severe anteversion of the femoral neck, a narrow canal, and a more posterior location of the greater trochanter, are commonly encountered. (Reproduced with permission from Masonis JL, Patel JV, Miu A, et al: Subtrochanteric shortening and derotational osteotomy in primary total hip arthroplasty for patients with severe hip dysplasia: 5-year follow-up. *J Arthroplasty* 2003;18(suppl 1):68-73.)

Contraindications

Because it often occurs bilaterally, the severely dysplastic, high-riding hip is associated with a bilateral Trendelenburg "waddling" gait, which may be minimally symptomatic. Patient education and delaying surgery until symptoms and radiographic progres-

Table 1 Results of THA in High Hip Dislocations

Author(s) (Year)	Number of Hips	Implant Type	Mean Patient Age (Range)	Mean Follow-up (Range)	Results	Comments
Masonis, et al (2003)	21	Both uncemented (S-ROM) and cemented (several designs) components	49 years (21–69)	5.8 years (2–11.2)	33% acetabular graft 91% femoral osteotomy union 3 dislocations No neurologic complications	All treated with subtrochanteric osteotomy
Stans, et al (1998)	70	Cemented components (several designs)	50 years (21–75)	16.6 years (5–23)	Aseptic loosening 33% acetabulum; 40% femur; Correlated with cup placement	All Crowe III dysplasia No shortening osteotomy
Anderson and Harris (1999)	20	All uncemented acetabular components All cemented femoral components	52 years (25–87)	6.9 years (5.3–8.5)	Acetabulum: no aseptic loosening or mechanical failure Femur: 1 component aseptic loosening	No shortening subtrochanteric osteotomy
Reikeraas, et al (1996)	25	4 cemented femoral components 21 uncemented femoral and acetabular components	54 years (17–67)	5 years (3–7)	Subtrochanteric osteotomy 1 nonunion 1 malunion No mechanical loosening	

sion are evident prevents unnecessary surgery. A history of septic arthritis (remote or recent) is a relative contraindication to arthroplasty. Any active chronic remote site infections should be treated preoperatively. Similarly, absent or severely compromised abductor muscle function is a poor prognosticator for success with THA.

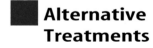

Alternative Treatments

Few practical alternatives exist for this challenging degenerative problem. Early recognition and treatment in childhood may delay or avoid eventual arthroplasty by restoring the hip to its anatomic center and improving congruency and femoral head coverage. Periacetabular and femoral osteotomy, although promising in a

minimally dysplastic hip, is contraindicated in the degenerative high dysplastic hip. A Chiari osteotomy may be a useful alternative in a low dysplastic degenerative hip with less than 2 cm of superior head migration; however, in high dysplasia it is not a suitable option. Resection arthroplasty (Girdlestone procedure) combined with appropriate soft-tissue releases for pain relief and hygiene may be beneficial in nonambulatory, low-demand patients with cerebral palsy or other similar disorder and a symptomatic high dislocation with degenerative changes. A hip fusion is rarely indicated with the current techniques available for hip arthroplasty.

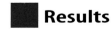

Results

Table 1 summarizes the results of THA in high hip dislocations in several re-

cent series. We recently reported that a total of 21 of 142 THAs for developmental dysplasia of the hip (DDH) required a subtrochanteric shortening osteotomy at the time of hip replacement. Of the 19 patients with Crowe III and IV DDH, 16 were women and 3 were men (mean age, 49 years). A direct lateral approach was used in 13 hips and a posterolateral exposure in 8. The mean follow-up was 5.8 years (range, 2 to 11 years). All sockets were uncemented (mean size, 44 mm; range 40 to 48 mm) and reconstructed at the anatomic hip center. One third of the sockets had less than 70% host bone coverage and required a femoral head bulk autograft fixed with cancellous screws. The mean distal translation of the anatomic hip center was 58 mm. The femoral component was cemented in 10 hips and uncemented in 11 hips. Twenty 22-mm heads and one 26-mm head were used. Nine strut femoral allografts were used to augment the osteotomy site for added stability. The mean femoral shortening osteotomy length measured 35 mm of bone resection (range, 20 to 70 mm). Improvement in Harris Hip scores (32 to 74 points), limp, and use of assistive devices for walking was significant. Six revisions were performed in this group in five patients. Two nonunions (91% healing rate) occurred at the osteotomy site, requiring bone grafting and strut allograft augmentation. Surgical revision was required in three hips: (1) one for recurrent dislocation (direct lateral approach used for primary surgery), (2) one for polyethylene failure, and (3) one for aseptic loosening of a precoated stem (34 months). Importantly, no neurologic complications occurred. These results compare favorably with the other limited series in the literature for THA performed in patients with high dysplasia. The nonunion rate and repeat revision rates are similar to other published series, whereas the rate of neurologic complication is improved.

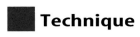

Technique

Exposure
DDH is practically classified into three categories: dysplasia, low dislocation, and high dislocation using the criteria of Hartofilakidis and associates. Using the system of Crowe and associates, high dislocation is further classified as Crowe types III and IV based on the extent of proximal migration of the femoral head relative to the teardrop. The significant difference between Crowe III and Crowe IV dysplasia is that in Crowe III hips the femoral head has eroded a portion of the superolateral acetabulum, whereas in Crowe IV hips this host bone remains intact and improves host bone coverage of the acetabular implant when the hip is restored at the true anatomic hip center. Crowe III hips may require structural

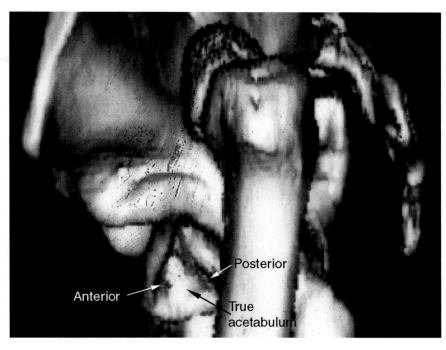

Figure 2   Preoperative three-dimensional CT sagittal reconstruction showing the complex anatomy of the high-riding dysplastic hip. Note that the femur is dislocated posteriorly and superiorly. (Reproduced with permission from Masonis JL, Patel JV, Miu A, et al: Subtrochanteric shortening and derotational osteotomy in primary total hip arthroplasty for patients with severe hip dysplasia: 5-year follow-up. *J Arthroplasty* 2003;18(suppl 1):68-73.)

autograft or allograft more frequently than Crowe IV hips. An AP view of the pelvis, a true lateral view of the acetabulum, and a frog-lateral view of the proximal femur are usually sufficient for preoperative templating. Judet views and CT may be useful adjuncts to assess column integrity; three-dimensional CT reconstructions may be helpful in appreciating the pelvic anatomy in the severely dysplastic and previously osteotomized acetabulum or femur (**Figure 2**).

In severely dysplastic DDH, underdevelopment of the entire pelvis occurs. The underdeveloped acetabulum is characteristically shallow, lateralized, anteverted, and deficient anteriorly, laterally, and superiorly. If a prior pelvic osteotomy has been performed, the anatomy may be even more distorted. Occasionally, the acetabulum may be retroverted or deficient posteriorly (eg, in association with cerebral palsy). Crowe III dyspla-

sia is associated with a superolateral acetabular defect, and coverage of an uncemented implant may require structural autograft. Similarly, the dysplastic proximal femur may have undergone prior osteotomy, have retained hardware, and may be ectatic with a distorted canal from remodeling. A small femoral head, excessive femoral neck anteversion and coxa valga, and a posteriorly displaced greater trochanter are common findings. The femoral canal is often narrow and twisted, with excessive bowing and a smaller mediolateral than anteroposterior diameter. The metaphyseal flare is often lost, narrowing to a tight isthmus.

Soft-tissue abnormalities require careful consideration. These patients have dysplastic soft tissues, including the fascia lata, which may compromise soft-tissue closure. The abductor musculature typically is underdeveloped and may have a horizontal or

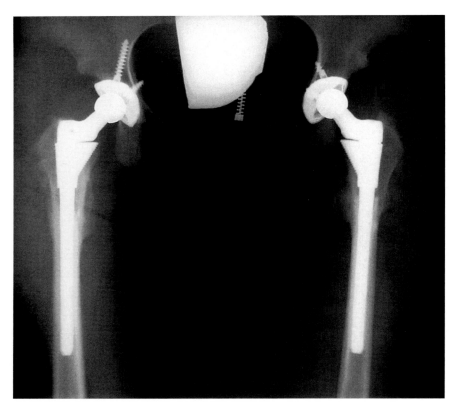

Figure 3 AP radiograph shows reconstruction using a modular uncemented stem-through-sleeve femoral component design with a subtrochanteric shortening femoral osteotomy. The acetabulum has been reconstructed bilaterally using an uncemented cup with screws at the level of the anatomic (true) hip center. The subtrochanteric osteotomy has united bilaterally. (Reproduced with permission from Masonis JL, Patel JV, Miu A, et al: Subtrochanteric shortening and derotational osteotomy in primary total hip arthroplasty for patients with severe hip dysplasia: 5-year follow-up. *J Arthroplasty* 2003;18(suppl 1):68-73.)

even reverse obliquity of vector pull. Similarly, the short external rotators, piriformis, and gluteus minimus may be absent or dysplastic. Capsular hypertrophy and redundancy with an hourglass constriction is typical. Psoas hypertrophy, and shortened hamstring, rectus femoris, and adductor muscles may require release. The sciatic nerve is also dysplastic, often tethered from prior surgery, and has dysplastic vascularity. The femoral nerve exits more superolaterally than normal and may be at risk from medial retractors. The profunda femora artery becomes proximally displaced, subjecting it to potential injury or laceration at the inferior margin of the acetabulum—a region usually free of major arterial structures.

Previous incisions from pelvic or femoral osteotomy are frequently encountered. An anterior Smith-Peterson incision is commonly used for a previous pediatric acetabular osteotomy, and a direct lateral incision may be present from a previous femoral osteotomy. The severely dysplastic hip may be approached from either the direct lateral or posterolateral approach, or from a combination of the two (which is our preferred method). Transtrochanteric and trochanteric slide approaches may also be used but normally are not necessary.

Visualization and palpation of sciatic nerve tension during the approach is important. Dissection of the nerve is not recommended to avoid further devascularization. Incising

into the capsule and passing a finger down through the hourglass constriction to the inferior aspect will localize the anatomic hip center. Excision of redundant and thickened capsule may be required to mobilize the proximal femur. Femoral shortening is frequently required; we prefer the subtrochanteric shortening osteotomy. Release of the psoas, rectus, and gluteus maximus insertion may also be required to mobilize the proximal femur.

Bone Preparation: Acetabulum

Whenever possible, we prefer to reconstruct the socket at or near the anatomic acetabulum in the highly dysplastic hip (**Figure 3**). This location usually provides the best host bone support and allows medialization of the anatomic hip center for improved biomechanics. The acetabulum is reconstructed before the femur because insertion of the acetabular implant influences limb length, femoral reconstruction, and the need for a shortening osteotomy.

In a high-riding DDH, care must be taken to identify the true acetabulum. This is best accomplished by following the ligament of teres from proximal to distal, which will lead the surgeon to the fovea of the true acetabulum. Errors can occur at this point because the true acetabulum often is extremely small, and it is possible to misidentify either the sciatic notch or the obturator foramen as the site of the true acetabulum. If in doubt, an intraoperative radiograph should be obtained.

Once the true acetabulum is identified, a blunt retractor is placed anteriorly, and a second blunt retractor is placed inferiorly. Removing fat and osteophytes from the foveal region identifies the medial wall of the acetabulum. A 2.5-mm drill can be used to make a drill hole through the medial wall, and a depth gauge can be used to determine the thickness of host bone available for medialization with reamers and to avoid medialization beyond the medial wall. Reaming is usually begun with a small-sized reamer in reverse and extends to the medial wall. The host acetabulum is frequently anteverted, a factor that must be considered when reaming. A deficient anterior wall and column may require preferential posterior reaming to obtain adequate host coverage of the implant. Similarly, the pelvis is frequently flexed as a result of pelvic tilt and compensated lordosis of the lumbar spine. The flexion of the pelvis must be considered when implanting the acetabular component because insufficient anteversion of the implant may occur.

Careful attention to cup abduction is also important because a vertical cup may predispose to wear and instability. The acetabular bone in a high-riding DDH is normally very osteopenic; thus, it is easy to inadvertently overream. We use the anterior and posterior columns as a landmark when inserting the trial component and ensure that the component is not excessively anteverted.

Prosthesis Implantation: Acetabulum

The columns serve as an excellent landmark to assist in anatomic positioning of the acetabular component. We prefer uncemented acetabular fixation and use a modular uncemented porous-coated acetabular implant with multiple screw holes to increase the options for screw fixation in the often poor-quality bone, which may incompletely cover the implant. Extra-small standard off-the-shelf acetabular implants (38- to 46-mm diameter) are frequently required. Smaller femoral heads (22 and 26 mm) are necessary to maintain adequate polyethylene thickness.

In Crowe III hips, superolateral coverage may be deficient; thus, a technique using a controlled medial wall protrusio "cotyloplasty" (controlled comminuted fracture) to en-

hance coverage occasionally may be helpful to increase medialization. Progressive medial migration of the implant and loss of medial bone support for future reconstruction have been reported as concerns with this technique. When bringing the hip center down to or near the anatomic location, optimizing host bone coverage of the component is the goal. Reamings are saved for packing around any uncovered region of the acetabular implant and later for the subtrochanteric osteotomy site. Frequently in Crowe III dysplastic hips, host bone coverage will be inadequate despite these methods.

The decision to reconstruct the acetabulum at a high hip center or augment coverage at or near the anatomic hip center with bulk autograft using the femoral head must be made before reaming at the anatomic hip center. We prefer reconstruction at the anatomic hip center and use the femoral head autograft to provide coverage if more than 30% of the implant will be uncovered. Improved results with structural bone grafting have been reported when the hip center is restored to its anatomic position, the graft supports less than 30% to 40% of the cup, and posterosuperior host bone support is provided and/or maintained. If the coverage by host bone is greater than 70%, cancellous autograft is packed around the uncovered region of the shell to act as a flying buttress graft and to provide host bone stock for future revision, thereby facilitating the use of another uncemented cup at future revision surgery. If the femoral head is used as an autograft, fixation with large cortical or cancellous screws is preferred.

The advantages of using a high hip center, including adequate host bone coverage and the decreased need for a shortening femoral osteotomy, are offset by problems with this technique. A smaller cup, the lack of host bone restoration for future reconstruction, limited bone available for screw fixa-

tion, vertical cup orientation with abnormal biomechanics, and impingement in flexion (anterior inferior iliac spine) or extension (ischial tuberosity) are concerns. Lateralization of the cup must be avoided in reconstruction using a high hip center because increased aseptic loosening of both femoral and acetabular implants may occur secondary to abnormal stresses transferred through the implant-bone interface.

Bone Preparation: Femur

The problems associated with femoral reconstruction and preexisting abnormal anatomy may be compounded by previous intertrochanteric or subtrochanteric osteotomy. Once the acetabulum has been reconstructed, the femur is prepared. In patients with high degenerative dysplasia (Crowe III and IV), a shortening procedure is often required to avoid overlengthening the limb and associated neurologic complications. In high dislocation, a femoral shortening osteotomy is safer, especially when the acetabulum has been brought down to the anatomic hip center. Lengthening of more than 2 to 2.5 cm may be associated with neurologic compromise. Lengthening of more than 4 cm or 6% of the length of the limb (whichever is less) should be avoided; we strictly avoid lengthening more than 2.5 cm.

Prosthesis Implantation: Femur

Methods of femoral reconstruction without shortening subtrochanteric osteotomy are detailed in chapter 16. In high-riding DDH, we prefer a subtrochanteric shortening osteotomy, which allows for relocation of the head within the true acetabulum, in all cases. Other methods such as greater trochanteric osteotomy with proximal femoral resection create a narrow strip of femur, require cemented DDH stems, and are associated with greater trochanteric union problems. In contrast, the subtrochanteric shortening transverse osteotomy is reproducible and allows correction of rotation, preserves the metaphyseal bone for implant fixation, and avoids problematic trochanteric fixation and complicated advancement techniques. When a shortening subtrochanteric osteotomy is performed, we prefer uncemented fixation with a modular system that allows proximal metaphyseal support, distal fluted fixation, and anteversion adjustment (a stem-through-sleeve design), such as the S-ROM (DePuy, Warsaw, IN). Uncemented extensively porous-coated implants with a narrow proximal metaphyseal flare also may be used if the metaphyseal flare of the implant can be fitted in the proximal femur. Cemented femoral fixation is also an acceptable alternative; for these patients, a short, straight DDH-type implant is required. The use of cement in combination with an osteotomy raises concern about this technique because the rate of nonunion may be increased at the osteotomy site.

The incision is a direct lateral incision longitudinally that allows for access to both the anterolateral and posterolateral hip.

We ordinarily expose the femoral neck through a direct lateral (Hardinge) approach. Alternatively, some surgeons use a posterior approach. The neck is usually significantly anteverted, and we dislocate the hip anteriorly, expose the head and neck, and then perform the neck cut via the anterolateral exposure. The sciatic nerve and shaft external rotators are then identified posteriorly. The rotators are released and tagged for later repair. The acetabulum is then exposed. We frequently prepare the femur at this stage (ream and place the cone body implant). Once the femur is reamed, we perform the subtrochanteric osteotomy. The proximal osteotomy fragment may then be retracted superiorly, giving excellent exposure of the acetabulum.

Careful preoperative planning is required to select the location of the osteotomy and determine the amount

of bone to be resected at the time of subtrochanteric shortening. We recommend a low neck resection in which the femur is prepared to receive a stem-through-sleeve design femoral component (**Figure 4**). Before making the osteotomy, the femur is reamed and prepared to receive the proximal cone. The femur is underreamed by 1 mm because once the osteotomy is made and the shortening performed, the anterior bowing of the femur is frequently eliminated. Failure to underream the femur may result in inadequate fixation in the distal fragment.

The definitive proximal cone body implant (sleeve) is seated in the proximal fragment before making the osteotomy. The osteotomy is then carefully performed using rotational landmarks drawn longitudinally along the femur and protecting the sciatic nerve. A trial head and neck segment, with the appropriate stem, is then inserted through the sleeve in the proximal fragment, and the hip is reduced into the acetabulum. The amount of overlap between the proximal and distal fragments is a guide to the amount of bone that needs to be removed during the shortening osteotomy. A second transverse osteotomy is made distally, removing the necessary amount of bone. We generally start by resecting somewhat less bone than we anticipate will be required (eg, 4 cm instead of 5 cm); more bone may always be resected, if necessary. When the resection is complete, the appropriately sized femoral stem is inserted across the osteotomy site. Distal fixation must be firm to achieve adequate torsional stability.

At the time of trial reduction, the amount of anteversion correction is assessed. It is very important that anteversion of the neck segment relative to the stem be confirmed and marked on the trial implants. Once the osteotomy is reduced, the use of adjunctive osteotomy fixation usually is not necessary, assuming adequate axial and torsional stability have been

achieved with the stem. On occasion, however, we use the resected bone divided in a coronal fashion as an onlay strut autograft at the osteotomy site (**Figure 5**). If the shortened segment is small, cortical strut allograft may be used instead of autograft. This allograft can be fixed proximally and distally with cerclage wires or cables. In addition, the cancellous reamings from the acetabulum may be packed around the osteotomy site as autograft.

Assessing intraoperative limb length is critically important during this procedure. The distance to bring the femoral head center down to the true acetabulum and the amount of shortening performed at the osteotomy site must be templated and assessed intraoperatively. Measurement with a limb-length caliper referenced off of a pin in the iliac crest is useful for assessing the lengthening of the proximal fragment. The overall lengthening may then be determined by the distance from the caliper pin to the proximal fragment minus the femoral osteotomy segment length. Despite a femoral shortening procedure, the leg is usually lengthened.

Assessments of hip stability and abductor tension, however, are the most important. Sciatic nerve tension must also be assessed. The trial reduction is performed with the knee flexed, and tension in the nerve is evaluated as the knee is gradually extended. A baseline examination of this tension before dislocation of the hip during the approach is important. If in doubt, a wake-up test with hip flexed and knee extended may be necessary, but this step is rarely required. If this test is planned, however, both the patient and anesthesiologist must be informed of this possibility before the induction of anesthesia.

Wound Closure

The vastus lateralis is repaired to the cuff preserved at the vastus ridge. The gluteus minimus and capsular layer

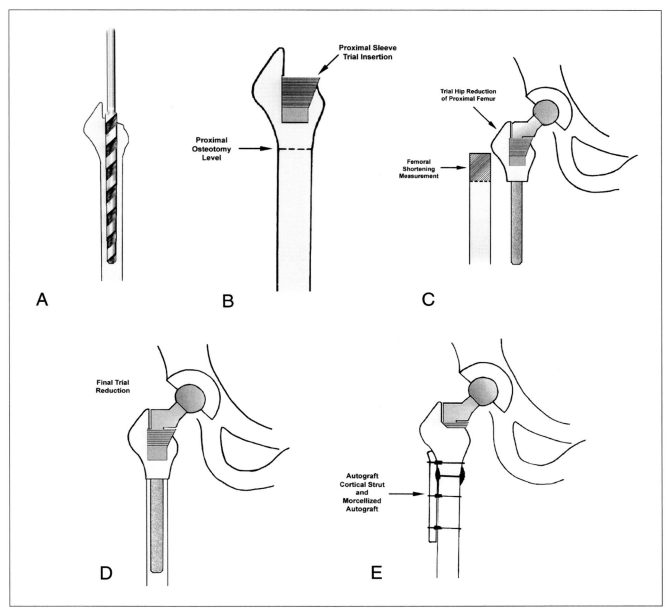

Figure 4 Reconstruction of the femur using a stem-through-sleeve implant. **A,** Intramedullary reaming of the femoral canal with straight (blunt-tipped) reamers is performed before acetabular reconstruction. The canal is underreamed by 1 mm with respect to the final implant stem diameter. **B,** Proximal reaming of the metaphyseal sleeve is performed, and a trial sleeve is inserted before the osteotomy is performed. A longitudinal mark is made on the lateral aspect of the femur for rotational reference. The transverse subtrochanteric osteotomy is then made 2 cm below the distal aspect of the trial metaphyseal sleeve. The trial stem is inserted through the sleeve, and a trial head is placed on the neck. **C,** The proximal fragment is reduced into the hip joint. The amount of overlap at the osteotomy site between the proximal and distal bone fragments is used to determine the amount of femoral shortening necessary. **D,** The distal fragment is then shortened, and the trial stem is inserted across the osteotomy site to reduce the osteotomy. Rotational alignment is reestablished. The hip is reduced with the trial femoral implants and assessed for stability and sciatic nerve tension. The amount of anteversion using the trial components is noted for the final implant anteversion. **E,** The final femoral components are inserted, and the osteotomy site augmented with cancellous autograft bone. The shortened cortical segment of osteotomized bone may be divided and applied as a strut autograft to augment stability at the osteotomy site. However, the stem must provide adequate distal rotational stability and avoid relying on the strut autograft alone to stabilize the construct. If the shortened segment is small, a cortical strut allograft may be used instead of autograft. (Reproduced with permission from Masonis JL, Patel JV, Miu A, et al: Subtrochanteric shortening and derotational osteotomy in primary total hip arthroplasty for patients with severe hip dysplasia: 5-year follow-up. *J Arthroplasty* 2003;18(suppl 1):68-73.)

are closed with a running bioabsorbable suture. The anterior one-third cuff of the gluteus medius is repaired to its tendinous insertion onto the trochanter with interrupted nonabsorbable suture. The fascia and skin are closed in routine fashion.

Postoperative Regimen
Toe-touch weight bearing is allowed immediately on the first postoperative day and maintained for at least 6 weeks (6 to 12 weeks), or until radiographic union at the osteotomy site is confirmed. Physical therapy proceeds in a standard regimen. Postoperative thromboembolic prophylaxis is routine. Clinical and radiographic follow-up occurs at 6 weeks and 3 months to assess osteotomy union and progression of weight-bearing status.

▮ Avoiding Pitfalls and Complications

Nonunion of the subtrochanteric transverse osteotomy occurs infrequently, but it may become symptomatic and cause additional problems. Nonunion is usually secondary to inadequate fixation at the osteotomy site and may imply inadequate rotational distal fixation. Rarely, this may lead to implant fracture or periprosthetic fracture. Management includes revision of the stem (longer stem or larger diameter) to achieve stability, autograft cancellous bone grafting at the osteotomy site, and augmentation with strut cortical onlay allografts with cable fixation. Compression plating across the osteotomy site may also be effective. Greater trochanter nonunion has been problematic with greater trochanteric osteotomy and sequential proximal femoral resection, and thus we avoid this technique.

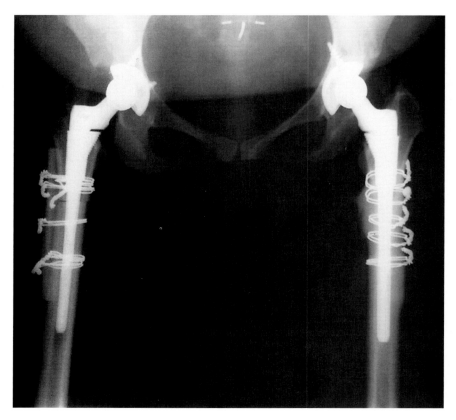

Figure 5 The subtrochanteric shortening osteotomy fragment may be divided longitudinally and used as a strut autograft to augment the osteotomy junction. AP radiograph at 3-year follow-up shows incorporation of the autogenous strut graft in the left hip and a lateral strut allograft and medial cancellous autograft packed around the osteotomy site in the right hip.

Dislocation rates of 5% to 11% have been reported to occur in association with THA in the severely dysplastic hip. Multiple anatomic, implant, and soft-tissue factors must be balanced intraoperatively. With the use of 22- or 26-mm femoral heads, trial reductions with the implants to confirm stability intraoperatively is emphasized.

Partial or complete sciatic or femoral nerve dysfunction is a more common complication of DDH surgery, especially with limb lengthening of more than 4 cm. Increased neurologic complications (up to 15%) have been reported in many series. Complete palsy may warrant a return to surgery, repeat assessment for compressive hematoma or nerve tension, and

consideration for further shortening if the surgeon believes there is still undue tension on the nerve. The use of a wake-up test, somatosensory-evoked potentials, and electromyographic monitoring remain controversial, and the effectiveness of the latter may be operator dependant. Care when passing cerclage cables or wires and when placing anterior retractors (femoral nerve) must also be emphasized.

Polyethylene wear and osteolysis, especially in younger active patients undergoing hip replacement for degenerative DDH, is a concerning yet common problem. Early identification of wear and osteolysis, with appropriate and timely management, is important.

References

Anderson MJ, Harris WH: Total hip arthroplasty with insertion of the acetabular component without cement in hips with total congenital dislocation or marked congenital dysplasia. *J Bone Joint Surg Am* 1999;81:347-354.

Crowe JF, Mani VJ, Ranawat CS: Total hip replacement in congenital dislocation and dysplasia of the hip. *J Bone Joint Surg Am* 1979;61:15-23.

Hartofilakidis G, Stamos K, Karachalios T, Ioannidis TT, Zacharakis N: Congenital hip disease in adults: Classification of acetabular deficiencies and operative treatment with acetabuloplasty combined with total hip arthroplasty. *J Bone Joint Surg Am* 1996;78:683-692.

Masonis JL, Patel JV, Miu A, et al: Subtrochanteric shortening and derotational osteotomy in primary total hip arthroplasty for patients with severe hip dysplasia: 5-year follow-up. *J Arthroplasty* 2003;18 (suppl 1):68-73.

Reikeraas O, Lereim P, Gabor I, Gunderson R, Bjerkreim I: Femoral shortening in total hip arthroplasty for completely dislocated hips: 3-7 year results in 25 cases. *Acta Orthop Scand* 1996;67:33-36.

Sanchez-Sotelo J, Berry DJ, Trousdale RT, Cabanela ME: Surgical treatment of developmental dysplasia of the hip in adults: II. Arthroplasty options. *J Am Acad Orthop Surg* 2002;10:334-344.

Stans AA, Pagnano MW, Shaughnessy WJ, Hanssen AD: Results of total hip arthroplasty for Crowe type III developmental hip dysplasia. *Clin Orthop* 1998;348:149-157.

Coding

CPT Codes		Corresponding ICD-9 Codes		
27130	Arthroplasty, acetabular and proximal femoral prosthetic replacement (total hip arthroplasty), with or without autograft or allograft	711.45 714.30 715.35 718.6 733.42	711.95 715.15 716.15 720.0 808.0	714.0 715.25 718.5 733.14 905.6
27132	Conversion of previous hip surgery to total hip arthroplasty, with or without autograft or allograft	715.15 718.2 733.14 996.4	715.25 718.5 733.42 996.66	715.35 718.6 905.6 996.77
27165	Osteotomy, intertrochanteric or subtrochanteric including internal or external fixation and/or cast	715.15 732.1 736.32 754.32 755.61	715.25 733.81 754.30 754.33 755.62	715.35 736.31 754.31 754.35 755.63
22 modifier	Unusual procedural services			

CPT copyright © 2004 by the American Medical Association. All Rights Reserved.

Chapter 18

Total Hip Arthroplasty: Protrusio Acetabulum

Michael H. Huo, MD

▊ Indications

The principal indications for total hip arthroplasty (THA) in patients with protrusio acetabuli are pain and deterioration of functional capacity. Progressive ankylosis leading to associated symptoms similar to the sequelae of hip fusion is another indication.

Primary or idiopathic protrusio acetabuli is an uncommon disease characterized by bulging of the acetabulum into the pelvic cavity. It has been postulated that it results from some degree of chondrodystrophy of the triradiate cartilage of the acetabulum. Secondary protrusio acetabuli has been attributed to many causes (**Table 1**). The common pathway, regardless of etiology, appears to be weakness of the medial acetabular bony support followed by (1) the principal joint reaction force vector being directed more medially than normal, (2) resultant medial migration of the hip center, and (3) increased progression once the vector has migrated medially to the ilioischial line of the pelvis. All of the contributing factors leading to the development of protrusio acetabuli must be identified.

Standard AP and lateral radiographs of the pelvis and affected hip(s) are used to establish the diagnosis. Most authors use the center-edge angle measurement as the principal criterion. A measurement greater than 40° is considered diagnostic. Others use protrusion medial to the ilioischial (Köhler's) line and/or violation of the teardrop (medial wall of the acetabulum) as diagnostic criteria (**Figure 1**). The severity of the protrusio acetabuli can be graded as follows: (1) mild: < 5-mm protrusion beyond Köhler's line; (2) moderate: 6- to 15-mm protrusion; and (3) severe: > 15 mm.

Laboratory studies are dictated by the associated medical etiologies. Infection and neoplasm always should be considered possible causes of the deformity. Additional imaging techniques can include CT and MRI. A CT scan can more accurately define the integrity of the anterior and posterior walls and columns of the acetabulum, which is critical in planning placement of the acetabular cup. MRI may be of particular use if neoplasia is considered.

━━━━━━━━━━━■

Table 1 Causes of Secondary Protrusio Acetabuli

Infectious	Genetic
Bacterial	Ehlers-Danlos syndrome
Tuberculosis	Marfan syndrome
	Sickle cell disease
Inflammatory	**Neoplastic**
Rheumatoid arthritis	Hemangioma
Juvenile rheumatoid arthritis	Metastasis
Ankylosing spondylitis	Neurofibromatosis
Psoriatic arthritis	
Metabolic	**Traumatic**
Paget's disease	Acetabular and pelvic fractures
Hyperparathyroidism	Iatrogenic fracture during surgery
Osteogenesis imperfecta	Radiation-induced osteonecrosis of the acetabulum
Ochronosis	

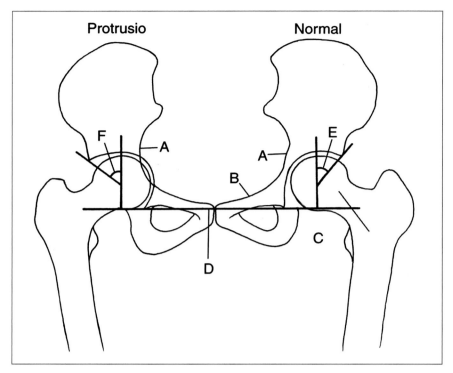

Figure 1 Radiographic landmarks used in the diagnosis of protrusio acetabuli. A = ilioischial (Köhler's) line. B = iliopectineal line. C = acetabular wall. D = interteardrop line. E = normal center-edge angle. F = abnormal center-edge angle indicative of protrusio acetabuli. (Reproduced from McBride MT, Muldoon MP, Santore RF, Trousdale RT, Wenger DR: Protrusio acetabuli: Diagnosis and treatment. *J Am Acad Orthop Surg* 2001;9:79-88.)

Contraindications

Contraindications for THA in patients with protrusion acetabuli are similar to those for other diseases. Active infection is an absolute contraindication. Relative contraindications include neuropathic conditions, significant myopathy, deficient or paralytic hip abductor mechanism, advanced medical comorbidities that are not correctable, morbid obesity, and a psychosocial profile that is risky for patient compliance.

Alternative Treatments

Maximizing medical management for pain control, physical therapy to maintain hip motion, and use of assistive devices for walking are the principal nonsurgical management options. Surgical treatment options differ for skeletally immature and mature patients. The focus of this chapter is on adults; thus, closure of the triradiate cartilage coupled with proximal femoral osteotomy are not discussed.

Surgical options are limited in adult patients. Resection arthroplasty and arthrodesis, as well as valgus femoral osteotomy, have been used. The clinical experience reported in the literature is limited. Most authors agree that osteotomy should not be performed in patients older than age 40 years or in patients with advanced arthritic changes. Prosthetic hip arthroplasty is the surgical option of choice in older patients. Hemiarthroplasty using a bipolar-type design coupled with acetabular bone grafting has been

reported to be unsuccessful in that progression of the protrusio acetabuli continued in many patients. THA remains to be the most clinically efficacious treatment. The critical technical challenge in THA is to restore the hip rotation center more laterally. Historically, the clinical outcome has been poorer with cemented cups if the hip rotation center was not restored to within 5 mm of the desired position.

Results

Most of the reported clinical results of THA in protrusio acetabuli have been with cemented fixation (**Table 2**). Sotelo-Garza and Charnley reported no difference in outcome between THAs done for protrusio acetabuli and THAs done for osteoarthritis at a mean follow-up of nearly 5 years. Ranawat and associates reported the results of 35 THAs done with cemented fixation. In 17 hips, the hip center was not lateralized; at a mean follow-up of 4.3 years, 16 of the 17 hips failed as a result of loosening. The critical value was 10 mm or less to the desired hip center position. There have been very few reports of uncemented fixation in protrusio acetabuli.

Technique

Exposure
THA can be performed through all routine surgical exposures. On occasion, the transtrochanteric approach, which offers wide exposure to access the acetabulum and facilitates hip dislocation, may have added advantages. Lateral and distal transfer of the trochanter may be beneficial in restoring the proper biomechanics of the hip abductor mechanism. Moreover, trochanteric transfer through this ap-

proach will add to hip stability, especially in collagen disorders (Ehlers-Danlos and Marfan syndromes) and paralytic conditions.

Dislocating the femoral head may be difficult because of the protrusio position, especially if progressive ankylosis is associated with soft-tissue contractures. Forceful dislocation maneuvers may result in fracture of the femur. Osteotomy of the femoral neck in situ may be necessary to mobilize the proximal femur. The femoral head can then be removed using a corkscrew type extraction device (as in femoral neck fractures) or in segments. Every effort should be made to preserve as much of the femoral head as possible to be used as graft for the medial defect.

Bone Preparation and Prosthesis Implantation
ACETABULAR RECONSTRUCTION
Wide exposure is imperative to identifying the proper landmarks of the acetabulum. Retractors should be placed over the anterior wall, around the transverse acetabular ligament inferiorly, and around the ischium to define the posterior wall. The superior rim of the acetabulum should be carefully defined as well. All soft tissues must be removed from the medial wall to expose the bony bed of the acetabulum. Acetabular preparation is more difficult in the presence of extensive marginal osteophytes. The definitions of the borders of the acetabular walls must be based on visualization of the anatomy and evaluation of the preoperative radiographs. Well-defined borders are critical to placement of the cup.

A small-diameter reamer or power burr is used to remove any remaining articular cartilage and soft tissues from the protrusio segment of the medial wall to allow for bone graft incorporation. The anatomic acetabular fossa can then be reamed using sequential reamers. The cup is reamed until a chamfered rim of peripheral

Table 2 Results of THA in Protrusio Acetabulum

Author(s) (Year)	Number of Hips	Implant Type	Mean Patient Age (Range)	Mean Follow-up (Range)	Results
Ranawat, et al (1980)	35	Stem: cemented Cup: cemented	50 years (N/A)	4.3 years (3–7)	66% satisfactory Loosening: 1 cup, 3 stems
Wilson and Scott (1993)	22	Stem: 59% cemented Cup: bipolar	46 years (19–78)	4.3 years (3–6.3)	95% satisfactory 23% bipolar migration
Rosenberg, et al (2000)	36	Stem: cemented Cup: cemented + impaction grafting	57 years (20–79)	12 years (8–18)	94% satisfactory 90% implant survival at 12 years
Matsuno, et al (2000)	15	Stem: uncemented Cup: uncemented cage	62 years (48–79)	4.5 years (2–7)	100% satisfactory 0% implant failure

N/A = Not Applicable

bone is machined that will provide good support for the cup. Reaming too medially with small reamers can create a reamed cylinder rather than a chamfered core of supportive bone. A trial cup is inserted to confirm the proper position and anteversion of the cup and also to assess the adequacy of cup fixation. An intraoperative AP radiograph helps assess proper placement of the cup compared with the contralateral hip. Moreover, this radiograph can be used to assess whether limb length has been restored by scrutinizing the vertical distance between the lesser trochanter and the transischial line.

Bone grafting of the medial defect is an integral part of the surgical technique. The resected femoral head can be used either in bulk or in particulate form (**Figure 2**). Incorporation of either form of bone graft has been predictably successful. The temporal sequence of incorporation is generally faster with morcellized graft than with bulk form. Cemented fixation of the acetabular cup is infrequently used in THA today. Revision THA using impaction grafting in the acetabulum and a cemented all-polyethylene cup

is reported to have predictable success and good medium-term durability. Cemented fixation of the cup may be considered in the rare situation in which either a protrusio ring or a pelvic reinforcement cage is used. The mechanical advantage of metallic reinforcement devices is that they transfer load away from the deficient medial wall onto the acetabular rim, in particular the superior ilium. This stress transfer has been shown to improve the distribution of biomechanical forces around the cup and the underlying cement mantle. These reinforcement devices are valuable in selected acetabular deficiencies encountered during revision surgery; however, their application is rarely required in uncomplicated primary or secondary protrusio acetabuli.

Currently, the most common surgical technique is to use a porous-coated cup design relying on rim fit (**Figure 3**). The medial defect is packed with morcellized autograft from the resected femoral head. The acetabular reaming technique is described above. Caution should be exercised to avoid excessive reaming of the acetabular walls that provide es-

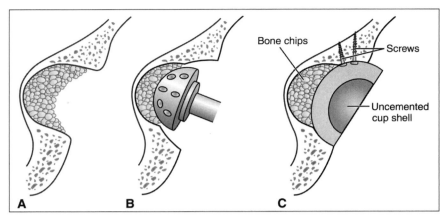

Figure 2 Bone grafting technique of acetabular reconstruction in protrusio acetabuli. Corticocancellous bone chips can be molded to fit the defects and the metal socket by placing the chips (**A**), reaming with the reamer 1 to 2 mm smaller than the socket chosen and rotated in reverse (**B**), and placing the cup into the defect with secure rim contact (**C**). (Adapted with permission from Vail TP, McCollum DE: Complex primary acetabular replacement, in Callaghan JJ, Rosenberg AG, Rubash HE (eds): *The Adult Hip*. Philadelphia, PA, Lippincott-Raven, 1998, vol II, pp 1183-1196.)

sential mechanical support of the cup. Supplemental screw fixation should be considered because the acetabular shell is not as well supported by strong host bone medially. Proper placement of the cup offers good contact with the acetabular dome where screws can be inserted to improve rotational stability. Some cup designs offer a slightly larger rim diameter (so-called dual geometry type) than the dome diameter. These designs can offer even greater

press-fit stability of the shell, although there may be a greater risk of fracture of the acetabular walls at insertion.

A variety of acetabular articulations is available, including the following: (1) a routine polyethylene liner with or without an elevated rim, depending on the amount of anteversion desired; (2) a lateralized liner that provides even further lateralization of the hip rotation center; (3) an offset liner that provides both lateralization

and inferior placement of the hip rotation center; (4) a ceramic or metal articulation if hard-on-hard coupling is desired; and (5) a constrained liner if hip stability is marginal. Fortunately, hip stability generally is not a clinical concern because lateralization of the hip rotation center increases the soft-tissue tension from the preoperative anatomy.

FEMORAL RECONSTRUCTION

Techniques of femoral canal preparation and stem insertion are similar to those in routine THA if no previous femoral osteotomy was done. A stem design with increased offset may be desirable to minimize femoral-pelvic impingement, especially if a short neck length is necessary to equalize limb length. If desired, a larger femoral head size (32 or 36 mm) can be selected (provided that the outer diameter of the acetabular shell so permits) to achieve greater hip motion free of prosthetic impingement. Deformity from a previous femoral osteotomy can present a considerable technical challenge. The options in this situation are (1) use of a smaller stem with cemented fixation to accommodate the deformed proximal femoral anatomy; (2) selected use of corrective osteotomy coupled with a

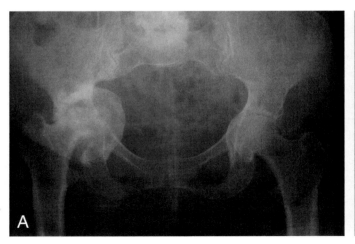
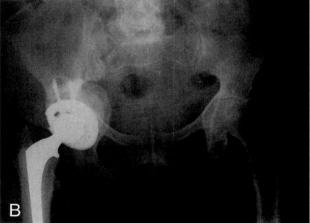

Figure 3 Preoperative (**A**) and postoperative (**B**) AP radiographs of a patient who underwent THA for protrusio acetabuli.

cylindrical, tapered, or wedged design; or (3) use of a modular femoral stem design that offers different combinations for proximal and distal fit of the altered femoral anatomy.

Postoperative Regimen

In most patients postoperative rehabilitation is routine. If the protrusio was severe and extensive bone grafting was required, or if the quality of acetabular bone support was marginal, toe-touch weight bearing may be recommended for 6 to 8 weeks postoperatively.

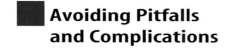

Avoiding Pitfalls and Complications

A key goal of THA in patients with protrusio acetabuli is to avoid inadequate restoration of the hip rotation center that was present before surgery. Thus, it is important to place the acetabular cup in a position lateral to the hip center. The new hip center adds to the challenge of equalizing limb length. Proper seating of the femoral stem is important to avoid contributing to excessive lengthening of the leg. Overlengthening can poten-

tially result in sciatic neuropathy. The surgeon must eliminate bony impingement by restoring femoral offset and resecting marginal osteophytes. Adductor tenotomy may be indicated if there are excessive contractures around the hip joint. Moreover, antibiotic and thromboembolic prophylaxis should be initiated, similarly to routine THA. Prophylaxis against heterotopic ossification should be considered in patients with soft-tissue dissection, particularly in hips with hypertrophic arthritic changes.

 ## References

Lachiewicz PF: Rheumatoid arthritis of the hip. *J Am Acad Orthop Surg* 1997;5:332-338.

Matsuno H, Yasuda T, Yudoh K, et al: Cementless cup supporter for protrusio acetabuli in patients with rheumatoid arthritis. *Int Orthop* 2000;24:15-18.

McBride MT, Muldoon MP, Santore RF, Trousdale RT, Wenger DR: Protrusio acetabuli: Diagnosis and treatment. *J Am Acad Orthop Surg* 2001;9:79-88.

Ranawat CS, Dorr LD, Inglis AE: Total hip arthroplasty in protrusio acetabuli of rheumatoid arthritis. *J Bone Joint Surg Am* 1980;62:1059-1065.

Rosenberg WW, Schreurs BW, de Waal Malefijt MC, Veth RP, Slooff T: Impacted morsellized bone grafting and cemented primary total arthroplasty for acetabular protrusion in patients with rheumatoid arthritis: An 8- to 11-year follow-up study of 36 hips. *Acta Orthop Scand* 2000;71:143-146.

Wilson MG, Scott RD: Bipolar socket in protrusio acetabuli: 3-6 year study. *J Arthroplasty* 1993;8:405-411.

Coding

CPT Codes		Corresponding ICD-9 Codes		
27130	Arthroplasty, acetabular and proximal femoral prosthetic replacement (total hip arthroplasty), with or without autograft or allograft	711.45 714.30 715.35 718.6 733.42	711.95 715.15 716.15 720.0 808.0	714.0 715.25 718.5 733.14 905.6
27132	Conversion of previous hip surgery to total hip arthroplasty, with or without autograft or allograft	715.15 718.2 733.14 996.4	715.25 718.5 733.42 996.66	715.35 718.6 905.6 996.77

CPT copyright © 2004 by the American Medical Association. All Rights Reserved.

Chapter 19
Total Hip Arthroplasty: Paget's Disease

Richard Iorio, MD
William L. Healy, MD

◼ Indications

Paget's disease of bone is a metabolic disorder of unknown etiology that is characterized by an increase in bone turnover. A pathologic increase in the number and cellular activity of osteoclasts and osteoblasts causes a disorganized bone structure characterized by trabecular hypertrophy, osteosclerosis, and cystic degeneration, which results in the unique radiographic appearance of pagetoid bone.

Paget's disease can present as a monostotic or polyostotic process. Patients with Paget's disease may experience bone pain as a result of deformity, fracture, neoplastic degeneration, or degenerative joint disease. The disorder is more common in Europe and North America, with an incidence of 2% to 4% in patients who are older than 40 years. Paget's disease may be asymptomatic for extended periods before symptoms develop. More than half of symptomatic patients report joint dysfunction at the time of diagnosis. Degenerative hip disease will develop in up to half of patients with Paget's disease. Total hip arthroplasty (THA) can be a predictably successful surgical treatment for a painful, degenerative hip secondary to Paget's disease.

Patients with Paget's disease who report pain about the hip joint require careful evaluation so that all potential causes of pain, other than degenerative hip disease, are considered. Active Paget's disease, characterized by high metabolic bone turnover, stress fracture, lumbar spinal compression with neurologic sequelae, and sarcomatous degeneration of Paget's disease can cause pain about the hip. Localized enlargement of the proximal femur or acetabulum with accompanying osteosclerosis is indicative of Paget's disease of the hip. If the origin of pain in a patient with Paget's disease remains in doubt, intra-articular injection of local anesthetic under fluoroscopy can differentiate the origin of the pain.

Degenerative disease associated with Paget's disease of the hip can be very painful. Accompanying bone deformity complicates the surgical management of hip osteoarthritis in these patients. Medically optimized patients with chronic hip pain caused by degenerative disease are candidates for THA. In the femur, coxa vara, diaphyseal bowing, fractures of the femoral neck or shaft, and a distorted, sclerotic, medullary canal are commonly seen. Enlargement of the pelvis, cavitary cystic degeneration, acetabular protrusio, and hypervascularity can be present on the acetabular side.

———◼

◼ Contraindications

Paget's disease can present with variable phases of bone resorption due to hyperactive osteoclasts and new bone formation as a result of a proliferation of osteoblasts. The active lytic phase of bone resorption is associated with vascular proliferation, and this phase of hypervascularity may be associated with bone pain. THA performed on pagetic bone during the hypervascular phase may be associated with increased intraoperative blood loss, increased bone-related pain postoperatively, and increased risk of bone resorption about the hip implants postoperatively.

The extent of pagetic lytic activity can be assessed with a bone scan. Serum alkaline phosphatase concentration is an indicator of bone formation, and urinary hydroxyproline excretion is an indicator of bone resorption. These biochemical markers correlate with the extent of disease found on the bone scan. Thus, preoperative medical management of the active phase of Paget's disease may decrease the risk of complications.

Sarcomatous degeneration of pagetic bone is seen in less than 1% of patients. If bone changes become rapidly destructive and increasingly painful and are associated with cortical erosions and an accompanying soft-tissue mass, sarcomatous degeneration must be considered.

———◼

Table 1 Results of Cemented Total Hip Arthroplasty for Paget's Disease of the Hip

Author(s) (Year)	Number of Hips	Implant Type	Mean Patient Age (Range)	Mean Follow-up (Range)	Results
Merkow, et al (1984)	21	N/A	68.6 years	5 years (2-11)	18 of 21 excellent or good results; 2 revisions
McDonald and Sim (1987)	52	N/A	69.9 years	8.8 years (3-15)	39 of 52 excellent or good results; 9 revisions
Ludkowski and Wilson-MacDonald (1988)	37	N/A	71.5 years	7.8 years (1-18.4)	26 of 37 excellent or good results; 0 revisions
Sochart and Porter (2000)	98	N/A	67.4 years	10.4 years (5.5-20)	81 of 98 excellent or good results; 8 revisions

N/A = Not Applicable

Table 2 Results of Uncemented Total Hip Arthroplasty for Paget's Disease of the Hip

Author(s) (Year)	Number of Hips	Implant Type	Mean Patient Age (Range)	Mean Follow-up (Range)	Results
Hozack, et al (1999)	5	N/A	68	5.8 years (4.8-8.8)	All had excellent or good results
Kirsch, et al (2001)	20	N/A	72	6 years (4.8)	18 of 20 excellent or good results; 0 revisions
Parvizi, et al (2002)	19	N/A	71.3	7 years (2-15)	16 of 19 excellent or good results; 0 revisions

N/A = Not Applicable

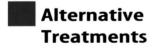

Alternative Treatments

Medical management of Paget's disease includes calcitonin, pliamycin, gallium nitrate, and bisphosphonates. Patients with bone pain secondary to Paget's disease who fail to respond to anti-inflammatory or pain medications are candidates for antiresorptive therapy. Bone deformity, risk of fracture, and preparation for surgery are indications for drug therapy. A decrease in bone turnover measured by a decrease in biochemical markers al-

ters the natural history of the disease and may preclude the need for intervention if pain and deformity are prevented. Treatment of pagetic bone in the resorptive phase may decrease vascularity of the diseased bone and decrease the incidence of bone-related pain and postoperative bone resorption status following THA.

Severe varus deformity of the proximal femur and bowing of the femoral shaft are commonly seen in patients with Paget's disease of the hip. These deformities can result in malalignment with subsequent abnormal

stress on the hip joint, stress fracture, impingement, and limited range of motion. When malalignment results from pagetic involvement of the femur and articular cartilage in the hip joint shows no signs of degeneration, corrective osteotomy may be an alternative to THA. Metaphyseal osteotomies heal significantly faster than diaphyseal osteotomies in the presence of Paget's disease.

Nonsurgical treatment of degenerative arthritis associated with Paget's disease is the same as for idiopathic osteoarthritis and may include anti-inflammatory agents, activity modification, and gait aids.

Results

THA for degenerative hip disease secondary to Paget's disease has been successful with cemented (**Table 1**) and uncemented (**Table 2**) hip implants. However, failure rates with cemented implants are higher than those seen in primary THA for patients with osteoarthritis. Hypervascularity, bone resorption, and bone deformity can affect the endurance of THA. Bone deformity and the unpredictability of bone ingrowth makes routine implantation of uncemented femoral implants controversial (**Figure 1**). Even though the studies listed in the tables may not be comparable, the reported revision rates at intermediate-term follow-up are lower for uncemented implants than for cemented implants.

Technique

Exposure

Paget's disease of the hip in the absence of femoral deformity can be approached as any other routine THA with an anterolateral, posterior, or tro-

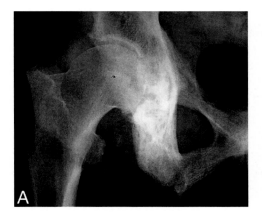

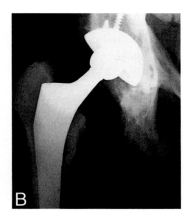

Figure 1 **A,** AP radiograph of Paget's disease of the hip with degenerative joint disease. **B,** Postoperative AP radiograph of an uncemented THA for Paget's disease of the hip.

chanteric osteotomy approach. Coxa vara or bowing of the femur may make entrance to the femoral canal more difficult than in other patients. In the pagetic hip with coxa vara, osteotomy of the greater trochanter has been advocated as a means to facilitate dislocation of the hip and also as a method to access the femoral canal. Additionally, advancement of the greater trochanter improves the biomechanics of the pagetic hip with coxa vara. The incidence of nonunion of a trochanteric osteotomy after THA for Paget's disease has been reported to be 13%.

Acetabular protrusio can be encountered in the pagetic hip. Acetabular protrusio combined with coxa vara can make dislocation difficult. Care must be taken to remove osteophytic bone around the acetabulum before dislocation is attempted. If the combination of acetabular protrusio and coxa vara is severe, in situ femoral neck osteotomy must be considered prior to dislocation and/or trochanteric osteotomy to facilitate dislocation and avoid fracture.

Bone Preparation

Hypervascularity can cause excessive bleeding; thus, preoperative medical treatment of active Paget's disease may minimize active bleeding, which subsequently facilitates evaluation of the bone-implant interface.

The acetabulum in patients with Paget's disease is often enlarged and may be medialized. Reaming to expand the periphery without deepening the socket is advised to avoid causing added protrusio. Cystic changes also can be encountered with pagetic bone; these may be curetted to remove fibrous tissue and grafted with host-bone reamings.

Preparation of the femoral canal depends on eradication of fibrous pagetic tissue and the ability to shape the sclerotic, enlarged femoral canal. Broaches may not be able to safely penetrate sclerotic bone; thus, high-speed burrs or rotary reamers may be necessary. Intraoperative fluoroscopic evaluation may help with proper placement of the trial femoral component.

Prosthesis Implantation

In the acetabulum, the inability to produce a dry acetabular bone interface may preclude the successful implantation of a cemented cup. Long-term follow-up of uncemented acetabular implants has yet to be reported in patients with Paget's disease; however, intermediate-term follow-up appears promising. Sclerotic acetabular pagetic bone may be at risk for fracture with underreaming technique. We prefer uncemented fixation of the acetabulum with supplemental screw fixation

when hemispherical contact can be maintained.

Bowing of the femur may necessitate osteotomy to allow implantation of the femoral stem (**Figure 2**, *A*). Proximal femoral osteotomy for coxa vara and multiple diaphyseal osteotomies for femoral bowing have been reported with both cemented (**Figure 2**, *B* and **2**, *C*) and uncemented techniques. Healing after diaphyseal osteotomies can be protracted in these femurs. Attempts to avoid osteotomy and use a customized curved cemented femoral stem to match the femoral geometry in Paget's disease have failed because of subsequent periprosthetic fracture.

If cement is used for femoral fixation in association with an osteotomy, care must be taken to prevent cement intrusion into the osteotomy sites, which will impair healing. Strut grafting may be a valuable adjunct to osteotomy.

We prefer uncemented fixation for femoral implants. If an osteotomy is necessary to accommodate the prosthesis, then a metaphyseal osteotomy spanned by a modular implant and supported with adjunctive fixation and strut grafting is advisable. If multiple diaphyseal osteotomies are necessary, then long-stem femoral cemented fixation may be a more stable construct. An attempt should be made to bypass all pseudofractures with the femoral prosthesis. Alternatively, pseudofractures may be supported by strut grafts and/or adjunctive fixation. Struts can also be invaded by pagetic bone as they revascularize and probably are best supported by an intramedullary femoral stem.

Wound Closure

Wound closure following THA in this patient group is done in a routine manner. However, because excessive blood loss is common with the preparation of pagetic bone, meticulous technique is required to minimize blood loss and prevent hematoma. Blood salvage

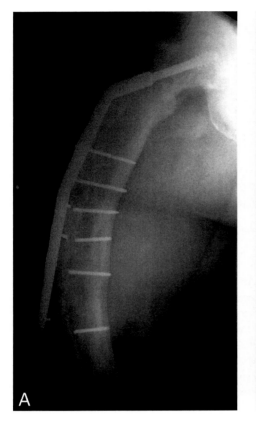

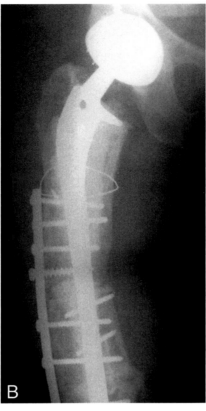

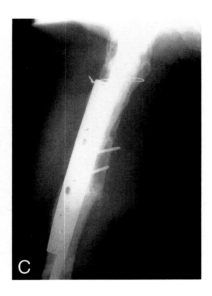

Figure 2 A, Paget's disease of the hip with varus bowing of the femur, coxa vara, and failing fixation of a previous femur fracture. Postoperative AP **(B)** and **(C)** lateral radiographs of a patient with Paget's disease with multiple diaphyseal osteotomies of the femoral shaft and a cemented femoral long stem implant with lateral plate stabilization of the osteotomies.

techniques may be helpful when hypervascular bone is encountered.

Postoperative Regimen
Protected weight bearing following osteotomy in conjunction with THA is recommended until evidence of radiographic union is present. Increased pain or increased bone resorption due to active disease can be prevented with calcitonin or bisphosphonates to prevent stress fractures or periprosthetic resorption.

Heterotopic ossification can occur in up to 52% of patients with Paget's disease who undergo THA. Prophylaxis with either a nonsteroidal anti-inflammatory regimen or perioperative irradiation is recommended.

■ Avoiding Pitfalls and Complications

Excessive intraoperative bleeding can be minimized by treating patients with active disease and hypervascularity with a preoperative medical regimen.

Varus positioning of the femoral component, which leads to early failure, can be avoided by checking the intraoperative position of trial components with fluoroscopy or an intraoperative radiograph. If trochanteric osteotomy or power tool reaming of sclerotic Paget's bone fails to provide a femoral shape, which correctly positions the implant, femoral osteotomy may be necessary to properly position the stem.

Osteotomy of the femoral diaphysis is prone to nonunion; thus, care must be taken to obtain adequate bone-to-bone contact and prevent cement intrusion into the osteotomy site. Strut grafts need to be augmented with either intramedullary or plate fixation to ensure that long-term bone reinforcement is provided.

Symptomatic heterotopic ossification can cause significantly decreased functional hip scores in patients with Paget's disease compared with unaffected control subjects. Therefore, heterotopic bone prophylaxis for these patients is strongly recommended.

References

Alexakis PG, Brown BA, Hohl WM: Hip replacement in Paget's disease. *Clin Orthop* 1998;350:138-142.

Hozack WJ, Rushton SA, Carey C, Sakalkale D, Rothman RH: Uncemented total hip arthroplasty in Paget's disease of the hip: A report of five cases with five-year follow-up. *J Arthroplasty* 1999;14:872-876.

Kirsch G, Kligman M, Roffman M: Hydroxyapatite-coated total hip replacement in Paget's disease. *Acta Orthop Scand* 2001;72:127-132.

Ludkowski P, Wilson-MacDonald J: Total hip arthroplasty in Paget's disease of the hip: A clinical review and review of the literature. *Clin Orthop* 1988;255:160-167.

McDonald DJ, Sim FH: Total hip arthroplasty in Paget's disease. *J Bone Joint Surg Am* 1987;69:766-772.

Merkow RL, Pellicci PM, Healy DP, Salvati EA: Total hip replacement for Paget's disease of the hip. *J Bone Joint Surg Am* 1984;66:752-758.

Namba RS, Brick GW, Murray WR: Revision total hip arthroplasty with correctional femoral osteotomy in Paget's disease. *J Arthroplasty* 1997;12:591-595.

Parvizi J, Frankle MA, Tiegs RD, Sim FH: Corrective osteotomy for deformity in Paget disease. *J Bone Joint Surg Am* 2003;85:697-702.

Parvizi J, Schall DM, Lewallen DG, Sim FH: Outcome of uncemented hip arthroplasty in patients with Paget's disease. *Clin Orthop* 2002;403:127-134.

Sochart DH, Porter NL: Charnley low friction arthroplasty for Paget's disease of the hip. *J Arthroplasty* 2000;15:210-219.

Coding

CPT Codes		Corresponding ICD-9 Codes		
27130	Arthroplasty, acetabular and proximal femoral prosthetic replacement (total hip arthroplasty), with or without autograft or allograft	711.45 711.95 714.0 714.30 715.15 715.25 715.35 716.15 718.5 718.6 720.0 733.14 733.42 808.0 905.6		
27132	Conversion of previous hip surgery to total hip arthroplasty, with or without autograft or allograft	715.15 715.24 715.35 718.2 718.5 718.6 733.14 733.42 905.6 996.4 996.66 996.77		
27165	Osteotomy, intertrochanteric or subtrochanteric including internal or external fixation and/or cast	715.15 715.25 715.35 732.17 733.81 736.31 736.32 754.30 754.31 754.32 754.33 754.35 755.61 755.62 755.63		

CPT copyright © 2004 by the American Medical Association. All Rights Reserved.

Chapter 20

Total Hip Arthroplasty After Acetabular Fracture

Mark C. Reilly, MD
Joel M. Matta, MD

Indications

Total hip arthroplasty (THA) following acetabular fracture can be a relatively uncomplicated procedure, but many patients present special difficulties such as retained implants from previous surgery, acetabular bone defects, acetabular nonunion, acetabular and innominate bone deformities, impaired musculature, heterotopic ossification, and infection.

As with THA for other situations, the indications for surgery are related primarily to the severity of hip pain rather than the radiographic appearance. Typically, the need for surgery is dictated by the severity of the patient's pain; however, at times it is best to proceed expeditiously with the arthroplasty. For example, in the case of failed posterior wall fixation, the femoral head will subluxate, and rapid bony wear will ensue. In these patients, the femoral head and neck may be a useful source of autograft; therefore, performing THA before the femoral head is completely destroyed is important.

Contraindications

Although patients may be unhappy with hip function following acetabular fracture, the problem may not always be best solved by THA. Painful loss of hip motion may be the result of heterotopic ossification or, uncommonly, femoral head or acetabular malunion. The patient may be unhappy because of a limp. Although an abnormal gait may be caused by osteoarthritis, it also may be caused by inadequate musculature, joint contracture, neurologic deficit, or pelvic deformity in the presence of a preserved hip joint.

THA is not indicated when the patient's primary complaints are unlikely to be solved by the procedure. The surgeon must rule out possible hip infection before considering THA, when appropriate.

Alternative Treatments

Treatment of symptomatic posttraumatic osteoarthritis following acetabular fracture differs from treatment of other types of hip arthritis. With posttraumatic osteoarthritis, the patient population is frequently younger and expects a more active and demanding lifestyle. Surgical options such as intertrochanteric osteotomy, periacetabular osteotomy, or arthrodesis still play a considerable role in delaying or obviating the need for THA in a young patient because of the inherent risks associated with THA for a lifetime of multiple revision surgeries. Similarly, reduction and fixation of an acetabular malunion or nonunion may provide symptomatic relief or long-term preservation of the hip joint if the arthritic destruction is in its early stages.

Results

In most published series of THA after fracture of the acetabulum, the incidence of femoral complications is similar or equal to that of primary THA, whereas the incidence of radiographic loosening, symptomatic loosening, and revision of the acetabular component is significantly higher. These problems occur in the young, predominantly male, patient population and in association with large segmental and cavitary bone deficiencies. Preliminary series have reported fewer instances of symptomatic loosening with uncemented acetabular components compared with cemented components. **Table 1** summarizes recent results of THA after acetabular fracture.

Table 1 Results of THA After Acetabular Fracture

Author(s) (Year)	Number of Hips	Implant Type	Mean Patient Age (Range)	Mean Follow-up (Range)	Results
Bellabarba, et al (2001)	30	Uncemented	51 years (26–86)	63 months (24–140)	10-year survivorship, 97%
Berry and Halasy (2002)	34	Uncemented	49.7 years (19–78)	10–16 years (8 of 33 followed 12 years)	9 of 25 revised, 36% revision rate
Huo, et al (1999)	21	Uncemented	52 years (23–78)	65 months (48–104)	Mechanical failure rate, 19% acetabulum, 29% stem
Romness and Lewallen (1990)	55	Mixed	48.7 years	7.5 years	Acetabular loosening, 52.9% Femoral loosening, 29.4%
Weber, et al (1998)	66	Uncemented (20) Cemented (44) Hybrid (2)	52 years (19–80)	9.6 years (2–20)	10-year survivorship 78% Age < 50 years Weight > 80 kg or large defect were associated with increased risk for revision

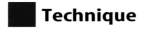

Technique

Preoperative Planning

Before THA is considered, a thorough history and physical examination is necessary to identify the severity and location of the pain. Intra-articular anesthetic injection of the hip may be helpful if the source of pain is unclear. A history of the injury, treatment, and any perioperative complications is also required. Evaluation of the patient's gait, range of motion, and muscle strength must also be included.

Radiographic evaluation should include an AP view of the pelvis and lateral view of the hip. A 45° oblique (Judet) view and CT may be helpful when there is substantial bone loss, bone deformity, or a possible persistent nonunion. A careful understanding of the bony anatomy, along with identifying the location of retained implants and any heterotopic bone is necessary. The AP pelvis templating radiograph generally best identifies limb-length discrepancy. If reduction of the acetabular fracture has resulted in cranial displacement of the innomi-

nate, the discrepancy must be measured from an intact anatomic landmark such as the midline of the sacrum.

The radiographic appearance of the femoral head may appear smaller than expected. Discerning the cause of this discrepancy is important preoperatively, regardless of whether it is osteonecrosis or, more commonly, wear of the femoral head against a fracture malunion or intra-articular hardware. Wear of the femoral head is also often associated with acetabular bone defects.

Exposure

Following either surgical or nonsurgical treatment of an acetabular fracture, the standard approach used for THA can be used. There are exceptions, but the hip usually tolerates new incisions even in the presence of scars. The approach also may be dictated by the presence of nonunion, malunion, or bony defects. The need to remove implants or resect heterotopic bone also may influence the approach at times.

The Kocher-Langenbeck, or posterior, approach is the best approach

when a posterior acetabular bone defect needs to be reconstructed with bulk graft, a previous posterior approach was used, or prior posterior implants need to be removed. However, patients may have impaired musculature or neurologic deficit associated with the previous surgery, and THA through a posterior approach may be associated with an increased risk of posterior hip dislocation. In this situation, consideration should be given to measures that improve hip stability such as increased femoral offset, hooded or constrained acetabular liners, and trochanteric advancement.

We prefer the "short" Smith-Petersen approach, also described by Heuter. With this approach, the interval of the Smith-Petersen is followed distal to the anterior superior iliac spine. Advantages of this approach include preservation of muscle attachments to the bone and an increased resistance to dislocation. The potential disadvantages are more difficult femoral access and the need for a specialized fracture table. The anterior approach can be extended more proximally along the iliac crest for exposure of the

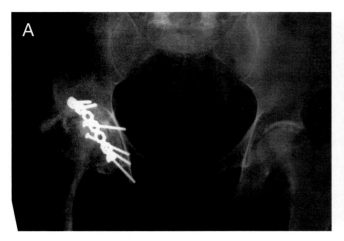

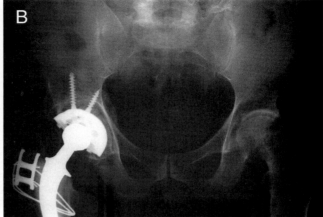

Figure 1   A 28-year-old man undergoes open reduction and internal fixation of a multiply fragmented posterior wall acetabular fracture. **A,** AP radiograph of the pelvis obtained 11 months later reveals articular incongruity and heterotopic ossification bridging from the trochanter to the acetabulum. **B,** AP radiograph obtained 22 months after reconstruction shows acetabular component ingrowth and no recurrence of heterotopic bone. A trochanteric osteotomy was used to protect the abductors during heterotopic ossification resection.

pelvis on the inner or outer table of the iliac wing. This exposure may be useful for addressing bone problems or for removal of implants placed through an ilioinguinal approach. The Smith-Petersen approach can also be continued to make the extended iliofemoral approach. This latter approach provides excellent access to the pelvis for reconstruction of pelvic and acetabular deformities or deficiencies at the time of arthroplasty. It is not necessary to detach the abductors from the femur, as is done for acute acetabular fractures. The removal of the femoral head and neck provides sufficient access to the posterior column.

Bone Preparation
PRIOR FRACTURE IMPLANTS
We prefer to remove fracture fixation before or at the time of THA. At times, this necessitates two incisions or even two-stage surgery. Dormant bacteria can be harbored adjacent to old implants; thus, removal of the hardware allows for a thorough evaluation of the fracture site and frozen section biopsy before prosthesis implantation. Patients requiring THA after acetabular fracture may be quite young, and removal of the fracture fixation provides an opportunity to identify and débride

any avascular bone, define the extent of any bone defect, and reconstruct the acetabulum without interference.

Cutting off screws inside the joint that are encountered during reaming leaves particulate metal debris that may contribute to third-body wear. Retained screw remnants may fret against the backside of the acetabular component and also contribute to wear debris. In addition, it is not always possible to appropriately graft around the retained hardware.

Removal of plates and screws is not necessarily easy. The radiographs must be understood and constantly referenced during the removal. Intraoperative fluoroscopy is often helpful. Specialized instruments for removing broken and stripped screws should always be available. In any given patient, the benefits of hardware removal must be weighed against the risks of extra soft-tissue dissection. Intraoperative cultures and frozen section biopsy specimens should be obtained from around the fracture fixation to minimize the chance of missing residual infection.

HETEROTOPIC OSSIFICATION
Heterotopic ossification may complicate the surgical treatment of acetabu-

lar fractures. The amount of heterotopic bone that forms in the hip abductors is often minimal, and the bone easily can be resected during THA, if it leads to impingement and contributes to instability. Small foci of heterotopic bone that do not affect stability of the hip replacement can be ignored; however, extensive heterotopic bone may interfere with the surgical approach or may surround neurovascular structures. In these circumstances, the bone may need to be removed before the femoral head is resected. The previously placed implants will serve as a landmark to guide the surgeon to the native cortical surface of the ilium and help prevent the inadvertent removal of normal cortical bone. Concomitant resection of heterotopic bone at the time of arthroplasty may be associated with impaired abductor musculature and thereby an increased risk of hip dislocation (**Figure 1**).

ACETABULAR BONE DEFECTS
Acetabular bone defects are often present following fracture and may be the result of initial fracture malreduction, loss of fracture reduction, or avascular acetabular bone, either traumatic or iatrogenic. Defects may also

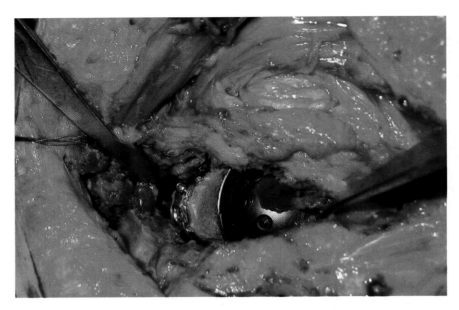

Figure 2 Intraoperative photograph shows posterior acetabular bone defect reconstruction. Note the acetabular component, femoral head autograft, and reconstruction compression plating. Screw augmentation of the acetabular component also has been performed.

be created when a worn or irregular femoral head abrades the acetabular bone. These defects are most commonly seen in the posterior wall and column of the acetabulum. Posterior wall defects may be caused by loss of reduction of the posterior wall fragments. The resulting subluxation generally brings the femoral head into contact with the posterior plate fixation, which causes a sudden destruction of the femoral head and additional destruction of the posterior column bone, often in the first few weeks after failure of fracture fixation.

Surgical devascularization of the posterior wall during reduction may also result in wall fragments that do not heal. This situation typically presents as a sudden destruction of the femoral head that occurs between 3 and 6 months after injury. Careful evaluation of the Judet view will often reveal the subtle subluxation of the femoral head that precedes its destruction, as well as the displacement of the posterior wall fragment(s).

Although it is tempting to treat posttraumatic acetabular bone defects with large or revision components and

techniques, affected patients are usually younger, have a higher activity level, and demand more of their arthroplasty than the typical revision THA patient. Therefore, special care is needed to reconstruct bone defects and use autogenous bone grafting to improve the bone stock of the pelvis, anticipating the probability of future surgeries throughout a patient's lifetime.

A posterior acetabular bone defect can be treated by using a femoral head autograft. After the fracture hardware is removed and any avascular acetabular bone or nonsupported, nonunited posterior wall fracture fragments are thoroughly débrided, the acetabular rim and posterosuperior bone are reconstructed. After removing the remaining cartilage from the femoral head, the femoral head and neck autograft is contoured to fit the defect. An attempt is made to orient the compressive trabeculae of the head and neck in such a way as to maximize the support of the acetabular component. The graft may be held in place with a quadrangular clamp placed through the greater sciatic notch and is provisionally fixed in place with interfragmentary screws

directed toward the quadrilateral surface. The graft/native acetabulum is then reamed and the reamings collected for morcellized graft. The acetabular component is inserted and secured with screw fixation.

Next, the femoral head autograft is buttressed by a plate that is contoured to provide compression of the graft against both the host bone and the acetabular component. The rigid compression plating of the graft may increase the healing potential between the innominate bone and the graft and may also increase the initial stability of the acetabular component, allowing for improved bony ingrowth in the nongrafted areas (**Figure 2**). If a significant portion of the cup is supported by the autograft, consideration should be given to using an acetabular component with additional support.

Anterior column defects are usually found in association with unreduced fracture, malunion, or nonunion of anterior column fractures. If the defect is constrained, it can be appropriately filled with morcellized or bulk autograft taken from the patient's femoral head and performed through an arthroplasty approach without the use of supplemental fixation. Large segmental defects may require structural grafting to allow for stable placement of the acetabular component. Fixation of the autogenous femoral head into the defect can be performed with a pelvic brim plate and interfragmentary screw fixation and done through the same incision as the arthroplasty if the Smith-Petersen approach is used. If this approach is used, however, structural stability of the femoral head graft is difficult to achieve, and the surgeon should be prepared to use an acetabular component that will achieve stability through iliac and ischial fixation.

With acetabular malunion or nonunion involving the anterior column fracture, reduction of the innominate bone should be considered before insertion of the acetabular

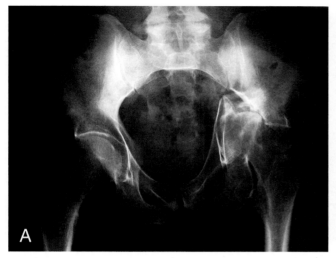

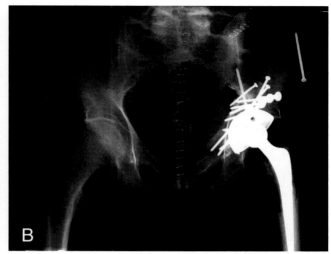

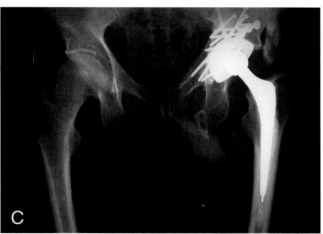

Figure 3 **A,** Preoperative AP radiograph of a nonunion/malunion of a T-shaped acetabular fracture with femoral head wear. **B,** Postoperative AP radiograph shows an osteotomy and partial reduction of the T-shaped fracture performed through a midline rectus splitting approach to the rami and quadrilateral surface, as well as an extended Smith-Petersen approach for the completion of the osteotomy, reduction, fixation, and arthroplasty. **C,** Arthroplasty at 2-year follow-up shows stable components and healed innominate bone.

component. Although reduction may frequently require osteotomy of united portions of the fracture, reduction of the innominate bone decreases the size of the acetabular bone defects and ensures a reconstruction with a hip center that is closer to the normal anatomic position. Attempting to implant an acetabular component without first addressing the malunion may increase the need for bulk grafting, decrease the surface area of the cup that is in contact with host bone, and make it difficult to avoid impingement between the femur and pelvis resulting from the medialization of the hip. Stable acetabular fixation can be achieved before insertion of the acetabular

component and the ingrowth of the cup can be maximized (**Figure 3**).

Prosthesis Implantation

Uncemented acetabular implants are most commonly selected for use in reconstruction following acetabular fracture. Although the defects in the innominate bone may be similar to those seen in revision surgery, the vascularity and density of the bone are often much more favorable. Because acetabular fractures typically occur in patients younger than those who undergo THA for degenerative causes, revision cemented components and cage reconstructions may not be ex-

pected to have the desired longevity and survivorship.

Screw augmentation of the acetabular component is almost always recommended, except in patients who are free of bone defect or deformity. When a significant portion of the acetabular component is in contact with graft, specialized acetabular components may be useful. Commercially available components that allow fixation of the acetabular component to the ilium, ischium, or obturator foramen can be useful to help achieve initial stability of the acetabular component. Use of these specialized components may improve bone ingrowth from the remaining portions of vascu-

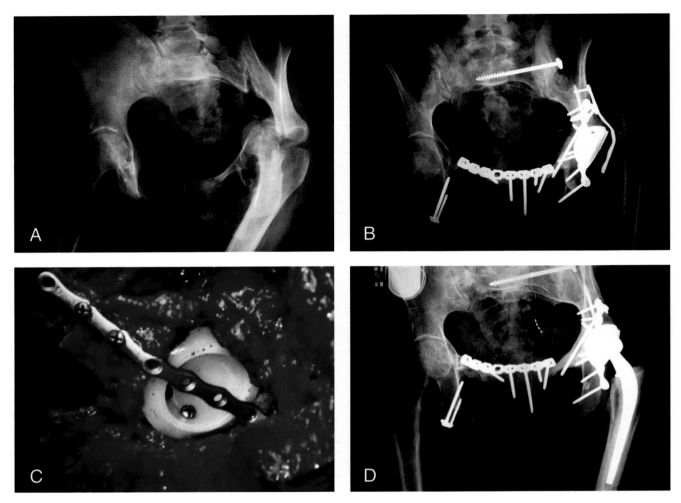

Figure 4 **A,** Severe pelvic deformity, including malunion/nonunion of a T-shaped acetabular fracture, ipsilateral sacroiliac dislocation, and contralateral rami fractures, that requires a two-stage procedure. **B,** In the first stage, the pelvic ring and acetabular deformities are reduced, grafted, and stabilized. The acetabular component is inserted, and femoral head autograft is used. No femoral component is inserted to allow the acetabular ingrowth to proceed in the absence of femoral forces. **C,** Intraoperative photograph shows placement of a protection plate across the acetabular component to prevent dislodging of the acetabular component during healing and ingrowth. The liner is later exchanged in the second stage when the femoral component is inserted. **D,** Postoperative AP radiograph after the second stage. The hip adduction tends to improve as abductor function recovers. The ischial ramus nonunion is asymptomatic.

larized native acetabulum and may also protect the acetabular reconstruction over time as the autograft resorbs and remodels.

Nonunion of a transverse fracture or nonunion of the anterior and/or posterior column can occur after acetabular fracture. These nonunions need to be stabilized with plate fixation before acetabular components can be implanted. In some patients, stabilization can be done at the time of THA, but in selected patients, such as those with large bone defects

and mobile nonunion, a two-stage THA may be considered. During the first stage, the acetabulum is reconstructed by reducing and fixing the nonunion. The femoral head and neck are used as autograft, and the acetabular shell is implanted. The femur is left as a resection arthroplasty, and a plate can be placed over the acetabulum to guard the shell from femoral contact. The absence of joint reactive force allows the acetabulum to heal and the cup to achieve bony ingrowth in a situation when its stability is more tenu-

ous than normal. After 8 to 12 weeks, the nonunion and graft have healed, and the acetabular liner and femoral component are implanted during the second stage (**Figure 4**).

Wound Closure

Standard wound closure is used. We prefer using drains, particularly if extensive pelvic dissection or reconstruction has been performed. Closing the wound might be difficult, especially if the fracture deformity has resulted in significant medialization of the femur that is corrected at the time of reconstruction.

Postoperative Regimen

Postoperative management usually does not significantly differ from that of a standard primary THA, but a delay in full weight bearing is recommended if the acetabular component is seated into a large area of grafted defect. Patients are instructed about total hip precautions appropriate to the surgical approach.

External beam radiation therapy may be considered very selectively after THA to prevent heterotopic bone formation, but we prefer to avoid it after reconstruction of bone defects or repair of fracture nonunion. In known cases of compromised abductor muscle function, postoperative abduction bracing may be considered.

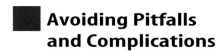

Avoiding Pitfalls and Complications

The most common complications following THA after acetabular fracture are dislocation and aseptic loosening. During placement of the acetabular component in these patients, there may be no bony landmarks available to help determine appropriate cup position. Patient positioning should be carefully considered preoperatively; in these patients, use of an intraoperative positioning guide may be helpful. Intraoperative radiographs or fluoroscopy can be used to confirm good acetabular component position. Aseptic loosening cannot be entirely avoided, but careful attention to removal of all avascular bone, grafting of acetabular defects, augmentation of the acetabular components as needed, and reconstruction of large pelvic deformities or deficiencies may reduce the rate of aseptic loosening to an acceptable level.

References

Bellabarba C, Berger RA, Bentley CD, et al: Cementless acetabular reconstruction after acetabular fracture. *J Bone Joint Surg Am* 2001;83:868-876.

Berry DJ: Total hip arthroplasty following acetabular fracture. *Orthopedics* 1999;22:837-839.

Berry DJ, Halasy M: Uncemented acetabular components for arthritis after acetabular fracture. *Clin Orthop* 2002;405:164-167.

Huo MH, Solberg BD, Zatorski LE, Keggi KJ: Total hip replacements done without cement after acetabular fractures: A 4- to 8-year follow-up study. *J Arthroplasty* 1999;14:827-831.

Jimenez ML, Tile M, Schenk RS: Total hip replacement after acetabular fracture. *Orthop Clin North Am* 1997;28:435-446.

Romness DW, Lewallen D: Total hip arthroplasty after fracture of the acetabulum: Long-term results. *J Bone Joint Surg Br* 1990;72:761-764.

Weber M, Berry DJ, Harmsen WS: Total hip arthroplasty after operative treatment of an acetabular fracture. *J Bone Joint Surg Am* 1998;80:1295-1305.

Coding

CPT Codes		Corresponding ICD-9 Codes		
20680	Removal of implant; deep (eg, buried wire, pin, screw, metal band, nail, rod, or plate)	716.15 733.82 996.4	728.12 905.1 996.67	733.81 905.6 996.78
27036	Capsulectomy or capsulotomy, hip, with or without excision of heterotopic bone, with release of hip flexor muscles (ie, gluteus medius, gluteus minimus, tensor fascia latae, rectus femoris, sartorius, iliopsoas)	716.15 733.81 905.6 996.78	728.12 733.82 996.4	728.13 905.1 996.67
27130	Arthroplasty, acetabular and proximal femoral prosthetic replacement (total hip arthroplasty), with or without autograft or allograft	716.15 733.82 996.4	728.12 905.1 996.67	733.81 905.6 996.78
27132	Conversion of previous hip surgery to total hip arthroplasty, with or without autograft or allograft	716.15 733.82 996.4	728.12 905.1 996.67	733.81 905.6 996.78

CPT copyright © 2004 by the American Medical Association. All Rights Reserved.

Chapter 21
Total Hip Arthroplasty After Hip Fusion

Mark J. Spangehl, MD

Indications

Arthrodesis of the hip remains a viable option for young adults with unilateral hip disease. It allows for long-term pain relief and provides adequate function for individuals who may not yet be candidates for total hip arthroplasty (THA). However, the disability resulting from a fused hip may, over time, require conversion of an arthrodesed hip to a THA.

Long-term sequelae of a fused hip include an increased incidence of low back, ipsilateral knee, and contralateral hip pain related to degenerative joint disease in those joints because of the increased stress placed through the joints juxtaposed to the fused hip. Additionally, patients with a fused hip expend more energy during gait and eventually may desire conversion to a more mobile hip.

Conversion of an arthrodesed hip to a THA is most commonly indicated for patients with disabling back pain. Additional indications include increasing knee pain or contralateral hip pain secondary to degenerative joint disease, a malpositioned arthrodesis resulting in functional disability, or a painful pseudarthrosis. Whether conversion of a fused hip is indicated before ipsilateral knee replacement remains controversial. Even in the absence of the above indications, patients may seek conversion of an arthrodesed hip to a mobile hip replacement as they

become less willing to accept the inconvenience that an arthrodesed hip places on activities of daily living.

Contraindications

Absolute contraindications to conversion of an arthrodesed hip are similar to those of primary or revision THA, specifically, active or suspected infection and poor overall health. Relative contraindications include the following: a young patient in whom the hip is fused in an acceptable position (20° of flexion, 5° of external rotation, neutral abduction/adduction), particularly if the patient plans to return to heavy labor; severely distorted anatomy that would preclude restoring near-normal biomechanics or place the THA at high risk of failure; and poor or absent abductor musculature.

Electromyography to assess gluteal muscle function is of limited value preoperatively because it does not correlate well with postoperative abductor function. Postoperative abductor muscle function can be estimated by preoperative palpation of contracting abductor musculature and, more importantly, by intraoperative assessment of the muscles. The intraoperative assessment correlates well with return of postoperative abductor function. Even severely atrophied muscle can recover acceptable function if it

appears otherwise intact and healthy (ie, vascular and red).

Additionally, patients who expect complete or near complete symptom relief in surrounding joints or a normal functioning hip replacement must be advised about realistic outcomes of this surgery.

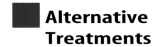
Alternative Treatments

Alternatives to conversion of an arthrodesed hip depend on treatment of the symptomatic joint or joints around the fused hip. Failed nonsurgical management of low back pain is the most common reason for conversion. Surgical treatment of mechanical low back pain should not be considered until after conversion of a fused hip is performed. Surgical management prior to conversion of a fused hip is much less likely to be successful because of the ongoing stress placed through the lumbar spine as a result of the fused hip. Pain relief in the ipsilateral knee or contralateral hip is less predictable after conversion of a fused hip, and surgical treatment, either before or after conversion of the fused hip, may be required depending on the pathology and the severity of symptoms in those joints.

Table 1   Results of THA After Hip Fusion

Author(s) (Year)	Number of Hips	Implant Type	Mean Patient Age (Range)	Mean Follow-up (Range)	Results
Joshi, et al (2002)	208	Cemented Charnley low-friction arthroplasty	51 years (20–80)	9.2 years (2–26)	96% 10-year, 90% 15-year survival 79% minimal pain or pain free 83% good to excellent function 8 sciatic, 7 femoral nerve palsies 28 heterotopic ossification; no significant stiffness 5 dislocations, 3 infections, and 9 trochanteric nonunions Better results with spontaneous or more than 15 years at time of fusion
Hamadouche, et al (2001)	45	Various	55.8 years (28–80)	8.5 years (5–21)	91% 10-year survival Walking improved 2 to 3 years 96% no pain Less back pain in 22 of 37 Less knee pain in 10 of 15 50% used cane
Kreder, et al (1999)	40	Various	58.5 years (N/A)	2.5 years (N/A)	High complication rate 10% deep infection 10% revision; 5% Girdlestone procedure within 4 years
Reikeras, et al (1995)	46	Various	58 years (N/A)	8 years (5–13)	76% good to excellent result 85% satisfied (hips fused at a younger age or shorter duration were more satisfied) 74% required walking aid 15.2% revision rate

N/A = Not Applicable

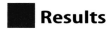# Results

Conversion of an arthrodesed hip to a mobile hip is usually undertaken to relieve pain in surrounding joints and to improve function and gait efficiency. Therefore, results can be categorized as pain relief in the surrounding joints, function and presence of pain in the converted hip, survival of the converted THA, and general patient satisfaction (**Table 1**).

Pain Relief in the Surrounding Joints

Low back pain is the most common complaint after long-standing hip fusion and thus the most common indication for surgery. Most patients (between 60% and 95%) report significant improvement in low back symptoms after surgery. However, pa-

tients must also be advised that up to one third of those who undergo surgery may not experience any improvement in their symptoms because of advanced degenerative changes. Pain relief in other surrounding joints is less predictable and depends on the primary pathology of the affected joint. Patients with degenerative changes may eventually require surgery in those joints. Ipsilateral knee pain was improved in only one third of patients in one series. Other authors have reported somewhat more favorable results with decreased knee pain in 10 of 15 patients in whom knee pain was present prior to conversion. Five patients in this series required total knee arthroplasty after conversion. Similarly, relief of contralateral hip pain depends on the extent of degenerative changes present within the hip.

Function and Presence of Pain in the Converted Hip

Patients are generally pleased with the function of the converted hip, accepting somewhat inferior results compared with routine primary THA in exchange for increased mobility and function. Despite this level of satisfaction, factors such as muscle strength, the need for assistive aids for walking, and range of motion are less satisfactory in converted hips compared with primary THA. Abductor muscle strength can continue to improve for years after surgery, with some authors noting improvement for up to 3 years following conversion. Despite this fact, a substantial number of patients require assistive aids for walking and continue to limp after conversion. A number of recent studies report that the need for a walking aid ranged from 46% to 62%. Other authors have reported that between 12% (5 of 41) and 74% (34 of 46) of patients required more walking aid support postoperatively. Reduced range of motion is also more common after conversion compared with after routine primary THA, with average flexion arcs reported between 76° and 88°.

Limb-length discrepancy usually improves after conversion. The side of the fusion generally is the shorter limb, and conversion improves the discrepancy. The ability to equalize limb length depends on the preoperative discrepancy, the amount of bony deficiency (although this usually can be compensated with contemporary implants), and the amount of scarring and ability to release soft tissues without excessively lengthening the limb, which places the femoral or sciatic nerves at risk. A number of series have reported an improvement in limb-length inequality, with an average lengthening of approximately 2.5 cm without complications. The presence of pain in the converted hip is generally small, but again somewhat more common than after routine primary THA. In a large series of 208 conversions, 79% of patients were pain free or had minimal pain. In another series of 45 conversions, 96% of patients were pain free postoperatively in the converted hip.

Survival of the Converted Total Hip Arthroplasty
Survival of the converted hip replacement shows variable results depending on the series reported (**Table 1**). Excellent survival results were recently reported in a large series of 208 conversions. The authors reported 96% survival at 10 years and 90% at 15 years with revision for any reason as an end point. Another recent study of 45 consecutive conversions demonstrated a 10-year survival of 91%. Other reports have been less encouraging, with one series reporting a mechanical failure in 11 of 60 hips that had undergone surgical fusion at 9- to

15-year follow-up, and another reporting a 15% (7 of 46) failure rate with similar follow-up. The authors of the latter study attribute most of the failures to the use of inferior prostheses.

Overall Patient Satisfaction
Despite a less predictable outcome compared to primary THA, the common occurrence of a limp, and the need for assistive aids for walking in many patients, overall patient satisfaction is high. Patients are generally happy with mobility in the converted hip and the improved function that generally occurs as a result. Various studies have reported patient satisfaction ranging from approximately 72% to 93%.

Some authors have noted that male sex, older age at time of fusion, longer duration of fusion, age at conversion (< 50 years of age), multiple surgeries, fusion because of sepsis, and surgical arthrodesis were risk factors for poorer clinical outcome. Better results are generally reported in patients who are older at the time of conversion, had a spontaneous fusion, and whose abductors were in relatively good condition.

———————————————■

■ Technique

Conversion of an arthrodesed hip to THA is a technically demanding procedure. The important technical considerations include (1) ensuring adequate exposure with maintenance or restoration of abductor function, (2) removing hardware if present, and (3) carefully identifying bony landmarks to ensure proper implant position. The appropriate equipment, apart from that required for the implants, should be readily available. Metal cutting burrs, broken screw extractors, and fluoroscopy may be required to remove hardware or identify

bony landmarks. Additionally, the surgeon should be familiar with the technique that was used to arthrodese the hip because this may influence the exposure and need for bone removal, particularly with extra-articular arthrodeses. Preoperative CT is often helpful to identify anterior and inferomedial bone bridges and to show the status of the abductor muscles.

Exposure
The patient should be in a lateral decubitus position, although a supine position is often favored in Europe. The type of skin incision made is dictated by the previous incisions and the need for hardware removal. If no incision is present, then a lateral incision centered just distal to the tip of the trochanter and curving posteriorly at the proximal end is used. Any hardware overlying the trochanter and proximal femur is removed. If a previous trochanteric osteotomy was performed at the time of fusion and hardware is beneath the trochanter, then a classic trochanteric osteotomy is required (**Figure 1**). Otherwise, a trochanteric slide with retraction anteriorly generally provides adequate exposure and reduces further violation of the abductors. A short extended osteotomy may be performed to facilitate closure and healing of the osteotomy. A more formal or longer extended osteotomy may be required if deformity in the proximal femur needs to be corrected. If a trochanteric fragment is absent, then a lateral approach with elevation of the anterior half of the remaining abductor or scar tissue, continuous with the anterior portion of the vastus lateralis, can be used. Soft tissues are then further cleared from the arthrodesis and proximal femur, identifying the femoral neck. If a bony bridge exists between the femur and ischium, the bridge is osteotomized prior to osteotomy of the femoral neck. Care should be taken to protect the sciatic nerve in this region. The femoral neck is then

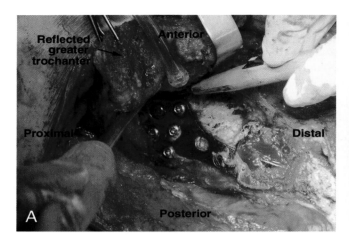
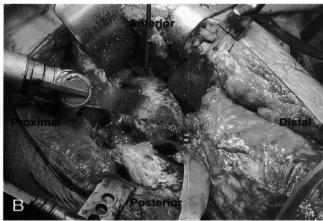

Figure 1 **A,** A classic trochanteric osteotomy was used to facilitate removal of the hardware. The plate was beneath the trochanter. **B,** Intraoperative photograph showing the femoral neck osteotomy. Retractors are placed anteriorly and posteriorly, and the osteotomy is performed just proximal to the superior aspect of the trochanteric osteotomy. (Courtesy of Dr. Clive Duncan, University of British Columbia, Vancouver, BC.)

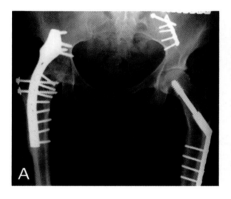

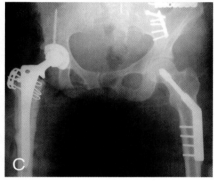

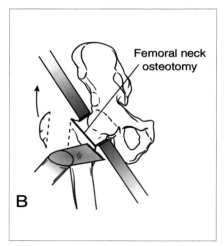

Figure 2 **A,** AP radiograph showing right-sided hip fusion using a cobra plate. Note that the greater trochanter was reattached over the lateral aspect of the plate. **B,** Once the fusion mass is exposed, the superior and inferior aspects of the femoral neck are identified (retractors are placed superiorly and inferiorly), and the femoral neck is osteotomized. Landmarks that can be used for the femoral neck cut include the trochanteric osteotomy site (proximal aspect), the lesser trochanter, or screw holes from removed hardware. **C,** Postoperative radiograph showing an extensively porous-coated implant that was used because of some metaphyseal distortion and to bypass the removed plate. (Courtesy of Dr. Clive Duncan, University of British Columbia, Vancouver, BC.)

ing and identification of bony landmarks (either the greater or lesser trochanter), a revised and definitive femoral neck cut is then performed to provide additional room to prepare the acetabulum. An intraoperative radiograph should be obtained if there is any doubt as to the location or level at either the initial osteotomy or the definitive femoral osteotomy.

Bone Preparation

Bone preparation is begun on the acetabular side. The inferior aspect of the acetabulum is the most critical landmark to be identified but may be difficult because of the bone overlying the floor of the acetabulum. Identifying the superior aspect of the obturator foramen and then placing a hooked retractor around the most inferior portion of the acetabulum will locate this area of the acetabulum. Prior to reaming, the anterior and posterior walls must also be identified for proper placement of the reamer. A blunt retractor carefully placed over the anterior wall is often helpful in maintaining exposure and orienting the surgeon to the anterior wall (**Figure 3**). Once this is accomplished, the acetabulum is carefully deepened and widened with successive reamers. Of-

osteotomized, somewhat more proximally than the anticipated final cut, followed by further release of soft tis-

sues around the proximal femur, which will improve exposure (**Figure 2**). Based on the preoperative templat-

ten, especially in cases of spontaneous fusion, as the acetabulum is deepened, soft tissue (transverse acetabular ligament or remnants of the ligamentum teres) is recognized in the floor of the acetabulum. Careful attention to the thickness of the anterior and posterior walls is also necessary during preparation of the socket. An intraoperative radiograph is helpful early in the preparation of the socket to ensure proper position of the reamer in the superoinferior plane (**Figure 4**). Additionally, with severe distortion of the anatomy, placement of a Kirschner wire as a marker prior to obtaining a radiograph will assist in orientation. Once the acetabulum is prepared, a trial socket is inserted. The femur is then prepared according to the type of implant to be used.

Prosthesis Implantation

Prosthetic selection depends on the patient's bone quality, the presence of any cortical defects or stress risers related to hardware removal, the amount of deformity in the proximal femur, and steps, if any, taken to address the deformity. The patient's age and activity level and the surgeon's general preference or philosophy regarding implant fixation are also factors in the selection of the prosthesis.

On the acetabular side, uncemented fixation can be used, as would be the case in primary or revision THA. In cases of distorted anatomy or defects in bone, autogenous bone graft from the femoral head and supplemental screw fixation may be required. On the femoral side, implant choice and fixation varies according to what is outlined in the paragraph above. An uncemented implant is generally favored because most patients undergoing conversion are younger (< 70 years) and/or have bone of sufficient quality to support stable fixation with an uncemented implant. Distal fixation may be necessary if the proximal metaphyseal bone is distorted or significantly compromised

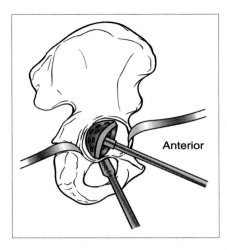

Figure 3 The inferior aspect of the acetabulum must be identified for proper orientation prior to reaming. A blunt retractor may be placed beneath the teardrop. The anterior and posterior aspects are also identified for orientation in the coronal plane.

by prior hardware or deformity (**Figure 5**). If an extended trochanteric osteotomy is required during exposure because of deformity, then distal fixation also is preferred. Additionally, if a long plate was removed from the proximal femur, the presence of multiple stress risers and the likelihood of stress-shielded bone under the plate make a long-stemmed uncemented implant that bypasses the stress risers desirable. Occasionally, the femur may have significant disuse osteopenia making stable fixation with an uncemented implant difficult and a cemented stem more appropriate (**Figure 6**). If cemented fixation is used, care should be taken to avoid cement at the trochanteric-osteotomy interface.

A large femoral head and liner (32 mm or larger) or constrained acetabular liner may be considered if the abductors are absent or if the patient is at high risk for postoperative instability.

Prior to final component implantation, a trial reduction is performed to determine the appropriate neck length for soft-tissue tension and limb lengths. Palpation of the sciatic

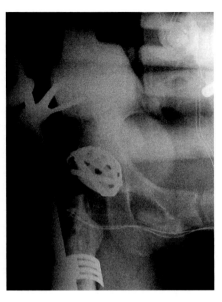

Figure 4 Intraoperative radiograph of the patient shown in Figure 1 confirming proper position of the reamer. (Courtesy of Dr. Clive Duncan, University of British Columbia, Vancouver, BC.)

nerve should follow to ensure that it is mobile with the hip slightly flexed and the knee extended. If excess tension on the nerve is noted, the neck length or position of the femoral component may need adjustment. The risk of stretching the sciatic nerve likely depends on both the amount of shortening and patient age at the time of arthrodesis. Although the extremity that is being converted will be short relative to the opposite side in most cases, excessive lengthening (more than 2 to 3 cm) should be avoided because of concern about nerve injury and difficulties in trochanteric reattachment.

Wound Closure

Prior to wound closure, the hip should be placed through a range of motion in the positions of risk for dislocation and carefully inspected for bony impingement. Potential areas of bony impingement should be removed. The converted hip will lack the usual motion of a primary THA immediately after conversion; however, over time this usually improves. The increase in motion may result in bony impinge-

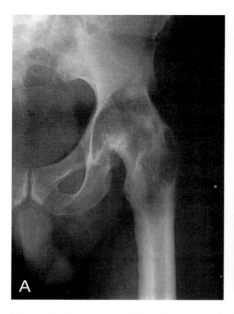 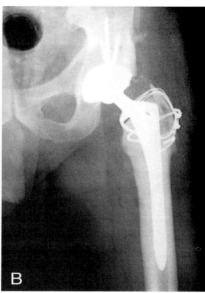

Figure 5 Preoperative **(A)** and postoperative **(B)** radiographs showing relative osteopenia in the metaphyseal region of the fused left hip. Note the relatively narrow femoral canal and thick cortical bone, making an extensively porous-coated implant an appropriate choice. (Courtesy Dr. Daniel Berry, Mayo Clinic, Rochester, MN.)

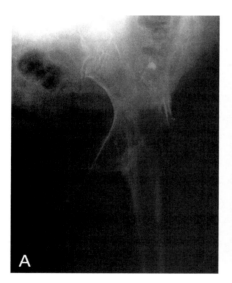 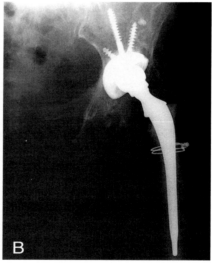

Figure 6 Preoperative **(A)** and postoperative **(B)** radiographs showing conversion of a fused hip to a hybrid THA. Note the greater trochanter is poorly defined and part of the fusion mass. An anterolateral approach was used in this patient. Note the relative osteopenia of the femur, making a cemented stem more appropriate in this case. (Courtesy Dr. Paul Kim, University of Ottawa, Ottawa, Ontario.)

overly shortened) may be sutured to the proximal femur. Alternatively, the tensor fascia lata may be sutured to the trochanter or proximal femur.

An adductor tenotomy or psoas tendon release may be required if hip abduction is limited, or if there is a persistent flexion deformity and shortening of the limb is not desired or would leave the hip unstable.

Postoperative Regimen
Weight bearing after conversion depends on the adequacy of trochanteric fixation, the type of implants used, and the surgeon's philosophy regarding weight bearing after primary THA. In patients with good trochanteric fixation, partial weight bearing may be allowed; however, if the quality of fixation is in doubt, then weight bearing should be delayed until 6 to 8 weeks postoperatively. Active abduction is delayed until 8 weeks after surgery to allow for adequate trochanteric or abductor healing.

Most patients who undergo conversion of an arthrodesed hip to a mobile hip replacement will have stiffness and lack the usual motion seen after primary THA and may be at decreased risk for early dislocation. However, patients with severely deficient or absent abductors may be at increased risk for dislocation and should be braced in a hip abduction orthosis, restricting flexion and adduction for 6 to 12 weeks.

Routine antibiotics and thromboembolic prophylaxis are indicated. Prophylaxis against heterotopic ossification is not routinely required. However, if the arthrodesis occurred spontaneously or if the patient is at risk for heterotopic bone formation (see chapter 33), then prophylaxis with either radiation therapy or anti-inflammatory drugs is needed.

ment; hence, there is a need to remove potential areas of impingement at the time of conversion.

The trochanteric osteotomy is then closed with wires or cables. A claw or grip device can be avoided if a short extended osteotomy is used. Alternatively, a wire technique may be used. If the trochanter is absent, then the abductors (if present and not

◼ Avoiding Pitfalls and Complications

Complications after conversion of an arthrodesed hip to THA are similar to those after primary THA performed for degenerative joint disease. However, the incidence of complications is greater than that seen after routine THA. The incidence of infection is higher, with reported rates ranging from 1.4% to 13%. Nerve palsy is also more common after conversion; one large series reported an incidence of 7% (15 of 208 hips), with an almost equal number of femoral and sciatic nerve palsies. The overall incidence of dislocation does not seem to be substantially higher after takedown of arthrodesis, which may be related to the fact that the average range of motion is less than that of primary THA. However, patients with very deficient or absent abductors may be at increased risk for dislocation. In the same large series of 208 conversions, four of five dislocations occurred in patients who were younger than age 15 years at the time of hip fusion. The authors concluded that the underdeveloped abductors increased the risk of dislocation.

Trochanteric nonunion has been reported to be as high as 14% after conversion, although most series report a lower incidence (approximately 5%). The use of a trochanteric slide while maintaining the vastus lateralis attachment, or a short extended trochanteric osteotomy allowing wire or cable fixation of the proximal lateral cortex while maintaining the soft-tissue attachments, may reduce the occurrence of trochanteric nonunion.

Heterotopic bone formation was reported in 13% of patients in one large series. No prophylaxis against heterotopic bone formation was used in any of these patients. Only 3 of 28 hips had Brooker class III heterotopic bone, the remainder having less, but no patients reported any functional limitations.

——————◼

◼ References

Hamadouche M, Kerboull L, Meunier A, Courpied JP, Kerboull M: Total hip arthroplasty for the treatment of ankylosed hips: A five- to twenty-one-year follow-up study. *J Bone Joint Surg Am* 2001;83:992-998.

Joshi AB, Markovic L, Hardinge K, Murphy JC: Conversion of a fused hip to total hip arthroplasty. *J Bone Joint Surg Am* 2002;84:1335-1341.

Kreder HJ, Williams JI, Jaglal S, Axcell T, Stephen D: A population study in the Province of Ontario of the complications after conversion of hip or knee arthrodesis to total joint replacement. *Can J Surg* 1999;42:433-439.

Panagiotopoulos KP, Robbins GM, Masri BA, Duncan CP: Conversion of hip arthrodesis to total hip arthroplasty. *Instr Course Lect* 2001;50:297-305.

Reikeras O, Bjerkreim I, Gundersson R: Total hip arthroplasty for arthrodesed hips: 5- to 13-year results. *J Arthroplasty* 1995;10:529-531.

Coding

CPT Codes		Corresponding ICD-9 Codes		
27130	Arthroplasty, acetabular and proximal femoral prosthetic replacement (total hip arthroplasty), with or without autograft or allograft	711.45 711.95 714.0 714.30 715.15	715.25 715.35 716.15 718.5 718.6	720.0 733.14 733.42 808.0 905.6
27132	Conversion of previous hip surgery to total hip arthroplasty, with or without autograft or allograft	715.15 715.25 715.35 718.2	718.5 718.6 733.14 733.42	905.6 996.4 996.66 996.77
Modifier 22	Unusual procedural services	998.9 V45.4		

CPT copyright © 2004 by the American Medical Association. All Rights Reserved.

Chapter 22

Total Hip Arthroplasty and the Deformed Femur

James V. Bono, MD
Matthew Olin, MD

◼ Indications

Total hip arthroplasty (THA) in the setting of proximal femoral deformity represents a unique challenge to arthroplasty surgeons. Proximal femoral deformity can be defined as any variation from normal anatomy that requires the surgeon to use advanced surgical techniques with special implants designed to accommodate a variety of conditions. The anatomy of the proximal femur, even in what may be considered straightforward primary conditions, often deviates from normal in cadaveric-based studies. The proximal femoral anatomy can become markedly distorted in a number of conditions, including developmental problems, previous surgical interventions, or as a result of trauma or bone pathology.

Classification of proximal femoral deformity has classically been based on etiologic principles, associating certain femoral pathology with particular disorders (ie, developmental dysplasia of the hip [DDH]). The American Academy of Orthopaedic Surgeons' classification system of femoral deformities is based on deficiencies, malalignment, stenosis, or discontinuities. More recently, Berry proposed a classification system based on anatomic location of deformity, with subclassifications for geometry and etiology. This classification system intends to direct surgeons to expectant pathologic conditions of the proximal femur and thus to potential implants and surgical techniques including but not limited to trochanteric or femoral osteotomies.

Once the abnormal proximal femoral anatomy is identified, careful preoperative templating and implant selection is critical to prepare for potential technical difficulties that may be encountered intraoperatively. Recognizing how certain deformities will affect exposure and bone preparation preoperatively will ease surgical decision making. Intraoperative fluoroscopy or radiographs may assist in canal preparation and can reduce the risk for canal perforation. The surgeon must also take into consideration basic arthroplasty principles of limb alignment, limb lengths, and hip biomechanics.

In isolated deformities of the femoral neck (ie, hyperanteversion seen in cases of DDH), surgical options include placing a monolithic proximally fitted stem anatomically or a smaller wedge-type stem or cemented stem in slight retroversion in relation to the neck. The former introduces a risk for posterior impingement and anterior instability, whereas the latter option introduces the risk of cement and stem failure. Another option is to make a lower and thus less conservative neck osteotomy and by-pass the deformity with a distally fit component. Finally, a modular two-piece stem could be used, maximizing the fit and fill concept while correcting for any version with final placement of the stem within the sleeve.

Deformity involving the greater trochanter can present as isolated trochanteric overhang or encroachment or be associated with proximal femoral varus deformity. In these cases, though becoming less popular, a trochanteric osteotomy or slide or subtrochanteric osteotomy can be used to facilitate the passage of a straight stem that is either proximally or distally supported. With a varus deformity, the osteotomy occurs at the apex of the deformity not only to allow for insertion of a straight stem but also to laterally displace the proximal fragment. The resulting lateralization of the trochanter provides greater soft-tissue tension of the abductors and ultimately improved function by virtue of a longer moment arm. A modular stem can also be used in this setting with reattachment of a well-vascularized trochanteric segment in a position that optimizes mechanics and reduces risk for impingement.

When evaluating deformities involving the metaphyseal or diaphyseal regions of the femur, surgeons are faced with some of the more difficult challenges. The etiology of deformities at these levels can be complex and

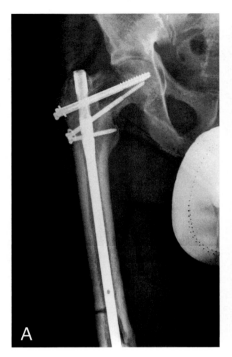

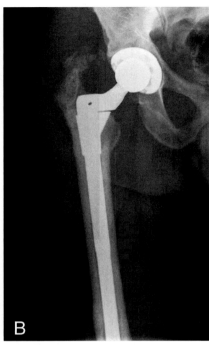

Figure 1   A, A 67-year-old merchant marine who sustained a basicervical fracture of the left hip and ipsilateral midshaft femoral fracture was treated initially with reconstruction nailing. **B,** His postoperative course was complicated by femoral neck and diaphyseal nonunion for which he underwent modular THA. Successful union of the diaphyseal fracture is noted postoperatively.

Figure 2   A, A 72-year-old woman who sustained a subtrochanteric fracture of the femur was treated with a reconstruction nail, resulting in nonunion. **B,** Bipolar hemiarthroplasty was performed in which the femoral head was used as bone graft.

most often will require osteotomy to correct the deformity and allow for passage of femoral components. These regions are the most common locations of deformities associated with prior intertrochanteric femur fracture and prior corrective osteotomies. The use of all varieties of femoral components has been reported, with or without an osteotomy. Though we have found that the anatomic and soft-tissue distortion seen in these complex cases often requires the off-the-shelf customization of a prosthesis available with a modular design, at the New England Baptist Hospital, the S-ROM (DePuy, Warsaw, IN) femoral stem has been the modular prosthesis of choice over the last 15 years (**Figure 1**). In our experience, when faced with this significant femoral deformity, the practical benefits of modularity far outweigh any theoretical disadvantages (**Figure 2**).

Contraindications

Contraindications in these cases do not differ from those for other primary or revision procedures. Patient selection and surgeon skill and experience are critical in determining the long-term success of these complex procedures. Patients indicated for primary THA with previous conditions often are younger and thus potentially more demanding on their components so careful preoperative discussion of goals must be outlined.

Alternative Treatments

Patients who undergo THA have had failed nonsurgical management or previous hip surgery for fracture or deformity correction; thus, these pa-

Table 1   Results of THA for Proximal Femoral Deformity

Author(s) (Year)	Number of Hips	Implant Type	Mean Patient Age (Range)	Mean Follow-up (Range)	Results
Holtgrewe and Hungerford (1989)	9 (6 revision, 3 primary)	Uncemented	N/A	47 months	Harris hip scores improved from 41 to 94 in primary cases; osteotomies healed in average 15 weeks
Mehlhoff and Sledge (1990)	27 (conversion from failed ORIF*)	4 hybrid 7 uncemented 16 cemented	65 years (35–90)	34 months	Harris hip scores improved from 33 to 81 in femoral neck fractures and from 29 to 78 in intertrochanteric fractures
Papagelopoulos, et al (1996)	31 (20 primary with osteotomy)	15 uncemented (proximally loaded and extensively coated) 5 cemented	51 years (24–82)	4.6 years	Harris hip scores improved from 51 to 77 in primary cases; osteotomy healed in average 30 weeks

N/A = Not Available
*ORIF = open reduction and internal fixation

tients have few options remaining other than joint replacement. In each anatomic location of proximal femoral deformity, prosthetic options have been outlined to present alternatives, depending on surgeon preference. However, in an effort to conserve as much native femoral bone stock as possible, surgeons may choose a surface replacement-type design. In addition, proximally loaded shorter stems, either press-fit or cemented, preserve distal bone while loading proximal bone and can be used with more distal deformities and can eliminate the morbidity associated with osteotomies.

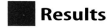

Results

Critical review of the literature reveals a paucity of comparative data on THA in the setting of proximal femoral deformity. With the exception of articles on hip dysplasia, most publications on deformed femora are case reports or small series of patients with certain deforming conditions or technical articles outlining techniques of osteotomies and their short-term outcomes. A summary of data from some of the more cited references is presented in **Table 1**.

The results of modular uncemented stems, which we prefer for most femoral deformity problems, were reported by Christie and associates for 125 hips, most without deformity. At 5.3 years 98% of patients had stable bone ingrowth; osteolysis proximal to the sleeve was present in only 7% of patients.

Technique

Preoperative Planning
Careful preoperative evaluation is critical so that implant selection will not compromise outcome. Use of straight, long stems in cases involving angular deformity may compromise either the trochanter or the femoral diaphysis with perforation or fracture. In these situations, subtrochanteric osteotomies are indicated. Osteotomies can be used to correct for high-riding dislocations in DDH, associated or isolated torsional deformities, or femoral malalignment from any number of causes. The surgeon must evaluate and plan for deformity apex, de-

termine whether a biplanar osteotomy will be required, and also determine the type of osteotomy required. Transverse subtrochanteric osteotomies at the apex of deformity, whether uniplanar or biplanar, are often the most reproducible; they allow for any shortening necessary, are inherently stable for early postoperative weight bearing, and allow for intraoperative adjustments to maximize deformity correction and hip mechanics (**Figure 2**).

The risk of nonunion is decreased if an osteotomy is performed at a site that is considered a "virgin" plane (ie, without previous soft-tissue stripping) and is loaded dynamically following surgery. A number of other technically demanding osteotomies have been described, including step-cut osteotomies, a double chevron osteotomy, and in situ transverse osteotomies with final implants in place. Surgeons should perform techniques in which they have training and are comfortable with to maximize the surgical outcome for the patient.

Exposure
In patients with femoral deformity, the need for corrective osteotomy is most often determined preoperatively. In some cases, however, it is an intraop-

erative decision. Exposure of the proximal femur, therefore, should be reserved for situations in which it is known to be necessary preoperatively, or in situations in which intraoperative cannulation of the proximal femur is unsuccessful. If a femoral osteotomy is needed, the incision is then extended distally over the femoral shaft. The tensor fascia is incised, and the vastus lateralis fascia is incised approximately 1 cm anterior to the linea. The fibers of the vastus lateralis are first swept off of the remaining fascia posteriorly, and then lifted superiorly from the femoral shaft. The perforating branches of the profunda femoris artery are divided and cauterized at a point 1 cm anterior to the linea to prevent retraction of the vessel with resultant uncontrolled bleeding. The periosteum is left undisturbed.

Bone Preparation

When using a modular stem, the proximal femur should be prepared, when possible, before completing the femoral osteotomy because once the osteotomy is made, control of the proximal femur is more difficult. The femoral deformity may preclude the use of conventional instruments in the proximal femur, requiring some modification of surgical technique, such as shortening or downsizing alignment rods. An assessment of distal femoral diameter is necessary preoperatively to select the size of the proximal sleeve. The orientation of the sleeve is dictated by anatomy of the proximal segment, taking advantage of existing bone stock. Once the proximal femur has been prepared, a trial sleeve is inserted, and the femoral osteotomy is completed. The osteotomy site is identified using existing bony landmarks. Rotational alignment is referenced by scoring the femur longitudinally using an oscillating saw or clear marking with electrocautery. If a modular stem is used, the proximal sleeve should be seated 1 to 1.5 cm above the osteotomy site to dynamize the os-

teotomy site. Curved retractors are placed anteriorly and posteriorly. The femur is lifted from the wound using a bone hook placed proximally, as opposed to lifting the limb from below; this allows for distraction of the femur from the soft tissues and neurovascular structures of the medial thigh. The osteotomy is then performed using an oscillating saw, preferably using a thin blade, multiple drill holes and osteotome, or a Gigli saw. The osteotomy site is cleared of soft tissue and adjusted as necessary to ensure maximum bone contact. Preparation of the distal fragment occurs with the use of straight reamers. A straight reamer is passed down the intramedullary canal to the point where cortical contact is achieved. Overreaming of the distal fragment results in loss of rotational control and should be avoided. However, an overzealous press-fit of the distal fragment can result in fracture of the distal femur.

With the femur properly aligned, the trial stem is placed within the trial sleeve, across the osteotomy site, and into the distal femur. The bony ends of the proximal and distal fragments can be trimmed to allow for better apposition. Adjustments in limb length can be made by shortening the distal segment of femur.

Prosthesis Implantation

The sleeve is inserted within the proximal fragment and impacted into position. If the proximal fragment is deemed to be excessively fragile, a prophylactic cerclage wire should be placed. The stem is then passed through the sleeve, across the osteotomy site, and into the distal fragment. Orientation of the stem is determined by its position in the distal fragment (ie, the version of the stem is determined by referencing the femoral shaft with the knee flexed, ignoring the position of the proximal fragment).

The fit into the distal femur should be tight enough to ensure

rotational control of the stem (by virtue of the distal flutes) and provide immediate stability but not so tight as to split the femur. In our experience, rotational control of the distal fragment as a result of the distal flutes of the stem obviates the need for oblique or step-cut osteotomy. A prophylactic wire about the proximal aspect of the distal fragment prior to insertion of the stem is often used and later removed. As stem insertion is near completion, the proximal fragment is rotated into position. If native alignment is acceptable, the proximal fragment is aligned anatomically with the distal fragment.

As mentioned previously, scoring of the femoral shaft longitudinally with a saw blade prior to osteotomy can be used as a rotational reference. If posterior or anterior impingement of the trochanter is detected, the proximal fragment can be rotated anteriorly or posteriorly, respectively. Final impaction of the stem locks in the rotation of the proximal fragment via the Morse taper between the sleeve (which controls the proximal fragment) and the stem (which controls the distal fragment). Final impaction of the stem also reduces the osteotomy site. At this time, rotational control of the osteotomy should be tested. If it is unstable, a femoral strut allograft is placed about the osteotomy and secured with cerclage wires above and below the osteotomy. Particulate bone graft can be placed about the osteotomy site (**Figure 3**).

A trial neck is then placed within the proximal sleeve. Reduction of the proximal fragment into the acetabulum is then attempted. If the reduction results in excessive soft-tissue tension, despite the use of a short neck and head, soft-tissue release (capsule ± psoas tendon) should be considered; advancement of the sleeve may jeopardize dynamic loading of the proximal and distal segments across the osteotomy site.

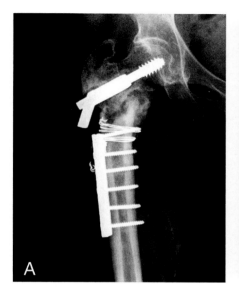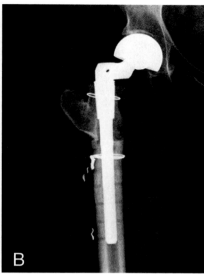

Figure 3 **A,** A 70-year-old woman underwent open reduction and internal fixation using a screw and side plate for a subtrochanteric fracture. The hardware subsequently failed as a result of nonunion. **B,** Bipolar hemiarthroplasty was performed using a modular prosthesis. The proximal sleeve was placed in the femoral neck, resulting in trochanteric advancement.

Wound Closure

The vastus fascia is reapproximated about the osteotomy site using interrupted or running absorbable suture. The gluteus maximus tendon, if divided, is repaired anatomically. Anatomic repair of the posterior capsule and external rotators also should be attempted. The wound is then irrigated and closed in layers. Drains are not typically used.

Postoperative Regimen

Immediate partial weight bearing is allowed because it allows the osteotomy site to be dynamized. A radiograph is obtained 6 weeks postoperatively. Callus formation is typically not seen at this point. However, if the implant has not shifted, and the patient is not experiencing pain, weight bearing as tolerated is permitted. By 3 months, healing of the osteotomy is usually apparent on radiographs. Remodeling of the femur is typically noted from 12 to 24 months postoperatively.

Avoiding Pitfalls and Complications

One of the most common pitfalls is failure to recognize magnification error during preoperative planning. Plain radiographs historically have not been standardized according to magnification. Depending on the size of a patient, a radiograph will either magnify a bone and joint (in large patients with more soft tissue) or decrease its apparent size (in thin patients). The surgeon must estimate the degree of over- or undermagnification to select an implant that is neither too large nor too small. The incorporation of a marker of known size may be of help in this regard. By calculating the difference between the size of the marker displayed on the radiograph and the actual size of the marker, the surgeon can identify the degree of magnification/minimization and compensate accordingly when selecting a prosthetic template and can be assured that all measurements are neither increased nor decreased artifi-

cially. Digital preoperative planning is evolving rapidly and may soon obviate this problem.

With trochanteric deformity in either a primary or revision setting, the anatomy of the trochanter is such that it impedes placement of a femoral stem in neutral position, and in a revision situation, it blocks the exit path of the stem that is to be revised. In this setting, the offending portion of the trochanter must be relieved, either by osteotomy or by lateralization of the trochanter. Lateralization of the trochanter involves forcing the axial reamer laterally, which decorticates the medial aspect of the trochanter and removes cancellous bone from within the trochanteric bed. The benefit of neutral stem positioning must be weighed against the risks of trochanteric sacrifice. Thinning of the trochanter by lateralizing the stem can weaken the bone, making it susceptible to intraoperative or postoperative fracture. Excessive lateralization can even cause avulsion of the abductor tendon insertion, a devastating complication. A potentially far greater and more common problem results from decortication of the trochanter, which exposes cancellous bone to polyethylene debris and can result in osteolysis. Alternatively, modest lateralization of the trochanter potentially avoids the complications as listed above but often results in varus positioning of the stem.

Unrecognized nuances of proximal femur deformity can result in disastrous consequences. If a straight femoral stem is selected, insertion will result in three-point fixation when placed into the curved proximal femur. The anterior cortex of the femur is the most proximal of the three points of fixation. Therefore, it should not be surprising that when the reamer is passed, the anterior cortex is the area in which the cortical bone is contacted first. Therefore, no matter what the template suggests, when cortical bone is exposed anteriorly with the reamer, it is time to stop. Further reaming beyond this point can only remove anterior cortex and will result in anterior cortical fenestration and perforation. One potential pitfall in treating a patient with a femoral deformity is that most radiographs are taken in only two planes, but deformities can be complex and not fully appreciated on two views. Understanding this potential added complexity in surgery is important.

When osteotomy is needed, the bone is weakened by the osteotomy and is thus at increased risk for fracture. Prophylactic wires or cables may reduce the risk of fracture during bone preparation and implant insertion.

———————■

References

Berry DJ: Total hip arthroplasty in patients with proximal femoral deformity. *Clin Orthop* 1999;369:262-272.

Bono JV, McCarthy JC, Lee J, Carangelo RJ: Fixation with a modular stem in revision total hip arthroplasty. *J Bone Joint Surg Am* 1999;81:1326-1336.

Carangelo RJ, Bono JV: Modularity in total hip arthroplasty: The S-ROM prosthesis, in Bono JV, McCarthy JM, Turner R (eds): *Revision Total Hip Arthroplasty*. New York, NY, Springer-Verlag, 1999.

Christie MJ, Deboer DK, Trick LW, et al: Primary total hip arthroplasty with use of the modular S-ROM prosthesis: Four- to seven-year clinical and radiographic results. *J Bone Joint Surg Am* 1999;81:1707-1716.

Holtgrewe JL, Hungerford DS: Primary and revision total hip replacement without cement and with associated femoral osteotomy. *J Bone Joint Surg Am* 1989;71:1487-1495.

McCarthy JC, Bono JV, Lee J: The difficult femur. *Instr Course Lect* 2000;49:63-69.

Mehlhoff MA, Sledge CB: Comparison of cemented and cementless hip and knee replacements. *Arthritis Rheum* 1990;33:293-297.

Papagelopoulos PJ, Trousdale RT, Lewallen DG: Total hip arthroplasty with femoral osteotomy for proximal femoral deformity. *Clin Orthop* 1996;332:151-162.

Perka C, Fischer U, Taylor WR, Matziolis G: Developmental hip dysplasia treated with total hip arthroplasty with a straight stem and a threaded cup. *J Bone Joint Surg Am* 2004;86:312-319.

Coding

CPT Codes		Corresponding ICD-9 Codes		
27130	Arthroplasty, acetabular and proximal femoral prosthetic replacement (total hip arthroplasty), with or without autograft or allograft	711.45 714.30 715.35 718.6 733.42	711.95 715.15 716.15 720.0 808.0	714.0 715.25 718.5 733.14 905.6
27132	Conversion of previous hip surgery to total hip arthroplasty, with or without autograft or allograft	715.15 718.2 733.14 996.4	715.25 718.5 733.42 996.66	715.35 718.6 905.6 996.77
27165	Osteotomy, intertrochanteric or subtrochanteric including internal or external fixation and/or cast	715.15 732.1 736.32 754.32 755.61	715.25 733.81 754.30 754.33 755.62	715.35 736.31 754.31 754.35 755.63

CPT copyright © 2004 by the American Medical Association. All Rights Reserved.

Chapter 23

Total Hip Arthroplasty After Failed Hip Fracture Fixation

Scott S. Kelley, MD

Indications

Complications of previous hip fracture surgery that can be indications for conversion to total hip arthroplasty (THA) include pain, a severe limp, significant limb-length discrepancy, and weakness (**Table 1**). The etiologies of these symptoms include malunion (**Figure 1**), nonunion (**Figure 2**), femoral head osteonecrosis, joint damage from failed internal fixation devices or degenerative arthritis, or any combination thereof.

THA in failed hip fracture fixation is known to be associated with higher dislocation rates; therefore, larger-head diameters (32 to 40 mm) should be considered, provided that adequate polyethylene thickness is maintained.

Contraindications

The most important contraindication to conversion to THA is a salvageable native hip in a young patient. Revision of failed internal fixation should be attempted whenever the native hip can be preserved. This situation is discussed in more detail in the next section.

For patients whose native hip is not salvageable, contraindications are similar to those for revision THA: un-

treated infection and poor medical condition. Even in these situations, conversion to THA can be considered provided that the patient's medical condition is stabilized and/or the infection is treated effectively. Infected nonunions of hip fractures, similar to infected implants, may require a two-stage procedure. Often this procedure involves reaming an infected, dead femoral head and creating a Girdlestone resection. Temporary spacers can be helpful in managing unstable intertrochanteric segments.

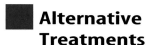

Alternative Treatments

There are three surgical alternatives to conversion to THA: partial hip arthroplasty, resection arthroplasty, and a repeat attempt at open reduction and internal fixation (ORIF). The choice depends on fracture location (femoral neck versus intertrochanteric), the status of the trochanter and abductors, the status of the hip articular cartilage, the viability of the femoral head, bone stock, fracture union (nonunion versus malunion), infection, and patient age.

Revision Open Reduction and Internal Fixation

Revision of failed internal fixation (for both intertrochanteric and femoral

neck fractures) should be attempted whenever the native hip can be preserved in a young patient. The presence of higher quality bone stock, undamaged articular cartilage, and a viable femoral head improves the success of repeat attempts at ORIF. Joint-preserving procedures also may need to incorporate trochanteric repair and/or bone grafting (vascularized versus nonvascularized). Fixation options include blade plate, dynamic hip screw, or femoral nail. Depending on the fracture orientation, variations of valgus osteotomy may be useful to improve compressive forces across the nonunion.

Partial Hip Replacement

The two most common modes of failure for femoral neck fractures, nonunion and osteonecrosis, are related. Osteonecrosis can contribute to nonunion, and nonunion can compromise head viability.

Patients with traumatic osteonecrosis may have localized and relatively asymptomatic involvement. When a patient is symptomatic, partial hip replacement is not a good option. Many surgical alternatives are available for idiopathic osteonecrosis; however, THA is often the best alternative for disabling traumatic osteonecrosis.

Conversion to a partial replacement for fracture nonunion (both intertrochanteric and femoral neck) may be a desirable alternative in elderly (low-demand) patients without hardware penetration into the joint. Partial replacement should be considered for patients at higher risk for medical complications associated with increased blood loss from acetabular reaming. The benefit of a reduction in dislocation risk with hemiarthroplasty compared to THA may have diminished with the use of larger femoral heads in THA.

Resection Arthroplasty (Girdlestone)

Resection arthroplasty may be considered as definitive treatment in the rare patient with recalcitrant infection or such severe medical problems that reconstruction with arthroplasty is not advisable. Pain relief typically is good, but function usually is poor. Most elderly, infirm patients who undergo resection arthroplasty will be able to walk only very short distances with two-arm support.

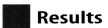

Results

Results of conversion THA in failed intertrochanteric fractures tend to be worse than those for femoral neck fractures (**Table 2**), most likely because of (1) persistent problems related to injury of the trochanteric/abductor mechanism and (2) more extensive involvement of the proximal femur. Definitive conclusions are elusive, however, given the paucity of studies describing outcomes in patients undergoing THA after internal fixation of an intertrochanteric fracture.

Serious intraoperative and postoperative complications have been described following conversion of intertrochanteric fracture to THA, specifically loss of fixation (loosening). In one study, loss of fixation was attributed to difficulties with distortion of the femoral neck-shaft angle, medial

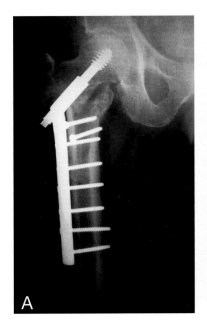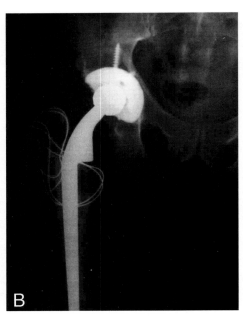

Figure 1 **A,** Preoperative AP radiograph of a 70-year-old man 10 months after ORIF of an intertrochanteric fracture who presented with a severe limp, abductor weakness, and fatigue pain with short distances. He required a 2-inch heel build up and had a fixed 30° external rotation malunion. **B,** Postoperative conversion THA radiograph shows correction of limb-length discrepancy and restoration of abductor position and length.

Table 1 Management Options for Failed Hip Fracture Fixation

Symptoms	Cause	Treatment
Pain	Infection	Hardware removal and antibiotics
	Soft-tissue irritation due to hardware	Hardware removal
	Nonunion	Repeat ORIF versus THA
	Malunion with impingement	Corrective osteotomy versus THA
Limp (painless)	Malunion	Corrective osteotomy versus THA
	Trochanteric nonunion with migration	Trochanteric fixation
Limb-length inequality, weakness	Malunion	Corrective osteotomy versus THA

displacement of the canal, and medial proximal bone loss. Dislocation occurred in 3 of 13 patients. This study also reported intraoperative difficulty with broaching and canal perforation caused by fracture malunion, which resulted in medialization of the shaft on the proximal fragment. Another

study reported increased intraoperative difficulty with THA after previous proximal femoral surgery, but in this series only 6 of 53 patients had a prior intertrochanteric fracture.

A recent study of 60 patients represents the largest series evaluating success of THA for salvage of failed

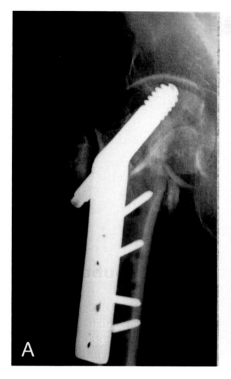 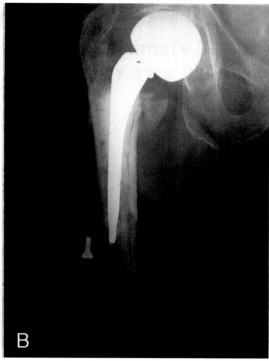 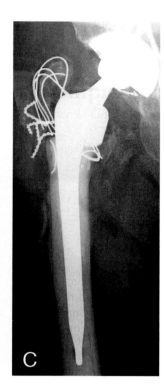

Figure 2 **A,** AP radiograph of a 72-year-old man 6 months after undergoing ORIF of an intertrochanteric fracture who presented with persistent pain and weakness. Failure of fixation led to subsequent conversion THA. **B,** AP radiograph following conversion THA demonstrates failure to correct the abductor mechanism, poor prosthetic position, and compromised cement technique. Note that the trochanter has healed in a lengthened, malunited position. The patient required revision to correct these problems. **C,** Postoperative AP radiograph after rerevision shows the trochanteric repair and improved prosthetic position and cement technique. The key elements affecting the clinical result are the restoration of abductor length (by trochanteric repair) and the quality of the cement technique.

Table 2   Results of Conversion THA

Author(s) (Year)	Fracture Type	Number of Hips	Implant Type	Mean Patient Age (Range)	Mean Follow-up (Range)	Complications	Survivorship (%)
Mehlhoff, et al (1991)	Femoral neck/ Intertrochanteric	14/13	Mixed: Cement, uncemented, hybrid	65 years (35–90)	34 months	1 infection 3 dislocations 0 revisions	100%
Haidukewych and Berry (2003)	Intertrochanteric	60	Mixed, including bipolar unipolar THA cemented uncemented	78 years (54–96)	5 months (2–15)	5 reoperations 1 dislocation	87.5% at 10 years
Mabry, et al (2004)	Femoral neck	84	Charnley	68 years (36–92)	12.2 months	9 dislocations	93% at 10 years 76% at 20 years

intertrochanteric hip fractures. Reported complications were low (five revisions), and implant survivorship was 87.5% at 10 years for revision as the end point. The authors reported that the most common musculoskeletal problem at follow-up was localized to the greater trochanter.

Other intraoperative difficulties with THA after internal fixation of proximal femur fractures have been described. Following fixation of intertrochanteric or subtrochanteric fractures, the femoral neck-shaft relationship can be distorted, and significant proximal bone loss and soft-tissue scarring can occur. These patients may have other neuromuscular disorders

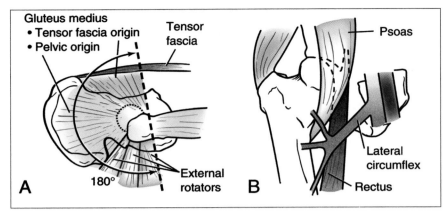

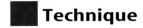

Figure 3 Anatomic considerations for the extensile trochanteric approach. **A,** Pertinent gluteus muscle anatomy. The muscle insertions onto the trochanter wrap 180° around from anterior to posterior. The origin of the anterior portion of the gluteus musculature from its attachment from the undersurface of the superficial fascia (tensor fascia) should be preserved. **B,** Pertinent deep anterior hip anatomy. Note the relationship of the ascending branch of the lateral circumflex to the iliopsoas tendon.

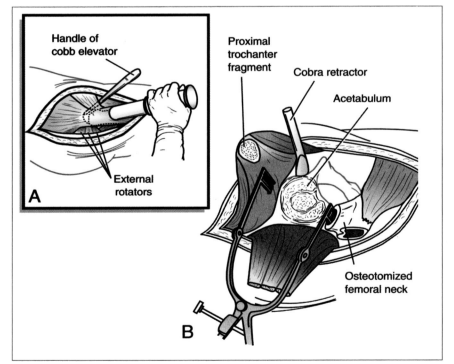

Figure 4 Aspects of the surgical exposure. **A,** A Cobb elevator is placed deep to the entire gluteus musculature and superficial to the hip capsule to orient the direction of a dome-shaped osteotome. The vastus lateralis should be elevated distally before the trochanteric cut at the level of its attachment. **B,** A self-retaining retractor is placed between the femur and gluteus muscle. Ideally, a Charnley (or modification) self-retainer should be used. The gluteus retraction can be aided by fastening a wet laparotomy sponge proximal and distal to the muscle (under the self-retainer).

and are often less healthy than patients undergoing elective hip replacement.

Technique

Exposure
Surgical approaches for conversion THA of failed femoral neck fixation are similar to those for primary THA. For most surgeons, this will be a variation of postero- or anterolateral surgical approaches. When a posterior surgical approach is used, careful attention to posterior soft-tissue repair may reduce dislocation risk. Hardware may be left in place until the hip is dislocated once to minimize risk of further fracture. For intertrochanteric fractures, especially those in which there is nonunion or malunion of the greater trochanter with residual trochanteric issues, extensile surgical approaches may be required (**Figure 2,** *C*). A trochanteric approach should strongly be considered in the presence of trochanteric nonunion or malunion. In the absence of residual trochanteric involvement, the surgical approach should be determined by the surgeon's expertise.

When an extensile trochanteric approach is used, I prefer the technique of Johnston. With this technique, a number of anatomic considerations need to be recognized: First, the anterior third of the gluteus musculature arises from the undersurface of the anterior superficial fascia (fascia lata). Second, the proximal muscle groups (gluteus and external rotators) attach 180° around the trochanter (**Figure 3,** *A*). This is of significance when mobilizing the trochanter. Either the entire external rotator group needs to be taken down or the anterior third of the gluteus needs to be detached. I prefer detaching the external rotators in a similar fashion to the posterior hip approaches. Third, the ascending branches of the lateral circumflex artery lie directly anterior to the interval between the iliopsoas and anteromedial hip capsule (**Figure 3**, *B*). Fourth, muscular insertion into the hip capsule is significant, particularly insertion of the gluteus minimus to the superior capsule. Lastly, the plane between the capsule and the overlying muscle is easiest to develop between the iliopsoas and the anteromedial hip capsule.

Exposure is through a lateral longitudinal incision, parallel to the femur down to the trochanter. The vastus lateralis is then elevated from the trochanteric ridge.

In patients with malunited trochanters, the trochanter is osteotomized using a broad (1.5-inch) dome osteotome. For migrated nonunions and fibrous unions, either a knife or sharp osteotome can be used to cut through the fibrous interface (**Figure 4**, *A*). Once the trochanter is broken free of its residual bony attachments, it is mobilized in two stages: first, it is preliminarily released posteriorly by releasing the attachment of the obturator externus; second, it is mobilized by sharp dissection from the capsule, from anterior to posterior.

This dissection is initiated from the anterior gateway vessels (branches from the lateral circumflex artery and vein). There are three branches off the lateral circumflex artery (ascending, transverse, and descending). The first branch of the femoral nerve travels with the transverse branch and usually can be preserved. The ascending vessels travel medial to the vastus lateralis (directly over the inferior border of the femoral neck) and can be suture ligated as a group (usually one artery and two veins). Directly under these gateway vessels lays the iliopsoas muscle (as it transitions to tendon) as it passes over the anteroinferior capsule (**Figure 3**, *B*).

The iliopsoas is easily elevated from the capsule with a Cobb elevator to where it passes over the superior pubic ramis. A cobra retractor can be

safely passed over the ramis for anterior retraction.

A broad deep retractor is used to facilitate sharp dissection between gluteus musculature and the capsule, from anterior to posterior. The external rotators will be released in the standard plane for a posterior approach, beginning superiorly from the piriformis and distally to the quadratus femoris (at the level of the lesser trochanter). This extensile exposure rarely requires release of the gluteus maximus. Next, the rotators and abductors are fully dissected free from the capsule.

I prefer to retain the capsule when performing hemiarthroplasty and resect it for THA.

Bone Preparation

Acetabular preparation is the same as for any other hip arthroplasty. Acetabular exposure can be facilitated by a self-retaining retractor between the femur and the abductor mechanism (**Figure 4**, *B*). Two problems may be encountered with acetabular preparation. First, the acetabular bone can be very weak, in part secondary to disuse osteoporosis. Second, hardware penetration may have created defects in the acetabulum.

Femoral preparation varies with the pathology that necessitated the surgery. The risk of intraoperative femoral fracture is increased during conversion THA as a result of osteoporosis, deformity, cortical defects (stress risers), and intramedullary sclerosis. Accommodating even the smallest prosthetic options may require reaming and rasping of the femur or removal of some sclerotic intramedullary bone with a power burr.

Generally, if the femur can be recanalized with reamers, it is not necessary to take down a nonunion or malunion, especially for cemented femoral components. The stable fixation provided with cemented components will facilitate healing. Because a perfect fit-fill is not necessary with ce-

mented components, a malunion usually can be left untouched, and the trochanter can be rotated into an anatomic position to correct associated muscle imbalance.

Prosthetic Implantation

Prosthetic fixation to bone continues to evolve. For the acetabulum, uncemented cups are most commonly used. Fixation of the femoral component is more controversial. Just as some surgeons use a hybrid hip for primary THA, a cemented femoral prosthesis is an option in conversion THA. I prefer cemented femoral fixation in patients older than age 60 years, and I carefully prepare the canal and plug all defects. In patients younger than age 50 years, I prefer to use an extensively coated ingrowth prosthesis. In patients between ages 50 and 60 years, I base prosthetic fixation on the patient's activity level and postfracture anatomy.

Standard primary femoral implants usually can be used when a failed femoral neck fracture is cemented to an arthroplasty. In contrast, conversion of intertrochanteric fracture is often facilitated by long-stemmed implants, calcar replacement implants, or implants with extra-long necks.

Calcar replacement of implants with extra-long necks facilitates management of proximal medial bone loss that is often present, helps restore limb length, and optimizes hip biomechanics and stability (**Figure 2**, *C*). Long-stemmed implants can bypass cortical defects left at the site of previous internal fixation devices. When cortical defects cannot be bypassed with a prosthesis, strut allografts can be considered.

CEMENTED

Care must be taken to prevent cement extrusion through old screw holes. Screw holes can be blocked by cutting (shortening) old removed screws (or new screws) and temporarily filling

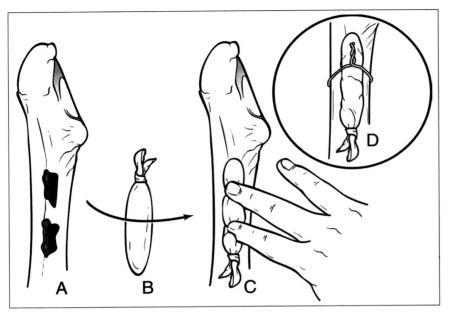

Figure 5 Cement plugging technique. **A,** The bone defects. **B,** The cement plug is created by injecting polymethylmethacrylate cement into the finger of a surgical glove, which then is tied off like a balloon. **C,** The doughy, latex-encased polymethylmethacrylate is pressed firmly into the defects and held until it polymerizes, leaving a custom-made mold of the bony defects. **D,** The mold can be wired in place temporarily with a single cerclage wire, or held in place by the surgeon, during the next steps of the operation. (Reproduced with permission from Slater, R, Morrison J, Kelley S: Custom-made molds that prevent cement extrusion through bone defects. *Clin Orthop* 1995;317:126-130.)

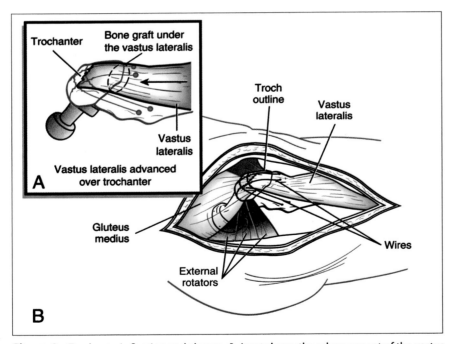

Figure 6 Trochanteric fixation and closure. **A,** Inset shows the advancement of the vastus lateralis over the repaired trochanter. Bone graft should be placed under this advanced muscle. **B,** The relationship of the gluteus muscle to the remaining structures (trochanter and vastus).

the hole during the cementing process. With broken screws, hollow mill drills may be required to remove screws and can potentially result in larger defects. Such defects can be contained with custom molds of cement plugs (**Figure 5**).

UNCEMENTED

For uncemented THA, use of prophylactic cable before implantation (preferably prior to rasping and trial implant placement) should be considered. I consider uncemented techniques for younger patients and for patients in whom bone deficiency may preclude optimal cement technique.

Wound Closure

Deep tissue closure begins with trochanteric fixation using a four-wire technique. I use an 18-gauge beaded cobalt-chromium wire. Trochanteric healing may be improved by including débridement of any fibrous tissue to bleeding trochanteric bone, autogenous bone grafting from the femoral head, imbrication of the vastus lateralis over bone graft, and use of wires facilitated by a fractional (fascial cut) lengthening of the vastus (**Figure 6**).

Postoperative Regimen

For patients without trochanteric fixation or other special considerations, gait training and mobilization identical to other primary THAs is initiated. If trochanteric fixation is performed, I recommend partial weight bearing (10% to 25% of body weight) for 6 weeks postoperatively. If trochanteric fixation was performed and/or hip stability is a concern, a hip guide brace may work for about 6 weeks. After 6 weeks, weight bearing can progress as tolerated. Either one cane or a crutch should be used for a minimum of 4 months to protect the trochanter from healing in a lengthened position.

Avoiding Pitfalls and Complications

THA in this patient population is associated with a higher frequency of both intraoperative and postoperative complications. Complications can be reduced by thorough preoperative evaluation of the patient's medical condition and by ruling out the presence of hip infection. Hip joint aspiration should be considered in patients with unexplained levels of pain, a history of wound problems, or radiographic evidence of a possible infection.

I prefer to avoid fracture revision from the second to the twelfth postoperative week after an internal fixation procedure (ie, the period of maximum inflammatory/vascularization phase). In situations in which the patient is incapacitated (ie, pain, weakness), the severity of the symptoms may dictate earlier intervention.

Intraoperative complications include an increased risk of fractures and increased blood loss from the more extensive dissection required to mobilize the femur and expose the acetabulum. Depending on the length of time after the index procedure, there will be variability in soft-tissue edema, soft-tissue planes, and the amount of callus and bone formation.

Postoperatively, increased dislocation, infection, weakness (**Figure 2**, *B*), and limb-length inequality are possible. These risks probably are inversely greater when the quality of the soft tissue and bone is poor.

The two most frequently overlooked concerns are weakness secondary to trochanteric problems and limb-length inequality. Patients often present with shortening, making residual shortening more of a problem than overlengthening. Mobilization of the femur with an extensile approach facilitates restoration of limb length. The extensile approach also allows the trochanter to be mobilized and restores abductor length (**Figures 1** and **2**). With an anterior or posterior approach, it may be more difficult to restore limb length and minimize hip biomechanics.

Recent interest in oversized femoral heads (> 32 mm) may decrease the risk of dislocation. In elderly patients with extensive disruption of anatomy, including the soft-tissue envelope, a constrained acetabular component may need to be considered. The advantage of large femoral heads in THA over hemiarthroplasty is the manufactured exact match (fit) between the articulating surfaces and possibly the likelihood of groin pain that can occur in some patients treated with hemiarthroplasty.

Diminished implant durability and increased complications are commonly associated with conversion THA of both failed intertrochanteric and femoral neck fractures. Failed intertrochanteric fracture management creates obvious problems for implant durability, but it is less obvious as to why this is also seen with femoral neck nonunions. One report speculated that THA could be less durable because of poor (acetabular and femoral) bone quality, holes in the femur at the sites of old fixation devices, and the inclusion of a subgroup of younger patients with unilateral hip disease (at risk for mechanical implant failure).

References

Haidukewych GJ, Berry DJ: Hip arthroplasty for salvage of failed treatment of intertrochanteric hip fractures. *J Bone Joint Surg Am* 2003;85:899-904.

Kelley SS, Johnston RC: Debris from cobalt-chromium cable may cause acetabular loosening. *Clin Orthop* 1992;285:140-146.

Mabry TM, Prpa B, Haidukewych GJ, Harmsen WS, Berry DJ: Long-term results of total hip arthroplasty for femoral neck fracture nonunion. *J Bone Joint Surg Am* 2004;86:2263-2267.

Mehlhoff T, Landon GC, Tullos US: Total hip arthroplasty following failed internal fixation of hip fractures. *Clin Orthop* 1991;269:32-37.

Slater R, Morrison J, Kelley S: Custom-made molds that prevent cement extrusion through bone defects. *Clin Orthop* 1995;317:126-130.

Tabsh I, Waddell JP, Morton J: Total hip arthroplasty for complications of proximal femoral fractures. *J Orthop Trauma* 1997;11:166-169.

Coding

CPT Codes		Corresponding ICD-9 Codes		
27132	Conversion of previous hip surgery to total hip arthroplasty, with or without autograft or allograft	715.15 718.2 733.14 996.4	715.25 718.5 733.42 996.66	715.35 718.6 905.6 996.77

CPT copyright © 2004 by the American Medical Association. All Rights Reserved.

Chapter 24

Total Hip Arthroplasty: Osteonecrosis of the Femoral Head

Bernard N. Stulberg, MD

Indications

For many years, controversy has surrounded the preservative treatments of femoral head osteonecrosis (ON). The goals of these various approaches include preserving the femoral head whenever possible or alternatively preserving hip function, relieving pain, and delaying arthroplasty. All are laudable goals, particularly for young, active patients, but they have resulted in a variety of operations on the femoral head that either alter its internal geometry (eg, decompression or bone grafting of various types) or alter the external geometry or that of the proximal femur (eg, varus, valgus, or rotational osteotomy). These procedures may make conversion to total hip arthroplasty (THA) more difficult and the ultimate results less satisfactory than if the proximal femur had been preserved. As written elsewhere, my preference is to confine most nonarthroplasty treatment options to limited surgical interventions (ie, decompression or decompression and grafting). This preserves proximal femoral geometry and ensures that the results of uncemented THA can remain predictable should limited interventions fail (**Figures 1** and **2**).

I currently prefer uncemented THA for most patients with a collapsed femoral head with proven cartilage fracture and sufficient symptoms to justify arthroplasty. In the University of Pennsylvania (Steinberg) classification, this condition is considered stage IV or higher and applies to all patients with a collapsed femoral head, regardless of previous treatment. The current state of the art suggests that in most cases THA is a more predictable option than hemiarthroplasty, a procedure that I have now abandoned. Femoral head hemiresurfacing is similarly less predictable. An uncemented arthroplasty should be considered for most younger patients with ON, but patients older than age 70 years with new-onset ON may benefit more from hybrid fixation techniques because their disease has likely developed as a result of arterial insufficiency. This

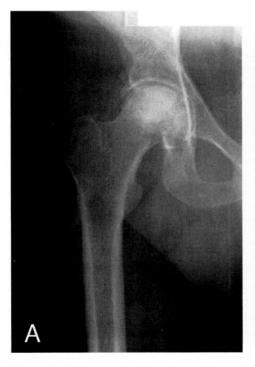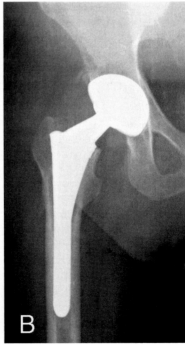

Figure 1 **A,** Preoperative AP radiograph 6 months following core decompression and grafting. THA was performed using contemporary uncemented THA with metal-on-metal bearing surfaces following unsuccessful right hip decompression and grafting. **B,** Postoperative AP radiograph obtained 3 years later.

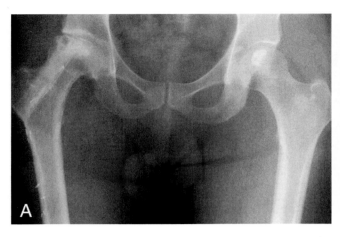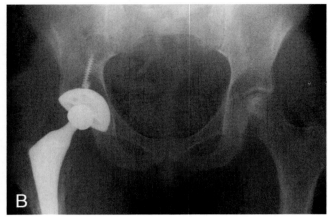

Figure 2 **A,** AP radiograph of the pelvis of a 38-year-old man who underwent vascularized fibular grafting of his right hip for stage IV ON. Further collapse occurred early after grafting, but the patient's symptoms were managed for 8 years before progressive arthritic changes led to recommendation for THA. **B,** Postoperative AP radiograph obtained 3 years after THA. Note that the vascular clips and remnant of fibula can be seen laterally.

chapter focuses on treatment of the young patient with ON.

Contraindications

The presence of active infection within the hip joint is an absolute contraindication to THA for ON. Relative contraindications include precollapse ON that is amenable to less invasive interventions or other preservative procedures and ON in the very young patient. THA also should be used with great caution in patients with hemophilia; in these patients, treatment must be based on the risks and benefits of intervention for each patient. Even though THA often represents the most predictable treatment for ON, there can be significant long-term consequences if the arthroplasty fails, and particularly if it fails repeatedly. Thus, patients and their families must be fully advised about the possible outcomes and should participate fully in the decision-making process. Given that THA still does not have a proven success rate of 40 years or more, patients should be counseled accordingly.

Alternative Treatments

This chapter focuses on arthroplasty options for ON and should be reviewed in conjunction with chapter 66 on Operative Indications for Osteonecrosis, which describes nonarthroplasty options for ON. In young patients, all options should be explored, but I believe that for end-stage ON uncemented THA provides the most predictable outcome. Alternatives to arthroplasty include hemiarthroplasty (either monopolar or bipolar), resurfacing hemiarthroplasty, or resurfacing THA (at present, available in the United States only through Investigational Device Exemption [IDE], given its present classification by the US Food and Drug Administration as a class III device) (**Figure 3**).

ON is a disease of the femoral head; therefore, it is very tempting to address only the femoral aspect of THA in these patients. However, several studies confirm that the acetabular cartilage is rarely normal in patients with collapse of the surface (stage IV or higher), and clinical experience suggests that hemiarthroplasty or resurfacing hemiarthroplasty is not as durable or as functional as THA.

The earliest experiences with THA raised doubts about cemented arthroplasty, and more recent studies raised concerns about uncemented acetabular components. Uncemented acetabular failures, however, seem to be similar for young patients with other diseases and suggest that the limitations are more the result of technology than the disease state. Current approaches to devices and bearing surfaces have addressed many of these shortcomings and make THA a better choice for most patients.

Results

Treatment of precollapse ON is significantly influenced by the size and location of the lesion (confirmed through appropriate staging) and the underlying disease state. The results of THA for ON, however, do not appear to be influenced by these factors but rather by the quality of the proximal femur (and thus initial fit and stability) and the acetabular component (**Table 1**).

ON may affect the geometry of the proximal femur. Because ON affects a heterogeneous population, in-

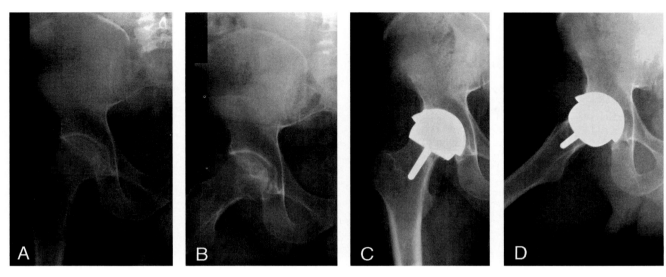

Figure 3 Preoperative AP **(A)** and frog-lateral **(B)** radiographs of 47-year-old man with ON treated by metal-on-metal resurfacing arthroplasty following failure of core decompression. Postoperative AP **(C)** and frog-lateral **(D)** radiographs show appropriate position of components with good bone apposition.

cluding women with systemic lupus erythematosus and men with alcohol-related ON, the geometry of the proximal femur varies widely. Both cemented and uncemented femoral component fixation have been described for treatment, but I believe that the uncemented interface for both acetabular and femoral components will provide a more durable fixation interface. Recent studies evaluating the effectiveness of uncemented THA for ON report less optimal acetabular results, similar to those reported in the non-ON population.

Technique

I prefer a posterolateral approach for most primary THAs because it allows excellent visualization of the proximal femur, the area in which geometric discrepancies are most likely to occur during arthroplasty and where there is greatest risk for fracture. It is particularly important to visualize the lateral cortex near the metaphyseal flare where endosteal buildup can occur. This buildup can interfere with seat-

ing a proximally loading and/or proximally filling device, and fracture can occur if a device is forced into varus. It is also important to visualize this area to avoid fracture or to identify a fracture if it occurs and to address it appropriately.

Exposure

The incision is centered over the greater trochanter, extending an appropriate amount cephalad and caudad to allow for sufficient exposure (ie, via a limited or mini-incision approach). The posterior aspect of the gluteus medius is identified, and the piriformis is visualized. Next, the interval between the piriformis and the gluteus minimus is identified, the minimus is elevated off of the capsule, and a retractor is placed superiorly. The piriformis and short external rotators are elevated off of the back of the greater trochanter by electrocautery in an attempt to preserve maximum length for later repair. If necessary, the quadratus femoris and tendinous insertion of the gluteus maximus can be divided at their insertions for additional exposure. The lesser trochanter must be either di-

rectly visualized or easily palpated to assist in determining the proper resection level. I do not separate the capsule and the short rotators. The capsule is divided superiorly over the femoral neck, and a trapezoidal flap of capsule and short external rotators is created for later repair. The hip is dislocated by flexion, adduction, and internal rotation, the femoral head is isolated, and the neck resection level measured. The femoral head and neck are resected, and the diseased head removed. Resecting the femoral head with a previously placed vascularized or nonvascularized fibular graft usually is not difficult, although the bone will be more sclerotic.

Bone Preparation

Preparation of the acetabulum is straightforward in patients with early femoral head collapse because there may be little deformity. In some cases, however, there is extensive inflammatory synovitis, which may result in marked periarticular osteopenia, and the bone can be quite soft. Removal of articular cartilage by curettage followed by very careful reaming will help to avoid overreaming and inad-

Table 1 Results of THA for Osteonecrosis

Author(s) (Year)	Number of Hips	Implant Type	Mean Patient Age (Range)	Mean Follow-up (Range)	Results*	Comments
Berend, et al (2003)	89	54 uncemented 8 cemented 27 NR	36 years (N/A)	9.2 years (5–15)	94.4% survival at 5 years 85.4% survival at 10 years	Proximal ingrowth stems (94.5%) Cemented stems failed (3 of 8 hips) Multiple revisions (8 of 16 hips)
Kim, et al (2003)	150	100 uncemented 50 cemented	47.3 years (26–58)	9.3 years (8–10)	98% overall survival at 10 years 100% survival free of loosening at 10 years	Increased UHMWPE wear rate Revisions (infection or fracture)
Lee, et al (2004)	71	40 uncemented bipolar 31 uncemented THA	44.1 years (18–73) 44.7 years (24–77)	8 years (6.1–10.7) 8.8 years (6.7–11.1)	d'Aubigne and Postel clinical scores 17.1 (bipolar) 17.9 (THA)	Significantly better clinical outcome with THA Survival N/A
Nich, et al (2003)	52	52 uncemented femur 39 cemented cups 13 uncemented cups	41 years (22–79)	16 years (11–23.7)	84.5% overall revision rate at 10 years 65% at 16 years 88.5% acetabular survival at 10 years 70.1% at 16 years 100% femoral survival at 10 years 96.7% at 16 years	Alumina-on-alumina No osteolysis 13 component revisions 3 acetabulum 2 femur (>10 years) 1 for infection
Schneider and Knahr (2004)	129 OA-72 ON-57	22 Mittelmeier 35 Zweymuller	NR All patients younger than 50 years	14 years 10 years	68% overall survival; 10 revised stems 93% overall survival; 0 revised stems	No difference between ON and other causes Included OA and ON in survival calculations

N/A = Not Available; NR = Not Reported; OA = Osteoarthritis
*Survival may vary by manuscript (all operations, survival of components)

vertent compromise of the posterior or medial wall of the acetabulum.

Retractors are placed around the acetabulum, with the femur brought anteriorly. After the labrum is excised, I generally use a large curette to remove remaining articular cartilage. I prefer to use a curette to remove the attachments of the pulvinar at the floor of the acetabulum and sweep them caudad to the transverse acetabular ligament. The soft tissues of the pulvinar can be quite inflamed in patients with ON of the femoral head,

and bleeding at the inferior aspect of this resection can be brisk. I use electrocautery to make the final transection. If necessary, the transverse acetabular ligament is excised. Reaming of the acetabulum is standard, and an uncemented acetabular component or shell is implanted.

Preparation of the femur is device specific but not substantially different from that of the patient with osteoarthritis, with a few exceptions. These exceptions include (1) prior surgery that alters the endosteal sur-

face and (2) geometric variations, including metaphyseal/diaphyseal mismatch, which may affect the choice of implant. I prefer proximally loading devices and thus am more attentive to endosteal buildup and proximal fit and fill (**Figure 1**). If an extensively coated implant is used, the surgical technique usually is routine.

Prosthesis Implantation

I ensure that the lateral flare of the metaphyseal-diaphyseal junction is free of excessive bone buildup and then stabilize a proximally coated implant according to the standard technique for that implant. Initial implant stability is mandatory for all uncemented implants and does not differ in these patients.

Wound Closure

With the posterior approach, an anatomic repair of the capsule and short external rotators is important. I use No. 2 nonbraided, nonabsorbable suture in the superior and inferior edges of the capsule and in the superior and inferior edges of the short external rotators using drill holes in the back of the greater trochanter. These sutures are tied with the hip in external rotation. A subcuticular skin closure is routine.

Postoperative Regimen

Weight bearing as tolerated with crutches is allowed immediately; I do not differentiate between cemented or uncemented THA in any age population. Most patients require at least a single walking aid by 6 weeks, although younger patients tend to be able to walk independently sooner. Appropriate education for proper hip positioning and strengthening is important and needs to be reinforced in this patient population.

■ Avoiding Pitfalls and Complications

Acetabular malposition and overreaming can occur in these patients. Component malposition is usually related to the difficulty of acetabular exposure, a consequence of a tight or muscular patient where circumferential visualization is challenging. Overreaming is particularly of concern in patients with substantial inflammation, hyperemia, and localized osteoporosis. To avoid overreaming, I remove cartilage to the subchondral bone and ream to just through the subchondral plate. I attempt to leave a combination of cancellous and subchondral bone to support the acetabular shell.

Endosteal buildup is expected in patients with previous core decompression alone, after decompression with augmentation or impaction grafting, and with use of fibular grafts (**Figure 2**). Femoral components that fit proximally will likely be forced into varus with reaming or broaching, which can lead to a fracture of the medial femoral neck that sometimes extends to below the lesser trochanter.

To avoid varus positioning, I confirm lateralization of the broach or reamer and use a curved rasp, Hall burr, or high-speed burr as necessary. These tools are needed if a fibular graft has been placed previously. When I use the burr, I am careful to avoid vi-

olating the lateral cortex. Preoperative assessment is helpful in determining the amount of graft that overhangs the central axis of the canal and is a guide in placing instruments appropriately. A large proximally filling implant (such as a custom implant) or a wedge implant will force the medial-lateral fit and may crack the femur if a lateral cortical hole or window has been previously used.

If an osteotomy has been used previously, a modular implant should be considered. These devices allow for use of power instruments to remove sclerotic bone and can aid in proper positioning of implants without the need for a repeat osteotomy of the proximal femur. These devices can also allow for adjustment of offset, rotation, and length without the necessity of extensive revision of the osteotomy.

In the early experience with uncemented THA for ON, metaphyseal-diaphyseal mismatch was a problem. Many contemporary systems now address these femoral shapes appropriately. However, given the inflammatory nature of involvement in some patients, there may be substantial metaphyseal breadth with a narrow diaphyseal diameter. Preoperative templating can help identify these hips. If the mismatch is substantial, a modular hip stem or a custom stem should be considered.

■ References

Berend KR, Gunneson E, Urbaniak JR, Vail TP: Hip arthroplasty after failed free vascularized fibular grafting for osteonecrosis in young patients. *J Arthroplasty* 2003;18:411-419.

Kim YH, Oh SH, Kim JS, Koo KH: Contemporary total hip arthroplasty with and without cement with osteonecrosis of the femoral head. *J Bone Joint Surg Am* 2003;85:675-681.

Lee SB, Sugano N, Nakata K, Matsui M, Ohzono K: Comparison between bipolar hemiarthroplasty and THA for osteonecrosis of the femoral head. *Clin Orthop* 2004;424:161-165.

Lieberman JR, Berry DJ, Mont MA, et al: Osteonecrosis of the hip: Management in the twenty-first century. *J Bone Joint Surg Am* 2002;84:834-851.

Nich C, Ali el-HS, Hannouche D, et al: Long-term results of alumina-on-alumina hip arthroplasty for osteonecrosis. *Clin Orthop* 2003;217:102-111.

Schneider W, Knahr K: Total hip replacement in younger patients: Survival rate after avascular necrosis of the femoral head. *Acta Orthop Scand* 2004;75:142-146.

Steinberg ME, Corces A, Fallon M: Acetabular involvement in osteonecrosis of the femoral head. *J Bone Joint Surg Am* 1999;81:60-65.

Stulberg BN: Osteonecrosis: What to do, what to do. *J Arthroplasty* 2003;18(suppl 1):74-79.

Coding

CPT Codes		Corresponding ICD-9 Codes		
27130	Arthroplasty, acetabular and proximal femoral prosthetic replacement (total hip arthroplasty), with or without autograft or allograft	711.45 714.30 715.35 718.5 733.42	711.95 715.15 720.0 718.6 808.0	714.0 715.25 716.15 733.14 905.6
27132	Conversion of previous hip surgery to total hip arthroplasty, with or without autograft or allograft	715.15 718.2 733.14 996.4	715.25 718.5 733.42 996.66	715.35 718.6 905.6 996.77

CPT copyright © 2004 by the American Medical Association. All Rights Reserved.

Chapter 25

Total Hip Arthroplasty: Metastases and Neoplasm

Mary I. O'Connor, MD

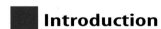

Introduction

Metastatic bone disease or primary bone tumor, whether benign or malignant, results in bone destruction. Although patients with metastatic bone disease are far more common, patients with primary bone tumors also present to the general orthopaedist. Neoplasm should be suspected in patients with progressive pain that is unrelieved by rest and is more pronounced at night. As much as 30% to 50% of trabecular bone can be lost before a lesion is visible on plain radiographs; thus, neoplasm should rank high as a differential diagnosis for patients with negative radiographs who do not respond to therapies appropriate for the working diagnosis. Furthermore, tumors that cause a permeative pattern of bone destruction (eg, lymphoma, Ewing's sarcoma) are often very difficult to identify on plain radiographs. Repeat radiography is recommended for patients with ongoing symptoms (particularly if progressive), and bone scintigraphy or MRI can also be considered.

Osteoarthritis, metastatic bone disease, and chondrosarcoma all commonly affect the elderly. A prior history of cancer should indicate the possibility of metastatic bone disease, particularly if the earlier cancer was a primary tumor with a tendency to metastasize to bone, such as lung, breast, prostate, kidney, and thyroid cancers.

The predilection of chondrosarcoma for the periacetabular region is well known.

Indications

After a bone tumor has been identified, a thorough diagnostic and staging evaluation is necessary before performing needle or open biopsy. Biopsies performed by nonspecialists are potentially hazardous, and patients suspected of having a primary bone sarcoma should be referred to an orthopaedic oncologist before any biopsy occurs. Tissue to confirm the diagnosis of bone metastasis can be obtained from patients with known metastatic bone disease during surgical treatment for impending or actual fracture.

Guidelines are less defined for patients with a history of carcinoma but without known metastases, or with a remote history of metastases. If multiple bone lesions develop in these patients, metastatic bone disease is a reasonable working diagnosis. Tissue for histologic confirmation can be obtained by needle biopsy or during surgical intervention. However, if these patients have a solitary bone lesion, primary bone sarcoma is still a consideration, particularly if the history of cancer is remote. If the general orthopaedist is not knowledgeable about the principles of needle or bone bi-

opsy, the patient should be referred to an orthopaedic oncologist.

Primary Bone Tumors

Benign bone tumors develop about the hip and often require excision or curettage and bone grafting. Patients with primary bone sarcomas are treated with wide en bloc resection followed by complex reconstruction. These procedures should be performed by an orthopaedic oncologist. However, the general orthopaedist will treat metastatic bone disease about the hip, and that treatment is the focus of this chapter.

Metastatic Bone Disease

Surgical treatment of metastatic bone disease about the hip is indicated for mechanical instability arising from actual or impending pathologic fracture and for symptomatic lesions that have not responded to medical treatment (ie, chemotherapy, bisphosphonates, radiation, hormones, and/or immunotherapy).

The goals of surgical intervention are to relieve pain, restore maximal function in the shortest possible time, prevent pathologic fracture, and avoid treatment-related complications. A patient's life expectancy should justify surgical treatment. Although there are no rigid guidelines, an expected survival of 3 to 6 months is appropriate for patients with acetabular metastases, with survival of

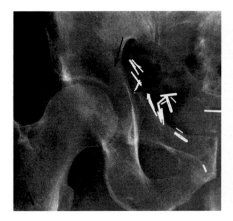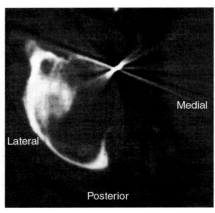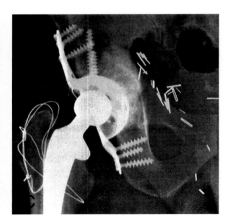

Figure 1 Metastatic prostate carcinoma in a 69-year-old man with progressive groin pain. **A,** AP radiograph suggests lucent change in the medial acetabular region. **B,** CT scan defines the area of bone destruction involving the medial wall. **C,** AP radiograph obtained after curettage and reconstruction with cementation, protrusio cage, and THA. The patient subsequently ambulated independently. (Reproduced with permission from O'Connor MI: Surgical management of metastatic disease of the pelvis, in Fitzgerald RH Jr, Kaufer H, Malkani AL (eds): *Orthopaedics.* St Louis, MO, Mosby, 2002, pp 1108-1115.)

2 to 3 months acceptable for patients with disease of the proximal femur. Selected patients with acute fracture and a shorter expected survival time may still be surgical candidates because of pain management and nursing care issues. Selected patients with a solitary metastasis from thyroid carcinoma or hypernephroma may be candidates for curative surgery (wide en bloc resection), but this is rare. These patients should be referred to an orthopaedic oncologist. A multidisciplinary approach to management of these patients is appropriate, with particular input from specialists in both medical and radiation oncology.

Periacetabular Metastases

Metastatic involvement can occur in any area of the pelvis, but periacetabular lesions are more likely to require surgical intervention because they result in pain and limited weight bearing. Destruction of the superior dome, medial wall, posterior column, or any combination thereof may lead to collapse of the articular surface, protrusio acetabuli, or acute fracture. The exact degree of bone destruction required for prophylactic intervention is not established. I routinely order CT and MRI in candidates for surgery. MRI

permits optimal assessment of soft-tissue extension of the tumor and other areas of metastases within the pelvis and sacrum, whereas CT better defines the degree of cortical bone compromise.

The extent of bone destruction in the periacetabular region determines the specific surgical technique. The following are goals of reconstruction: (1) to transfer weight-bearing stress away from the diseased bone to the remaining intact pelvis; (2) to avoid bone grafting and other procedures requiring osseous healing that may limit postoperative function in patients with limited life expectancy or who may require subsequent radiation therapy; and (3) to minimize the risk of postoperative complications.

Acetabular reconstruction of metastatic destruction typically involves thorough curettage of the tumor and diseased bone, placement of Steinmann pins or screws from within the defective bone into intact (generally superior) bone, filling of the defect with methylmethacrylate with incorporation of the pins or screws, placement of a protrusio acetabular implant (cage or ring), and total hip arthroplasty (THA). Small lesions may require only methacrylate and a pro-

trusio ring (**Figure 1**). Constrained liners to minimize the risk of postoperative dislocation should be considered. A Girdlestone procedure to eliminate the risk of life-threatening hemorrhage from intrapelvic displacement of the femoral head may be considered for patients who are not candidates for acetabular reconstruction. Limb shortening will develop and pain relief is variable. A saddle prosthesis may be used for reconstruction in patients with sufficient bone in the ilium but severe destruction of the acetabular columns.

Proximal Femur Metastases

Significant metastatic destruction of the femoral neck or intertrochanteric region places the patient at great risk of pathologic fracture. The exact degree of bone destruction required for prophylactic intervention is not well defined. Compromise of the medial cortex (including avulsion of the lesser trochanter) usually leads to fracture because the lateral cortex cannot withstand the compressive loads. Destruction of both the medial and lateral cortices should warrant surgical consideration. CT is helpful for determining the need for prophylactic intervention. In patients at clear risk of fracture, I recommend prophylactic surgical treatment. In patients who are not at clear risk of fracture, nonsurgical management such as radiation therapy, chemotherapy, protected weight bearing, and monitoring with repeat radiographs are appropriate to ensure stability of the bone.

The location and extent of bone destruction determine whether internal fixation or arthroplasty is selected. Compromise of the femoral head or neck is best treated with hip arthroplasty because internal fixation is not likely to achieve rigid fixation and tumor progression may lead to fracture or hardware failure. The choice of a hemiarthroplasty articulation versus a fixed acetabular component is based on the presence or absence of acetabular tumor involvement, the status of the acetabular cartilage, and the potential activity level of the patient. Bipolar or unipolar articulation is reasonable in low-demand patients lacking significant metastatic acetabular involvement and satisfactory acetabular cartilage (**Figure 2**). Acetabular micrometastases are not uncommon but often can be controlled with radiation therapy and other nonsurgical measures. A cemented acetabular component can be placed if metastatic involvement of the acetabulum is a concern. An uncemented acetabular component may be used if preoperative MRI does not reveal metastatic acetabular involvement. However, the component should be shielded from postoperative radiation therapy. I prefer an uncemented acetabular component in patients without evidence of acetabular tumor who have the potential to regain a high level of activity.

The femoral component should be cemented. Modern uncemented femoral components, including long-stemmed implants, are not appropriate for treatment of metastases in the proximal femur. Postoperative radiation therapy, which is required to control residual disease, and postoperative chemotherapy would likely pro-

hibit bone ingrowth into such a component. The location and extent of bone destruction determine the type of replacement component (standard, calcar-replacing, long-stemmed, or proximal femoral). The entire femur should be imaged preoperatively (plain radiographs with additional specialized imaging, such as bone scintigraphy). A calcar-replacement stem is indicated if the calcar is compromised. A long-stemmed femoral component should be used if metastatic foci are present elsewhere in the femur. A long-stemmed femoral implant should also be considered in patients with longer life expectancy (such as patients with breast carcinoma metastases) because it will prophylactically address most of the femur should additional metastases develop. However, cemented long-stemmed femoral components are associated with increased risk of embolization of marrow contents and cardiopulmonary events. To help vent medullary contents during cementation of the implant, a drill hole can be made into the distal femur.

Communication with the anesthesiologist is also important. For patients with known cardiopulmonary compromise and limited life expectancy, I use a standard or midlength femoral component, if adequate for the degree of bone destruction, to minimize the risk of an intraoperative event.

Metastatic involvement of the intertrochanteric region may be addressed with a calcar-replacing hip arthroplasty or a compression hip screw. For patients with intertrochanteric lesions but minimal compromise of the adjacent cortical bone, a compression hip screw with adjuvant methylmethacrylate can be considered. Using methylmethacrylate to fill metastatic defects and augment internal fixation is an off-label use of bone cement not approved by the US Food and Drug Administration. I prefer a calcar-replacing hip arthroplasty for

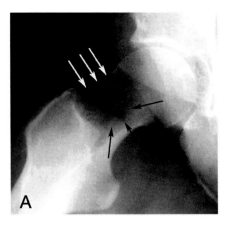

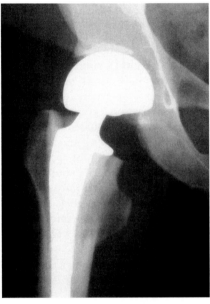

Figure 2 Multiple myeloma in a 67-year-old woman with hip pain and impending pathologic fracture. **A,** AP radiograph of the hip showing marked destruction of the femoral neck region. **B,** AP radiograph obtained after bipolar hip hemiarthroplasty. After postoperative radiation therapy, the patient ambulated with a cane until her death.

treatment of intertrochanteric lesions in patients with moderate to significant cortical involvement; failure of a compression hip screw can occur in such patients because of inadequate host bone. For patients with extensive destruction of the entire proximal femur, a proximal femoral replacement in combination with a bipolar or constrained acetabular component is used to minimize the risk of postoperative dislocation. Finally, in patients with metastatic lesions in the subtrochanteric region of the hip, prophylactic fixation with a reconstruction-type nail is typically the procedure of choice.

Contraindications

Sclerotic metastases pose less risk of fracture and typically are treated medically. Surgical intervention is not appropriate for patients with very short life expectancy or medical compromise that precludes surgery. Other surgical contraindications are the presence of any metastatic disease that would limit functional restoration (such as spinal metastases with epidural cord compression) and extensive bone destruction in the pelvis that prevents a mechanically sound reconstruction. Nonsurgical measures are appropriate if surgical goals (pain relief and maintenance or restoration of function) cannot be achieved.

Alternative Treatments

In addition to nonsurgical measures, embolization therapy is an alternative to surgical treatment of metastatic hip disease. In many vascular pelvic metastases (particularly hypernephroma, myeloma, and thyroid carcinoma), embolization is often performed on the day of surgery or the day before to prevent massive intraoperative hemorrhage. Embolization may also be used to decrease pain and slow disease progression in patients with vascular metastases who are not undergoing surgery. Serial embolizations may also be performed.

Results

Periacetabular Metastases
Surgical intervention has been reported to result in more tolerable pain with no loss of function for most patients and improved function for some. All studies, however, reported limited survival, with most noting a median postoperative survival of less than 12 months. The actual durability of the procedure was therefore difficult to determine. The presence of visceral metastases resulted in early death, with one recent study indicating a median postoperative survival of 3 months. Most reports included a perioperative death; the morbidity associated with complex procedures in these patients may be significant.

Proximal Femur Metastases
Surgical intervention typically reduces pain and maintains or restores ambulation. In general, more favorable results are achieved by treating impending rather than completed pathologic fracture. Patient mortality limits assessment of surgical results. In a series of patients who underwent surgery for femoral metastatic disease, survival rates were 35% at 1 year and 19% at 2 years for patients with impending fractures; survival rates for patients with completed fractures were 25% at 1 year and 10% at 2 years. Results of prosthetic replacement for pathologic or impending fractures of the hip have been favorable, with ambulation restored or maintained in most patients and the incidence of complications low.

Technique

I will not discuss all surgical techniques for metastatic disease of the hip region but will focus on two techniques: the modified Harrington tech-

nique of acetabular reconstruction and a proximal femoral replacement implant for reconstruction of extensive metastatic involvement of the proximal femur. Calcar-replacing femoral stems are detailed in chapter 54.

Acetabular Reconstruction
Any patient suspected of having a vascular metastasis should undergo preoperative embolization. The surgical approach should permit sufficient exposure to ensure thorough access to the lesion and placement of a protrusio device. A trochanteric osteotomy may be necessary, and, if performed, should be shielded from postoperative radiation therapy. After dislocation of the hip and femoral neck osteotomy, the gross tumor and involved bone are thoroughly curettaged. It is important to remove as much tumor as possible to minimize the risk of local disease progression that would result in fixation failure. Depending on the extent of the defect, reconstruction may include cancellous screws (or threaded Steinmann pins), methylmethacrylate, and a protrusio ring or cage. The principle is the transfer of weight-bearing stress to the intact proximal bone. Protrusio (or reinforcement) rings may be used for smaller lesions with intact anterior and posterior columns. For larger lesions, I favor a protrusio cage.

Screws or pins may be driven proximally from within the defect toward the sacroiliac joint for fixation into the strong, intact, posterior iliac bone. When the acetabular columns are compromised, screws or pins are placed in an antegrade fashion from the iliac wing distally into the superior pubic rami to reconstruct the anterior column and into the ischium to reconstruct the posterior column. A triangulation guide can be used for antegrade screw or pin placement. A portion of the precontoured protrusio cage should rest on intact host bone (at a minimum, the flanges should contact intact bone). Initial screws are drilled and measured for both the iliac and the ischial flange, and these screws and the cage are then removed. I cement the defect, incorporating any previously placed screws or pins, and then place the cage or ring. If necessary, mesh can be placed medially to prevent intrapelvic extrusion of cement.

The two initial flange screws are quickly replaced to provide initial fixation to the cage. Additional screws through the protrusion device are quickly inserted through the doughy cement into intact bone, with dome screws placed first. Flange screws are placed subsequently because they are typically placed into host bone. Because a protrusio cage typically is seated against the pelvis in a vertical fashion, particular attention is given to cementation of the polyethylene acetabular liner. The back surface of the liner is roughened for improved cement fixation, and a constrained liner is often used. If the protrusio cage is of sufficient size, an alternative technique is to cement a metal-backed acetabular component into the cage and then insert the liner in a standard fashion.

The patient is promptly mobilized postoperatively. Using a constrained acetabular liner makes bracing unnecessary. Patients are advised that an assistive device will be required for ambulation.

Proximal Femur Reconstruction

Reconstruction of a proximal femur with extensive metastatic destruction is best achieved with a proximal femoral replacement implant (**Figure 3**). This device allows immediate weight bearing and rehabilitation. An allograft prosthetic composite is not appropriate in patients with metastatic disease because prolonged protected weight bearing may be required, delayed union or nonunion of the allograft to the host bone may occur, and the allograft should be shielded from postoperative radiation therapy. With intact acetabular cartilage and

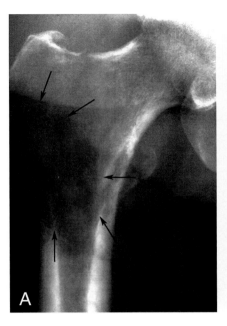 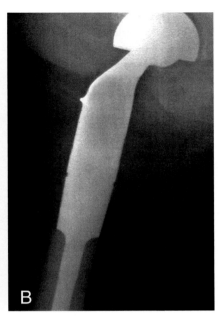

Figure 3 Metastatic breast carcinoma in a 48-year-old woman with severe hip and thigh pain. **A**, AP radiograph shows marked destruction of the proximal femur (arrows). **B**, AP radiograph obtained after resection of proximal femur and reconstruction with a proximal femoral replacement implant with a bipolar articulation. The patient was able to ambulate with a walker.

no significant metastatic compromise of the acetabulum, a bipolar articulation to the proximal femoral replacement is favored to enhance stability. A constrained liner should be considered if an acetabular reconstruction is performed. Intraoperative flexibility should be provided by a modular implant system.

A standard surgical approach to the hip is typically sufficient, with more distal extension used to access the mid- to proximal femur. The abductor tendons are preserved and, if possible, a portion of the greater trochanter is retained with the tendons. The rotational position of the femur is marked before hip dislocation as an aid during implant cementation. The hip is dislocated and the diseased portion of the proximal femur resected as en bloc as possible. The length of the resected segment is measured, if possible, to aid in selecting the proper length of the implant. The implant should be seated on solid cortical bone with no gross evidence of disease. The

canal is reamed for a 2-mm cement mantle. The intramedullary stem length should be 135 to 200 mm with an anterior bow, unless the resection level is distal to the mid-diaphysis. A trial reduction should be performed to assess limb length and hip stability. Care should be taken to avoid excessive limb lengthening, and the patient should be counseled preoperatively about a change in limb length. With a more proximal resection, a cement restrictor is used. For more distal resections, this plug may not be functional or necessary. Optimal cement technique is used to cement the implant in approximately 15° to 20° of anteversion.

Soft-tissue reconstruction is critical to optimal postoperative function. The acetabular capsule, iliopsoas tendon, and short external rotators are closed around the neck of the implant in a purse-string–like manner. The abductor tendon (or greater trochanter) is secured to the implant's trochanteric portion with nonabsorbable suture, and the vastus lateralis is reapproximated to the implant. The deep tissues should be sutured to completely enclose the implant.

Skin may be closed with staples or nonabsorbable suture. In patients at risk of delayed wound healing, such as those who have had radiation therapy, I close the skin with nylon sutures and retain these for 2 to 3 weeks to ensure proper healing. The surgeon should verify that satisfactory healing of the surgical site is present before postoperative radiation therapy begins. Radiation therapy, up to a dose of 3,000 cGy, typically starts 10 to 14 days after surgery.

Closed suction drains should be used because patients are at risk of postoperative hematoma. Antibiotic prophylaxis (typically a cephalosporin) should be administered while drains are in situ. I favor removal of drains 24 to 48 hours after surgery.

Current implant designs do not permit effective healing of host soft tissues to metal implants. However, with scarring of the deep soft tissues, satisfactory function can be obtained with sufficient postoperative healing and rehabilitation.

Patients are promptly mobilized postoperatively, and rehabilitation should emphasize ambulation. Range-of-motion and abduction exercises should not be performed for several months. Survival typically is not long enough for hip strength to develop, so a Trendelenburg gait is common and patients will use a cane. I try to avoid a hip abduction brace in these patients by using either a bipolar articulation or a constrained acetabular liner.

Avoiding Pitfalls and Complications

Failure to appreciate the extent of metastatic bone disease is a pitfall to be avoided. The surgeon should have good preoperative imaging studies and anticipate more bone compromise than indicated on those images (similar to debris-induced osteolysis). Thorough gross tumor removal should be performed, and weak, compromised, diseased bone should be removed. This technique minimizes the risk of local tumor progression that would compromise fixation and ultimately cause reconstruction to fail. This is particularly true with disease that does not respond to adjuvant therapies. Various implants and internal fixation devices should be available at the time of the procedure in case additional bone removal is necessary or fracture occurs.

Instability of the hip, particularly after complex acetabular reconstructions, can be minimized by appropriate positioning of the acetabular component, avoiding neck impingement, and using large-diameter femoral heads and constrained acetabular liners. For patients with metastatic bone disease and limited life expectancy, I favor using a constrained liner.

Planning and technique can minimize other complications. Extensive intraoperative blood loss can occur. Preoperative angiography with embolization is essential for vascular metastases, although substantial bleeding may occur even with embolization. Rapid tumor removal is critical, and bleeding usually subsides markedly thereafter. Problematic bleeding after tumor removal can be treated by placing a layer of bone cement to cauterize the bleeding bone.

Anesthesia personnel must be prepared for potentially severe intraoperative blood loss and sudden cardiopulmonary events. Fat embolization, particularly during preparation and cementation of a long-stemmed femoral component, can result in intraoperative cardiac arrest. The risk of embolism is minimized by slow reaming of the femoral canal with narrow, fluted reamers, frequent suctioning of the medullary contents from the canal, avoidance of a cement restrictor, distal venting of the medullary contents, and controlled insertion of the implant.

Patients with metastatic disease of the hip are at higher risk of deep vein thrombus. Postoperative prophylaxis with low molecular weight heparin is appropriate. Clear guidelines do not exist for duration of therapy in these patients. I routinely administer such prophylaxis for 2 weeks. However, in patients with additional risk factors (prior deep vein thrombosis), prophylaxis with low molecular weight heparin (or Coumadin) is extended to 6 weeks.

References

Marco RA, Sheth DS, Boland PJ, et al : Functional and oncological outcome of acetabular reconstruction for the treatment of metastatic disease. *J Bone Joint Surg Am* 2000;82:642-651.

O'Connor MI: Surgical management of metastatic disease of the pelvis, in Fitzgerald RH Jr, Kaufer H, Malkani AL (eds): *Orthopaedics*. St. Louis, MO, Mosby, 2002, pp 1108-1115.

Ward WG, Holsenbeck S, Dorey F, Spang J, Howe D: Metastatic disease of the femur: Surgical management. *Clin Orthop* 2003;415:S230-S240.

Wunder JS, Ferguson PC, Griffin AM, Pressman A, Bell RS: Acetabular metastases: Planning for reconstruction and review of results. *Clin Orthop* 2003;415:187-197.

Coding

CPT Codes		Corresponding ICD-9 Codes		
Surgical Treatment: Pelvis				
27049	Radical resection of tumor, soft tissue of pelvis and hip area (eg, malignant neoplasm)	171.3 733.14	171.6	172.7
27065	Excision of bone cyst or benign tumor; superficial (wing of ilium, symphysis pubis, or greater trochanter of femur), with or without autograft	213.6 733.22	733.20 733.29	733.21 756.54
27066	Excision of bone cyst or benign tumor; deep, with or without autograft	213.6 733.22	733.20 733.29	733.21 756.54
27070	Partial excision (craterization, saucerization), (eg, osteomyelitis or bone abscess); superficial (eg, wing of ilium, symphysis pubis, or greater trochanter of femur)	730.05 998.5	730.15	730.25
27071	Partial excision, deep (subfascial or intramuscular)	730.05 998.5	730.15	730.25
27075	Radical resection of tumor or infection; wing of ilium, one pubic or ischial ramus or symphysis pubis	170.6 730.15	198.5 998.5	730.05
27076	Radical resection for tumor, ilium, including acetabulum, both pubic rami, or ischium and acetabulum	170.6 730.15	198.5 998.5	730.05
27077	Radical resection for tumor, innominate bone, total	170.6 730.15	198.5 998.5	730.05
27226	Open treatment of posterior or anterior acetabular wall fracture, with internal fixation	808.0 808.53	808.1	808.43
27227	Open treatment of acetabular fracture(s) involving anterior or posterior (one) column, or a fracture running transversely across the acetabulum, with internal fixation	808.0 808.49	808.1 808.53	808.43
27228	Open treatment of acetabular fracture(s) involving anterior and posterior (two) columns, includes T-fracture and both column fracture with complete articular detachment, or single column or transverse fracture with associated acetabular wall fracture, with internal fixation	808.0 808.49	808.1 808.53	808.43

Coding Continued

CPT Codes		Corresponding ICD-9 Codes		
Surgical Treatment: Hip				
27125	Hemiarthroplasty, hip, partial (eg, femoral stem prosthesis, bipolar arthroplasty)	715.15 716.15 733.42	715.25 718.6 905.6	715.35 733.14
27130	Arthroplasty, acetabular and proximal femoral prosthetic replacement (total hip arthroplasty), with or without autograft or allograft	711.45 714.30 715.35 718.6 733.42	711.95 715.15 716.15 720.0 808.0	714.0 715.25 718.5 733.14 905.6
27132	Conversion of previous hip surgery to total hip arthroplasty, with or without autograft or allograft	715.15 718.2 733.14 996.4	715.25 718.5 733.42 996.66	715.35 718.6 905.6 996.77
27187	Prophylactic treatment (nailing, pinning, plating, or wiring), with or without methylmethacrylate, femoral neck and proximal femur	170.7 733.20	198.5 733.29	213.7
27236	Open treatment of femoral fracture, proximal end, neck, internal fixation or prosthetic replacement	733.14 820.03 820.13	820.00 820.10 820.8	820.02 820.12 820.9
27244	Treatment of intertrochanteric, peritrochanteric, or subtrochanteric femoral fracture; with plate/screw type implant, with or without cerclage	733.14 820.21 820.8	733.15 820.22 820.9	820.20 820.3
27245	Open treatment of intertrochanteric, peritrochanteric, or subtrochanteric femoral fracture; with intramedullary implant, with or without interlocking screws or cerclage	170.7 733.15 733.22 820.9	198.5 733.20 733.29	733.14 733.21 820.8

CPT copyright ©2004 by the American Medical Association. All Rights Reserved.

Chapter 26

Total Hip Arthroplasty: Inflammatory Arthritis and Other Conditions Affecting Bone Quality

Andrew A. Freiberg, MD

 ## Indications

Hip pathology in patients with inflammatory arthritis and other conditions affecting bone quality are unique to each diagnosis. The most common problem is arthritis with joint space loss, but displaced fracture of the femoral neck, femoral neck fracture nonunion, and osteonecrosis of the femoral head also may lead to total hip arthroplasty (THA) in these patients.

Marked pain and functional disability are the main clinical indicators for THA in patients with these conditions. Hip arthroplasty and major joint replacement have revolutionized the care of patients with inflammatory arthritis and become standard treatments. However, it is important to consider the risks and benefits of THA in patients with functional disabilities caused by multiple musculoskeletal problems. Many of the diagnoses discussed in this chapter are associated with serious medical conditions for which THA is a less well-established treatment. The risks of surgery are therefore greater, and medical management should be optimized before THA is considered.

Inflammatory arthritides often are associated with reduced bone quality because of disuse osteopenia linked to polyarticular joint disease and the effects of chronic corticosteroid treatment. Bone deficiencies are often present in patients with synovitis with periarticular bone erosion. Altered bone quality is present in many other conditions as well, ranging from weak, soft bone (in most patients) to sclerotic, brittle bone. The surgeon must decide whether a patient's bone quality is sufficient for a successful arthroplasty.

Contraindications

Any active infection (local, systemic, or distant) is a contraindication to THA, as is the inability to control systemic medical problems so that surgery can be performed safely. With some conditions, medical intervention can reduce the impact of systemic disease; therefore, THA should occur only after medical optimization. THA is contraindicated if the local bone quality of the proximal femur or acetabulum is so compromised that durability is unlikely to be achieved. Pharmacologic or other systemic treatment may be used to improve bone quality preoperatively if such treatment can provide a rapid enough benefit to be practical.

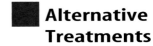 ## Alternative Treatments

THA poses excessive risk for some patients because of the possibility of systemic or surgical complications. Medical management is therefore the main treatment alternative to THA in patients with inflammatory disease. Synovectomy may be considered in young patients with well-preserved joint space and synovitis uncontrolled by pharmacologic treatment.

For most diagnoses (other than inflammatory disease), the main treatment alternative to THA is hip resection arthroplasty (Girdlestone procedure). It is reasonable to consider this procedure for some patients with severe pain who can tolerate surgery but who cannot undergo THA because of inadequate bone quality, risk of infection, or other concerns. However, patients should understand that the Girdlestone procedure usually provides good pain relief but poor functionality. Postoperatively, most patients can walk relatively short distances but require two-arm support. Careful consideration is necessary before suggesting resection arthroplasty in ambulatory patients with conditions that might preclude two-arm support, such as inflammatory arthritis, polyarticular arthritis, and/or compromised upper extremity function. Hip arthrodesis usually is not an option in patients with systemic disease for whom multiple lower extremity joint problems and bilateral hip disease are common.

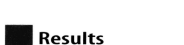

■ Results

Rheumatoid Arthritis
THA can produce dramatic pain reduction and some functional improvement, limited mainly by polyarticular disease, in patients with rheumatoid arthritis (RA). The durability of implants in patients with RA is controversial, and studies differ on whether durability is improved or reduced compared to the general population. Poor bone quality negatively affects durability, whereas reduced activity probably exerts a protective effect. Cemented and uncemented acetabular and femoral components have been used successfully, although there is an increased risk of late prosthetic infection in patients with RA.

Ankylosing Spondylitis
Most reports of THA in ankylosing spondylitis show reduced pain and improved function, partly as a result of improved hip mobility. The rates of aseptic loosening of cemented implants probably are somewhat higher for this diagnosis compared with rates for the general population. It is not yet known if selected use of uncemented implants can produce improved results. The degree to which this diagnosis increases the risk of heterotopic ossification remains controversial, with some studies demonstrating a high risk and others reporting much less.

Psoriatic Arthritis
Pain relief and functional improvement have been reported as a result of THA in patients with psoriatic arthritis. The risk of infection probably is increased, partly because of the potential for bacteremia associated with colonized skin lesions.

Systemic Lupus Erythematosus
THA may be required for either osteonecrosis of the femoral head or joint space loss. Although the results of THA in patients with lupus probably do not differ dramatically from the results in other age-matched patients, there may be an increased risk of infection for patients with lupus.

■ Technique

Rheumatoid Arthritis
I prefer to use uncemented acetabular components in patients with RA because aseptic loosening does not appear to be a problem. Acetabular protrusio is not uncommon in RA and is managed according to the principles discussed in chapter 18. Femoral fixation with cemented or uncemented implants is possible, with the implant choice being the surgeon's preference based on bone quality, bone geometry, and patient demographic factors. A small bone structure, especially of the femur, is common in patients with juvenile rheumatoid arthritis. It is important that preoperative templating ensure that there is an adequate range of implant sizes available at surgery.

The possibility of cervical spine instability, temporomandibular joint stiffness, and micrognathia should be carefully evaluated and optimally managed by the anesthesia team.

Ankylosing Spondylitis
Surgical exposure may be more difficult in patients with this diagnosis because of hip stiffness and large flexion contractures. Some surgeons prefer an anterior or anterolateral surgical approach when severe flexion contractures are present.

Implant fixation is performed according to surgeon preference, based on bone quality, bone geometry, and patient demographic factors.

Large flexion contractures usually can be improved with anterior capsulectomy. Severe adduction contractures occasionally require adductor tenotomy; the need for tenotomy can be determined at the conclusion of the procedure and can be performed percutaneously at the adductor origin from the pelvis. Because of the potential risk of heterotopic ossification, many surgeons use some form of heterotopic bone prophylaxis postoperatively (either radiation with uncemented component interface shielding or an anti-inflammatory agent) because it is necessary to optimize the hip range of motion in patients with stiff spines.

Psoriatic Arthritis
The most important treatment principle is to avoid skin incision through active psoriatic lesions, which are highly colonized by bacteria. Aggressive preoperative dermatologic treatment to rid the proposed incision area of psoriatic lesions also is recommended.

Systemic Lupus Erythematosus
Although osteonecrosis of the femoral head often is the indication for arthroplasty, and the acetabular cartilage may look normal, THA is recommended over hemiarthroplasty.

Other Miscellaneous Conditions Affecting Bone Quality
GAUCHER'S DISEASE
Gaucher's disease is a lysosomal storage disorder characterized by the accumulation of glucocerebroside in the reticuloendothelial system. It is associated with osteonecrosis of the femoral head and osteopenia.

Current reports in a modest number of cases suggest that THA can be successful in patients with Gauch-

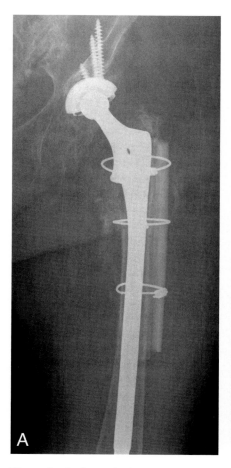

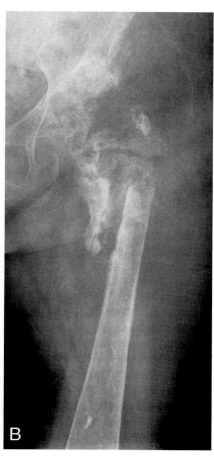

Figure 1 Radiograph of a 73-year-old woman following THA for osteonecrosis secondary to Gaucher's disease. The procedure was revised 5 years later because of aseptic loosening. **A,** A second revision was performed for recurrent dislocation, and deep infection developed postoperatively. **B,** Control of the infection could be achieved only after all implants and nonviable bone were removed.

er's disease. However, aseptic loosening and deep infections may compromise the long-term survival of the hip prosthesis (**Figure 1**). Limited results suggest that reduced bone ingrowth potential and infiltration by Gaucher cells may make uncemented implant fixation less successful, but the small number of reports precludes definite guidelines. I prefer to cement the femoral prosthesis in most of these patients because there are usually large femoral canals that cannot readily be treated with uncemented devices. I usually use uncemented, porous-coated titanium acetabular component implants, often with supplemen-

tal screw fixation. Impaction grafting may be considered for revision surgeries. The role of enzyme replacement therapy in these patients is not yet fully understood; it may be important in controlling systemic and local disease.

OSTEOPETROSIS
Osteopetrosis is a systemic disease characterized by osteoclast dysfunction and dense sclerotic bone with diminished or absent medullary canals. The most common indications for THA are degenerative arthritis and hip fracture nonunion. Reports indicate that THA can produce satisfactory re-

sults in patients with osteopetrosis without excessive risk of infection or periprosthetic fracture.

Surgical challenges principally relate to the sclerotic, brittle bone and its effect on bone preparation and implant fixation (**Figure 2**). Acetabular reaming can be performed with standard instrumentation. Femoral preparation frequently involves creation of a medullary canal; fluoroscopic guidance can help prevent femoral perforation. Cemented and uncemented sockets have been used successfully, although most reports of femoral fixation describe cemented implants, which are effective despite the presence of sclerotic bone.

OSTEOMALACIA
Osteomalacia is now uncommon because of improved nutrition and dietary supplementation of calcium and vitamin D. Demineralization may appear radiographically as blurring of the trabecular pattern in the metaphyseal/diaphyseal regions of long bones. Pathologic bowing of the femur and tibia occur late in the disease. An important clinical distinction is that osteoporosis is painless unless there are fractures, whereas osteomalacia often is associated with diffuse pain. THA should be delayed until correctable nutritional or physiologic causes have been addressed.

OSTEOGENESIS IMPERFECTA
Osteogenesis imperfecta is a type of bone dysplasia sometimes associated with dramatically deformed bones. It also frequently presents as multiple pathologic fractures. Osteoarthritis of the hip may develop in some patients. Common problems include a narrow, anterolaterally bowed femur and acetabular protrusio. Only a few cases of THA have been reported in patients with osteogenesis imperfecta, with mostly satisfactory results. One report of severe intrapelvic protrusio of a bipolar hemiarthroplasty suggests that hemiarthroplasty may be contraindi-

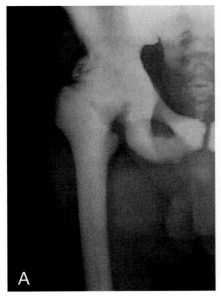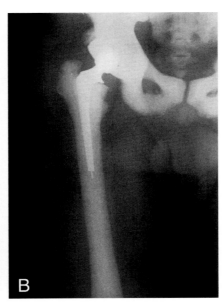

Figure 2 **A**, Preoperative AP radiograph of the right hip of a 47-year-old man with osteopetrosis and advanced osteoarthritis. **B**, AP radiograph obtained 4 years postoperatively shows that the implants are stable. (Reproduced with permission from Strickland JP, Berry DJ: Total joint arthroplasty in patients with osteopetrosis: A case report and review of the literature. *J Arthroplasty,* in press.)

cated because the abnormal pelvic bone may deform over time.

Insufficient information is available to provide definite treatment guidelines; however, it is recognized that weak bone can make uncemented components difficult to implant. Small bone size can require miniaturized or custom implants.

HEMOPHILIA
Hemophilia is associated with chronic synovitis, leading to arthritis. The development of arthropathy can be significantly delayed and even prevented with effective factor replacement therapy. However, some patients become candidates for THA because of end-stage arthritis.

Effective perioperative management of coagulopathy, sophisticated factor replacement protocols, and the help of hematology experts ensures that THA can be performed safely in most patients.

Patients who are HIV-positive may be candidates for THA if their CD-4 lymphocyte counts are adequate.

The use of protease inhibitors has been associated with the development of osteonecrosis of the hip. Because many of these patients are young, uncemented fixation should be considered if the bone stock can support it.

Patients with hemophilia have demonstrated substantial benefit from THA. However, both cemented and uncemented implants have a high rate of late aseptic loosening, and patients with hemophilia have a higher risk of postoperative and late hematogenous infection. Technical challenges include bone deformities, joint stiffness, and a smaller, weaker bone structure in some patients.

RENAL FAILURE
Renal failure is associated with reduced bone quality. Patients with renal failure may become candidates for THA because they have a displaced femoral neck fracture, osteoarthritis, or osteonecrosis (in some cases related to corticosteroid use in renal transplants).

THA results for patients with renal failure generally have been worse

than THA results in the general population, principally as a result of aseptic loosening and infection. Infection risk appears to be considerably higher in patients on chronic hemodialysis, probably because of transient bacteremia and immunosuppression. Results of THA in patients who have undergone renal transplantation are encouraging. However, many of these patients are young, and increased life expectancy means they may experience aseptic loosening and bearing-surface, wear-related implant failure. If possible, elective THA should be delayed in candidates for renal transplantation until after transplant surgery, when dialysis is not required.

No strict guidelines for implant fixation are available. Uncemented implants may be considered for young patients with adequate bone quality; intermediate results have been promising. The proximal femur can remodel in patients with renal disease, resulting in a large diameter femoral canal. When this occurs, I prefer a cemented stem over a large uncemented femoral stem. When using cemented implants in patients with high risk of infection, antibiotic-impregnated cement may be used. Poor bone quality increases the risk of intraoperative fracture during bone preparation, especially for uncemented implants. The risk of postoperative fracture is also increased.

PIGMENTED VILLONODULAR SYNOVITIS
Pigmented villonodular synovitis is a monoarticular synovial disease that can lead to advanced joint space destruction, an indication for THA. Thorough débridement of villonodular synovitis at arthroplasty is important because recurrence is possible (though uncommon), even after arthroplasty. Management of the large subchondral cysts typically present in end-stage disease is the main technical issue in these patients. In most patients, these cysts represent cavitary acetabular defects;

they can be treated with particulate cancellous bone grafting.

PAGET'S DISEASE

A complete discussion of THA in the context of Paget's disease is presented in chapter 19.

SICKLE CELL HEMOGLOBINOPATHIES

A complete discussion of THA in the context of sickle cell hemoglobinopathies is presented in chapter 28.

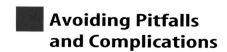

Avoiding Pitfalls and Complications

Many of the diseases described in this chapter are systemic disorders with associated medical problems. A multidisciplinary team approach, careful preoperative medical optimization, and intraoperative and postoperative medical treatment can reduce the risk of many medical complications.

An increased risk of infection is associated with many of these diagnoses. Antibiotic-impregnated cement can be used for implant fixation and may reduce the risk of early infection. Many patients with these diagnoses also have poor skin quality; thus, careful handling of the skin may reduce the risk of wound healing complications. Many patients with inflammatory disease who take immunosuppressive or disease-modifying agents can stop taking those agents for several weeks perioperatively, which may reduce the risk of wound and infection problems; however, the effectiveness of this regimen has not been proved. Patients on long-term corticosteroid treatment need appropriate perioperative stress steroid doses.

Most patients with these diagnoses are at increased risk of intraoperative bone fracture because of poor bone quality, bone deformity, or joint stiffness. The hip should be gently manipulated intraoperatively, especially during initial hip dislocation. Acetabular reaming and femoral instrumentation, especially for uncemented implants, should be performed cautiously because of the weakened bone. When bone deformity is present, intraoperative radiographs or fluoroscopy may be used to optimize implant position and reduce the risk of bone perforation.

References

Bhattacharyya T, Iorio R, Healy WI: Rate of and risk factors for acute inpatient mortality after orthopaedic surgery. *J Bone Joint Surg Am* 2002;84:562-572.

Boos N, Krushell R, Ganz R, Muller ME: Total hip arthroplasty after previous proximal femoral osteotomy. *J Bone Joint Surg Br* 1997;79:247-253.

Ilyas I, Moreau P: Simultaneous bilateral total hip arthroplasty in sickle cell disease. *J Arthroplasty* 2002;17:441-445.

Kelley SS, Lachiewicz PF, Gilbert MS, Bolander ME, Jankiewicz JJ: Hip arthroplasty in hemophilic arthropathy. *J Bone Joint Surg Am* 1995;77:828-834.

Lebel E, Itzchaki M, Hadas-Halpern I, Zimran A, Elstein D: Outcome of total hip arthroplasty in patients with Gaucher's disease. *J Arthroplasty* 2001;16:7-12.

Katsimihas M, Taylor AH, Lee MB, Sarangi PP, Learmonth ID: Cementless acetabular replacement in patients with rheumatoid arthritis: A 6 to 14 year prospective study. *J Arthroplasty* 2003;18:16-22.

Marco RAW, Sheth DS, Boland PJ, et al: Functional and oncological outcome of acetabular reconstruction for the treatment of metastatic disease. *J Bone Joint Surg Am* 2000;82:642-651.

Mears DC, Velyvis JH: Primary arthroplasty after acetabular fracture. *Inst Course Lect* 2001;50:335-354.

Panagiotopoulos KP, Robbins GM, Masri BA, Duncan CP: Conversion of hip arthrodesis to total hip arthroplasty. *Inst Course Lect* 2001;50:297-305.

Parvizi J, Schall DM, Lewallen DG, Sim FH: Outcome of uncemented hip arthroplasty components in patients with Paget's disease. *Clin Orthop* 2002;403:127-134.

Swanson KC, Pritchard DJ, Sim FH: Surgical treatment of metastatic disease of the femur. *J Am Acad Orthop Surg* 2000;8:56-65.

Thomason HC III, Lachiewicz PF: The influence of technique of fixation of primary total hip arthroplasty in patients with rheumatoid arthritis. *J Arthroplasty* 2001;16:628-634.

Coding

CPT Codes		Corresponding ICD-9 Codes		
27130	Arthroplasty, acetabular and proximal femoral prosthetic replacement (total hip arthroplasty), with or without autograft or allograft	711.45 714.30 715.35 718.6 733.42	711.95 715.15 716.15 720.0 808.0	714.0 715.25 718.5 733.14 905.6
27132	Conversion of previous hip surgery to total hip arthroplasty, with or without autograft or allograft	714.0 715.25 718.2 733.14 996.4	714.30 715.35 718.5 733.42 996.66	715.15 718.6 905.6 996.77

CPT copyright ©2004 by the American Medical Association. All Rights Reserved.

Chapter 27

Total Hip Arthroplasty in Obese Patients
Craig J. Della Valle, MD

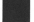 ## Indications

Obesity has been associated with degenerative joint disease of the hip; given the near-epidemic proportions of the population who fit the criteria for obesity, orthopaedic surgeons are encountering an increasing number of patients who have severe degenerative joint disease of the hip. Obesity is defined as a body mass index (BMI) of 30 to 40, with morbid obesity defined as a BMI greater than 40 (BMI is defined as weight in kilograms divided by height in meters squared).

Total hip arthroplasty (THA) is indicated for patients in whom nonsurgical treatment for end stage hip disease has failed. Although the main indications for THA are failure to achieve adequate pain relief and poor function, patients who have severe deformity or who show radiographic evidence of progressive acetabular bone loss also benefit from THA. The term "indications" represents the end point of a complex decision-making process undertaken by physician and patient that requires thoughtful consideration of the potential risks and benefits of THA. With obese patients, the question is whether the risks and benefits of THA are the same as those for patients of normal weight.

Obesity is a risk factor for perioperative morbidity. Medical comorbidities, such as diabetes mellitus, coronary artery disease, and pulmonary dysfunction are common in the obese population. A thorough preoperative evaluation by an internal medicine specialist or a primary care physician is critical to determine if the patient is an appropriate risk from a medical perspective and to identify medical conditions that might be managed preoperatively. Obese patients are also at increased risk for wound healing complications, which may be related to poor vascularity of the fatty subcutaneous tissues. In addition, evidence indicates that even nondiabetic obese patients have immune dysfunction.

Increased body weight places higher stress on the THA components and the fixation interfaces, which may lead to a higher rate of mechanical failure. Increased weight also heightens joint reaction forces that might lead to increased wear of the bearing surface. However, obese patients are typically less active than patients of normal weight, and obesity may therefore be protective in terms of bearing-surface wear. I have found that long-term complications such as osteolysis are actually inversely related to patient weight, presumably secondary to relative inactivity.

Unfortunately, few studies specifically address the outcomes of THA in obese patients. Despite the theoretical concerns outlined above, most of the available literature suggests that even morbidly obese patients have satisfactory outcomes, and rates of both orthopaedic and medical complications are similar if not equal to those for patients of normal weight. Although the available literature is affected by its poor statistical power because of the relatively small populations examined, the data suggest that THA can be quite successful in obese patients.

 ## Contraindications

There are no specific contraindications to THA in obese patients. However, extra precautions are needed to ensure that patients have been adequately evaluated by an internist or primary care physician to ensure that any existing medical comorbidities are managed preoperatively. The skin of obese patients is also prone to rashes; thus, the surgeon should make sure that the skin in the operative area is intact before proceeding with surgery.

Alternative Treatments

Nonsurgical treatment for degenerative hip joint disease typically consists of systemic medications (eg, acetaminophen and anti-inflammatory medications), activity modification, using as-

Table 1 Results of Total Hip Arthroplasty in Obese Patients

Author(s) (Year)	Number of Hips	Implant Type	Mean Patient Age (Range)	Mean Follow-up (Range)	Results
Chan and Villar (1996)	81	Not specified	69 years (range not given)	Not given	Mean improvement in quality of life no different than non-obese patients
Jiganti, et al (1993)	41	Not specified	65.9 years (range not given)	Not given	No higher risk of perioperative complications in obese patients
Lehman, et al (1994)	63	Uncemented femoral and acetabular components	50 years (17-72)	48 months (24-89)	Obesity not associated with increased risk of complications or failure
Soballe, et al (1987)	41	Cemented Lubinus cup and stem	70 years (28-89)	Minimum 5 years	Obese patients not at higher risk for complications or prosthetic loosening

sistive devices, and occasionally intra-articular injections of corticosteroids. Viscosupplementation has also been described for treating hip osteoarthritis but is not currently US Food and Drug Administration approved. I do not find physical therapy particularly helpful in treating degenerative joint disease of the hip. Significant weight loss typically is an unrealistic goal, but gastric reduction surgery may become an option for the morbidly obese. Nonsurgical treatment should be attempted in most patients prior to surgical intervention, but it is not without risks and these must be considered as well. Long-term use of nonsteroidal anti-inflammatory agents may result in significant morbidity, particularly in older patients. Furthermore, the natural history of hip osteoarthritis is poor, and an unnecessary delay in surgical intervention is equally inappropriate. Alternative surgical options to THA include osteotomy, resurfacing procedures, and arthrodesis, all of which have their own specific indications that are covered elsewhere in this book.

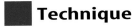

Results

Few studies have specifically examined the results of THA in obese patients or compared obese patients with patients of normal weight. The available literature suggests that obese patients enjoy excellent pain relief, an improved quality of life, and have good overall satisfaction. However, some studies cite decreased functional outcomes and also suggest that complication rates for orthopaedic and nonorthopaedic procedures do not differ significantly from those of normal-weight patients. However, a trend toward increased surgical time and greater blood loss has been identified in obese patients (**Table 1**).

Early studies documented a higher rate of femoral component fracture in larger patients, but more recent literature has not identified this as a substantial problem in obese patients, secondary to improvements in metallurgy and manufacturing techniques, including using forged alloy components. Similarly, earlier studies found aseptic loosening more common among patients of greater body weight when cemented components were used. More recent literature citing the use of uncemented components has not confirmed these findings, although the populations studied were small with little statistical power. No long-term studies are currently available to determine if using more modern components is associated with a higher rate of mechanical failure in the obese patient.

Technique

The surgical technique for THA in the obese patient follows the same principles as a standard THA. Patient size, however, may make certain aspects of the procedure more challenging. It is important to recognize the patient's obesity pattern. Men typically have a more truncal pattern of obesity, whereas women tend to accumulate adipose tissue in the lower extremities. Truncal obesity patterns create significant patient-positioning difficulties, but lower extremity obesity can be more challenging in terms of exposure, bone preparation, implant insertion, and wound closure.

Patient Positioning
Appropriate patient positioning requires special attention in the obese patient. Most positioning devices for stabilizing the pelvis in the lateral decubitus position rely on anchoring the

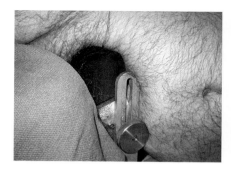

Figure 1 Anterior positioning device in an obese patient. Note that the soft tissue of the abdomen is in direct contact with the metallic portion of the device. The device must be appropriately padded to avoid injury to the overlying skin.

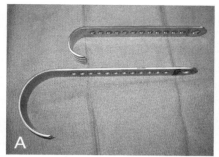
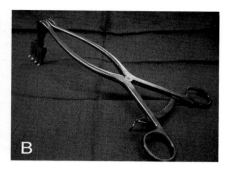

Figure 2 **A**, Standard (top) and deep (bottom) anterior blades of the Charnley-type retractor. The deep blades are needed for appropriate retraction in the obese patient. **B**, Large self-retaining retractor used for soft-tissue retraction in obese patients.

symphysis pubis anteriorly and the sacrum posteriorly. This can be very difficult in patients with truncal obesity. In some patients it may be impossible to obtain adequate pelvic stability, and in these situations a large beanbag may be necessary. In some patients it may be impossible to obtain adequate pelvic stability, as the large amounts of adipose tissue make it difficult to obtain rigid fixation against the bony pelvis anteriorly and posteriorly. For these patients, a beanbag may provide better stability by cradling the patient's entire body.

It is also important to ensure that the soft tissues of the anterior abdomen are not placed under excessive pressure. Because damage to the skin can occur, appropriate padding in this area is often needed (**Figure 1**). Malpositioning of the anterior stabilizer, inferior to the symphysis pubis, can also cause pressure in the femoral triangle, with the potential for disastrous complications secondary to neurovascular compromise. Because the symphysis pubis may be more difficult to palpate, such events may be more common in the obese patient. The surgeon must ensure that the pelvis is situated appropriately in both the coronal and transverse planes to avoid implant malposition. An axillary roll placed beneath the down chest helps

prevent excessive weight from being placed on the dependent chest and upper extremity. Padding the down leg is also recommended (particularly beneath the peroneal nerve at the knee) to avoid down-leg injury. Because surgical times are often increased in obese patients and their skin may be more prone to injury secondary to impaired blood supply, careful patient positioning is of the utmost importance.

Exposure

Surgical exposure can be a substantial challenge in the obese patient, particularly if there is excessive adipose tissue in the incision area. Generous incisions are often needed to obtain adequate visualization, and care must be taken with soft-tissue dissection to avoid compromising the vascularity of the soft-tissue envelope, which is already more fragile in obese patients. Deeper versions of the Charnley-type retractors commonly used in THA are often required (**Figure 2**, *A*), and large self-retaining retractors assist with obtaining adequate visualization (**Figure 2**, *B*). Whether using an anterior or posterior approach, the femur is often more difficult to retract to accomplish acetabular exposure, and release of a portion of the gluteus maximus insertion may be required.

Bone Preparation

Bone preparation in the obese patient is the same as for a standard THA in a

patient of normal weight. When reaming the acetabulum, it is important to avoid damage to the acetabular columns because the retracted femur may push the reamer into either the anterior or posterior column, depending on the surgical approach used. This phenomenon may be exacerbated in obese and more muscular patients where exposure can be more difficult. When preparing the proximal femur, the surgeon must be aware of the tendency to broach or ream in varus, which can be exacerbated in the obese patient. If a cemented femoral stem is selected, reaming of the femoral canal is avoided, and the largest broach that fits easily within the femoral canal is selected to allow for an appropriate cement mantle. If an uncemented femoral component is selected, axial and rotational stability of the broach is imperative to ensure adequate implant stability for bone ingrowth to occur.

In general, obese patients tend to have good bone quality in both the femur and acetabulum. Given the oftentimes greater difficulty with exposure, uncemented fixation is an attractive option for these patients. Although excellent results have been reported for both cemented and more modern uncemented femoral components, obese patients tend to have narrow femoral canals, further making uncemented fixation desirable.

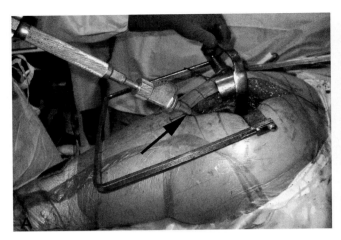 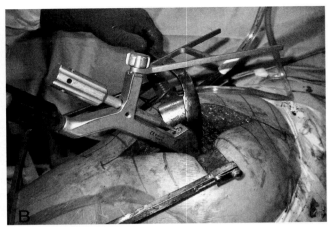

Figure 3 **A**, Straight acetabular component inserter can impinge on the soft tissues (arrow) of the thigh and lead to vertical component position in the obese patient. **B**, Offset acetabular component inserter avoids impingement on the soft tissues of the thigh and assists with appropriate component position.

Prosthesis Implantation

Prosthetic implantation is performed according to standard THA protocols to ensure optimal component alignment. Surgeons must keep in mind, however, that prosthetic implantation may be more difficult in the obese patient because of the problems obtaining exposure (as previously described). In particular, obese patients are at risk for vertical placement of the acetabular component because they may have a large amount of soft tissue over the lateral side of the hip that may cause a more vertical inclination of the acetabular insertion device (**Figure 3**). In these patients, using an offset insertion device can be quite helpful in obtaining appropriate acetabular component inclination. The typical landmarks used for acetabular component anteversion may also be altered in obese patients.

Femoral component insertion may also be difficult in the obese patient. If an uncemented femoral component is used, appropriate exposure of the proximal femur must be obtained to ensure adequate visualization during implant insertion so that fracture and malposition are avoided. Similar issues arise if a cemented device is used. Surgeons should also realize that intraoperative determina-

tions of limb length may also be more difficult in the obese patient, particularly if the down leg is used as a comparison because of increased pelvic tilt in obese patients lying in the lateral decubitus position. Multiple methods for determining limb length intraoperatively should be used to avoid excessive limb lengthening.

Wound Closure

Wound closure is a critical part of THA in the obese patient. With an anterolateral approach, the abductor musculature repair must be carefully crafted to ensure adequate postoperative function because the increased weight of obese patients may make them less tolerant of a poorly functioning abductor mass. With a posterior approach, careful soft-tissue repair decreases postoperative instability rates. The deep fascia must be closed meticulously. The superficial fascia should be closed in multiple layers to eliminate the dead space in this area and ensure adequate healing. Both deep and superficial drains may be helpful in this population to decrease the risk of wound healing complications. Studies of patients after total knee arthroplasty and general surgical and obstetrical procedures have identified delayed wound heal-

ing and skin problems as major concerns in obese patients. Therefore, extra care is required for wound closure.

Postoperative Regimen

Postoperatively, whether cemented or uncemented devices are used, patients are allowed to bear weight as tolerated using appropriate assistive devices (such as a walker or two crutches). I find that patients bear weight as tolerated regardless of what they are instructed to do, and obese patients have particular difficulty complying with protected weight bearing. Therefore, it is important that adequate intraoperative implant stability be achieved, and relying on the patient to protect the construct is not recommended. It should be noted that activities such as using a bedpan place much larger forces across the hip joint than are experienced with ambulation.

Deep venous thrombosis prophylaxis in some form should be used for all patients undergoing THA. The surgeon should be especially vigilant with obese patients because obesity is clearly a risk factor in thromboembolic complications. Early ambulation should be routine, along with some form of pharmaceutical prophylaxis and/or mechanical compression devices for the lower extremities. Total hip precautions are stressed for the first 3 months postoperatively. Patients with very large lower extremities may not be able to flex or adduct their legs adequately to induce instability, and there is no available literature to suggest that these patients are at higher risk for postoperative dislocations.

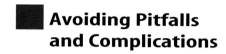

Avoiding Pitfalls and Complications

The main complications for which the obese patient may be at increased risk are medical in nature. Obesity is highly associated with hypertension, diabetes mellitus, coronary artery disease, and pulmonary disease. A thorough preoperative medical evaluation is imperative for obese patients, and an internal medicine specialist should be involved with perioperative patient care.

Surgical considerations for obese patients include precise patient positioning to ensure a stable, appropriately positioned pelvis and carefully using positioning devices to avoid damage to the soft tissues. The approach required to obtain appropriate exposure is often more extensive, and the surgeon must be aware of the propensity for vertical acetabular component positioning, particularly in patients with large amounts of adipose tissue in the lower extremity. Obese patients may also be at increased risk for local wound healing complications, and special care must be taken with wound closure. In addition, obese patients are at higher risk for decubitus ulcers, and additional nursing care should be specified to prevent such occurrences. Furthermore, obese patients are at increased risk for pulmonary complications and may require additional oxygen saturation monitoring in the perioperative period.

References

Chan CL, Villar RN: Obesity and quality of life after primary hip arthroplasty. *J Bone Joint Surg Br* 1996;78:78-81.

Jiganti JJ, Goldstein WM, Williams CS: A comparison of the perioperative morbidity in total joint arthroplasty in the obese and nonobese patient. *Clin Orthop* 1993;289:175-179.

Lehman DE, Capello WN, Feinberg JR: Total hip arthroplasty without cement in obese patients: A minimum two-year clinical and radiographic follow-up study. *J Bone Joint Surg Am* 1994;76:854-862.

Soballe K, Christensen F, Luxhoj T: Hip replacement in obese patients. *Acta Orthop Scand* 1987;58:223-225.

Stickles B, Phillips L, Brox WT, Owens B, Lanzer WL: Defining the relationship between obesity and total joint arthroplasty. *Obes Res* 2001;9:219-223.

Coding

CPT Codes		Corresponding ICD-9 Codes		
27130	Arthroplasty, acetabular and proximal femoral prosthetic replacement (total hip arthroplasty), with or without autograft or allograft	278.00 278.01 711.45 711.95 714.0 714.30	715.15 715.25 715.35 716.15 718.5 718.6	720.0 733.14 733.42 808.0 905.6
27132	Conversion of previous hip surgery to total hip arthroplasty, with or without autograft or allograft	715.15 715.25 715.35 718.2	718.5 718.6 733.14 733.42	905.6 996.4 996.66 996.77

CPT copyright © 2004 by the American Medical Association. All Rights Reserved.

Chapter 28

Total Hip Arthroplasty in Patients With Sickle Cell Hemoglobinopathy

Richard E. Grant, MD
Bonnie M. Simpson, MD

■ Indications

Sickle cell–related osteonecrosis of the hip is primarily a disease of African Americans of Central African ancestry. Osteonecrosis will develop in 23% to 30% of patients with sickle cell hemoglobinopathy (SCH) if they reach age 45 years, as opposed to 25% to 50% of patients presenting with sickle cell-thalassemia. A total of 54% of patients with hemoglobinopathy-induced osteonecrosis present with bilateral involvement.

Improved health care and a coordinated team approach have appreciably expanded the life expectancies of patients with SCH. Half of the patients with SCH are expected to survive into the fifth decade of life. Improved longevity within this patient population provides firm support for total hip arthroplasty (THA) for patients with debilitating sickle cell–induced end-stage osteonecrosis of the hip.

THA is indicated for patients with SCH presenting with intractable pain, advanced osteonecrosis (stage III-IV Ficat-Arlet/Steinberg; **Table 1**) with radiographic evidence of advanced femoral head collapse, and associated significant acetabular involvement. Radiographic evidence of hip joint deterioration is usually associated with restricted hip motion, antalgic gait, and difficulties with activities of daily living.

The radiographic progression of osteonecrosis beyond stage III-IV (Ficat-Arlet/Steinberg) appears to be directly related to femoral head necrotic volume, as assessed by a combination of MRI and orthogonal radiographs of the femoral head (**Figure 1**). Sickle cell osteonecrosis has a high probability of progressing to femoral head collapse with adaptive acetabular changes and associated loss of range of motion. Once hip osteonecrosis progresses to Steinberg stage IV, there is usually no expectation for clinical improvement without surgical intervention. The transition from a Steinberg stage II femoral head osteonecrosis to stage IV osteonecrosis takes an average of 30 months.

Table 1 Classification for Nontraumatic Osteonecrosis of the Hip

Stage	Description
Ficat	
I	Normal radiograph
II	Sclerosis, cystic normal contour
III	Subchondral fracture/collapse, normal joint space
IV	Acetabular changes, joint space
Steinberg	
I	Normal radiograph, normal MRI
II	Normal radiograph; abnormal MRI
III	Sclerosis and/or cyst formation, A, B, C
IV	Crescent sign, no flattening
V	Flattening, decreased joint space
VI	Advanced degenerative joint disease

■

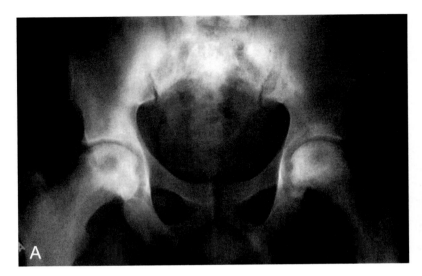
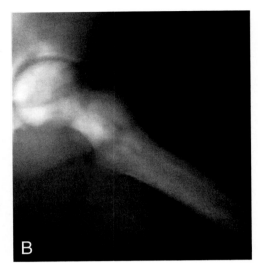

Figure 1   Preoperative AP **(A)** and lateral **(B)** radiographs of the pelvis and femur with intramedullary infarct with sclerosis in a patient with SCH.

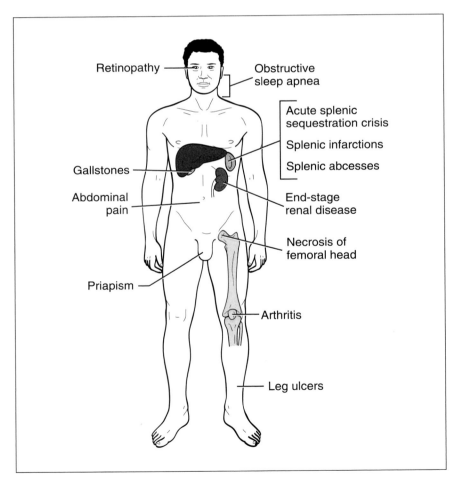

Figure 2   A review of systems is necessary to determine the extent of SCH-related comorbidities.

Contraindications

Contraindications include a history of severe pulmonary compromise (eg, uncontrolled pulmonary hypertension) and an anesthesiology evaluation that assigns the patient to a higher surgical risk category. Patients with SCH and a history of pulmonary disease have a higher incidence of postoperative acute chest syndrome. An extensive history of pulmonary problems should be evaluated by pulmonary function tests with a bronchodilator response analysis, especially if the patient has a history of asthma or an episode of acute chest syndrome or other pulmonary complications (**Figure 2**).

Surgery should be delayed in the patient with SCH presenting with active leg ulcers (**Figure 3**). Treatment for these patients should include a consultation with a plastic surgeon, débridement, and skin grafting. Surgery should likewise be delayed if the patient profile includes a hemoglobin level less than 10 g/dL or a hemoglobin S level greater than 30%. Vaso-occlusive crisis, active infection, fever, and dehydration are also relative contraindications for surgery.

Careful deliberation before proceeding to surgery is indicated in patients who are elderly, present with multiple-organ dysfunction, have a history of frequent hospitalization, have a history of frequent blood transfusions, or have alloimmunization.

Alternative Treatments

Femoral head-saving procedures generally have a poor prognosis in patients with SCH because of recurrent vaso-occlusion. Core decompression is an alternative treatment for just a few patients with osteonecrosis of the hip and SCH without femoral head collapse and without acetabular involvement or joint space narrowing. The prognosis for core decompression is directly related to the extent of femoral head involvement. If the combined arc of femoral head involvement is greater than 200° (as measured by AP and lateral views of the femoral head), as is frequently the case in SCH, the prognosis for success with core decompression is markedly compromised. Core decompression should not be performed in hips that have demonstrated a crescent sign or femoral head collapse.

Femoral head osteonecrosis in the patient with SCH is not associated with intraosseous hypertension. Because the patient with SCH continues to experience episodes of intraosseous sickling, recurrence of osteonecrosis and the certainty of future infarcts mitigate against the temporary effectiveness of core decompression. Cortical strut grafting and free vascularized grafts are a consideration; however, free vascularized fibula grafts can be associated with a significant degree of comorbidity and problems at the donor site. Patients with muscle pedicle bone grafting, cancellous grafts, and osteochondral allografts would like-

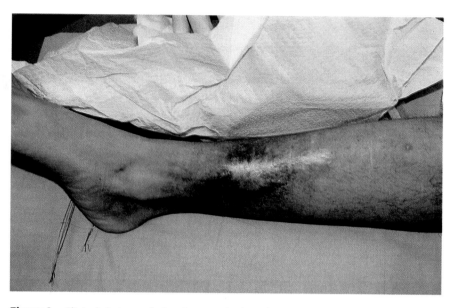

Figure 3 Clinical photograph showing a stasis ulcer. The presence of a stasis ulcer precludes immediate surgical treatment.

wise be subject to recurrent episodes of ischemia, infarction, and eventual biomechanical compromise.

Rotational or angular osteotomies have been associated with a reduction in impingement and correction of deformity. The angular or rotational osteotomy must be designed in such a way that it is able to deliver the osteonecrotic segment from the weight-bearing sector. Femoral head lesions with a combined osteonecrotic arc of less than 200°, as measured on both AP and lateral radiographs, are considered amenable to either rotational or angular osteotomies. However, the degree of involvement in the femoral head in the patient with SCH usually exceeds the 200° arc, and the femoral head will be subject to future infarcts by way of repeated crises.

Hemiarthroplasty has been applied to the treatment of patients with sickle cell–induced osteonecrosis of the hip. However, hemiarthroplasty in the patient with SCH is characterized by additional challenges, including a soft acetabulum, the association of increased osteolysis, and the possibility

of continued medial migration of the bipolar shell.

Girdlestone excisional arthroplasty has been considered in the patient with SCH. However, several researchers have pointed out the possibility of high oxygen demands, especially in patients presenting with bilateral disease requiring bilateral Girdlestone arthroplasty.

Hip arthrodesis for patients with SCH typically is avoided because these individuals usually present with bilateral hip disease.

Results

Success and failure depend on multiple factors, including technique, implant design, recognition of associated comorbidities, presence of acute or chronic concurrent infections, patient-specific factors, and osteolysis. The overall failure rate reported in the literature, especially for patients with a minimal clinic follow-up of 2 years or less, is 31% to 63%. There is a 34% probability of revision within

Table 2 Summary of Series of THA in Patients With SCH

Author(s) (Year)	Number of Hips	Implant Type	Mean Patient Age	Mean Follow-up	Results
Hanker and Amstutz (1988)	8 cemented THA	N/A	N/A	6.5 years	38% failure due to aseptic loosening; 25% failure due to septic loosening; 50% revision at 5 years
Hickman and Lachiewicz (1997)	16 uncemented THA	N/A	N/A	6 years	87% good to excellent results; 33% reoperation/revision rate; femoral osteolysis most common late complication
Moran, et al (1993)	22 (20 cemented, 2 uncemented) THA	N/A	N/A	5 years	38% failure of primary THA; 43% revision THA due to acetabular and femoral component loosening; aseptic loosening main mode of failure
Ilyas and Moreau (2002)	36 (18 bilateral uncemented bipolar) THA	N/A	N/A	5.7 years	94% good to excellent results; acetabular aseptic loosening in one patient, no femoral stem loosening; 2 postoperative sickle cell crises in two patients; infection in two patients; heterotopic ossification in two patients
Al-Mousawi, et al (2002)	35 patients	N/A	N/A	9.5 years	83% good to excellent results; six hips failed due to symptomatic aseptic loosening; six hips failed due to aseptic loosening; one late deep infection

N/A = Not Applicable

4.5 years. THA failure is usually caused by aseptic loosening, followed in close order by sepsis (**Table 2**).

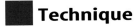

Technique

If THA is selected, the patient will require an extensive preoperative briefing for informed consent, which should include a lengthy discussion about the high risk-benefit ratio of THA. The treating surgeon should consider assembling a cohesive special interest team of consulting specialists representing hematology, anesthesiology, and intensive care. The clinical pathway should include specific roles for each specialty.

Meticulous preparation, planning, and careful templating are prerequisites. Fluoroscopy for intraoperative monitoring during reaming of the relatively sclerotic radiodense diaphysis will help with patients who

present with an obscure femoral intramedullary (IM) canal. Preparations for the use of a high-speed burr are well advised. Careful acetabular templating is needed with special attention to Köhler's line and the integrity of the acetabular radiographic teardrop.

Exposure and Surgical Considerations

Either a standard posterior approach or an anterolateral approach can be used for primary THA in patients with SCH. Meticulous preoperative positioning is essential to avoid circulatory stasis and perioperative stasis ulcers.

Venous access for hydration can take some time prior to surgery. The appropriate selection of perioperative antibiotics, in addition to perioperative analgesia, is important. Intravenous antibiotics, including a third-generation cephalosporin, are started preoperatively and continued for 48 hours perioperatively. Cefazolin, 1 g IV, is routinely administered preoperatively. Gentamicin should be added if the pa-

tient has a history of gram-negative infection. The dose of aminoglycoside should be adjusted according to the patient's preoperative BUN and creatinine levels. In patients undergoing revision THA that requires extensile exposure, the addition of allografts, and extensive internal fixation, extending the infusion of intravenous antibiotics past the recommended 48 hours may be considered.

Preoperative arterial blood gas measurements are advisable to assess preoperative pulmonary function; baseline echocardiography, and renal and liver function tests are especially important in patients with a history of abnormal chest radiographs or history of acute chest syndrome.

During surgery, the anesthesiology team must avoid hypothermia, hypoxemia, hypovolemia, hyperviscosity, and acidosis. The operating room should be maintained with an ambient temperature that encourages or maintains continuous normothermia. This can be accomplished either by manipulating the operating room ambient temperature or by using a supplemental forced air heating blanket positioned outside the operative field.

The patient should be maintained in a state of mild respiratory alkalosis (pH of approximately 7.45). In addition, 50% inspired oxygen should be maintained throughout the procedure. Estimated blood loss should be carefully monitored throughout the procedure. Central venous pressure monitoring can be helpful.

Some debate exists about the use of regional versus general anesthesia. Regional anesthesia reportedly encourages vasodilation. The debate about the use of general anesthesia centers on the use of chemicals such as halothane. Several studies have suggested that halothane might contribute to increased blood viscosity in patients with SCH.

At all times, the anesthesiologist and the surgeon should anticipate blood loss and aggressively replace it. Fluid shifts should also be anticipated. Pulse oximetry should be maintained throughout the procedure and in the perioperative and postoperative periods. The oxygen level should be maintained at 97%. Electrolyte status and urine output must be carefully monitored and adequately maintained. In addition to central venous pressure monitoring, the anesthesiologist must consider invasive hemodynamic monitors.

Intraoperative cultures of the femoral head are advised to detect pathogenic organisms. Bone cultures have been found to be much more effective than cultures of the periacetabular synovium. Intraoperative specimens should be obtained for definitive histopathology, culture and sensitivities, gram stain, and a survey of leukocyte concentration via high-powered microscopic field.

Bone Preparation

The acetabulum should be reamed carefully with frequent evaluation of

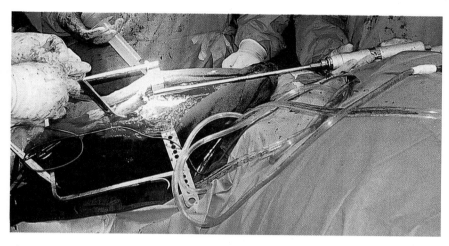

Figure 4 Use of a guidewire and flexible intramedullary reaming under fluoroscopic guidance.

the integrity of the medial acetabular wall. During acetabular reaming of the femur (**Figure 4**), the surgeon must consider the infarcted areas of soft bone alternating with islands of dense sclerosis. At times, a high-speed burr can be used to remove recalcitrant bony infarcts within the acetabulum bed.

Acetabular protrusio is often associated with osteopenia secondary to marrow hyperplasia. In cases of acetabular protrusio, the surgeon may plan uncemented cup fixation on the acetabular rim, supplemented with particulate allografting of the acetabular concavity. The hip center should not be left in a medial location. After culturing, the original femoral head is often used as a source of particulate autograft to correct protrusio. Autogenous bone can be supplemented with particulate allograft impacted against the medial acetabular border.

The medial graft serves to lateralize the center of hip rotation and allows the implanted socket to be placed in a more anatomic position, allowing for correct femoral offset and reduced impingement.

We prefer uncemented acetabular fixation in most cases. Once acetabular rim contact is established, socket fixation can be supplemented

with iliac screw fixation. Acetabular reinforcement rings or cages have been used in cases of extreme acetabular protrusio or combined cavitary and segmental acetabular deficiencies, as characterized by the AAOS classification system. The surgeon should also be aware of the tendency toward lengthening of the lower extremity as a result of lateralizing the hip center during cage or reinforcement ring implantation. If there is a limb-length discrepancy, a lower neck cut, modularity, or the use of a shorter neck may be considered.

Preparation of the femur can be very difficult in SCH. Compromised bony architecture of the metaphysis and diaphysis because of marrow hyperplasia, widening of the proximal femoral medullary canal, and very thin cortices also are frequently present. In patients who have extensive infarction of the femoral metaphyseal/diaphyseal region, a focus of dense sclerosis will be encountered, which extends from the femoral metaphyseal region throughout the extent of the diaphysis.

The severity of femoral canal stenosis helps determine how to prepare the femur (**Table 3** and **Figure 5**). During prosthetic implantation, the increased cortical fragility and the

Table 3 Grant-Simpson Classification of Femoral Diaphysis/IM Canal Patency According to Radiographic Findings in Patients With SCH

Grade	Radiographic Description of Femoral Metaphyseal/Diaphyseal Bone
I	Normal radiographic appearance of the femoral cortex and IM canal and metaphyseal region with a Dorr A and B calcar-to-canal ratio.
II	Thickening and increased relative radiodensity of the femoral cortex with < 25% compromise of the femoral IM canal. Evidence of scattered infarcts within the endosteum and cortical bone.
III	Thickening of the femoral cortex with ≥ 50% narrowing of the IM canal with scattered cortical and IM infarcts. Consider guidewire and flexible IM reaming with fluoroscopy.
IV	Complete obliteration of the IM canal. IM white out resembling osteopetrotic bone. Use of large burrs and drills designed to penetrate acrylic cement or carbide bit and end-cutting high-speed drill attachments.

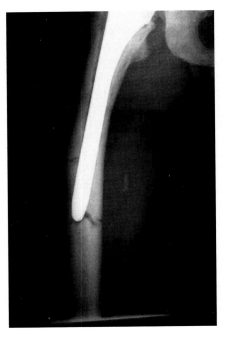

Figure 5 AP radiograph showing a pathologic diaphyseal fracture after implantation of an uncemented prosthesis.

possibility of inadvertent femoral diaphyseal perforations must be considered. Intraoperative spot views or fluoroscopy of the femur should be strongly considered during reaming and initial rasping when entering a canal with narrowing or bone infarcts.

If the femoral IM canal is obliterated by osteopetrotic infarcted bone, use of fluoroscopy should be considered throughout femoral preparation. Intraoperative perforation and fracture can occur during reaming, during femoral component insertion, or during both procedures. Reaming is risky in femurs with hyperplastic medullary canals, thin cortices, and scattered foci of sclerotic bone. Some clinicians recommend introducing a drill bit under fluoroscopy until it is possible to insert a guide wire for flexible reamers. In patients with extensive femoral canal obliteration, radiographic confirmation of guidewire placement is recommended to confirm proper position within the center of the femoral canal before flexible reaming and broaching. In addition, prophylactic wiring of the femur may protect against fracture or extension of small perforations in the femur.

Prosthesis Implantation

After the femoral canal is prepared, the prosthesis is inserted against the thinned cortices of the sickle cell femur, which can cause perforation, fracture, or both. The difficulty of seating an uncemented prosthesis into a femur containing areas of sclerotic bone has been described. Some clinicians recommend the use of smaller-sized femoral components to avoid perforation or fracture. Prevention, prompt recognition, and appropriate treatment of perforations and fractures are critical to the success of uncemented arthroplasty (**Figure 6**).

Cement fixation is a viable option for Grant-Simpson grade I and II femoral metaphyseal/diaphyseal bone types. However, the preoperative radiographs and intraoperative findings should confirm the presence of adequate trabecular bone to ensure adequate cement interdigitation into the cancellous interstices. In general we prefer to use uncemented femoral fixation in patients with SCH because of the presence of metaphyseal and diaphyseal sclerotic bone, which mitigates against the application of polymethylmethacrylate as a grouting agent. The absence of cancellous bone in the multiply infarcted femoral metaphyseal/diaphyseal regions or in the periacetabular or intra-acetabular area allows little chance for cement interdigitation within the cancellous bone interstices by virtue of standard cementing techniques that require pulsatile lavage, cement plugs, and pressurization. In addition, cemented arthroplasty has been associated with increased bleeding, leading to suboptimal preparation of cancellous bone and thermal necrosis. Surface replacement arthroplasty is associated with the same challenge of early failure because of recurrent sickle cell–induced osteonecrosis beneath the replaced femoral head surface.

Wound Closure

Traditional principles of wound closure must be followed, with meticulous care of soft tissue. In patients who have received multiple analgesic injections into the region of the proximal thigh, great care must be taken to avoid complete denudement of scar tissue from the tensor fasciae latae beyond 2 to 4 cm from the midline. Excessive stripping of the highly vascular subcutaneous granulation tissue from the tensor fasciae latae can precipitate postoperative dermal demarcation and wound necrosis.

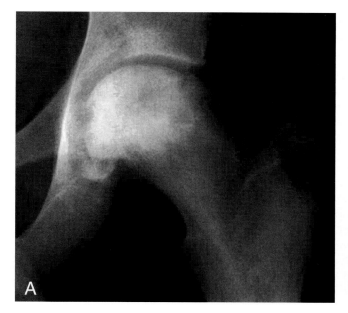
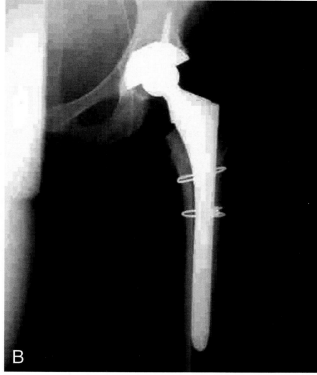

Figure 6 **A,** Preoperative AP radiograph of a proximal femur in a patient with SCH. **B,** Postoperative radiograph shows an uncemented prosthesis with proximal femoral cerclage cables.

Postoperative Regimen

Postoperative complication rates can be as high as 54%; therefore, a cohesive team of consultants is recommended for preoperative medical clearance and medical evaluation of hematologic involvement for the patient with SCH undergoing THA. In the postoperative period, the incidence of vaso-occlusive crisis can be 9%; therefore, it should be anticipated as a possibility in all patients. Postoperative prophylaxis for deep vein thrombosis should follow standard protocols, usually with warfarin or low molecular weight heparin; consultation with a hematologist may be helpful in some cases. Intense respiratory therapy is important to avoid postoperative atelectasis, especially if general endotracheal intubation and anesthesia are used. Adequate oxygenation helps avoid acidosis. The preoperative hemoglobin A level should be maintained at 30% or higher, and the preoperative hemoglobin S level should be maintained at

no more than 30% to 40%. This level is best achieved by a nonaggressive transfusion regimen. Hydroxyurea can be used if indicated but must be started 3 months preoperatively.

There is a 4% incidence of postoperative congestive heart failure. Key indicators of this complication are a history of respiratory distress and preoperative documentation of cardiomegaly. In these patients, the anesthesiologist and the surgeon must take great care to avoid fluid overload. In addition, there is a 4% risk of major transfusion reaction secondary to the presence of increased antierythrocyte antibodies and an abnormal immune system in the patient with SCH.

Intraoperative autotransfusion should be avoided. The cell saver subjects the relatively fragile and abnormal erythrocyte membranes to increased sickling and hemolysis. Excessive intraoperative blood loss can also result in postoperative wound hematoma and prolonged drainage from the hip wound. Postoperatively, plate-

let and serum calcium levels should be monitored carefully. Alloimmunization that occurs in a patient with SCH is usually directly proportional to the patient's transfusion history or a history of multiple transfusions.

In the recovery room, oxygenation, hydration, and pain control should be monitored carefully. Pulmonary function studies should be carefully monitored as well to detect and prevent acute chest syndrome. Acute chest syndrome is often associated with low total hemoglobin within 48 hours of surgery. Continued full intraoperative monitoring should be maintained in the recovery room. Pulse oximetry should also continue when the patient is in the recovery room. Several protocols include postoperative overnight observation in the surgical or mobile intensive care unit, as well as provisions for aggressive respiratory care. Postoperative rehydration with isotonic crystalloids and oral intake helps reduce blood viscosity and, therefore, prevents thrombogenesis and vascular occlusion. Increased hemoglobin viscosity occurs at Po_2 of 80 mm Hg.

Suggested pain management for the patient with SCH in the postoperative period includes a patient-controlled analgesic pump or epidural anesthesia, extradural analgesia, transdermal fentanyl patches, or ketorolac, a nonsteroidal anti-inflammatory agent. Ketorolac or other nonsteroidal anti-inflammatory drugs are preferred over morphine or meperidine, both of which are associated with respiratory depression.

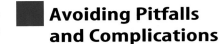

Avoiding Pitfalls and Complications

Many complications can be avoided by careful preoperative planning and a team approach to perioperative management, with appropriate specialists aiding in the care of different organ systems. Careful preoperative planning also helps the surgeon to anticipate technical challenges. Care during bone preparation and use of intraoperative imaging as needed can help reduce bone perforation and fracture and may improve implant fixation.

Postoperative complications can be classified as (1) sickle cell–related

complications, which include crisis, acute chest syndrome, or cerebral vascular accident, and (2) non-SCH–related complications. The latter include fever, infection, hemorrhage, thrombosis, embolism, or death. A third category includes complications such as transfusion reaction.

Late aseptic loosening of the acetabular femoral components has also been associated with cemented and uncemented components, but recently more favorable early results have been reported in patients undergoing uncemented THA.

References

Al-Mousawi F, Malki A, Al-Aradi A, et al: Total hip replacement in sickle cell disease. *Int Orthop* 2002;26:157-161.

Garden MS, Grant RE, Jebraili S: Perioperative complications in patients with sickle cell disease: An orthopedic perspective. *Am J Orthop* 1996;25:353-356.

Hanker GJ, Amstutz HC: Osteonecrosis of the hip in sickle cell diseases: Treatment and complications. *J Bone Joint Surg Am* 1988;70:499-506.

Hickman JM, Lachiewicz PF: Results and complications of total hip arthroplasties in patients with sickle-cell hemoglobinopathies: Role of cementless components. *J Arthroplasty* 1997;12:420-425.

Ilyas Y, Moreau P: Simultaneous bilateral total hip arthroplasty in sickle cell disease. *J Arthroplasty* 2002;17:441-445.

Moran MC, Huo MH, Garvin KL, Pellicci PM, Salvati EA: Total hip arthroplasty in sickle cell hemoglobinopathy. *Clin Orthop* 1993;294:140-148.

Soucacos PN, Beris AE, Malizos K, Koropilias A, Zalavras H, Dailiana Z: Treatment of avascular necrosis of the femoral head with vascularized fibular transplant. *Clin Orthop* 2001;386:120-130.

Coding

CPT Codes		Corresponding ICD-9 Codes		
27125	Hemiarthroplasty, hip, partial (eg, femoral stem prosthesis, bipolar arthroplasty)	715.15 716.15 733.42	715.25 718.6 905.6	715.35 733.14
27130	Arthroplasty, acetabular and proximal femoral prosthetic replacement (total hip arthroplasty), with or without autograft or allograft	711.45 714.30 715.35 718.6 733.42	711.95 715.15 716.15 720.0 808.0	714.0 715.25 718.5 733.14 905.6
27134	Revision of total hip arthroplasty; both components, with or without autograft or allograft	996.4	996.66	996.77
27137	Revision of total hip arthroplasty; acetabular component only, with or without autograft or allograft	996.4	996.66	996.77
27138	Revision of total hip arthroplasty, femoral component only, with or without autograft or allograft	996.4	996.66	996.77
27244	Treatment of intertrochanteric, peritrochanteric, or subtrochanteric femoral fracture; with plate/screw implant, with or without cerclage	733.14 820.21 820.30 820.8	733.15 820.22 820.31 820.9	820.20 820.3 820.32

Chapter 29

Total Hip Arthroplasty in Patients With Neurologic Conditions

Andrew I. Spitzer, MD

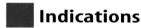 **Indications**

Neurologic disease has long been recognized as a significant risk factor for degeneration of the hip joint. However, management of the neuromuscular hip has primarily been the domain of the pediatric orthopaedic surgeon. Residual deformities from congenital neuromuscular diseases (eg, cerebral palsy and myelomeningocele) in which intrinsic muscle imbalance leads to subluxation or dislocation and adult acquired neurologic diseases (eg, stroke, Parkinson's disease, spinal cord or head injuries, multiple sclerosis, and Charcot arthropathy) and their associated muscle imbalances can either cause or be accompanied by degenerative hip disease. As the population ages and the prevalence of age-related neurologic disease rises, degenerative hip disease associated with neuromuscular disorders will become increasingly common. Total hip arthroplasty (THA) is the treatment of choice for these patients, and a strategy for managing the unique challenges that they present is mandatory for successful outcomes.

The indications for THA in patients with neurologic disease are similar to those for a patient with routine osteoarthritis, but the surgeon should consider whether the neurologic condition or associated medical condition could preclude a satisfactory result from THA. Radiographically confirmed degenerative disease of the hip joint accompanied by pain that has failed to respond to nonsurgical treatment (eg, nonsteroidal anti-inflammatory drugs, nutriceuticals, analgesics, physical therapy, intra-articular injection, activity modifications, weight loss, and assistive devices) and significant activity and functional limitations are the classic indications. Physical examination should confirm the hip as the source of pain.

Additional indications include progressive pain in the degenerated dysplastic, subluxated or dislocated hip, subcapital hip fracture with underlying arthritis or failed fixation with nonunion, malunion, or osteonecrosis (**Figure 1**), and painful arthritis that prevents comfortable positioning of the patient for perineal care or functional activities—sitting, standing, and ambulating.

A discussion between the surgeon and the patient and/or caregivers about realistic expectations is critical. Risks for postoperative complications such as dislocation in patients with severe muscle imbalance or spasticity or decubitus ulcers in patients with altered sensation or difficulty with independent mobilization must be weighed against the benefits of THA. Alternative surgical options, such as resection arthroplasty, interposition arthroplasty, and hip arthrodesis, as well as alternative emerging arthroplasty procedures such as hemiresur- facing or surface replacement arthroplasty may be considered, depending on patient needs, activity level, and expectations.

Contraindications

Absolute contraindications to THA in any patient include active or chronic infection in the hip joint and active or chronic distant infection, such as skin breakdown and/or decubitus ulcer. In addition, Charcot neuropathic arthropathy, although rare in the hip, is nearly an absolute contraindication to THA; the few results reported in the literature have been uniformly poor.

Relative contraindications specific to patients with neurologic disease must be individually assessed, considering potential complications, activity level, age, and medical risk. Significant abductor weakness from polio, myelomeningocele, stroke, or multiple sclerosis increases the risk of dislocation and may require constrained components or alternative treatments. Patient noncompliance, either because of unwillingness or inability, may substantially increase the risk for dislocation, particularly in the context of notable preexisting muscle imbalance, spasticity, paresis, or paralysis. Patients with minimal activity demands, who may be bedridden or

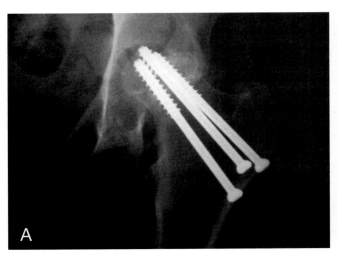
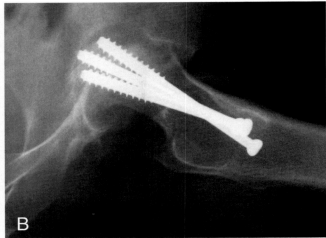

Figure 1 Preoperative AP (**A**) and lateral (**B**) radiographs of a patient with Parkinson's disease and failed internal fixation of a subcapital hip fracture. Note erosion of the acetabulum by screws protruding through the avascular femoral head.

nonambulatory, and who may have positioning requirements that place the hip at risk for dislocation may be best served with an alternative treatment approach. Young age, although traditionally considered a risk factor for early failure, is less of a concern in this population because of their relatively low activity level, which should foster longevity of the prosthesis. Medical risk should be carefully considered, however, particularly in elderly patients who have had a stroke or have a progressive neurologic disorder such as Parkinson's disease or multiple sclerosis. Any underlying medical problem should be addressed, and perioperative management should be designed to prevent cardiac, pulmonary, gastrointestinal, urinary, thromboembolic, and other general complications. Patients at high medical risk should be active participants in the surgical decision-making process.

Alternative Treatments

Nonsurgical management of osteoarthritis in these patients always should

be attempted before surgery is considered. However, when this approach fails, alternative surgical treatments include resection, with or without interpositional arthroplasty, and arthrodesis. Because bilateral hip involvement is common (as is spinal deformity and disease) in this population, arthrodesis is relatively contraindicated. Older patients with acquired neurologic disease or long-term sequelae of muscle imbalance without dislocation or subluxation may be potential candidates for arthrodesis, but THA often provides a more functional result and greater patient satisfaction. Resection arthroplasty is reserved for patients who are essentially bedridden or for patients who can, at most, be transferred to a sitting position, to permit comfortable positioning and to facilitate hygiene and perineal care. Complications include heterotopic ossification and recurrent pain.

Results

Of the very few studies that document THA in patients with neuromuscular disease (**Table 1**), all are case or series reports with variable follow-up. Nev-

ertheless, a number of important conclusions can be drawn. A well-performed THA in properly selected patients with neuromuscular disease can achieve a durable, long-term successful result. Surgical approach has not been proved to be associated with disparate dislocation rates. Careful positioning of the components is critical to avoid postoperative dislocation. Slight increase in acetabular anteversion may reduce postoperative dislocation, especially in patients who predominantly sit, such as those with severe cerebral palsy. Adductor tenotomy and other releases are frequently necessary to optimize range of motion and maximize the safe zone to avoid dislocation. Uncemented stems have not been studied in this patient population, but cemented stems have functioned well and demonstrated only rare prosthetic loosening. Finally, postoperative bracing is advised during soft-tissue healing to prevent dislocation.

Technique

The technical considerations surrounding THA in patients with a neurologic condition are based on the unique anatomic and functional abnormalities of this population. Significant muscle imbalance and spasticity can result in soft-tissue contractures of the anterior capsule and the powerful hip flexors and adductors. This, in turn, can result in substantial acetabular erosion, subluxation/dislocation, increased femoral anteversion, and coxa valga. Conversely, paresis or paralysis can result in growth disturbance in bone and disuse osteopenia. Each of these factors can increase the complexity of the surgical procedure, and if not meticulously addressed, may result in intraoperative complications, postoperative instability, and an overall unsatisfactory result. Therefore, as in any reconstructive procedure, preoperative planning is essential. A careful history, thorough physical examination, and complete radiographic evaluation are essential. Special imaging techniques, such as CT or MRI, may be necessary to fully understand the extent of the pathoanatomy. With all of this information, and after templating the radiographs, a surgical plan can be designed.

Exposure

The most important consideration when selecting the surgical approach is the familiarity and skill of the surgeon. Although the literature strongly indicates that the dislocation rate associated with THA in the general population is higher when a posterior rather than an anterior approach is used, most of the literature specific to THA for the neuromuscular hip does not support this conclusion. Nevertheless, specific precautions may reduce postoperative dislocation, regardless of approach, including careful soft-tissue repair posteriorly and secure soft-tissue and bony fixation for anterior and transtrochanteric approaches.

Tenotomies may be necessary as part of the primary approach to adequately expose the hip joint. Release

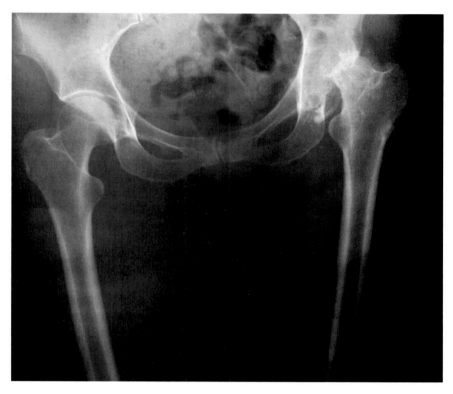

Figure 2 Preoperative AP pelvis radiograph of a patient with a severe adduction contracture.

of the reflected head of the rectus femoris insertion from the anterior superior acetabulum, the psoas tendon insertion from the lesser trochanter, and the anterior superior capsule can facilitate mobilization of the femur and exposure of the acetabulum and help to reduce preoperative flexion contractures. Subcutaneous adductor tenotomy for severe adduction contracture (**Figure 2**) should be delayed until the end of the procedure, when, with the patient supine, the degree of passive abduction can be adequately assessed. A minimum of 30° of passive abduction helps to maintain the hip in the safe zone.

Bone Preparation

The combination of the neurologic disease, the arthritic process, and the patient's decreased activity level often results in significant disuse osteopenia of the bones surrounding the neuromuscular hip. As such, preparation of

the bone should be performed gently to avoid overreaming and/or fracture.

The bone quality may permit uncemented fixation, but the available literature supports cemented fixation of both acetabular and femoral components. Hybrid fixation with an uncemented acetabular component and a cemented femoral component has also demonstrated efficacy in these patients but in smaller numbers.

Adjunctive screw fixation is advised for uncemented acetabular components to ensure component stability, and a broach-only technique for the femur is recommended to preserve the endosteal cancellous bone critical for cement intrusion, interdigitation, shear strength, and durable fixation.

Acetabular bone grafting, when necessary, should be performed using standard techniques, ensuring secure, stable osteosynthesis. Simultaneous corrective osteotomies of the femur should be avoided, however, because

Table 1 Results of THA in Patients With Neuromuscular Conditions

Author(s) (Year)	Patient Condition	Number of Hips	Type of Implant*	Patient Age (Range)	Mean Follow-Up (Range)	Results
Cameron (1995)	Polio	1	Uncemented components with a fully constrained socket	N/A	3 years	N/A
Cabanela and Weber (2000)	Mentally impaired	5	2 uncemented sockets All other components cemented	N/A	(5–15) years	Both uncemented sockets loosened
Ries, et al (1994)	Mentally impaired	11	Total or bipolar hip arthroplasty	62.3 years (49–73)	(2–7) years	NHigh complication rate: 5 reoperations (3 periprosthetic fractures, 1 deep infection, 1 thoracic decubitus, 6 urinary tract infections) Hospital costs, length of stay, and complications higher than mentally competent patients
Weber and Cabanela (1998)	Myelomeningocele	3	1 cemented THA 1 uncemented THA 1 cemented metal-backed acetabulum and uncemented long stem	45 years (28–54)	7.6 years (5–10)	3 anterolateral approach 3 dislocated 2 revised Poor results with pain in all patients
Skoff and Keggi (1986)	Mental retardation, Down syndrome, Cerebral palsy	12	Cemented and uncemented components Numbers of each not recorded	42 years (16–65)	3.5 years (0.33–7.1)	6 anterior, 3 lateral or posterior approach 1 revision for aseptic loosening at 4.5 years No major complications, with 100% good to excellent results
Koffman (1981)	Cerebral palsy	5	1 Sivash 2 Lagrange-Letournel (bilateral) 2 T28 Snapfit	33.8 years (21–57)	N/A	4 pain and/or loss of mechanical integrity 1 dislocation
Root and Bostrom (1998)	Cerebral palsy	15	All cemented components	31 years (16–52)	6.75 years (2.5–12)	2 posterolateral and 13 transtrochanteric approaches 11 tenotomies 13 postoperative hip spica cast (4 weeks) 3 dislocations 2 revisions 14 patients had complete pain relief Recommended increasing anteversion and inclination in patients who predominantly sit

N/A = Not Applicable

Table 1 (Continued)   Results of THA in Patients With Neuromuscular Conditions

Author(s) (Year)	Patient Condition	Number of Hips	Type of Implant*	Patient Age (Range)	Mean Follow-Up (Range)	Results
Buly, et al (1993)	Cerebral palsy	19	All cemented components	30 years (16–52)	10 years (3-17)	14 transtrochanteric and 5 posterolateral approaches 12 tenotomies 4 acetabular bone grafts 17 postoperative hip spica casts 2 dislocations 3 revisions (1 stem, 1 cup, 1 stem and cup) 17 patients reported pain relief and improved function 95% survivorship at 10 years for loosening, 86% for any reason
Weber and Cabanela (1999)	Cerebral palsy	16	12 all cemented components 2 all uncemented components 2 hybrid	48.5 years (22–79)	9.7 years (2.5–21)	8 anterolateral, 7 transtrochanteric, 1 posterior approaches 2 tenotomies 2 postoperative immobilization 1 revision for aseptic loosening at 13 years 3 other reoperations (1 trochanteric fixation, 1 heterotopic ossification removal, 1 tenotomy) 13 with significant pain relief
Staeheli, et al (1988)	Parkinson's disease and hip fracture	50	50 endoprostheses (44 unipolar, 6 bipolar) 19 cemented components 31 uncemented components	74 years (47–92)	7.3 years (2–??)	25 anterolateral, 20 posterior, 5 transtrochanteric approaches 5 tenotomies 1 dislocation 20% urinary tract infections, 10% decubitus ulcers, 10% pneumonia 20% mortality at 6 months
Weber, et al (2002)	Parkinson's disease	107	16 types of acetabular components (94 cemented, 13 uncemented) 17 types of femoral components (103 cemented, 4 uncemented)	72 years (57–87)	7 years (2–21)	56 anterolateral, 36 transtrochanteric, 12 posterior, 3 direct lateral approaches 8 tenotomies 2 postoperative braces 58 primary THAs, 49 revision THAs 6 dislocations, all in revisions 3 aseptic loosening (1 femur, 1 acetabulum, 1 femur and acetabulum) 5 other reoperations (1 trochanteric nonunion, 1 instability, 1 wire removal, 1 fracture, 1 infection) 93% good to excellent pain relief 6% mortality at 6 months 93% survivorship at 5 years High complication rate

*Prosthesis manufacturers are Sivash (DePuy, Warsaw, IN); Legrange-Letournel (Stryker-Howmedica Osteonics, Allendale, NJ); T28 Snapfit (Zimmer, Warsaw, IN)

the added complexity, the challenge of fixation, particularly when the femoral component is cemented, and the need for postoperative weight protection all potentiate postoperative complications and failure.

Prosthesis Implantation

Prosthesis implantation begins with templating the radiographs and choosing the prosthesis. Cemented acetabular cups have a documented track record in this patient population, whereas uncemented cups have shown promise. The reported success of the latter in a wide variety of patients with differing levels of bone quality suggests that these cups should also perform well in the neuromuscular hip. Acetabular deficiency may require bulk allograft reconstruction. Oblong cups, or even acetabular reconstruction rings and cages, may also be useful; however, no data on use of these implants in this setting are available.

Cemented stems should be applicable to most neuromuscular hips, and the published data certainly support their use in these patients. However, the pathoanatomy of the proximal femur in a patient with spastic cerebral palsy may resemble that of the dysplastic hip, with coxa valga and excessive anteversion. Cemented stems designed for use in the dysplastic femur may be necessary. In addition, although its use is not reported in the literature in the neuromuscular hip, a proximally modular stem, such as the S-ROM (DePuy, Warsaw, IN) is well suited to address these issues, offering adjustment of version and offset independent of component fixation.

The risk of postoperative dislocation in this population should lead surgeons to consider using innovative implants that were not available at the time the reported series were generated. A larger head diameter, coupled with cross-linked polyethylene, alternative bearing surfaces (metal-on-metal, ceramic-on-ceramic), or the re-

emerging use of surface replacement arthroplasty, should reduce the dislocation risk. Constrained articulations are also now available. These developments could extend the indications of THA in this patient population, enabling the excellent pain relief afforded by THA to be offered to more of these often very unfortunate patients. Nevertheless, premature loosening is a concern with the use of constrained articulations. Future study is required to understand the role of these newer implant technologies in this population.

Acetabular preparation begins by adequate circumferential exposure and identification of the intraoperative landmarks of the teardrop and the bony contributions to the acetabulum. Reaming should be attempted to prepare the acetabular bed in its anatomic location. A slightly high hip center is acceptable if length and stability can be established by femoral length and offset. Firm cancellous surfaces should be retained for cement interdigitation, and fixation holes should be placed in strategic locations in the ischium, pubis, and ilium.

For uncemented cups, the thickness of the anterior and posterior walls limits the extent of reaming; these are the critical areas for achieving press-fit fixation. Caution should be exercised when attempting to reduce the extent of a superior deficiency by reaming to a larger hemisphere; this may ream away the anterior and posterior walls and rims of the acetabulum and significantly compromise initial stability and long-term fixation.

Once the appropriate cup size is established, any deficiency should be assessed. Bone grafting or alternative devices should be considered if adequate cup coverage or stability cannot be obtained. Final implantation of the cemented or uncemented cup should proceed according to standard protocol. Screw augmentation for uncemented cups is advisable, particularly in relatively osteopenic bone and cer-

tainly when a constrained liner is contemplated.

Femoral preparation should be routine, regardless of stem type. Trial reduction should establish that stability is achievable and limb length is optimized with the available component options, such as offset, neck length, version, and head size. The need for additional constraint should be assessed at this point so that the appropriate acetabular insert can be selected before final insertion of the femoral stem.

Wound Closure

Once the prostheses have been implanted and the hip is stable, closure commences. Careful, secure repair of any bony or soft-tissue dissection that was necessary for exposure is imperative to maximize the potential of adequate healing and reduce the risk of postoperative dislocation. The wound should be closed in layers, ensuring that the fascia is tightly approximated and any dead space is eliminated in the subcutaneous tissues. Choice of skin closure technique is at the discretion of the surgeon. Adhesive dressings should be applied carefully to reduce shearing the skin and causing blisters.

After the dressing is applied, the patient is turned supine and abduction is assessed. If abduction to 30° is not easily obtained, a percutaneous adductor release is performed. The insertion of the adductors at the pubic tubercle is prepared and draped using sterile technique. Close to the pubis, directly over the tight tendons, a tiny stab incision is made with the tip of a No. 11 blade. The tip of the blade is rotated and angled to release the tight fibers until 45° or more of abduction is possible (**Figure 3**). Skin adhesives are applied, and the wound is covered with a small sterile dressing. Sutures are discouraged given the challenge of suture removal in this area.

Postoperative Regimen

The postoperative protocol in these patients may be predicated, in part, on the nature of the underlying disease. Assuming no intraoperative complications, precautions in the postoperative period are directed at avoiding catastrophic complications such as falling and dislocation. Disruption of bony or soft-tissue repair is also a concern, particularly in the noncompliant patient or in the patient with spasticity. Medical complications are anticipated and avoided.

Vigilance against infection is particularly appropriate in this population, particularly in patients with Parkinson's disease, in whom a higher incidence of postoperative infections has been documented. Aggressive pulmonary toilet is important to avoid atelectasis and pneumonia. Depending on the extent of neurologic involvement, aspiration precautions may also be appropriate. Urinary catheterization for a few days may be advisable to minimize the likelihood of urinary retention and subsequent infection, and bowel management should be aggressive to avoid painful constipation or impaction and possible resulting bacteremia. Surgical drains should be removed promptly, within 24 hours. Perioperative antibiotics should be continued until all indwelling catheters are removed.

Prophylaxis against thromboembolic disease should be administered according to surgeon protocol, considering any increased risk in the patient, such as anticipated prolonged immobilization, hypercoagulability risks, or family or personal history of a venous thromboembolic event. Choices include mechanical devices, antiplatelet agents, low molecular weight heparins, and warfarin.

Patients should be carefully but rapidly mobilized to minimize skin breakdown, pulmonary and urinary complications, venous thromboembolic disease, and to facilitate expeditious functional independence. Use of

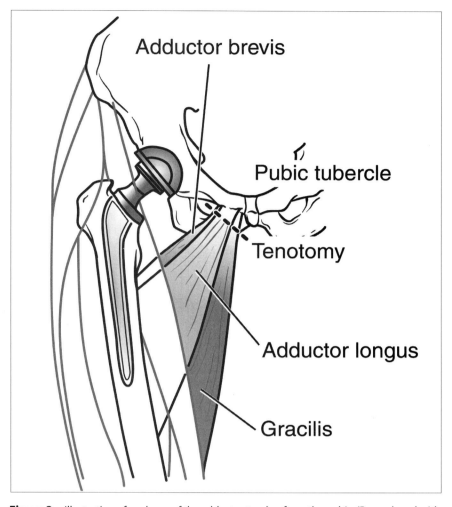

Figure 3   Illustration of a release of the adductor tendon from the pubis. (Reproduced with permission from Frassica FJ, Wenz JF, Sim FH: Parkinson's disease, in Morrey BF (ed): *Joint Replacement Arthroplasty*, ed 3. Rochester, MN, Mayo Foundation for Medical Education and Research, 2003, p 773.)

assistive devices for walking, which may be familiar and necessary in these patients because of underlying disease even after the hip has been rehabilitated, should be mandatory to improve ambulatory stability and avoid falls, fractures, and dislocations. Full weight bearing should be allowed, unless protection of a bony or soft-tissue repair or reconstruction is necessary.

The use of an abduction hip brace or a spica cast is individualized but should be strongly considered when there is a high risk of either postoperative dislocation or disruption of soft-tissue or bony repair. Use

of immobilization, although inconvenient to patients and caregivers, may improve the long-term prognosis and eventual success of the reconstruction by avoiding early complications.

Finally, returning the patient to a familiar environment is ideal, even though inpatient rehabilitation may benefit many of these patients and allow them to be truly ready to return home at an appropriate time. Caregivers should be thoroughly instructed in precautions and activity restrictions. Close follow-up should be arranged.

■ Avoiding Pitfalls and Complications

Avoiding complications is critical in this patient population, particularly because their underlying disease often places them at increased risk. The key elements of success involve proper patient selection and meticulous attention to technical detail and execution, as described throughout this chapter. A carefully managed postoperative regimen should complement these elements to avoid medical complications, falls, fractures, and dislocations and optimize the rehabilitative results.

————■

■ Acknowledgment

I would like to acknowledge Denise Paige, CPC for technical assistance with the Coding Section.

■ References

Buly RL, Huo M, Root L, Binzer T, Wilson PD Jr: Total hip arthroplasty in cerebral palsy: Long-term follow-up results. *Clin Orthop* 1993;296:148-153.

Cabanela ME, Weber M: Total hip arthroplasty in patients with neuromuscular disease. *Instr Course Lect* 2000;49:163-168.

Cameron HU: Total hip replacement in a limb severely affected by paralytic poliomyelitis. *Can J Surg* 1995;38:386.

Koffman M: Proximal femoral resection or total hip replacement in severely disabled cerebral-spastic patients. *Orthop Clin North Am* 1981;12:91-100.

Ries MD, Wolff D, Shaul JA: Hip arthroplasty in mentally impaired patients. *Clin Orthop* 1994;308:146-154.

Root L, Bostrom MPG: The neuromuscular hip, in Callaghan JJ, Rosenberg AG, Rubash HE (eds): *The Adult Hip*. Philadelphia, PA, Lippincott-Raven, 1998, pp 493-506.

Skoff HD, Keggi K: Total hip replacement in the neuromuscularly impaired. *Orthop Rev* 1986;15:154-159.

Staeheli JW, Frassica FJ, Sim FH: Prosthetic replacement of the femoral head for fracture of the femoral neck in patients who have Parkinson disease. *J Bone Joint Surg Am* 1988;70:565-568.

Weber M, Cabanela ME: Total hip arthroplasty in patients with cerebral palsy. *Orthopedics* 1999;22:425-427.

Weber M, Cabanela ME: Total hip arthroplasty in patients with low-lumbar-level myelomeningocele. *Orthopedics* 1998;21:709-713.

Weber M, Cabanela ME, Sim FH, Frassica FJ, Harmsen WS: Total hip replacement in patients with Parkinson's disease. *Int Orthop* 2002;26:66-68.

Coding

CPT Codes		Corresponding ICD-9 Codes		
27125	Hemiarthroplasty, hip, partial (eg, femoral stem prosthesis, bipolar arthroplasty)	715.15 716.15 733.42	715.25 718.6 905.6	715.35 733.14
27130	Arthroplasty, acetabular and proximal femoral prosthetic replacement (total hip arthroplasty), with or without autograft or allograft	711.45 714.30 715.35 720.0 808.0	711.95 715.15 716.15 733.14 905.6	714.0 715.25 718.6 733.42
27132	Conversion of previous hip surgery to total hip arthroplasty, with or without autograft or allograft	715.15 718.2 733.42 996.66	715.25 718.6 905.6 996.77	715.35 733.14 996.4
27134	Revision of total hip arthroplasty; both components, with or without autograft or allograft	996.4	996.66	996.77
27137	Revision of total hip arthroplasty, acetabular component only, with or without autograft or allograft	996.4	996.66	996.77
27138	Revision of total hip arthroplasty; femoral component only, with or without allograft	996.4	996.66	996.77
27236	Open treatment of femoral fracture, proximal end, neck, internal fixation or prosthetic replacement	733.14 820.03 820.13	820.00 820.10 820.8	820.02 820.12 820.9

CPT copyright © 2004 by the American Medical Association. All Rights Reserved.

SECTION 3
Complications After Total Hip Arthroplasty

Chapter 30
Management of the Unstable Total Hip Arthroplasty

Paul F. Lachiewicz, MD

▰ Indications

Hip dislocation remains a frequent and very disabling complication after both primary and revision total hip arthroplasty (THA). The surgical approach in primary THA has been related to the rate of dislocation, with a prevalence of less than 1% reported with the direct lateral or anterolateral approach. However, the rate of dislocation with the posterior approach also can be less than 1% if there is appropriate repair of the posterior capsule and external rotator tendons.

Patient factors related to an increased risk of dislocation have been reported to be female sex, patient age older than 70 (or 75) years, and a preoperative diagnosis of osteonecrosis and acute femoral neck fracture. Surgical factors include surgeon volume and experience, acetabular or femoral component malposition, soft-tissue or bony impingement, a skirted modular femoral head, severe polyethylene wear, and large-diameter ($\geq$ 62-mm) acetabular components combined with small (22- and 28-mm) femoral heads.

Dislocation is more common following revision THA, with prevalences reported from 10% to 25%. Factors implicated include soft-tissue deficiency, nonunion of the greater trochanter, limb-length discrepancy, and the use of a large, long-taper revision femoral component. A very high

rate of dislocation has been reported with isolated acetabular revisions and polyethylene liner exchange procedures for acetabular component wear.

The indications for acetabular component revision for recurrent dislocation are (1) acetabular component malposition (0° anteversion or any retroversion for posterior dislocation [**Figure 1**]; > 20° anteversion for anterior dislocation; abduction angle > 55°); (2) loosening or angular shift of the component; and (3) severe polyethylene wear. The indications for femoral component revision for recurrent dislocation are femoral component malposition and loosening with or without subsidence. Whether a well-fixed femoral component with a large taper or one that requires a modular femoral head with a "skirt" should be retained to equalize limb length is controversial and requires careful intraoperative judgment concerning range of motion and impingement. Femoral offset needs to be evaluated to determine if femoral component revision is necessary to establish adequate soft-tissue tension and stability. In some cases, trochanteric advancement can be used instead of femoral component revision to obtain adequate soft-tissue tension.

The indications for modular revision (ie, use of an elevated liner and a larger femoral head) have not been firmly established and continue to evolve. To be considered for modular

(or "dry") revision, the components must be well fixed and positioned within the acceptable ranges; components should have known good long-term results, and modular components of various sizes should be available.

The indications for soft-tissue augmentation have not been firmly established but should include the absence of or an irreparable posterior hip capsule-short external rotator complex in an otherwise well-positioned THA that has recurrent dislocations.

Indications for any constrained acetabular component include recurrent dislocation resulting from soft-tissue insufficiency (capsular or abductor musculature) that is not amenable to repair or augmentation; chronic nonunion of an osteotomy of the greater trochanter, with severe and irreparable loss of abductor muscle function; cognitive dysfunction or dementia; neurologic motor disorder (previous stroke or parkinsonism); late dislocation without component loosening or malposition; and failure of modular component exchange or posterior capsule allograft augmentation. An alternative to a constrained liner is a tripolar arthroplasty. In this situation, a large bipolar head articulates with a large acetabular component. This construct may be a better option for younger, more active patients.

In rare cases, revision to a bipolar prosthesis may be necessary. This

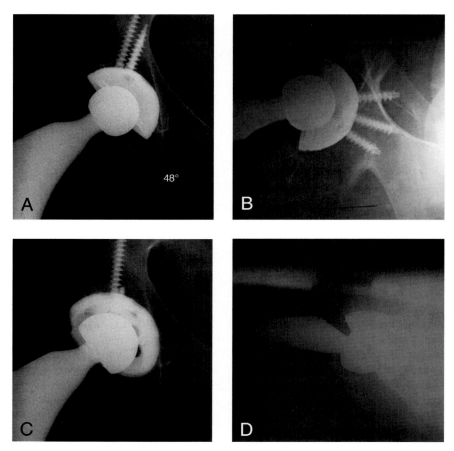

Figure 1 **A,** AP radiograph of a 67-year-old woman who underwent a primary THA for osteonecrosis and had recurrent posterior dislocations. The acetabular abduction angle measures 48°. **B,** Cross-table lateral view shows little anteversion. **C,** Postoperative radiograph after acetabular revision. The acetabular abduction angle measures 38°. **D,** Cross-table lateral view shows approximately 20° anteversion. The femoral head size was increased from 28 to 32 mm.

rent dislocation is contraindicated in an active healthy patient with reasonable acetabular bone structure.

A specific contraindication to the use of any constrained component is acetabular component loosening or malposition. In this situation, it is imperative to revise the acetabular component. A constrained liner may be implanted into this new acetabular component if required for intraoperative stability. The technique for using constrained liners in existing well-fixed, well-positioned acetabular shells involves cementing the polyethylene liner into the existing shell.

Alternative Treatments

The treatment of an early postoperative dislocation after either a primary or revision THA is closed reduction, with the patient under intravenous sedation in the emergency department or under general or regional anesthesia in the operating room. In the case of a first-time dislocation, range of motion in the reduced hip is examined to determine the safe zone of motion, followed by use of a hip abduction brace or hip spica cast for 6 weeks to limit range of motion and encourage soft-tissue healing. However, the efficacy of this type of immobilization in preventing recurrent dislocation has not been proved in a prospective randomized study. If the hip is extremely unstable after reduction and the cause of the dislocation is obvious, the patient should be advised that revision may be necessary. In several studies, the risk of recurrence after an early dislocation is approximately 33% to 40%. Rarely, an open reduction may be required if the dislocation cannot be reduced closed with the patient under general anesthesia.

In some patients a first dislocation occurs 5 years or more after a

type of revision should be limited to elderly, debilitated patients with recurrent dislocations and a loose acetabular component. There must be insufficient bone to revise to a constrained acetabular liner.

Contraindications

Dislocation associated with an acute avulsion of an osteotomy of the greater trochanter or an acute fracture of the greater trochanter should be treated by closed reduction and surgical repair or advancement. However,

repair of a chronic nonunion of the greater trochanter usually will be unsuccessful.

The contraindications for modular revision include component malposition that contributed to dislocation, loosening of one or both components, abductor muscle insufficiency or chronic nonunion of the greater trochanter, history of a cognitive disorder (eg, dementia) or neurologic motor disorder (eg, stroke, parkinsonism), and inadequate intraoperative stability. The contraindications for soft-tissue augmentation are the same as for modular revision. Revision to a bipolar prosthesis for recur-

THA. The risk factors include the female sex, previous subluxations, substantial trauma, and new-onset cognitive or motor neurologic impairment. Radiographic factors associated with late dislocation are polyethylene wear greater than 2 mm, implant loosening with migration or a change in position, and initial malposition of the acetabular component. In one such series of late dislocations, 7% of hips required an open reduction after closed reduction was unsuccessful. The late dislocation recurred in 55% of all hips, and 61% of the recurrent dislocations required another operation. Despite this prognosis, I recommend closed reduction and immobilization with a hip orthosis following a first-time late dislocation.

Results

Overall results of surgical treatment for recurrent dislocation by revision of one or both components have been historically poor. In one study from the Mayo Clinic, a failure rate of 31% after attempted surgical correction of hip instability was reported.

There are only three published reports of the results of modular exchange for recurrent dislocation (**Table 1**). In two studies using this approach, 10 of 13 patients (72%) and 14 of 17 patients (82%), respectively, had no further dislocations. However, in another study, this approach was unsuccessful in 16 of 29 patients (55%). Modular exchange should be considered judiciously in the treatment of recurrent dislocation and only if the components are well aligned. One situation in which modular exchange has been generally successful is the patient with a large-diameter (≥ 62-mm) acetabular component combined with a small (22-, 26- or 28-mm) femoral head. The use of a very large (36- or 40-mm) femoral head combined with a highly cross-linked polyethylene liner may increase the success rate of mod-

Table 1 Results of Modular Revision for Dislocation

Author(s) (Year)	Number of Hips	Implant Type	Mean Patient Age (Range)	Mean Follow-up (Range)	Results
Toomey, et al (2001)	14	10 DePuy* AML 4 others	59.3 years (26-79)	5.8 years (2.8-11.8)	10 no dislocation 2 one dislocation 1 recurrent dislocation 1 lost to follow-up
Earll, et al (2002)	29	17 DePuy* 3 Biomet† 5 Osteonics‡ 1 Howmedica§ 2 Zimmer‖ 1 Wright¶	64 years (22-90)	55 months (34-122)	13 no dislocation 16 redislocation (9 recurrent)
Lachiewicz, et al (2004)	23	All Zimmer	*Primary* 59.5 years (32-80) *Revision* 54 years (40-64)	*Primary* 4 years (2-7) *Revision* 3 years (2-5)	*Primary* 14 no dislocation 1 one dislocation 2 recurrent dislocation *Revision* 3 no dislocation 2 recurrent dislocation

*DePuy, Warsaw, IN †Biomet, Warsaw, IN
‡Osteonics, Allendale, NJ §Howmedica, Rutherford, NJ
‖ Zimmer, Warsaw, IN ¶Wright, Arlington, TN

ular component exchange for recurrent dislocation.

Soft-tissue augmentation was successful in 6 of 10 patients (60%) in one study and all three patients in another study. This procedure may be combined with modular component exchange in selected patients.

Although conversion to bipolar arthroplasty involves removal of a well-fixed acetabular component, the results, in terms of stability, have been very good with absence of dislocation in one small series of patients. However, these patients have variable amounts of groin pain and disability, as well as lower hip scores. Over time, these components invariably migrate into the pelvis.

The results of constrained components are device specific. The reported failure rates of the S-ROM (DePuy, Warsaw, IN) constrained component range from 9% to 33%, with

failure due to acetabular component loosening, liner dissociation, breakage or disengagement of the metal constraining ring, or dissociation of a modular femoral head from its trunnion. The rate of repeat dislocation with the tripolar constrained device has been reported to be only 4%, but there was also definite loosening of the acetabular component in 6% of patients and of the femoral component in 6%. In the largest study of the tripolar component, the patient population consisted of predominantly elderly, debilitated women, and the surgeons were willing to accept the increased risk of wear, osteolysis, and component loosening with the device to achieve a stable hip. In the future, new and improved designs of constrained acetabular liners may increase the use of this approach for recurrent dislocation.

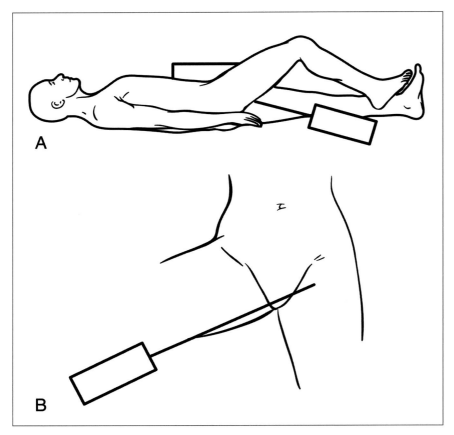

Figure 2 Cross-table ("shoot-through") lateral radiograph of the hip used for evaluation of the acetabular component. The contralateral hip is flexed (90°, if possible) **(A)** and the x-ray beam is directed with slight caudocephalad angulation to a cassette located lateral to the patient's hip **(B)**. (Adapted with permission from Towers JD: Radiographic evaluation of the hip, in Callaghan JJ, Rubash H, Rosenberg A (eds): *The Adult Hip*. Philadelphia, PA, Lippincott-Raven, 1998, p 336.)

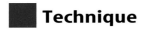 **Technique**

Preoperative Planning

A careful evaluation of the patient and his or her components is required prior to reoperation for recurrent dislocation. The patient should be evaluated and treated, if possible, for any cognitive dysfunction or neurologic motor disorder. Limb length, range of hip motion, and abductor muscle function should be carefully examined. The components should be evaluated for loosening or migration by comparison of serial radiographs, if possible. The abduction angle of the acetabular component should be measured on an AP pelvis radiograph. An-

teversion of the acetabular and femoral components can be estimated using a cross-table lateral view (**Figure 2**) or with the methods described by Ghelman, or Ackland and associates, respectively. Comparison of the offset of the replaced and native hips and an anteversion study of the femoral component may be helpful if malposition of the femoral component is suspected. The reason for early dislocation can be identified in approximately two thirds of patients. Instability may be secondary to acetabular component malposition (**Figure 1**, *A* and *B*), femoral component malposition, limb-length discrepancy (shortening), damage or absence of capsule, inadequate femoral offset (**Figure 3**,

A), bone or prosthesis impingement (**Figure 3**, *B* through *E*), or trochanteric avulsion or nonunion. In the study of late dislocation, a clinical factor could be identified in only 25% of patients and a radiographic factor in only 34% of patients. To maximize the choice of surgical approaches for recurrent dislocation, the reason for dislocation must be identified.

Exposure

WELL-FIXED ACETABULAR COMPONENT
An acetabular component that has been placed in retroversion or excessive anteversion often requires revision. An adequate soft-tissue exposure is necessary to completely visualize the circumference of the acetabulum. Skeletization of the proximal femur may be necessary to allow for mobilization of the femur to ensure proper exposure to the acetabular component.

MODULAR REVISION
The availability of modular acetabular and femoral components has provided another possible treatment method for recurrent dislocation. This involves retention of well-fixed and well-positioned components, along with acetabular polyethylene liner and modular femoral head-neck exchange.

SOFT-TISSUE AUGMENTATION
Another new approach involves the use of an Achilles tendon-bone allograft to replace or augment a deficient posterior hip capsule in patients with recurrent dislocation, despite well-positioned components. Exposure is through the posterior approach.

Prosthesis Implantation

WELL-FIXED ACETABULAR COMPONENT
If a well-fixed acetabular component must be removed because of retroversion or excessive anteversion, then it is safest to remove the component with the Explant system (Zimmer,

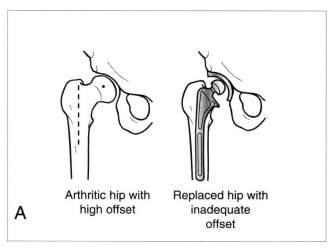

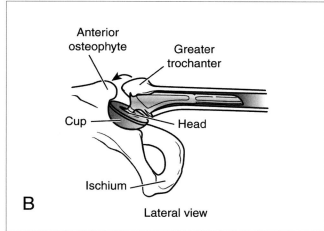

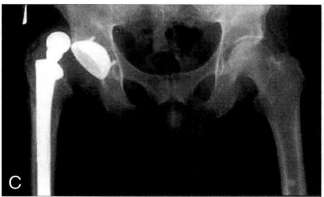

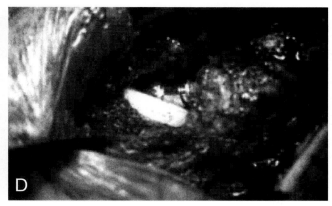

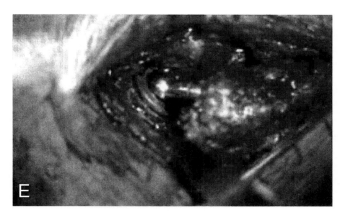

Figure 3 **A,** If the THA femoral component provides less than the preoperative offset, recurrent dislocation may occur as a result of soft-tissue laxity or impingement. **B,** In a THA with properly positioned components, bone-to-bone or bone-to-prosthesis impingement anteriorly may lead to posterior dislocation. With internal rotation, the trochanter hits against the anterior bone rim or osteophyte, and the femoral head is pushed posteriorly. **C,** AP radiograph showing anterior dislocation that occurred with extension and external rotation consistent with impingement of the skirted head on the elevated rim liner. Intraoperative photographs confirm impingement (arrow) of the skirted head on the elevated rim liner **(D)**, which was not present with a neutral liner **(E)**. (C, D, and E reproduced from Barrack RL, Thornberry RL, Ries MD, Lavernia C, Tozakoglou E: The effect of component design on range of motion to impingement in total hip arthroplasty. *Instr Course Lect* 2001;50:275-280.)

Warsaw, IN). A more detailed description of this device can be found in chapter 39. After reimplantation of a new acetabular component, potential sources of soft-tissue and bony impingement should be identified. The posterior capsule should be repaired if a posterior approach was used. With the recent development of cross-linked polyethylene liners, it is now possible to use thinner polyethylene liners with larger femoral heads. Jumbo femoral heads (size 36- to 38-mm) can increase stability because the increased femoral head-neck ratio reduces impingement. However, the thinner polyethylene liners may be a problem in active patients.

MODULAR REVISION

With this procedure, the acetabular polyethylene liner is usually changed from "neutral" to one with an elevated rim (10° or 20°) positioned in the direction of the dislocation. The femoral head size is usually increased from 22, 26, or 28 mm to 32 mm (**Figure 4**) or larger (36- or 40-mm femoral heads

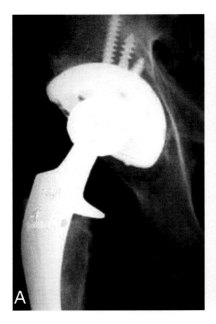
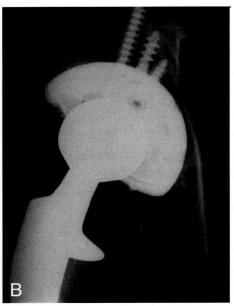
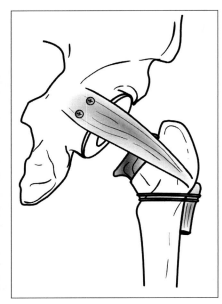

Figure 4 **A,** AP radiograph of an 80-year-old man who had a primary THA for osteoarthritis using a standard 28-mm liner and a "short-plus" neck. He had nine posterior dislocations between 6 and 18 months postoperatively. Using the method of Ghelman, the acetabular component was in 27° of anteversion. **B,** A modular revision was performed with placement of a 10° elevated rim liner in the posterosuperior quadrant, a 32-mm femoral head, and a medium (3.5-mm longer) neck. He had no further dislocation at 3-year follow-up. (Reproduced with permission from Lachiewicz PF, Ellis JN, Soileau ES: Modular revision for recurrent dislocation of primary or revision total hip arthroplasty. *J Arthroplasty* 2004;19:424-429.)

Figure 5 The calcaneal end of the Achilles tendon allograft is fixed to the posterosuperior acetabulum with two screws, and the tendinous portion is fixed to the femur with a soft-tissue restraint and cables. (Adapted with permission from Lavigne MJF, Sanchez AA, Coutts RD: Recurrent dislocation after total hip arthroplasty. Treatment with an Achilles tendon allograft. *J Arthroplasty* 2001; 16(suppl):13-18.)

are available from some manufacturers). The neck length is increased slightly to provide increased soft-tissue tension, provided that this increase does not require the use of a skirted component. Sources of soft-tissue or bony impingement should be removed. Range of motion should be evaluated intraoperatively with the modular components (or trial components) in place so that the hip is stable in maximum flexion, in full extension with external rotation, and in at least 45° of internal rotation with the hip in 90° of flexion and maximum adduction. The posterior capsule should be repaired or augmented, if possible.

SOFT-TISSUE AUGMENTATION

The segment of os calcis is trimmed and fixed to the posterosuperior acetabulum with two 3.5-mm titanium cancellous bone screws. The tendon allograft is attached to the femur just

below the flare of the greater trochanter with a soft-tissue cable device (**Figure 5**). The graft is tensioned to prevent any internal rotation. The wound is closed in standard fashion.

CONSTRAINED COMPONENTS

Presently, two constrained THA devices have been approved by the US Food and Drug Administration and have data published on their results. They are the S-ROM constrained liner (Poly-Dial; DePuy) (**Figure 6**, *A*) and the tripolar constrained liner (Stryker-Howmedica Osteonics, Rutherford, NJ) (**Figure 6**, *B* and *C*). Other constrained liners have been used in clinical trials or are in development. With the S-ROM component, the constraint is derived from extra polyethylene in the rim, which deforms to more fully capture the femoral head implant. A metal locking ring provides increased constraint. The Stryker-Howmedica

Osteonics component is a tripolar device: a polyethylene inner liner covered with a chrome-cobalt shell articulates with another polyethylene liner, which is inserted into a standard acetabular shell. The inner liner accepts a 22-, 26-, or 28-mm femoral head, with a locking ring identical to the ring in a bipolar prosthesis. With both constrained components, the range of the motion is much less and the forces at the joint will be transferred to the acetabular and femoral bone interfaces (**Figure 7**). In general, constrained components should only be used when the acetabular component is in an acceptable position.

Postoperative Regimen

Postoperatively, a prefitted hip orthosis that limits the range of motion to 70° flexion is worn for 6 weeks.

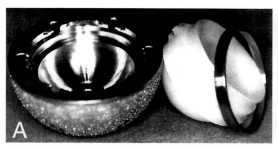
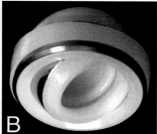
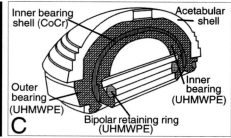

Figure 6 **A,** The S-ROM constrained acetabular component. (Reproduced with permission from Kaper BP, Bernini PM: Failure of a constrained acetabular prosthesis of a total hip arthroplasty: A report of four cases. *J Bone Joint Surg Am* 1998;80:561-565.) **B,** The Stryker-Howmedica Osteonics constrained acetabular liner. **C,** Illustration showing the tripolar nature of the device. UHMWPE = ultra high molecular weight polyethylene, CoCr = cobalt chrome. (Courtesy of Stryker-Howmedica Osteonics, Rutherford, NJ.)

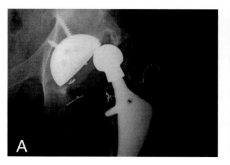
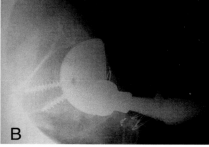
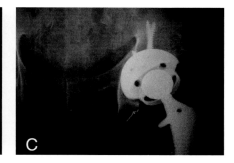

Figure 7 Preoperative AP **(A)** and lateral **(B)** radiographs of an 80-year-old man with a chronic dislocation of a revision THA. There is a trochanteric nonunion, and the acetabular component is malpositioned (0° anteversion). **C,** The acetabular component was revised (26° anteversion, 38° abduction) and a constrained liner (locking ring type) was used. The greater trochanter could not be repaired.

Avoiding Pitfalls and Complications

A dislocated hip prosthesis must be treated expeditiously, if possible. The hip may be reduced in the emergency department with the patient under intravenous sedation. However, dissociation of modular components (femoral head off the taper) and disruption of component fixation have been reported with forceful reduction maneuvers. Therefore, spinal anesthesia or general anesthesia with intravenous muscle relaxation is strongly recommended for reduction of a dislocated hip if there are concerns about the adequacy of the sedation. The hip should be put through a range of motion after reduction to determine the safe zone of motion and for prognostic purposes. Although immobilization has not been proved to lower the risk of recurrent dislocation, I strongly recommend placement of a hip orthosis or hip spica cast after a first-time dislocation to rest the soft tissue and avoid early recurrence. I also recommend a prophylactic hip orthosis after certain revisions that have a particularly high rate of early postoperative dislocation. These revisions include isolated acetabular revision through the posterior approach and liner ex-change for osteolysis and after reimplantation for infected THA.

Complications resulting from the use of constrained acetabular components may be decreased by avoiding placement into metal acetabular shells with less than optimal position or when the fixation of the acetabular shell is suspect or compromised by extensive pelvic osteolysis. Failure of a constrained component usually requires an open reduction or another revision, and patients should be advised about this possible complication.

▉ References

Alberton GM, High WA, Morrey BF: Dislocation after revision total hip arthroplasty: An analysis of risk factors and treatment options. *J Bone Joint Surg Am* 2002;84:1788-1792.

Earll MD, Fehring TK, Griffin WL, et al: Success rate of modular component exchange for the treatment of an unstable total hip arthroplasty. *J Arthroplasty* 2002;17:864-869.

Grigoris P, Grecula MJ, Amstutz HC: Tripolar hip replacement for recurrent prosthesis dislocation. *Clin Orthop* 1994;304:148-155.

Knoch MV, Berry DJ, Harmsen WS, Morrey BF: Late dislocation after total hip arthroplasty. *J Bone Joint Surg Am* 2002;84:1949-1953.

Lachiewicz PF, Kelley SS: The use of constrained components in total hip arthroplasty. *J Am Acad Orthop Surg* 2002;10:233-238.

Lachiewicz PF, Soileau ES, Ellis JN: Modular revision for recurrent dislocation of primary or revision total hip arthroplasty. *J Arthroplasty* 2004;19:424-429.

Lavigne MJF, Sanchez AA, Coutts RD: Recurrent dislocation after total hip arthroplasty: Treatment with an Achilles tendon allograft. *J Arthroplasty* 2001;16(suppl):13-18.

Toomey SD, Hopper RH Jr, McAuley JP, Engh CA: Modular component exchange for treatment of recurrent dislocation of a total hip replacement in selected patients. *J Bone Joint Surg Am* 2001;83:1529-1537.

Coding

CPT Codes		Corresponding ICD-9 Codes		
27091	Removal of hip prosthesis; complicated, including total hip prosthesis, methylmethacrylate with or without insertion of spacer	996.4	996.66	996.77
27134	Revision of total hip arthroplasty; both components, with or without autograft or allograft	996.4	996.66	996.77
27137	Revision of total hip arthroplasty; acetabular component only, with or without autograft or allograft	996.4	996.66	996.77
27138	Revision of total hip arthroplasty; femoral component only, with or without allograft	820.20 996.66	905.6 996.77	996.4
27248	Open treatment of greater trochanteric fracture, with or without internal or external fixation	820.20 820.09 996.66	820.30 905.06 996.77	820.8 996.4
27253	Open treatment of hip dislocation, traumatic, without internal fixation	820.20 835.03 835.13 996.66	835.01 835.11 905.6 996.77	835.02 835.12 996.4
27265	Osteotomy, intertrochanteric or subtrochanteric including internal or external fixation and/or cast	715.15 731.0 736.31 754.31 754.35 755.63 996.4	715.25 732.1 736.32 754.32 755.61 820.20 996.66	715.35 733.81 754.30 754.33 755.62 905.6 996.77
27266	Closed treatment of post hip arthroplasty dislocation; requiring regional or general anesthesia	820.20 996.66	905.6 996.77	996.4
Modifier 22	Unusual procedural services			

Management of the Infected Total Hip Arthroplasty

Arlen D. Hanssen, MD

 ## Indications

The primary etiologies of a painful hip replacement include aseptic loosening, synovitis secondary to wear debris, extra-articular soft-tissue inflammation, or referred pain from the lumbar spine. Patients with infected hip wounds occasionally have a draining sinus tract and associated cellulitis. However, because of the large soft-tissue envelope surrounding the hip joint, most patients present with well-healed incisions, making detection of swelling or joint effusion impossible. Although some patients may have painful, restricted range of motion, many experience a surprisingly small increase in aggravated pain during hip joint examination.

Pain at rest is the most common presenting symptom. Persistent pain always suggests the possibility of infection. Other indications include prolonged wound drainage or antibiotic treatment for healing difficulties. Purulent drainage, although rare, confirms the presence of infection. Formal débridement of a draining wound to obtain deep tissue cultures is occasionally required to diagnose infection. Subacute or chronic infections are often insidious, and systemic signs of infection are usually absent. Laboratory tests are recommended to diagnose chronic infection-associated pain.

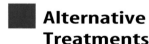

 ## Contraindications

In patients with chronic infection, débridement with retention of the prosthesis universally fails. Resection arthroplasty is a better choice for patients who have had multiple failed reimplantations. Although a direct exchange technique is advocated by some, I believe it is contraindicated in almost all patients, particularly those with resistant organisms.

Implantation of a new prosthesis is the most desirable method of treatment for most patients. The potential for improved functional outcome with a new prosthesis must be carefully balanced against the disadvantage of a higher reinfection rate compared with a definitive resection arthroplasty. Contraindications to reimplantation include persistent or recalcitrant infection, medical conditions that preclude multiple reconstructive procedures, and severe local soft-tissue damage or systemic conditions that predispose to reinfection.

Alternative Treatments

Basic treatment objectives include eradicating infection, alleviating pain, and restoring function. Six basic treatment options are available: antibiotic suppression, open débridement, resection arthroplasty, arthrodesis, implantation of another prosthesis, and hip disarticulation. A summary of approaches to treating an infected total hip arthroplasty (THA) is shown in a treatment algorithm (**Figure 1**).

Antibiotic suppression is rarely indicated and should be used only when prosthesis removal is not feasible (usually because a medical condition precludes surgery), the microorganism is susceptible to an oral antibiotic that the patient can tolerate without serious toxicity, and the prosthesis is well fixed and functional.

Débridement with prosthesis retention is indicated for acute fulminant infection in the immediate postoperative period or for late hematogenous infection of a securely fixed and previously functional prosthesis. Débridement usually is not successful when performed more than 2 weeks after the onset of symptoms, and débridement for chronic infection universally fails. Implants should be well fixed, and the causative organism(s) should be susceptible to antibiotics that the patient can tolerate. Prosthesis removal is generally required in the presence of organisms such as methicillin-resistant staphylococci.

Girdlestone resection arthroplasty is a highly successful method of eradicating infection and usually provides pain relief. However, most patients undergoing this procedure re-

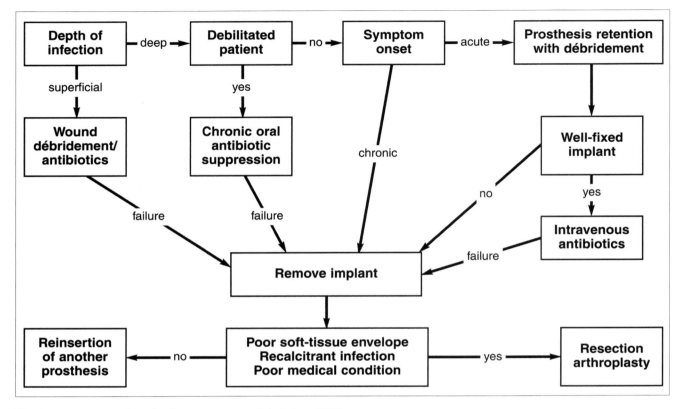

Figure 1 Treatment algorithm for management of the infected THA.

quire use of ambulatory aids, have a Trendelenburg gait, fatigue easily, experience hip instability, and have a substantial limb-length discrepancy.

Hip arthrodesis for the infected THA is rarely indicated or accepted by the patient.

Implantation of another prosthesis after a failed THA provides the patient with markedly better functional recovery. Two-stage reimplantation protocols allow observation of patient response to treatment and assessment for recurring infection once antibiotics are discontinued. The disadvantages of this approach include the hardships experienced by patients during the interval without a prosthesis, the costs of a second surgical procedure, and the technical difficulties associated with delayed prosthesis implantation. Direct exchange techniques are usually precluded by the magnitude of bone loss and the in-

creasing prevalence of drug-resistant organisms. Direct exchange has a lower success rate than two-stage reimplantation, but some authors still advocate this technique. The indications, as outlined by these authors, include an organism exquisitely sensitive to antibiotics, a well-vascularized soft-tissue envelope, and minimal bone loss.

Hip disarticulation is indicated for life-threatening infection, severe loss of soft tissue and bone stock, and vascular injury. Its use in the treatment of an infected hip is rare.

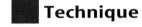

Results

An 85% to 90% success rate generally can be expected when performing a two-stage reconstruction (**Table 1**).

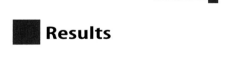

Technique

Classifying the Infection

The first step in treatment is to establish and classify the infection according to symptom onset and duration. The four infection categories are (1) positive intraoperative culture, (2) early postoperative infection, (3) acute hematogenous infection, and (4) late chronic infection.

Patients with positive intraoperative cultures are best treated with 4 to 6 weeks of intravenous antibiotics. Some patients with early postoperative or late hematogenous infections may be treated with open débridement and prosthesis retention. Patients with late chronic infection generally require removal of the infected implant, unless they cannot undergo further surgery.

No laboratory test is completely sensitive to and specific for a diagnosis of infection. A white blood cell count is not helpful in identifying infection. An erythrocyte sedimentation rate (ESR) of more than 30 to 35 mm/h and a C-reactive protein (CRP) level of more than 10 mg/L are abnormal and warrant further investigation. The CRP level returns to normal much faster than the ESR; thus, the CRP level is a more sensitive indicator of infection, particularly in the early postoperative period.

Plain radiographs are usually normal in patients with late hematogenous infection in the immediate postoperative period. However, obtaining these radiographs is essential because the status of prosthesis fixation is an important variable in the management decision process. Routine aspiration of a painful THA is not indicated, although it should be used selectively in patients with a history of wound healing problems, radiographic changes, and elevation of either ESR or CRP. Aspiration is one of the best preoperative tools available to document the presence of infection because it identifies the offending organism(s), thus allowing for more specific direction of the antibiotics used in the cement spacers and administered parenterally in the immediate postoperative period.

Additional imaging studies are rarely required to diagnose an infected THA. The technetium Tc 99m (^{99m}Tc) scan has been recommended as an initial screening tool because it is very sensitive, but it is also nonspecific. A negative scan suggests that infection is unlikely, but a positive scan may indicate that additional scintigraphic studies should be ordered.

Exposure

Many aspects of surgical débridement are similar, regardless of treatment approach. In general, old incisions are used to expose the hip. If the prior incision is invaginated, it is usually advisable to excise the scar and any adjacent sinus tracts so that the skin

Table 1 Results of Treatment of Infected Total Hip Arthroplasty

Type of Procedure	Antibiotic-loaded Bone Cement (ABLC)	Prosthesis Fixation	Success Rate
Direct exchange	N/A	Plain cement	60%
Direct exchange	N/A	ABLC	83%
Two-stage	No	Plain cement	82%
Two-stage	No	ABLC	90%
Two-stage	Yes	Uncemented	92%
Two-stage	Yes	ABLC	92%

N/A = Not Applicable

and subcutaneous tissue layers are well vascularized and will heal readily. Antibiotics are withheld until tissue specimens are obtained from the pseudocapsule and the bone-prosthetic interfaces of both components.

The goal of débridement is to remove all necrotic tissue and foreign material yet maintain the vascular supply of the bone and associated soft tissues. When possible, it is advisable to use the previous surgical approach to facilitate suture removal and minimize additional devascularization. The use of extensile surgical exposures, such as the extended trochanteric osteotomy, is increasingly common and facilitates removal of well-fixed implants while helping to maintain vascularity of the proximal femur.

Bone Preparation

A thorough resection of the pseudocapsule is necessary to expose the acetabulum, and it is important to carefully look for retained cement if either the existing or prior cup was cemented. This step is accomplished by reaming the acetabulum and carefully looking for cement fragments in the inferior aspect of the foveal region. Intraoperative radiographs are helpful in identifying and localizing cement fragments. For uncemented cups with screws, I burr the holes to adequately débride the screw tracts. After implant removal and débridement, a decision regarding reimplantation is made.

Most patients will be reimplantation candidates.

Prosthesis Implantation

A construct that will deliver high-dose local antibiotics is usually advised. Using antibiotic-loaded cement beads is strongly discouraged because removing these beads from the femoral canal or the periacetabular region can be extremely difficult (**Figure 2**).

Structural antibiotic-loaded cement spacers can be fabricated in a variety of ways. I prefer to use a standard cement gun and create a gently tapered dowel that can be easily extracted from the femoral canal at reimplantation. These dowels are used in patients with mild or moderate femoral bone loss. I prefer this method primarily because, in the presence of these dowels and in the absence of patient weight bearing, the endosteal surface of the femur undergoes a process of bony spicule formation and cancellization that facilitates the use of antibiotic-loaded cement for femoral fixation. However, if a PROSTALAC (Prosthesis of Antibiotic Loaded Acrylic Cement, DePuy, Warsaw, IN) implant is used, the sclerotic endosteal surface of the femoral canal essentially requires an uncemented femoral implant at the time of reconstruction. I typically mix 2 g of vancomycin and 2.4 g of gentamicin per 40 g of bone cement to create the dowel, and the same amount of cement and antibiotics to create a cup spacer for the acetabular fossa (**Figure 3**). The use of the acetabular spacer markedly eases exposure of the acetabulum at the time of reimplantation.

Wound Closure

When performing an extended trochanteric osteotomy, I use several 18-gauge cerclage wires to stabilize the osteotomy at wound closure because

use of large sutures results in insufficient fixation.

Postoperative Regimen

Patients are mobilized postoperatively as soon as possible. Traction is discouraged. Once intravenous antibiotic therapy is completed, I prefer to wait 6 to 8 weeks to assess the patient's response to treatment. No antibiotics are administered during this time. I monitor the ESR and CRP at 6 and 12 weeks, respectively. If hematologic parameters have improved, I proceed with reimplantation at 3 months without preoperative aspiration or other imaging modalities. This requires intraoperative judgment and consultation with an experienced pathologist to determine whether reimplantation is safe.

I like to use a cemented femoral component fixed with antibiotic-loaded bone cement when possible, using 1 g of vancomycin and 1.2 g of gentamicin per 40 g of acrylic cement. If the patient is young and has good bone stock, or the quality of bone stock precludes the use of a cemented

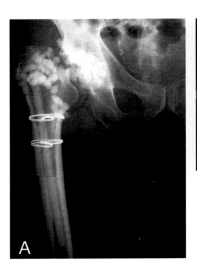
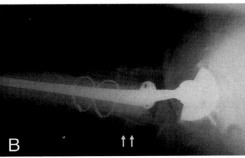

Figure 2 **A**, AP radiograph showing cerclage wires used to fix an extended trochanteric osteotomy performed for exposure and removal of a well-fixed femoral component. Note the antibiotic-loaded cement beads in the acetabular fossa and the surrounding soft tissues. Using beads is discouraged because their removal is very difficult after 6 weeks. **B**, Postoperative lateral radiograph of hybrid reimplantation prosthesis. The arrows show two antibiotic beads that were not found at reimplantation.

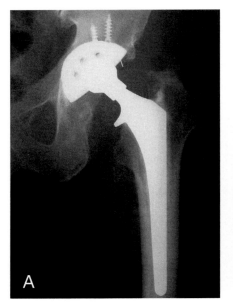
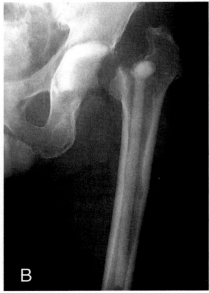
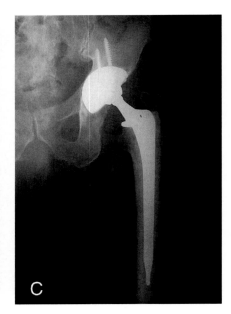

Figure 3 **A**, Preoperative AP radiograph of a chronically infected hybrid THA. **B**, AP radiograph of hip resection arthroplasty with intramedullary antibiotic-loaded cement dowel and acetabular cup spacer. **C**, Postoperative AP radiograph of hybrid reimplantation THA using antibiotic-loaded bone cement for femoral fixation.

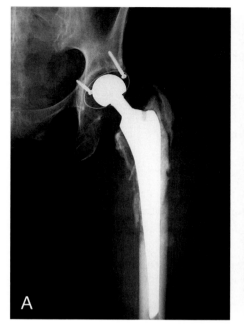
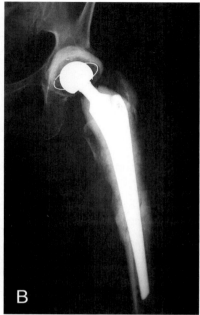
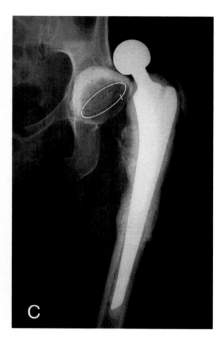

Figure 4   **A**, AP radiograph of chronically infected revision THA with severe proximal femoral bone loss. **B**, AP radiograph of an articulated antibiotic-loaded spacer (made by sterilizing the old implant and coating it with antibiotic cement) implanted for severe segmental femoral bone loss. **C**, AP radiograph of dislocated articulated spacer.

femoral component, then an uncemented femoral device is used. Uncemented hemispheric shells can usually be used on the acetabular side. The use of an abduction brace is strongly recommended because hip instability is a significant problem for these patients.

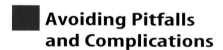

Avoiding Pitfalls and Complications

Intraoperative frozen tissue sections are a valuable tool for diagnosing infection and are most useful when preoperative evaluation results are unclear. Tissue samples should be obtained from the most inflamed areas and examined by a pathologist experienced in the interpretation of such specimens. Gram stain should not be used in intraoperative decision making because it is often more confusing than helpful.

Antibiotic-loaded cement is traditionally recommended to minimize the risk of reinfection in prosthesis fixation. The use of high-dose antibiotic-loaded cement spacers is also helpful and has allowed successful uncemented fixation at the time of reimplantation. However, the optimal duration of treatment with intravenous antibiotics for infected THA has not been definitively established. Current recommendations range from 4 to 6 weeks of treatment.

Identifying the infecting organism and a thorough débridement are critical to successfully treat an infected THA. A thorough débridement is essential but difficult to quantify and assess.

I reserve the articulated antibiotic-loaded spacer implant for the treatment of patients with severe femoral bone loss (**Figure 4**). This hip prosthesis facsimile has a thin polyethylene acetabulum and modular stainless steel femoral endoskeleton that are coated with antibiotic-loaded cement and serve as a local antibiotic delivery system while maintaining limb length and anatomic relationships. This prosthesis prevents contracture of the soft tissues and facilitates safe exposure at reimplantation. In the presence of good acetabular bone stock, hip instability can be reduced with a snap-fit articulation between the femoral prosthesis and acetabular polyethylene. It is difficult to use these prosthetic designs in patients with poor acetabular bone stock, and hip stability remains a significant issue.

■ References

Garvin KL, Hanssen AD: Infection after total hip arthroplasty: Past, present, and future. *J Bone Joint Surg Am* 1995;77:1576-1588.

Masterson EL, Masri BA, Duncan CP: Treatment of infection at the site of total hip replacement. *Instr Course Lect* 1998;47:297-306.

Spangehl MJ, Younger AS, Masri BA, Duncan CP: Diagnosis of infection following total hip arthroplasty. *Instr Course Lect* 1998;47:285-295.

Tsukayama DT, Estrada R, Gustilo RB: Infection after total hip arthroplasty: A study of the treatment of one hundred and six infections. *J Bone Joint Surg Am* 1996;78:512-523.

Ure KJ, Amstutz HC, Nasser S, Schmalzried TP: Direct-exchange arthroplasty for the treatment of infection after total hip replacement: An average ten-year follow-up. *J Bone Joint Surg Am* 1998;80:961-968.

Younger AS, Duncan CP, Masri BA: Treatment of infection associated with segmental bone loss in the proximal part of the femur in two stages with use of an antibiotic-loaded interval prosthesis. *J Bone Joint Surg Am* 1998;80:60-69.

Coding

CPT Codes		Corresponding ICD-9 Codes		
27030 (includes 11040-4)	Arthrotomy, hip, with drainage (eg, infection)	711.05 996.66-041.00-041.9	730.25 998.5	958.3
27090	Removal of hip prosthesis (separate procedure)	996.4	996.66-041.00-041.9	996.77
27091	Removal of hip prosthesis; complicated, including total hip prosthesis, methylmethacrylate with or without insertion of spacer	996.4	996.66-041.00-041.9	996.77
27132	Conversion of previous hip surgery to total hip arthroplasty, with or without autograft or allograft	715.15 718.2 733.14 996.4	715.25 718.5 733.42 996.66	715.35 718.6 905.6 996.77
27134	Revision of total hip arthroplasty; both components, with or without autograft or allograft	996.4	996.66-041.00-041.9	996.77
27284	Arthrodesis, hip joint (including obtaining graft)	715.15 718.2 718.8 808.49 808.8	715.25 718.4 808.0 808.53 808.9	715.35 718.6 808.43 808.59 905.6
27286	Arthrodesis, hip joint (including obtaining graft); with subtrochanteric osteotomy	714.0 715.35 718.6 808.43 808.59	715.15 718.2 718.8 808.49 808.8	715.25 718.4 808.0 808.53 808.9
27295	Disarticulation of hip	170.7 228.0 890.0	171.6 228.1 890.1	198.5 785.4 905.9

CPT copyright © 2004 by the American Medical Association. All Rights Reserved.

visions, limb lengthening ranged from 0.04 to 5.8 cm. A total of 66 hips were lengthened more than 2 cm, and the one sciatic nerve palsy that occurred was secondary to laceration of the nerve. Other reports have not found a significant correlation between limb lengthening and nerve palsies. These results suggest that nerve palsy should not routinely be attributed to excessive tension from limb lengthening. Unfortunately, there are no guidelines that enable the surgeon to predict the amount of lengthening that can be achieved safely.

Significant bleeding associated with wound hematoma and neuropathy has been reported as long as 3 weeks following THA. The bleeding episodes are almost universally associated with anticoagulation. This is not surprising, however, because most patients undergoing THA receive some form of anticoagulation, and bleeding may occur even though the anticoagulation therapy has been administered properly. Therefore, hematocrit and coagulation parameters should be monitored. A low hematocrit combined with abnormal coagulation parameters and swelling in the thigh or buttock suggest of an expanding hematoma. CT or ultrasound may be useful in confirming the presence of a hematoma, regardless of when it develops.

A clinically significant wound hematoma usually presents as increasing buttock and/or thigh pain. Nerve palsy may not be apparent initially but may develop over 12 to 24 hours. Patients with buttock and or thigh pain associated with a hematoma should be monitored for systemic signs of crush syndrome. In addition to compromising the sciatic nerve, pressure from the hematoma may disrupt circulation to the muscles of the gluteal compartment, resulting in rhabdomyolysis, myoglobinuria, and decreased renal function.

True peroneal palsy can occur in association with THA. Although initial neurologic function may be clinically normal, neurologic dysfunction may develop within 5 days postoperatively as a result of tight bandages and/or other type of compression of the peroneal nerve at the level of the fibular neck. Patients generally respond well once the offending agent is addressed and generally have good function at 6 months.

In most patients, the cause of the nerve palsy is really not known and is the subject of speculation. The most common scenario is that of an apparently uncomplicated THA in which the patient awakens from surgery with a loss of sensory or motor function, or both, in the surgically treated extremity.

Intraoperative Monitoring

Several studies have failed to clearly document that intraoperative cortical SSEP monitoring of sciatic nerve function during THA reduces the prevalence of nerve palsy. The advantage of spontaneous EMG over cortical SSEP monitoring is that spontaneous EMG records muscle activity moment by moment, which allows corrective action to be taken immediately, whereas cortical SSEPs record an averaged impulse over a defined period of time. Spontaneous EMG is more specific to certain kinds of trauma, such as direct trauma with cautery, but not sensitive to changes with time, such as stretching. The efficacy of this technique has not been conclusively established.

Treatment

Most nerve palsies are managed nonsurgically, and in most cases some level of function returns. However, hematomas, definite overlengthening of the extremity, or nerve compression by a screw or component should be excluded as the cause of the nerve palsy. Surgical evacuation of the hematoma, shortening of the extremity by exchange of the femoral head, or revision of the femoral component and removal of the screws or components causing the impingement are necessary as soon as possible. If a nerve has been transected, it should be repaired in the early postoperative period.

When a neuropathy is discovered, a formal consultation with neurology is helpful. The neurologist can validate the physical findings, assist in localization of the nerve injury (often through electrodiagnostic studies), and help identify any treatable causes of peripheral neuropathy. A thorough electrodiagnostic evaluation includes evaluation of the innervation of the short head of the biceps. This is the only muscle in the thigh to receive innervation from the peroneal division of the sciatic nerve. Denervation of this muscle indicates nerve injury in the proximal thigh in what may otherwise appear to be a peroneal nerve injury at or below the knee.

I am unaware of any published reports describing the effectiveness of imaging studies such as CT or MRI for the localization of nerve injury, either acutely or subacutely, after THA. However, I find that these modalities can detect hematomas, localized compression, and localized swelling of a major nerve. Thus, I believe it is reasonable to consider these modalities in an effort to identify a treatable cause of a neuropathy. However, there are insufficient data to evaluate the impact of these imaging studies on treatment and outcome.

Another risk factor for nerve palsy associated with THA may be concurrent spinal stenosis. In one report, 21 patients with spinal stenosis and a history of back and leg pain without weakness before THA exhibited a foot drop postoperatively. Spinal imaging studies in these patients showed high-grade spinal stenosis. Sixteen of the 21 patients were treated by lumbar decompression. Six of these patients recovered completely, and six showed some improvement. Without surgery, patients did not improve.

Minimizing edema in the nerve fibers is of theoretical benefit, but there is no scientific basis or documented efficacy for the use of steroids or osmotic agents to teat a nerve palsy after THA. When a nerve palsy is diagnosed in the immediate postoperative period, release of tension on the nerve may help restore function. When treating a sciatic nerve palsy, the hip should be extended and the knee flexed over the side of the bed to reduce tension on the nerve. The opposite position would be desirable for minimizing the risk of femoral neuropathy. Treatment of any coexisting causes of peripheral neuropathy would be theoretically beneficial.

As soon as a diagnosis of nerve palsy is established and the patient's condition allows, the surgeon should discuss the problem with the patient. An educated patient is the best ally in maximizing recovery. The nursing staff and physical therapists should be advised of the nerve injury, and additional exercises should be prescribed to strengthen weakened muscles and stretch uninjured antagonists to prevent joint contracture. The patient should be fitted with appropriate orthotics as soon as possible to allow physical therapy to proceed. A knee immobilizer or similar removable brace to hold the knee in extension will allow safe ambulation in the presence of a femoral neuropathy. An ankle-foot orthosis can facilitate ambulation in patients with sciatic neuropathy. The patient should learn to examine sensory impaired skin regions daily. If dysesthesias are present, treatment with a tricyclic antidepressant or tetracyclic antidepressant may be of some benefit, although the associated orthostatic hypotension or other anticholinergic side effects may outweigh the benefits in some patients.

There are no absolute indications for repeat surgery (exploration) and only anecdotal experience. Good outcomes have been reported with nonsurgical management. With input from the patient, the surgeon must weigh all the variables and individualize treatment based on the overall clinical condition of the patient and the relative risks and benefits of repeat surgery in each case.

Outcomes

The outcomes of a nerve palsy associated with THA are variable. One study reported that 41% of patients had complete or essentially complete nerve function, whereas 44% of patients had a mild persistent deficit. Complete recovery of function occurred within 2 years postoperatively. In this study, the prognosis for neurologic recovery was related to the degree of nerve damage. All patients who retained some motor function immediately postoperatively, or recovered some motor function within 2 weeks of surgery (indicative of a lesser degree of nerve injury), made a good recovery. Approximately 15% of patients in this study had a poor outcome characterized by weakness that limited ambulation and/or persistent dysesthesias. None of the patients with severe dysesthesia had a good recovery.

Although I am not aware of any study that directly compares outcome with type of nerve(s) injured, in my experience patients with femoral nerve injuries have a better prognosis. This difference in outcome may be a function of the distance that the nerve must regenerate to reach the motor end plates. The distance to the motor end plates is substantially less for the femoral nerve; thus, successful reinnervation after high-grade injury is more likely in patients with femoral nerve damage than in those with sciatic nerve damage. Early return of motor function or the presence of partial nerve or motor deficits generally are associated with higher rates of recovery. In contrast, a poor prognosis is associated with a dense palsy with no return of function within 2 weeks postoperatively.

———————————■

■ Vascular Injuries

Prevalence

Vascular injuries associated with THA are rare with a prevalence of less than 0.3%. Risk factors include revision THA, intrapelvic migration of the acetabular component, infection, left-sided surgery, and female sex. Acute injuries may present as bleeding during surgery; delayed complications include postoperative hemorrhage or hematoma, ischemia due to arterial occlusion, embolism, thrombosis, false aneurysm, or arteriovenous fistula. Patients may report symptoms associate with these complications, specifically cardiovascular reactions due to blood loss, pain due to ischemia, or pressure from a false aneurysm.

Vessels at Risk

The extrapelvic structures at risk principally are the common femoral vessels, the profundus femoral vessels and their branches, and the medial and lateral circumflex arteries. Blunt damage from placement of retractors and intraoperative retraction appear to be the principal causes for the damage, especially retractors placed around the anterior rim of the acetabulum (femoral artery and vein) and around the femoral neck (medial and lateral circumflex artery).

The external iliac artery and vein, the obturator vein and artery, and the inferior gluteal vessels are at risk during THA. The external iliac vessels and the obturator vessels can be damaged by anterior and inferior retractors or by the removal of an acetabular component that has migrated medially. With the use of screws for fixation of uncemented prostheses and revision cages, the most common mechanism of injury is intrapelvic screw placement.

The quadrant system was introduced to help the surgeon with intraoperative orientation of safe zones for screw placement (**Figure 2**). The ac-

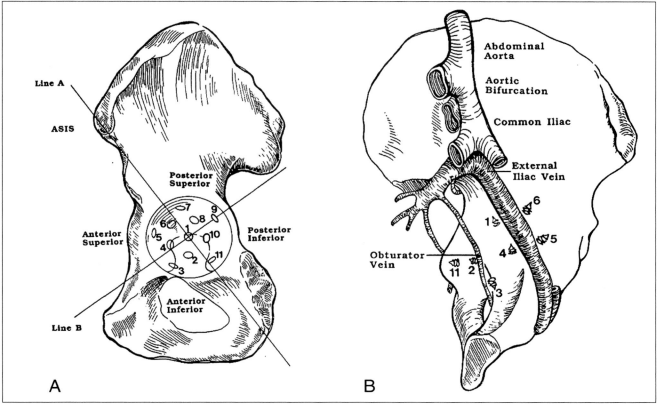

Figure 2 **A,** Acetabular quadrant system. **B,** Principal vessels inside the pelvis. (Reproduced with permission from Wasielewski RC, Cooperstein LA, Kruger MP, Rubash HE: Acetabular anatomy and the transacetabular fixation of screws in total hip arthroplasty. *J Bone Joint Surg Am* 1990;72:501-508.)

etabulum is divided into anterior and posterior halves by a line originating from the anterior superior iliac spine. A perpendicular line divides each half into a superior and inferior quadrant. The intrapelvic structures adjacent to the anterior quadrants include the external iliac vessels and the obturator vessels. Located opposite to the posterior inferior quadrant are the inferior gluteal and the internal pudendal vessels. The posterior superior quadrant is considered the safest zone for screw placement because it consists of the greatest bone depth for secure screw fixation. It should be recognized that the superior gluteal vessels are located beyond this quadrant.

Diagnosis

Retroperitoneal or intrapelvic bleeding usually is not visually apparent in the field of dissection. Intrapelvic bleeding from a major vessel should be high in the differential diagnosis if an acute sustained drop in blood pressure occurs during THA, particularly after screw placement.

Treatment

If a potential vessel injury is suspected, an immediate consultation with a vascular or general surgeon is necessary. Most surgeons do not have expertise in the management of a major arterial injury; thus, the practical goal for the surgeon is to reduce the acute bleeding. In the operating room, temporizing methods include packing off of the bleeding vessel from the remainder of the wound or placing a clamp around the surrounding tissue, if not on the actual vessel or lumen. Prompt, adequate volume replacement can prevent vascular collapse. A laparotomy may be necessary to control life-threatening retroperitoneal or intrapelvic bleeding by applying direct pressure to the source of bleeding. Arterial bleeding can be reduced by pressure to the aorta (below the renal arteries) or on the iliac artery. Localized packing of venous bleeding, with or without thrombostatic agents, can reduce acute blood loss. Embolization can stop retroperitoneal or intrapelvic bleeding, given the availability of this modality and that the patient is stable enough to be transferred to an angiography suite.

■ Acknowledgment

Thanks to Dr. Christian Heisel for his assistance in the review and editing of this manuscript.

■ References

Barrack RL, Butler RA: Avoidance and management of neurovascular injuries in total hip arthroplasty. *Instr Course Lect* 2003;52:267-274.

Lewallen DG: Neurovascular injury associated with hip arthroplasty. *Instr Course Lect* 1998;47:275-283.

Nercessian OA, Piccoluga F, Eftekhar NS: Postoperative sciatic and femoral nerve palsy with reference to leg lengthening and medialization/lateralization of the hip joint following total hip arthroplasty. *Clin Orthop* 1994;304:165-171.

Schmalzried TP, Noordin S, Amstutz HC: Update on nerve palsy associated with total hip replacement. *Clin Orthop* 1997;344:188-206.

Coding

CPT Codes		Corresponding ICD-9 Codes		
26990	Drainage, hematoma, hip	998.11 998.2 902.53 956.0 956.9	998.12 904.0 902.54 956.1	998.13 904.2 959.6 956.3
27134	Revision of total hip arthroplasty; both components, with or without autograft or allograft	996.4	996.66	996.77
27138	Revision of total hip arthroplasty; femoral component only, with or without allograft	996.4	996.66	996.77

CPT copyright © 2004 by the American Medical Association. All Rights Reserved.

Chapter 33

Management of Heterotopic Ossification

Vincent D. Pellegrini Jr, MD

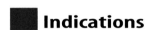 **Indications**

Risk Factors

Heterotopic ossification is the process by which aberrant bone is formed in the soft tissue arising from the capsular tissues or skeletal muscle in close proximity to a joint. This pathologic process most often occurs about the hip and is typically incited by surgical procedures such as total hip arthroplasty (THA), fixation of acetabular fractures, pelvic osteotomy, and intramedullary nailing of femoral shaft fractures. Heterotopic ossification also occurs about other joints, such as the shoulder, elbow, and knee, and after nonsurgical events such as head injury, cerebrovascular accident, and burns. Nonetheless, it is clinically seen most often as ectopic bone formation in the abductor musculature after THA. Factors intrinsic to the patient, injury to the abductor musculature, surgical approach, hemorrhage, and bone debris remaining in the soft tissues all contribute to the overall risk of heterotopic ossification in any individual patient.

As a radiographic phenomenon without accompanying symptoms, heterotopic ossification has been reported to occur in as many as 90% of patients who have undergone THA. In this setting, it is seen as small islands of bone in the soft tissues about the hip or as bony outgrowths from the margin of the acetabulum or tip of the greater trochanter, measuring less than 1 cm in length. However, in 8% to 10% of patients, ectopic bone formation after THA occurs to such an extent or in such a location that it results in pain and restricted motion. In the most extreme cases, the resulting pain and stiffness replace those that prompted the patient to seek surgery in the first place and may actually negate the beneficial effect of the THA.

Patients believed to be at increased risk for heterotopic bone formation should receive some form of prophylaxis; in my experience this constitutes approximately 20% of those undergoing THA. Classically, these high-risk patients include those with a diagnosis of hypertrophic osteoarthritis and prominent marginal osteophytes (**Figure 1**), diffuse idiopathic skeletal hyperostosis, or ankylosing spondylitis, and those in whom heterotopic bone has formed after a previous procedure or injury about the hip. Nearly all patients in whom heterotopic bone has formed after surgery about the hip will develop bone again, usually to a greater degree, after reoperation on the involved hip or primary operation on the contralateral hip. Men are generally twice as likely as women to form heterotopic bone, but in women in these risk categories ectopic bone develops at rates comparable with those of men. It is increasingly recognized that central nervous system disorders, specifically Parkinson's disease, spinal cord injury, and perioperative cerebrovascular accident, also predispose patients to heterotopic ossification about the hip.

The surgical approach to the hip also affects the risk of heterotopic ossification, reflecting the extent to which the abductor musculature is violated or injured during the procedure. The transgluteal or modified Hardinge approach is credited with the highest rate of severe ossification, followed by the transtrochanteric, anterolateral, and posterolateral approaches; the posterolateral approach has the lowest rate of heterotopic ossification after THA. Similarly, after acetabular fracture repair, the ilioinguinal approach has the lowest incidence of heterotopic bone formation, followed by the posterolateral, transtrochanteric (**Figure 2**), and extended iliofemoral approaches; the extended iliofemoral approach strips the abductors from the iliac wing and has the greatest risk of heterotopic ossification.

Pathophysiology

The cellular mechanism of heterotopic ossification remains unclear. Essential to this issue is the question of the anatomic origin of the pluripotential mesenchymal cells participating in the process of bone formation within the soft tissues. Transformation of local cells into bone-producing elements has been proposed by many investigators. Trauma to muscle leads to hemorrhage, muscle degeneration, and proliferation of perivascular connective tissue, culminating in the production of heterotopic bone. Studies in an animal model using tritium-labeled thymidine and uridine have shown that local soft-tissue fibroblasts adjacent to an implanted demineralized bone fragment were induced to transform into pluripotential mesenchymal cells that differentiated into osteoblasts. Pluripotential mesenchymal cells are ubiquitous in the soft tissues about the hip, and it is postulated that these cell lines may be induced to undergo atypical differentiation into osteogenic stem cells capable of participating in the process of heterotopic ossification. Maturation of these cells down either osteoblastic or chondroblastic stem cell lines could then lead to the formation of ectopic bone.

Other investigators have postulated that distant migratory hematopoietic stem cells may be essential to inducing local connective tissue elements to form heterotopic bone. Pluripotential mesenchymal cells and osteocytes are liberated from the marrow space of the ilium and femoral canal during THA and are likely present in the local hematoma. They may contribute to the process of heterotopic ossification, either directly by bone formation or indirectly via stimulation of local cells to express osteogenic phenotypes. Distant hematopoietic stem cells transported to the wound as

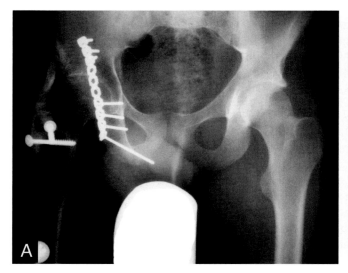

Figure 1 AP radiograph of a 66-year-old man with primary osteoarthritis and diffuse hypertrophic skeletal hyperostosis. The whiskering of periosteal new bone about the ischial tuberosity and iliac crest is evident. Stigmata of enthesopathy are seen as calcification in the tendinous insertion of the iliopsoas on the lesser trochanter.

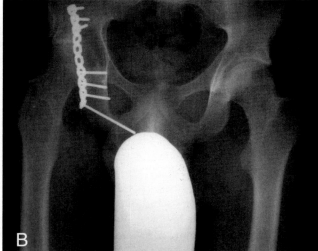

Figure 2 AP radiographs of a 16-year-old boy following open reduction and internal fixation of an acetabular fracture he sustained in a motor vehicle accident. **A**, Grade IV heterotopic ossification occurred postoperatively despite prophylaxis with indomethacin (25 mg administered three times a day for 2 weeks). The hip was functionally ankylosed. **B**, Radiograph obtained 6 months after surgical excision of the heterotopic bone and prophylaxis with a single dose of 800 rad. Ectopic bone did not recur, and an excellent clinical result was achieved.

part of the normal response to surgical injury also possess the capability to mature along osteogenic cell lines under the influence of mitogenic stimuli in the wound environment.

In 1975, it was postulated that three requisite conditions must be met to allow heterotopic bone formation: (1) the presence of an inducing agent, (2) an osteogenic precursor cell, and (3) an environment conducive to osteogenesis. Several bone morphogenic proteins exist, and bone dust recovered from patients who formed heterotopic bone has been shown to stimulate proliferation of isolated bone progenitor cells in culture sixfold more than similar material extracted from patients who did not form heterotopic bone. Histomorphometric and biochemical data have shown that heterotopic bone contains more than twice as many active osteoclasts and has a rate of appositional new bone formation nearly three times that of normal age-matched bone. A stimulatory protein isolated from heterotopic bone has been shown to induce both osteoprogenitor cell proliferation and collagen synthesis.

Regardless of the site of origin of the pluripotential mesenchymal cells, heterotopic ossification seems to be clearly dependent on cellular differentiation down osteoprogenitor cell lines. Ionizing radiation is known to exert its greatest influence on rapidly dividing cells by interfering with the normal production of nuclear deoxyribonucleic acid. It has been demonstrated in mice that differentiation of pluripotential mesenchymal cells into osteoblasts began 16 hours after fracture of the femur and peaked at approximately 32 hours. In the resulting model, the critical events of cellular differentiation occurred during the immediate postoperative period. A similar chronology may be extrapolated to the sequence of heterotopic ossification, even though the actual ectopic bone is not detectable radiographically for several weeks after surgery. There-

fore, to be most effective, it seems essential that irradiation or other prophylactic measures be administered early during the postoperative period to prevent osteoblastic differentiation of pluripotential mesenchymal stem cells, effectively arresting osteoid and subsequent heterotopic bone formation during the initial phases of cellular reorganization.

Radiographic Staging

A radiographic classification system is most commonly used to describe the pattern and extent of ossification on the AP pelvic radiograph. In stage I, islands of bone appear in the soft tissues; in stage II, bone spurs arise from the pelvis or proximal femur with 1 cm or less between adjacent bone surfaces; in stage III, bone spurs arise from the pelvis or proximal femur with more than 1 cm between adjacent bone surfaces; and in stage IV, confluent bone bridges the pelvis and proximal femur and there is apparent bony ankylosis of the hip.

Further description of the radiographic extent of ossification correlates with the degree of functional impairment attributed to the ectopic bone formation. The grading system describes the proportion of the area involved in the triangle defined by the base of the greater trochanter, the anterior iliac spine, and the inferior aspect of the ischium. Grade A bone involves 33% or less of this area, grade B involves 34% to 66%, and grade C involves 67% to 100%. Greater extent of involvement correlates with more clinically significant limitation of motion about the hip.

Clinical Presentation

Vague discomfort or frank pain in the region of the hip is believed to be the direct result of the inflammatory process involved in heterotopic ossification. It is characteristically present at rest, is unaffected by activity, and often interferes with sleep. This pain typically occurs during the first 6 months

after surgery and spontaneously resolves as the activity of the process subsides and the radiographic appearance of the bone matures. The extent of radiographic ossification varies and is difficult to assess because the symptoms often occur before the bone is well mineralized; ultimately, grade III or IV bone formation is apparent in patients with clinically bothersome symptoms. Nonsteroidal anti-inflammatory drugs (NSAIDs) or nonnarcotic analgesics are the cornerstone of treatment.

Greater trochanteric bursitis may occur in association with apparently small bone spurs (stage II) originating from the base or lateral surface of the greater trochanter. Although not extensive, the strategic location of these spurs at the prominence of the greater trochanter beneath the iliotibial band may provoke troublesome irritation of the bursa located in this area. These symptoms are aggravated by postoperative gluteal abductor weakness secondary to disuse during a prolonged period of arthritic disease before surgery. Effective treatment typically consists of NSAIDs and a gluteal abductor strengthening program. Occasionally, a steroid injection into the region of the bursa and the offending bone spur is necessary to break the cycle of symptoms. Symptoms usually resolve over a period of several months, but the bursitis associated with these spurs of ectopic bone can be particularly troublesome and refractory to the usual treatment measures. A series of several steroid injections may be indicated and, rarely, surgical removal of the spurs might be considered in conjunction with postoperative measures to prevent recurrence.

Stiffness about the hip is the most problematic consequence of heterotopic ossification after THA and is typically present only when grade III or IV bone is evident on the radiograph. Most commonly, the surgeon finds it remarkable that rather promi-

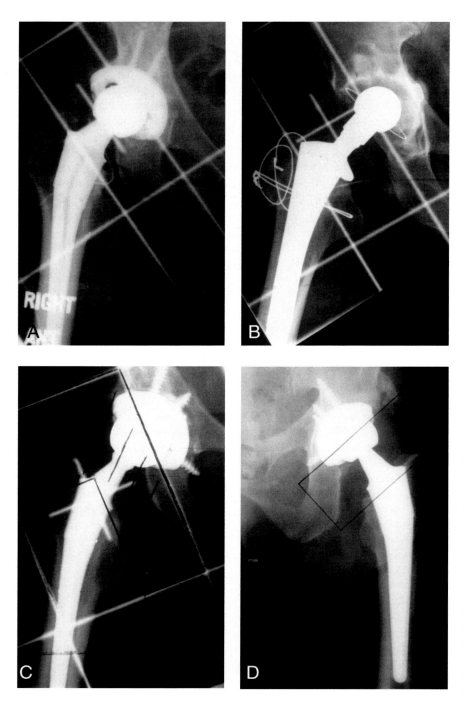

Figure 3 Radiation treatment portals used for prophylaxis of heterotopic ossification are shown. **A**, Primary THA with obliquely oriented limited field portal aligned parallel to the iliac crest and acetabular component. **B**, Revision THA with obliquely oriented limited field portal with modified "L" configuration to exclude the site of trochanteric osteotomy. **C**, A modified L-shaped treatment portal to include the lateral trochanteric ridge in a patient with diffuse idiopathic skeletal hyperostosis to reduce risk of ectopic bone in this area leading to local bursitis. **D**, Extra-field ossification is evident outside the treatment portal along the iliac wing after a single dose of limited-field 800 rad prophylaxis. This was not functionally significant.

nent radiographic ossification is accompanied by a measurable decrease in range of motion with comparatively little, if any, functional restriction in most patients. The degree of loss of range of motion necessary to compromise function varies by patient and depends on the patient's needs for mobility during daily activities along with the severity of arthritic disease on the adjacent joints and low back. Even though the lumbar spine is most often called on to compensate for a stiff hip, high-grade heterotopic ossification is most problematic in patients with concurrent lumbar spondylosis and spinal stenosis. Typical limitations occur secondary to limited rotation and flexion of the hip, restricting sitting ability, donning of shoes and socks, and foot hygiene. Neither medication nor injection therapy is effective in restoring range of motion once radiography shows evidence of ectopic bone or there is clinical restriction of motion. Although relatively few patients seek surgery to restore lost mobility secondary to heterotopic ossification after THA, surgical excision of the offending bone is the only effective intervention once restricted motion is clinically evident. Surgery is rarely indicated when less than radiographic stage III or IV ossification is present. Moreover, adjunctive prophylactic measures and radiation or NSAIDs in conjunction with surgical excision are essential to prevent postoperative recurrence of bone formation to the same or an even greater degree. Thus, the development of effective prophylaxis has appropriately attracted even more attention than the surgical management of this problem.

Contraindications

Contraindications to prophylaxis depend on the specific modality used for prevention. Although external-beam irradiation in doses less than 3,000 rad delivered over 3 weeks has not been shown to result in local formation of sarcoma, patients receiving treatment specifically for heterotopic ossification have only recently been followed long enough (and not yet in sufficient numbers) to permit this analysis. More specifically, in one series, radiation-induced sarcoma of bone was not observed for as long as 25 years after more than 1,000 rad was administered in the treatment of patients with childhood cancers. Typically, radiation-induced sarcoma has a latency period of 20 to 25 years. Considering that longer life expectancy provides greater opportunity for development of this complication, younger patients (particularly those younger than age 40 years) present a relative contraindication to radiation prophylaxis. Women of childbearing age should not receive radiation prophylaxis for heterotopic ossification. Patients who have received previous radiation therapy for a cancer diagnosis, such as Hodgkin's disease, require special consideration to avoid a cumulative effective radiation dose in the toxic range. NSAIDs should be avoided in patients with a history of peptic ulcer disease; previous gastrointestinal bleeding is a specific contraindication to this form of prophylaxis. In one study, more than one third of patients receiving indomethacin prophylaxis for heterotopic ossification after THA experienced gastrointestinal symptoms that precluded completion of the prescribed 6-week course.

Both external-beam irradiation and NSAIDs have been shown in the laboratory to delay bone ingrowth into uncemented devices intended for biologic fixation. Radiation fields have been successfully limited to exclude prosthetic hip implants (**Figure 3**), such that devices 1 cm outside the intended treatment portal receive less than 5% of the prescribed dose delivered to the specified area. In contrast, indomethacin has a systemic effect from which the hip prosthesis cannot

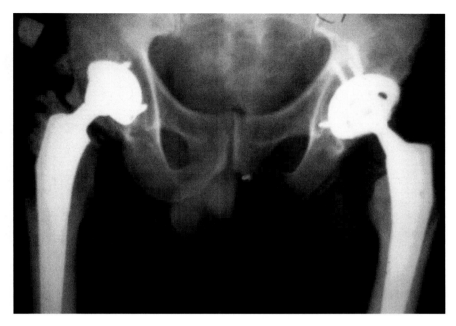

Figure 4 AP radiograph of a 65-year-old man with hypertrophic osteoarthritis and diffuse skeletal hyperostosis. Grade III heterotopic ossification is evident after THA on the right hip with no prophylaxis. No heterotopic ossification is evident after subsequent THA on the left side with a single dose of limited-field 800 rad prophylaxis administered on the second postoperative day.

be effectively protected. Nonetheless, no clinical THA failures have been attributed to lack of component fixation related to either irradiation or indomethacin prophylaxis for heterotopic bone formation.

Alternative Treatments and Results

Recognition of the early initiation of osteoblastic cell differentiation at the time of surgical insult, coupled with the understanding that this process is not easily arrested once begun, has made prevention the cornerstone of management of heterotopic ossification. External-beam irradiation and NSAIDs, particularly indomethacin, are the most thoroughly studied and widely used interventions for prophylaxis. Bisphosphonates have been used for this purpose. However, their

use was abandoned after recognition that these agents only delay heterotopic ossification by blocking mineralization of osteoid matrix, which proceeds normally after discontinuation of the drug.

External-beam irradiation is my preferred method of prophylaxis and has been shown to be effective in single doses of 700 or 800 rad, provided treatment is delivered before the fifth postoperative day. Despite other complicating medical conditions, the patient is typically treated on the first or second postoperative day (**Figure 4**). A single-dose regimen of 550 rad has been shown to be ineffective. Historically, divided doses of 2,000 and 1,000 rad have been delivered in 10 and 5 fractions, respectively, but single-dose regimens have demonstrated comparable efficacy and rendered fractionated treatment obsolete because of greater ease of treatment. Preoperative single-dose administration of 800 rad within 6 hours of surgery has been shown to provide efficacy comparable with post-

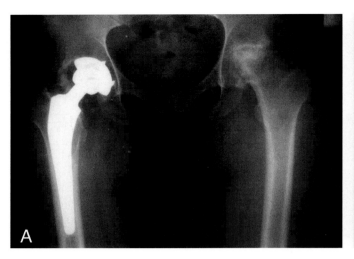
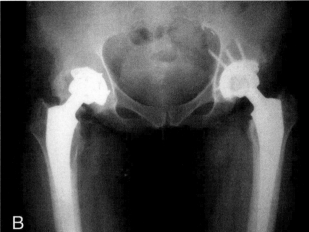

Figure 5 AP radiographs of a 55-year-old woman with Hodgkin's disease and osteonecrosis of both hips after receiving chemotherapy protocol, including high-dose prednisone. The patient was not thought to have risk factors for heterotopic ossification after THA. **A**, Grade IV heterotopic ossification with ankylosed hip occurred after THA. **B**, AP radiograph obtained after contralateral THA with a single dose of limited-field 800 rad prophylaxis administered 4 hours preoperatively. An excellent clinical result was achieved.

operative treatment and greater patient convenience and comfort while eliminating the complications associated with patient transport (eg, dislocation) soon after THA (**Figure 5**). Limited treatment fields, usually an obliquely oriented rectangular portal centered over the joint space and oriented parallel to the acetabular component, have effectively excluded the ingrowth of hip components from the adverse effects of the radiation and eliminated concern regarding impaired bone ingrowth into the device (**Figure 3**, *A*). Addition of a small lateral treatment area over the greater trochanter, converting the rectangle into an L-shaped treatment portal, has reduced the incidence of greater trochanteric bursitis associated with extra field ossification at the vastus lateralis ridge (**Figure 3**, *C*). Radiation prophylaxis has nearly eliminated clinically significant (grades III and IV) heterotopic ossification while reducing the occurrence of grade I and II ectopic bone to 10% to 20% in high-risk patients studied.

Similarly, indomethacin has been shown to be effective in reducing the prevalence of heterotopic ossification compared with control agents. Historically, 6 weeks of indomethacin at doses of 25 mg administered three times a day effectively prevented clinically meaningful heterotopic bone formation. This dose administered for 7, 10, or 14 days has been shown to be effective in eliminating grade III and IV ossification while reducing the occurrence of grade I and II bone to less than 10% in patients studied. Conversely, a higher daily dose of 150 mg (50 mg three times a day) administered over only 3 days has been shown to be ineffective in preventing ectopic bone formation. Although prospective controlled clinical trials have failed to demonstrate a statistically significant difference between single-dose postoperative radiation and indomethacin administered in a divided daily dose of 75 mg in preventing heterotopic ossification after surgery about the hip, as much as a twofold greater efficacy has been observed with radiation prophylaxis (**Figure 2**).

![■]
■ Complications

Adverse events associated with prophylactic regimens directed against heterotopic ossification have been few. Although the risk of radiation-induced malignancy is always present, no cases have been reported in association with doses as low as those used for heterotopic ossification prophylaxis. No wound complications of any kind have been observed about the hip, including skin erythema, pigmentation, and delayed wound healing. Parenthetically, increased skin pigmentation has been observed about the elbow after radiation prophylaxis for heterotopic ossification after takedown of posttraumatic bony ankylosis.

NSAIDs in general, and indomethacin in particular, are associated with gastrointestinal bleeding complications. This propensity for bleeding is further exaggerated perioperatively in the patient population undergoing THA and having preexisting comorbidities. Concurrent use of NSAIDs with pharmacologic agents for prophylaxis of venous thromboembolic disease further complicates the management of bleeding complications in these patients. One study noted a doubling of the rate of bleeding complications in patients receiving both indomethacin for prevention of heterotopic ossification and warfarin for prophylaxis of deep vein thrombosis after THA.

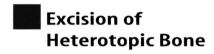

Excision of Heterotopic Bone

Indications

Once heterotopic bone is apparent on radiographs of the hip, nonsurgical measures are ineffective in retarding progression of bone formation or removing or clearing the bone from the hip area. Surgical excision of heterotopic bone about the hip is rarely necessary. Severe restriction of functional range of motion is the primary indication for surgery. In its mildest form, this may consist of difficulty in reaching the feet for personal hygiene and dressing; in more severe cases, inability to sit secondary to bony ankylosis of the hip may occur. Problems with sitting posture and balance that adversely affect the ability to independently achieve a transfer may pose a serious threat to functional independence in patients with spinal cord or head injury. Infrequently, impingement of heterotopic bone may contribute to recurrent instability of the THA and require surgical excision. More commonly, however, the patient with heterotopic ossification about the hip has restricted range of motion with a stable prosthetic hip joint, and other reasons for the instability should be sought.

The timing of surgical excision of heterotopic bone is a matter of ongoing discussion. Based on a high rate of recurrence when excision is undertaken at an earlier interval, conventional wisdom has held that 12 to 24 months should pass before an attempt is made to excise the ectopic bone. The bone scan and serum alkaline phosphatase levels traditionally have been used to monitor activity of the pathologic process of bone forma-

tion; it has been recommended that surgical excision be deferred until these studies return to normal, often 2 years after the index operation. With increasing appreciation of the necessity and efficacy of adjunctive measures, such as perioperative irradiation or indomethacin to reduce the recurrence of heterotopic ossification, the importance of an extended period of waiting for maturation of the ectopic bone before attempting excision is less clear. A 6-month interval before excision may be more reasonable; it allows radiographic maturation of the bone sufficient to judge its extent and may encourage formation of the surrounding fibrous membrane that facilitates blunt dissection during the surgical procedure.

Finally, it should be emphasized that pain about the hip is not an indication for excision of radiographically apparent heterotopic bone. The pain associated with heterotopic ossification occurs while the inflammatory process is active and the bone is immature. Other sources for continued pain about the hip should be sought when the heterotopic bone is radiographically mature and metabolically quiescent, as judged by the serum alkaline phosphatase levels and bone scan. Clinical results have generally been poor when the primary indication for excision of ectopic bone about the hip has been pain.

Contraindications

Lack of radiographic maturation sufficient to determine the extent of heterotopic bone, and thus, the correct surgical approach, is a relative contraindication to its surgical removal. Similarly, because the procedure is accompanied by considerable blood loss, coagulopathies should be corrected and anticoagulants reversed before undertaking such an operation.

It should be clearly understood by the patient and the surgeon that pathologic ectopic bone arises most commonly from the gluteal abductor

muscle mass. Therefore, the larger the amount of heterotopic bone, the smaller is the amount of functional abductor muscle that remains to stabilize the hip. The implication is that excision of large amounts of heterotopic bone is accompanied by a risk of destabilizing the hip and imparting a gluteal limp secondary to weak and inadequate remaining abductor muscle mass. The patient should be apprised of this risk preoperatively and must be willing to use a cane indefinitely or until the abductor strength is regained in exchange for regaining range of motion. Unwillingness of the patient to use a cane postoperatively, especially when one was not needed before surgery, is a relative contraindication to surgical excision of the heterotopic bone that stiffens and stabilizes the hip.

Technique

Preoperative CT is helpful in defining soft-tissue structures that are displaced by the mass of ectopic bone and are therefore at risk during the dissection, particularly when the bone is medial to the hip center. Most commonly, the ectopic bone displaces adjacent structures and does not invade neighboring soft-tissue planes; a fibrous plane usually exists at the periphery of the bone mass that facilitates blunt dissection of the ectopic bone. Sharp dissection of the bone mass should be avoided.

The surgical approach used for excision of heterotopic bone is most commonly the same approach used for the index procedure that resulted in the bone formation. Blunt dissection of normal structures at the periphery of the ectopic bone resulting in isolation of the pathologic bone mass should be the surgical strategy. An elevator is the instrument of choice in dissecting the periphery of the ectopic bone. Final separation and removal of the bone mass may require a mallet and osteotome. Radical circumferential excision of the hip capsule or

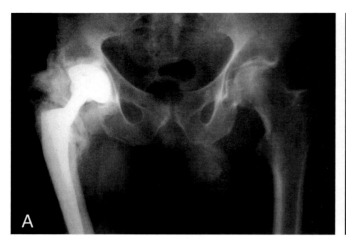 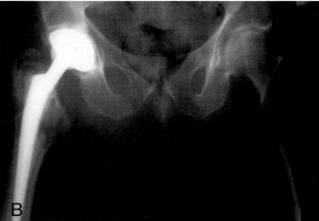

Figure 6   AP radiographs of a 68-year-old man with Parkinson's disease who was thought not to have risk factors for heterotopic ossification after THA. **A**, Grade IV heterotopic ossification with ankylosed hip occurred after THA. **B**, AP radiograph obtained 6 months after surgical excision of the heterotopic bone and prophylaxis with a single dose of expanded-field 800 rad. Ectopic bone did not recur and an excellent clinical result was achieved.

pseudocapsule usually is necessary to maximize improvement in range of motion.

Adjunctive radiation or indomethacin treatment is essential to avoid reactivation of the process of heterotopic ossification; without some form of effective prophylaxis recurrence is almost guaranteed, often to a greater extent than that which prompted the effort at excision. I prefer radiation (**Figure 6**). If ectopic bone is excised without concurrent revision of the arthroplasty and if well-fixed components are retained, an expanded field of radiation is used. This rectangular treatment field extends from a proximal point cephalad to the acetabulum to a distal point at the midshaft of the femoral component and includes a symmetric area medial and lateral to the hip center, encompassing the abductor musculature. Such an expanded field minimizes the risk of ectopic bone recurrence at the margins of the treatment portal, as is occasionally seen after primary radiation prophylaxis after THA.

Excision of heterotopic bone, accompanied by expanded field radiation or indomethacin prophylaxis, reliably provides an increase in functional range of hip motion but does not restore normal mobility. Published results report an average increase in flexion range of 34° to 45° and approximately 25° of abduction. The greatest functional gain is evident in those hips with the most severe preoperative limitation in motion. Pain is not reliably relieved by excision of the heterotopic bone.

Complications

Recurrence of ectopic bone is the most common complication, especially in the absence of adjunctive measures such as indomethacin or irradiation.

Recovery of less than full range of motion is the rule and reflects the dense connective tissue that replaces the excised bone mass, even in the absence of recurrence of ossification.

Gluteal abductor weakness is a common occurrence after this procedure if a large amount of bone (and replaced abductor muscle mass) is excised. Use of a cane is often necessary for 6 to 12 months postoperatively, if not indefinitely. In severe cases, instability of the prosthetic hip may result.

Massive blood loss from the raw surfaces of the excised ectopic bone is common, and liberal transfusion of blood in conjunction with crystalloid is the rule to prevent problematic hypovolemia. Nerve palsy and blood vessel injury may result from difficult dissection of soft tissue or removal of ectopic bone encircling these structures.

———————————————————■

References

Brooker AF, Bowerman JW, Robinson RA, Riley LH Jr: Ectopic ossification following total hip replacement: Incidence and a method of classification. *J Bone Joint Surg Am* 1973;55:1629-1632.

Burd TA, Lowry KJ, Anglen JO: Indomethacin compared with localized irradiation for the prevention of heterotopic ossification following surgical treatment of acetabular fractures. *J Bone Joint Surg Am* 2001;83:1783-1788.

Chalmers J, Gray DH, Rush J: Observations on the induction of bone in soft tissues. *J Bone Joint Surg Br* 1975;57:36-45.

Cobb TK, Berry DJ, Wallrichs SL, Ilstrup DM, Morrey BF: Functional outcome of excision of heterotopic ossification after total hip arthroplasty. *Clin Orthop* 1999;361:131-139.

Coventry MB, Scanlon PW: The use of radiation to discourage ectopic bone: A nine-year study in surgery about the hip. *J Bone Joint Surg Am* 1981;63:201-208.

DeLee J, Ferrari A, Charnley J: Ectopic bone formation following low friction arthroplasty of the hip. *Clin Orthop* 1976;121:53-59.

Healy WL, Lo TC, DeSimone AA, Rask B, Pfeifer BA: Single-dose irradiation for the prevention of heterotopic ossification after total hip arthroplasty: A comparison of doses of five hundred and fifty and seven hundred centigray. *J Bone Joint Surg Am* 1995;77:590-595.

Kjaersgaard-Andersen P, Schmidt SA: Total hip arthroplasty: The role of antiinflammatory medications in the prevention of heterotopic ossification. *Clin Orthop* 1991;263:78-86.

Knelles D, Barthel T, Karrer A, Kraus U, Eulert J, Kolbl O: Prevention of heterotopic ossification after total hip replacement: A prospective, randomised study using acetylsalicylic acid, indomethacin and fractional or single-dose irradiation. *J Bone Joint Surg Br* 1997;79:596-602.

Pellegrini VD Jr, Gregoritch SJ: Preoperative irradiation for prevention of heterotopic ossification following total hip arthroplasty. *J Bone Joint Surg Am* 1996;78:870-881.

Pellegrini VD Jr, Konski AA, Gastel JA, Rubin P, Evarts CM: Prevention of heterotopic ossification with irradiation after total hip arthroplasty: Radiation therapy with a single dose of eight hundred centigray administered to a limited field. *J Bone Joint Surg Am* 1992;74:186-200.

Schneider DJ, Moulton MJ, Singapuri K, et al: Inhibition of heterotopic ossification with radiation therapy in an animal model. *Clin Orthop* 1998;355:35-46.

Tonna EA, Cronkite EP: Autoradiographic studies of cell proliferation in the periosteum of intact and fractured femora of mice utilizing DNA labeling with ^{3}H thymidine. *Proc Soc Exp Biol Med* 1961;107:719.

van der Heide HJ, Koorevaar RT, Schreurs BW, van Kampen A, Lemmens A: Indomethacin for 3 days is not effective as prophylaxis for heterotopic ossification after primary total hip arthroplasty. *J Arthroplasty* 1999;14:796-799.

Warren SB, Brooker AF: Excision of heterotopic bone followed by irradiation after total hip arthroplasty. *J Bone Joint Surg Am* 1992;74:201-210.

Coding

CPT Codes		Corresponding ICD-9 Codes		
27036	Capsulectomy or capsulotomy, hip, with or without excision of heterotopic bone, with release of hip flexor muscles (ie, gluteus medius, gluteus minimus, tensor fascia latae, rectus femoris, sartorius, iliopsoas)	343.0 343.3 728.12 (if pre-THA)	343.1 343.9 728.13 (if post-THA)	343.2 718.45 781.2 905.1
Modifier 22	Unusual procedural services			

CPT copyright © 2004 by the American Medical Association. All Rights Reserved.

Chapter 34

Management of Periprosthetic Fractures

William Jiranek, MD

Indications

Fractures adjacent to hip implants are a relatively uncommon complication of total hip arthroplasty (THA), but treatment of these fractures is often quite difficult and associated with a high complication rate. Most periprosthetic fractures require some type of surgical management. These fractures can be divided into two major anatomic classifications: (1) femoral fractures and (2) acetabular fractures.

Several authors have identified risk factors for periprosthetic femoral fractures. Patients at risk for intraoperative fracture include (1) those with rheumatoid arthritis, metabolic bone disease, or other bone weakening disease; (2) those who require revision surgery; and (3) those with abnormal femoral geometry. Patients at risk for postoperative fracture include (1) those with osteoporosis and thinned cortices; (2) those with cortical perforation (particularly those near the tip of the stem); and (3) those with osteolysis or a loose femoral component.

Results

The results of treatment are summarized in **Table 1** but generally are considered to be quite variable, and de-pendent on proper diagnosis and meticulous surgical technique. Non-surgical treatment is successful only with nondisplaced fractures. In some series, strut grafts have been as successful as plate fixation for type B1 fractures. With types B2 and B3 fractures, most authors report better results from extensively coated uncemented femoral components than for cemented or proximally coated uncemented components. All series of femoral fractures treated with revision of the femoral stem have reported relatively high levels of subsequent loosening of the revision stem at relatively short-term follow-up. Most reported periprosthetic acetabular fractures have been treated with revision of the acetabular component.

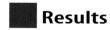
Femoral Fractures

Vancouver Classification
Most of the common classification systems categorize femoral fractures in the context of anatomic location, degree of comminution, fixation of the prosthesis, and quality of the host bone. Secondary variables include patient activity level and the timing of the fracture as it relates to the arthroplasty. All classification systems divide the femur into three regions: (1) the peritrochanteric region (type A or type 1); (2) the proximal diaphysis to the tip of the stem (type B or type 2); and (3) the area distal to the tip of the stem (type C or type 3). The Vancouver classification is described here given its validated ability to guide treatment of these challenging clinical situations (**Figure 1**).

In the Vancouver system, proximal-type femoral fractures are considered to be type A; fractures of the greater trochanter (A_G) and lesser trochanter (A_L) are A subtypes. Fractures at or just distal to the stem are considered to be type B fractures, with three subtype categories. B_1 fractures occur at or just below the stem, with the stem well fixed. B_2 occurs at or just below the stem, with the stem loose. B_3 occurs at or just below the stem, with very poor bone stock in the proximal femur. Type C fractures occur well below the tip of the femoral stem, thus allowing for conventional treatment.

Fractures of the Greater Trochanter

INDICATIONS
Type A_G fractures are most commonly associated with osteolysis or a fall. However, these fractures also can occur with preparation or implantation of the femoral component. The degree of displacement dictates the type of treatment. Symptomatic treatment with crutches and limited abduction is recommended if the fractures are nondisplaced. If the fracture is displaced

Table 1 Results of Treatment of Periprosthetic Femur Fractures

Author(s) (Year)	Number of Hips	Implant Type	Mean Patient Age	Mean Follow-up	Results
Springer, et al (2003)	118, all type B fractures	Cemented (42) Prox CL (28) Ex CL (30) APC (18)	68 years	5.4 years	16 repeat revisions (13 loose) 90% survival 5 years 80% survival 10 years Best results with Ex CL
Ko, et al (2003)	12, all type B2 fractures	Tapered flute	75 years	5 years	100% union
Berry (2003)	8, all type B3 fractures	Tapered flute	68 years	1.5 years	100% union 100% stable implant
Wang and Wang (2000)	15, 7 type B1, 2 type B2, 4 type B3, 2 type C	9 ORIF 6 long stem	61 years	2.5 years	100% union 93% good results
Tadross, et al (2000)	9, all type B1 fractures	ORIF, plate	77 years	1.2 years	33% satisfactory results 66% varus failure
Logel, et al (1999)	10, all type B1 fractures	Allograft struts (3)	65 years	4 years	90% union by 6 months
Siegmeth (1998)	42, all type B1 fractures	Plate	69 years	3 years	10% failure (3 plates loose, 1 varus failure)
Jukkala-Partio, et al (1998)	75, all type B fractures	40 revision stem 35 plate fixation	N/A	1.6 years	5 nonunions, 20 reoperations (revision stem) 9 nonunions, 27 reoperations (plate fixation)
Lewallen and Berry (1997)	97 (60% type B2, 25% type B3)	Cemented, Prox CL, Ex CL	N/A	N/A	85% fracture healing
Beals and Tower (1996)	93	15% cemented 34% uncemented 23% plates 28% nonsurgical	N/A	N/A	32% excellent results 16% good results 52% poor results

Prox CL = proximally coated uncemented, Ex CL = extensively coated uncemented, APC = allograft prosthetic composite, ORIF = open reduction and internal fixation, N/A = Not Applicable

more than 1 cm, surgical treatment is recommended because of the risk of nonunion, a painful abductor lurch, or increased torsional force on the femoral stem, which has been associated with loosening (**Figure 2**). On occasion an unstable fracture of the greater trochanter will occur during placement of a proximally coated stem. In this situation, it may be necessary to change to a diaphyseal fitting uncemented stem to obtain adequate fixation, and the greater trochanter can be repaired with wires or a claw-type device.

Type A_G fractures that occur more than 5 years after initial arthroplasty are usually the result of weak-ened bone due to osteolysis. They are often insufficiency fractures that have no clear precipitating traumatic episode; thus, the development of activity-related lateral hip pain in a patient with osteolysis that affects the trochanter should raise the index of suspicion for this type of fracture (**Figure 3**, *A*). A bone scan also can be helpful to identify the fracture (**Figure 3**, *B*). This fracture type requires surgical treatment to prevent migration of the trochanter and significant disability (**Figure 3**, *C*).

CONTRAINDICATIONS
The major contraindication to surgical repair of these fractures is inade-quate bone stock. In addition, if diagnosis is delayed, the trochanteric fragment has migrated proximally, and there is poor-quality bone stock, then nonsurgical treatment may be prudent. However, the patient must be advised that he or she may always limp and could require a cane for ambulation.

ALTERNATIVE TREATMENTS
The degree of fracture displacement determines treatment. If the fracture is nondisplaced or displaced less than 1 cm, then treatment may consist of limited weight bearing with support (ie, crutches or a walker) and possibly with an abduction brace. In this sce-

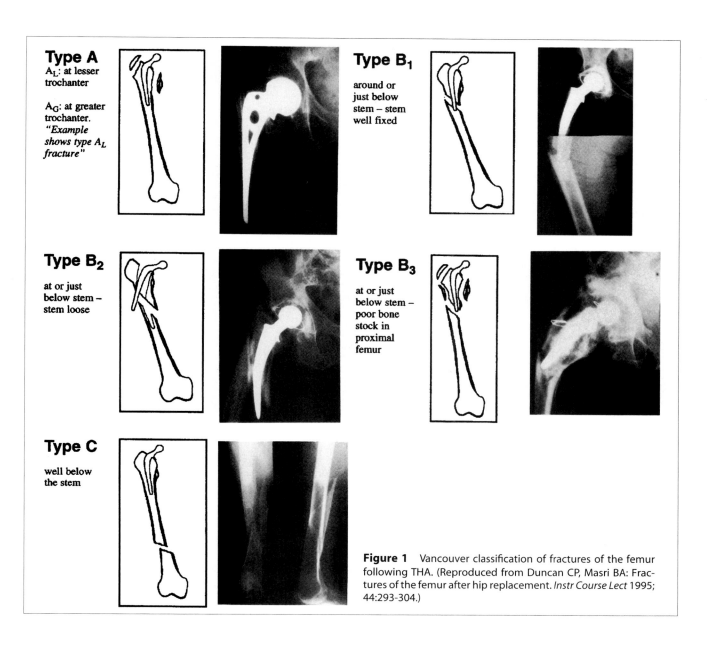

Type A

A$_L$: at lesser trochanter

A$_G$: at greater trochanter. *"Example shows type A$_L$ fracture"*

Type B$_1$

around or just below stem – stem well fixed

Type B$_2$

at or just below stem – stem loose

Type B$_3$

at or just below stem – poor bone stock in proximal femur

Type C

well below the stem

Figure 1 Vancouver classification of fractures of the femur following THA. (Reproduced from Duncan CP, Masri BA: Fractures of the femur after hip replacement. *Instr Course Lect* 1995; 44:293-304.)

nario, the patient needs close follow-up to confirm that proximal migration of the trochanter has not occurred. Weight bearing can be gradually increased as pain subsides and healing is noted on plain radiographs. Ambulation with support may be necessary for as long as 3 to 4 months.

TECHNIQUE

These fractures are fixed with 16- or 18-gauge wire or cables, a passing device to place wires around the femur, a fracture reduction forceps to reduce the trochanter to the femoral bed, and a wire or cable-tightening device. If the fracture is secondary to osteolysis, then an adequate supply of bone graft should be available. Allograft bone prepared by a tissue bank to a consistent size (3- to 5-mm cancellous chips) can save time in the operating room. In addition, the surgeon should be prepared to exchange the polyethylene acetabular liner, and backup acetabular and femoral components should be readily available in the event that the osteolysis is more significant than anticipated.

Exposure The surgical technique is similar to a standard trochanteric repair during revision surgery except that the prosthesis is well fixed; thus, the femoral canal cannot be accessed to place fixation wires.

Bone Preparation If the femoral stem is well fixed, the trochanter may be fixed with a trochanteric clamp or a modified four-wire tech-

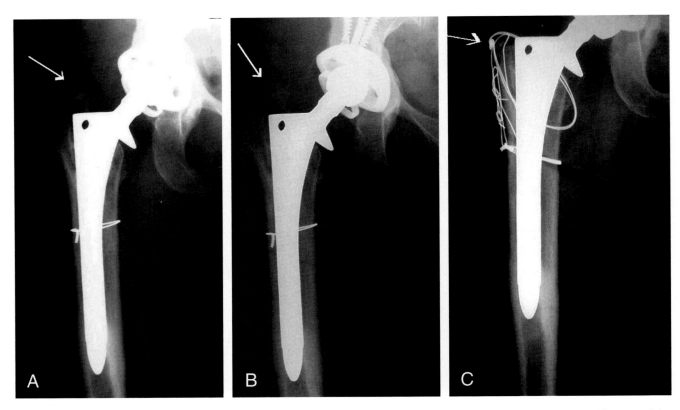

Figure 2 **A,** AP radiograph of a 48-year-old woman who fell 5 years after revision right THA shows a minimally displaced fracture of the greater trochanter (type A$_G$) (arrow). **B,** After 6 weeks of protected weight bearing, the fracture displaced further (arrow), and the patient had a symptomatic limp. **C,** AP radiograph showing the result after open reduction of the trochanteric fracture using a distal cerclage wire to anchor the vertical wires (arrow).

nique. The trochanteric bed should be débrided first, and bone graft added after the trochanter has been stabilized. The horizontal wires should be looped just above the lesser trochanter, or if the calcar is deficient, through drill holes in the lesser trochanter. If the proximal trochanter is still reasonably thick, transverse holes can be made in the trochanter with a 2-mm drill, a 14-gauge needle can be passed from posterior to anterior, and the wire can be passed through the needle. The wires can then be tightened posteriorly. If the trochanter is quite thin, trochanteric mesh can be placed on the lateral surface of the trochanter and the wires run through the mesh and then tightened to more evenly distribute the load.

If the trochanter is not fractured, then it may be prophylactically stabilized with horizontal wires or cables (**Figure 3**, *C*). If the trochanter has migrated or is unstable, vertical and horizontal wires are necessary (**Figure 2**, *C*). The vertical wires of the modified four-wire technique are tethered distally by a cerclage wire placed around the femoral shaft 6 cm below the base of the fracture. Pointed fracture reduction forceps can then be used to reduce the trochanter, with one point around the distal cerclage wire and the other around the trochanter. If the fracture is old, the trochanter has usually migrated proximally and anteriorly; therefore, the trochanteric fragment must be fully mobilized for the repair to be successful.

Wound Closure Standard closure is performed with the leg abducted on a Mayo stand, and the leg is maintained in abduction during trans-

fer to the hospital bed to minimize tension on the repair.

Postoperative Regimen Postoperatively, the patient should be placed in a hip orthosis in at least 15° of abduction for 6 weeks, with touchdown weight bearing and no active abduction for 2 months.

PREVENTING PITFALLS AND COMPLICATIONS

The most common complication is failure of the fixation wires and nonunion/migration of the trochanter. Failure of the fixation hardware is common and may be managed with observation unless the trochanter has migrated. Patients should be kept on protected weight bearing until radiographic evidence of healing. Lateral radiographs are particularly helpful for this assessment. In some patients

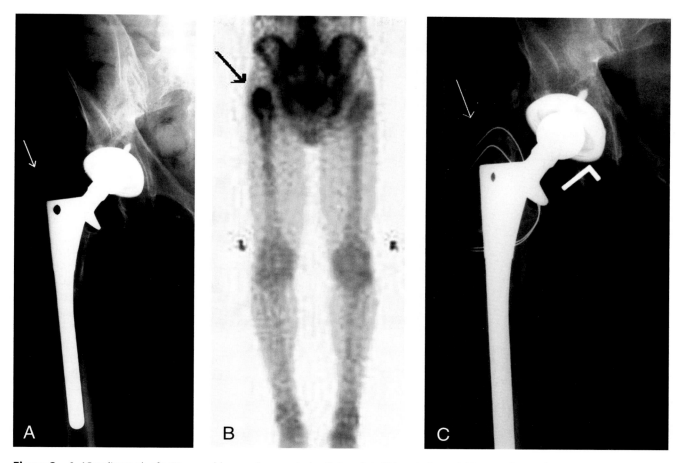

Figure 3 **A,** AP radiograph of a 45-year-old man who reported activity-related hip pain (arrow) 10 years after undergoing primary THA. **B,** A bone scan demonstrating intense uptake in the trochanter (arrow), greater than would be expected with osteolysis alone. **C,** AP radiograph after grafting and fixation of the trochanter. Because the trochanter was not displaced, only two horizontal wires were necessary for fixation (arrow).

the fractures will not heal, but there will be a stable fibrous union.

Fractures of the Lesser Trochanter
INDICATIONS
Surgical treatment is less commonly indicated for type A_L fractures because displacement does not result in as much disability as in type A_G fractures. Type A_L fractures have two subtypes: a vertical split in the calcar (hoop fractures) and horizontal fractures.

Vertical fractures almost always occur intraoperatively, but they can also occur postoperatively in a fall with an axial load. They are related to excessive hoop forces, commonly associated with insertion of uncemented femoral components, and should be repaired in all cases. Fractures identified within the first postoperative month probably involve a loose prosthesis, which may or may not become stable. Uncemented prostheses that have subsided more than 1 cm and cemented prostheses that have changes in the proximal cement mantle are at significantly higher risk of symptomatic loosening and will probably require revision. Fractures that occur more than 3 months after the prosthesis is implanted are often stable and require only protected weight bearing during the healing process.

CONTRAINDICATIONS
If these fractures occur postoperatively, generally they can be treated nonsurgically unless a substantial piece of medial cortex is attached.

ALTERNATIVE TREATMENTS
In very rare instances, if there is displacement of the lesser trochanter with severe proximal bone loss and a loose stem, then revision with a calcar replacement prosthesis or a proximal femoral replacement may be necessary. If a fracture occurs during prosthetic preparation or implantation, treatment usually consists of wire fixation and impaction of the prosthesis. In rare instances the proximal bone may no longer support a proximally coated prosthesis, and an extensively porous-coated prosthesis may be necessary.

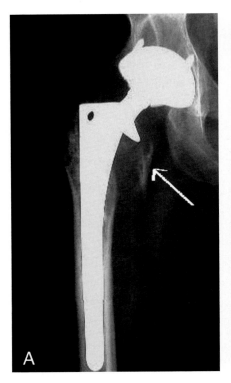
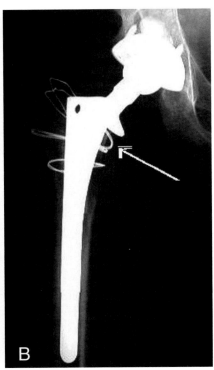

Figure 4 **A,** AP radiograph of a 41-year-old man who reported significant medial groin pain 12 years after undergoing uncemented THA shows a displaced fracture of the lesser trochanter (type A$_L$) (arrow). **B,** AP radiograph after grafting and fixation (arrow) of the lesser trochanter.

TECHNIQUE

These fractures are repaired with 18-gauge stainless steel wire or cables, wire passers, and tightening devices. This equipment should be part of the inventory of any operating room in which uncemented THA is performed.

If a vertical fracture is identified during insertion of an uncemented femoral prosthesis, it can be managed by removing the hoop stress (ie, backing out the broach or prosthesis), passing a double-looped 18-gauge wire above the lesser trochanter, and tightening laterally in the region of the vastus tubercle. If the fracture extends beyond the lesser trochanter, the second wire should be passed just below the lesser trochanter. Wire twists or cable clamps should be positioned along the posterior aspect of the lateral femur to minimize postoperative trochanteric irritation. Postop-

eratively, the patient is allowed partial weight bearing with support for 6 weeks.

Horizontal fractures occur through an avulsion mechanism, most commonly through osteolytic lesions (**Figure 4**). Thus, radiographs should be scrutinized for other areas of lysis and excessive polyethylene wear, both of which may indicate the need for revision surgery. Materials for repair are similar to what was needed for hoop fractures, specifically 18-gauge wire or cables, a wire passer, a tightener, and pointed reduction clamps to facilitate reduction of the lesser trochanter, which has usually migrated proximally and medially.

Exposure The hip can be approached from an anterolateral or posterior approach, depending on the approach previously used. Scar tissue should be taken down on both the anterior and posterior sides of the femur.

The lesser trochanter is most easily reduced with the leg in as much external rotation as possible.

Bone Preparation One double-looped 18-gauge wire should be passed above the lesser trochanter and tightened laterally. A second wire can be placed through a drill hole in the lesser trochanter if additional fixation is needed. If possible, particulate bone graft can be packed into the fracture site. However, care must be taken to avoid particulate material in the hip joint, which can cause third-body wear.

Wound Closure Standard wound closure is performed with the leg in abduction. The vastus lateralis fascia and the iliotibial band must be carefully repaired to avoid adhesions.

Postoperative Regimen Postoperatively, the patient should be placed on protective weight bearing and should avoid active hip flexion or straight leg raising for at least 6 weeks.

Type B1 Fractures
INDICATIONS

These fractures often involve the lesser trochanter and calcar femoris and usually are caused by a significant fall or trauma. If the fracture is nondisplaced or minimally displaced and the prosthesis shows no signs of loosening, the patient can be treated with protected weight bearing for at least 6 weeks. A hip orthosis with a long thigh piece can help protect the fracture and decrease pain and is recommended. Once there is evidence of fracture healing, weight bearing may be advanced.

If the fracture is displaced but the femoral stem appears well fixed, surgical stabilization is usually warranted to prevent subsequent loosening and excessive cantilever stresses on the femoral stem. Stabilization usually can be accomplished with cerclage wires with either metallic plate or strut graft allograft augmentation, if needed (**Figure 5**).

The materials needed to fix these fractures include fracture clamps (pointed reduction forceps, Verbrugge clamps), an 18-gauge wire or cable, wire passers, and 8-in × ¾-in frozen cortical allograft bone struts or metallic fracture plates. At least three of these allograft struts should be ordered from the tissue bank prior to surgery. The advantages of metallic plates include greater tensile and compressive strength and the ability to be attached with screws distal to the prosthesis. The advantages of allograft struts are the potential for biologic incorporation, less potential for fretting and corrosion, and less stress shielding. Frozen struts have much better mechanical properties than freeze-dried struts. However, even the most rigid constructs have a certain amount of micromotion; therefore, I prefer large-diameter monofilament wire to braided small-diameter multifilament cables to minimize the potential for fretting, debris formation, and breakage.

CONTRAINDICATIONS

Surgical treatment is almost always necessary with displaced fractures. Traction is inconvenient for the patient and leads to malunion or nonunion.

ALTERNATIVE TREATMENTS

Because surgical treatment is necessary for displaced fractures, nonsurgical treatment with casts, braces, or traction is rarely successful.

TECHNIQUE

Exposure Using a lateral approach, expose the femur by splitting the vastus lateralis and then inspect the femoral component. Unless there is a problem at the articulation, the hip joint does not need to be exposed.

Bone Preparation Pass three to four double-looped 18-gauge stainless steel wires on either side of the fracture and then align two allograft cortical struts (approximately 200-mm long) along the medial and lateral aspects of the femur. It may take some work to align the graft on the medial

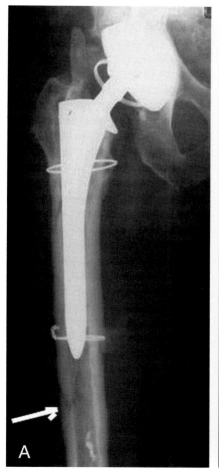 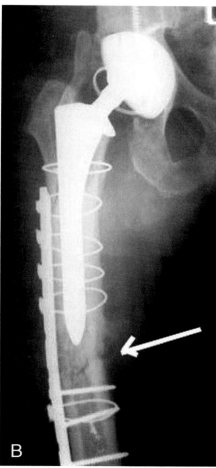

Figure 5 **A**, AP radiograph of a 55-year-old man who fell 6 years after uncemented THA, sustaining a Vancouver type B1 fracture of the femur (arrow). **B**, Treatment of the fracture with a metallic plate attached with screws and cerclage wires. Optimal fixation should include an anterior medial strut graft to counteract large varus moment (arrow).

side of the femur, but it is worth the extra effort. Reduce the fracture and apply fixation clamps, then tighten the wires around the allografts. Verbrugge clamps work well to clamp proximally and distally. Alternatively, a plate clamp approach can be used in which a plate is applied to the lateral side of the femur with screws distal to the prosthesis and attached with cerclage wires or cables at the level of the prosthesis. Many manufacturers make versions of this type of plate. This plate can be augmented with a strut allograft placed medially.

Wound Closure A standard wound closure can be performed. The

vastus lateralis fascia and iliotibial band should be closed in separate layers.

Postoperative Regimen Postoperatively, the patient is allowed touchdown weight bearing on the affected limb for 6 weeks. A hip orthosis with a thigh piece that extends to the knee will help reduce forces at the fracture during the healing process.

AVOIDING PITFALLS AND COMPLICATIONS

The goals of this procedure are to create a stable femoral construct in which the fracture fragments will heal. Therefore, the critical aspects of this procedure include careful handling of

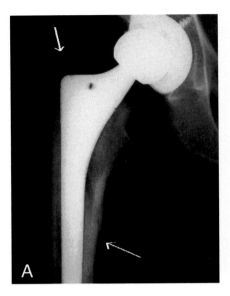
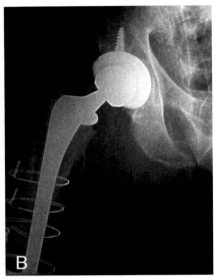

Figure 6 A 61-year-old man reports severe left thigh pain as a result of a fall 3 months after undergoing uncemented THA. **A**, AP radiograph shows a Vancouver type B2 periprosthetic fracture. Note that there is subsidence of the stem; the arrows show the proximal and distal extent of the fracture. **B**, AP radiograph after removal of the loose prosthesis, open reduction with strut grafts, and cementing of a 180-mm prosthesis.

the soft tissue and stabilizing the fracture so it can heal.

First, adequate radiographs need to be obtained to ascertain the fracture pattern and the stability of the acetabular and femoral components. During the exposure of the fracture, the soft-tissue envelope must be preserved to avoid devascularization of the fracture fragments that could impede healing.

When using either strut grafts or a plate/clamp device with a strut graft, the wires must be carefully placed around the femur to avoid damage to the soft-tissue or neurovascular structures. A wire passer should be used. The strut grafts can be placed anteriorly and laterally, and the fracture site should be grafted with morcellized autograft or allograft bone.

Type B2 Fractures
INDICATIONS
These fractures occur at or just below the femoral stem, and the stem is loose but the quality of the femur is good (**Figure 6**). These fractures usually require revision with a long-stemmed

femoral component. Uncemented stems are technically easier to implant in this situation. Cemented fixation is possible but technically difficult. The advantages of a cemented implant include immediate stability, full weight bearing, and the ability to incorporate antibiotics into the cement.

The technique and fixation choice depend on the fracture pattern and the stability of the open reduction. If the reduction can be stabilized with allograft struts or a temporary metal plate (cerclaged or clamped to the femur) sufficiently to allow manipulation, reaming, and broaching of the femur, then revision can be performed with standard techniques.

CONTRAINDICATIONS
If a stable reduction cannot be achieved, however, cemented fixation is contraindicated. In this situation, rigid fixation needs to be achieved by diaphyseal fixation in the distal fragment; once fixation is achieved, the proximal fragments are wired to the final prosthesis.

TECHNIQUE
Careful surgical planning is critical to successfully treat these fractures. Both cemented and uncemented prostheses of sufficient length to span the fracture should be readily available. A full complement of revision instruments is necessary, including high-speed burrs and cement osteotomes. At least three strut grafts should be ordered from a tissue bank, preferably precut to the needed dimensions. A full complement of fracture reduction clamps is also necessary, and fracture plates can be helpful for temporary fixation. In addition, 18-gauge wire or cables should be available, as should devices to pass and tighten these wires. If cemented fixation is elected, nozzles of sufficient length to deliver the cement to the tip of the long-stemmed femoral component are necessary. Fiber-reinforced gloves are also helpful to protect against sharp fracture fragments and wire tips.

Exposure An extensile exposure is required, but the distal portion of the femoral stem is usually accessed though the fracture site. A trochanteric or extended trochanteric osteotomy will further weaken a compromised femur and thus is not indicated. The hip is then exposed; note that generally less manipulation is required through a posterolateral approach. The hip should then be dislocated using a bone hook, ensuring that twisting of the femur is limited. If the femoral component is loose, it often can be removed manually or with gentle retrograde pressure on the tip of the stem. Once the stem is removed, the acetabular component should be completely exposed. At this point, a decision about whether to retain or revise the cup should be made. If necessary, the cup should be revised at this time.

Bone Preparation The fracture site is addressed next, first by splitting the vastus lateralis (ie, in the middle so that perforating vessels can be identified and coagulated) to a point at least 10 cm below the tip of the fracture. The condition of the distal fragment should then be evaluated, and a decision made about whether the fragment will support distal uncemented fixation. The canal should be fully opened, which often requires a high-speed burr to contour sclerotic bone or cement fragments. Cement should be removed from the distal fragment. If the quality of the proximal femur is good and the fracture can be reduced to reconstitute a reasonable proximal tube, then cemented fixation is possible. The distal fragment should be controlled securely using bone-holding clamps. If cemented fixation is elected, the canal should be cleared without extensive reaming.

Once the distal fragment is prepared for either uncemented or cemented fixation, the proximal fragments can be approached in either a retrograde or an antegrade fashion, or both if the clinical situation warrants. All retained cement and neocortex should be removed from the endosteum using revision osteotomes and high-speed burrs.

Prosthesis Implantation Next, a trial femoral prosthesis (of sufficient length to bridge the fracture) is inserted to serve as a stent during reduction. The fragments are then reduced as anatomically as possible. Three double-looped 18-gauge wires are then placed proximal and distal to the major fracture line (more wires may be necessary if the fracture extends in a spiral fashion). Two fresh frozen cortical strut grafts (measuring at least 8-in long and ⅝-in long) are then fitted along the lateral and anterior aspects of the femur spanning the fracture, and the cerclage wires are tightened between the grafts. A trial reduction can then be attempted to assess proper height of the femoral component and joint stability. The femur can then be manipulated into position for insertion of the final femoral component.

All contracted soft tissue, including the anterior capsule, should

be released prior to manipulation into the final position before the trial implant is removed. The final femoral component should be of sufficient length to reach at least two cortical diameters below the end of the fracture, but the strut graft should extend at least two cortical diameters below the tip of the new stem. The new stem can then be cemented in place using modern cement technique. Any cement that extrudes through the fracture sites may be removed prior to final set.

Uncemented fixation should be considered if the distal femur is of sufficient quality to allow diaphyseal fixation, particularly if the proximal femur is of good quality but comminuted. After any acetabular work is finished, attention should be turned to the distal femur. Grasping the femur with bone-holding forceps, the surgeon should ream the distal canal with straight reamers if a straight, extensively coated stem is planned and with flexible reamers if a curved stem is planned. A trial femoral component can be used to judge height, and once the final stem is implanted, the fracture fragments can be reduced and wired to the final stem. A strut graft should be placed along the medial side of the femur to decrease cantilever forces on the femoral stem.

Wound Closure A meticulous wound closure is necessary. The vastus lateralis fascia, along with the fascia at the iliotibial band and gluteus minimus, must be identified and repaired.

Postoperative Regimen Postoperatively the patient is allowed touch-down weight bearing for 6 weeks. Over the next 6 weeks weight bearing is slowly increased, but the patient needs to walk with support until the fractures are healed.

AVOIDING PITFALLS AND COMPLICATIONS
The critical aspects of this procedure include careful handling of the soft tis-

sue, appropriate selection of the implant, stabilizing the femoral component, and producing a stable THA at the end of the procedure.

Although the stem may be loose it must be removed carefully to avoid proximal propagation of the fracture. If the stem was originally cemented in place, the cement from the proximal femur must be removed to avoid fracture at the greater trochanter during component removal. For a loose uncemented stem, flexible osteotomes should be used proximally to completely free the stem to avoid a fracture.

All cement fragments and fibrous tissues need to be removed from the distal femur. If the cement column is well fixed distally, an ultrasound device may be useful to prevent perforation of the femur.

Selection of the appropriate implant is also critical to a successful reconstruction. A number of stems should be available for uncemented fixation. The surgeon needs to determine if an extensively porous-coated straight or curved stem will be satisfactory or if distal fluted taper fixation (Wagner-type prosthesis) is required. A cemented prosthesis should not be used if an adequate bone tube cannot be reconstituted.

The femoral trial component must be placed carefully down the canal and in appropriate version to avoid fracture. If the appropriate size or length of the implant is of concern, then intraoperative radiographs should be obtained with the femoral and strut grafts in place. This will aid the surgeon in selecting the appropriate size implant. It is also advisable to test the hip joint at this point.

These procedures require extensive soft-tissue dissection, and, therefore, patients are at increased risk for dislocation. The manufacturer of the acetabular shell should be identified preoperatively, and all of the different femoral head sizes and neck lengths available should be determined and

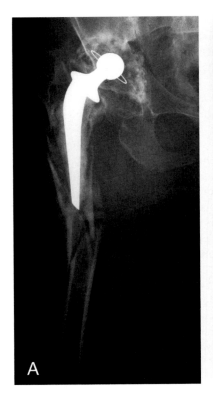

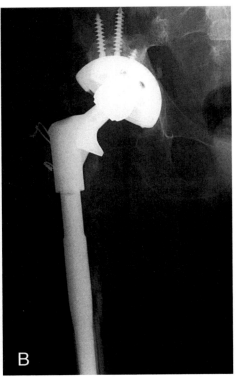

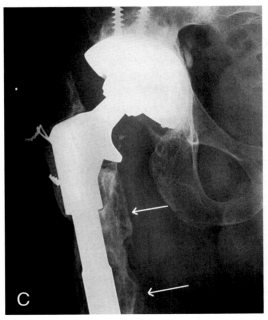

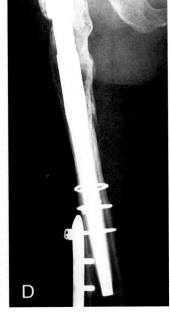

Figure 7 **A,** AP radiograph of a 36-year-old man who fell 16 years after undergoing THA shows a type B3 fracture with proximal bone loss and a loose stem. **B,** An early postoperative radiograph shows limited fracture fixation following long stem revision using a titanium distally tapered stem. **C,** AP radiograph of the proximal femur 2 years postoperatively shows a stable prosthesis and fracture healing. Marked bone reconstitution can be seen (arrows). **D,** AP radiograph of the distal femur 2 years postoperatively shows that the femoral component is stable. Note the presence of a distal plate that was used to treat a separate supracondylar femur fracture above a knee arthroplasty that occurred concurrently with the periprosthetic fracture about the hip. (Courtesy of Daniel Berry, MD, and the Mayo Clinic Foundation, Rochester, MN.)

ordered. If the acetabular component has been in place for a while then the polyethylene liner should be exchanged. If there is concern about the quality of the soft tissues, then the use of a hip abduction orthosis for 6 weeks should be considered.

Type B3 Fractures

INDICATIONS
Virtually all of these fractures require revision of the femoral component. If the proximal femur itself is deficient but the bone distal to the fracture is of good quality, then distal fixation with a bypassing uncemented prosthesis is the best option. If the quality of the distal femur is poor or the diameter of the femur is too large to support extensively coated cylindrical fixation, another option is to use a Wagner-type long tapered stem (**Figure 7**). Every attempt should be made to restore the structural support of the proximal femur to prevent a late cantilever fracture of the femoral stem. Occasionally this can be accomplished by cerclaging the fragments with strut allografts; however, in cases of severe bone loss, either a tumor-type prosthesis (for low-demand patients) or an allograft-prosthetic construct (APC) is required for the proximal femur.

ALTERNATIVE TREATMENTS
Another possibility is impaction grafting, although this is a technically difficult option because considerable stability of the open reduction is required to allow manipulation of the femur and impaction of bone graft, which is quite difficult in comminuted fractures.

TECHNIQUE
Exposure The femur is exposed through a long lateral or posterolateral approach. The loose prosthesis is then removed and the distal femur exposed.

Bone Preparation At this time, the surgeon must determine whether the quality and diameter of the femur will support cylindrical fixation or if distal fluted taper fixation is required. If preliminary reaming suggests that a stem can be well fixed in the distal fragment and the proximal bone can be augmented sufficiently with strut grafts to provide reasonable proximal support for the prosthesis, then a long-stemmed monoblock or modular uncemented stem can be used.

If proximal bone cannot be augmented, then an APC should be used. Consultation with the local tissue bank is important to ensure that a femoral allograft is available that is the proper side (ie, right or left) and is as large or larger than the native femur. A separate table is used to prepare the allograft, which should be thawed at the start of the operation.

Prosthesis Implantation After the distal femur is prepared, a trial prosthesis is placed in the distal femur using a length that restores the desired limb length. The hip is reduced and the needed length of the allograft is assessed. The distal allograft femur can then be cut with a step cut using a lateral tongue of approximately 6 cm. The host distal femur is then cut to accept this tongue, ensuring that the rotation of the femur will be correct.

Next, the allograft femur can be reamed and broached to accept the new femoral prosthesis. Most authors recommend cementing the stem into the allograft. The resulting APC can then be press-fit into the host distal femur. Several authors suggest that once the step cut is engaged the autograft bone (either from the iliac crest or from reamings of the distal femur) should be packed into the junction to aid incorporation of the graft with the host. Once this is completed, two allograft struts can be wired across the lateral and anterior aspects of the femur to protect the junction. It is critical to save the proximal fracture fragments whenever possible. These fragments can be wired around the proximal femoral allograft to enhance healing at the graft-host junction. In

addition, the original abductor mechanism with the bony attachment needs to be preserved so that it can be wired down to the allograft.

Postoperative Regimen Patients should be kept on protected weight bearing for at least 6 weeks. A hip orthosis with a long medial thigh sleeve can also protect the graft-host junction during initial healing.

AVOIDING PITFALLS AND COMPLICATIONS
The complications associated with type B2 and B3 fractures are quite similar. Careful handling of the proximal soft tissue is critical to avoid devascularization of the fracture fragments. An extensive array of implants (eg, uncemented, calcar replacement, proximal femoral replacement, long-stemmed cemented) and graft materials (femoral struts and a proximal femur) should be available to treat these complex periprosthetic fractures.

Large femoral heads should be available to create a stable construct at the end of the procedure.

Type C Fractures
INDICATIONS
These fractures occur far enough below the stem that they can be treated with standard open reduction and internal fixation (**Figure 8**, *A*). Low-energy, nondisplaced fractures can be treated with protected weight bearing and close follow-up. A hip orthosis with a thigh piece that extends to the knee can help stabilize the fracture and is recommended. Unfortunately, most type C fractures are displaced. Displaced fractures can be treated with skeletal traction, but the costs of extended hospitalization and the morbidity associated with prolonged bed rest make this option unattractive.

In most patients with type C fractures, the femoral stem is well fixed, making revision to a longer stem difficult; thus, open reduction and internal fixation is the best approach. Screw fixation usually is not

possible proximally given the presence of the femoral stem, which often requires cerclage fixation.

TECHNIQUE
Surgical treatment involves open reduction and internal fixation, and most fractures may be treated with a locking plate or a blade plate. In some patients, the fracture will extend high enough that either unicortical fixation (locking plate) or a plate/clamp device is required. Several manufacturers make plates that can accept wires or cables through holes or grooves in the plate and thus allow the plate to be attached to the femur over the stem. A full complement of fracture reduction clamps are needed, as are wires or cables for cerclage fixation.

Exposure In general, the patient is placed on either a radiolucent table or a fracture table. I prefer a fracture table because a support is placed beneath the thigh but the leg is free, and it is easier to use fluoroscopic guidance. An incision is made at the central aspect of the distal femur through the fascia and down to bone. The fracture is not exposed. The locking plate or blade plate is slid along the femur from distal to proximal. Proximal and distal screws are placed to attain appropriate limb length. Either percutaneous or open technique may be used to place the screws. The reduction and screw placement are then verified with fluoroscopy. Unicortical screws can be used if necessary with a locking plate. A blade plate or supracondylar screw also can be used for fracture fixation. If the patient had no antecedent pain before the fracture occurred and the femoral component appears well fixed, the hip is not exposed.

Bone Preparation Most type C fractures can be fixed with standard fracture techniques using locking plates, compression plates, blade plates, or dynamic compression screws as the fracture dictates. The fracture site usually does not have to

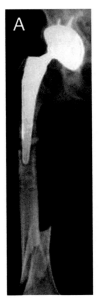
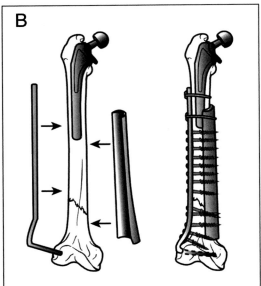
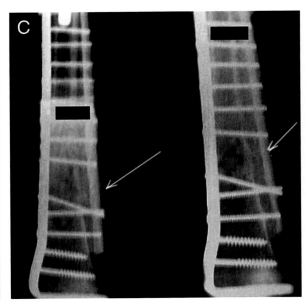

Figure 8 **A,** AP radiograph of a 75-year-old man who sustained a type C fracture as a result of a fall. **B,** Fixation technique using a spanning blade plate laterally and a cortical strut allograft placed along the medial femur. The plate and the strut graft may be stabilized using proximal and distal Verbrugge clamps, and the medial strut can be fixed with the same cortical screws used for the plate, or it can be attached with cerclage wires. **C,** Postoperative AP radiographs at 5 weeks (left) and 21 months (right) showing progressive incorporation of the strut graft with the host bone (arrows).

be exposed. To avoid creating a bridge zone between the tip of the femoral stem and the tip of the internal fixation in fractures lower in the femur, the internal fixation device should be extended at least 5 cm proximal to the tip of the prosthesis, or the gap should be bridged with struts.

Occasionally a high type C fracture will occur. The key principle in treating high type 3 fractures is restoring the medial buttress. Generally, placing a cortical strut graft on the medial side of the femur is easier than placing a metal plate (**Figure 8**, *B*). Once the fracture site is exposed to a level of at least 10 cm proximally and distally, a metal plate can be placed on the lateral aspect of the femur, the fracture reduced, and then the plate secured with fracture reduction clamps proximally and distally. The plate can be provisionally fixed with a few unicortical 4.5-mm screws proximally and distally. This will stabilize the fracture while a medial strut graft is aligned along the medial femur, centered at the medial fracture line (**Fig-**

ure 8, *C*). The graft can be held with Verbrugge clamps while additional transfixing screws can be placed through the plate, across the femur, and through the strut graft. Alternatively, medial and lateral strut grafts can be used to span the fracture and can be attached with cerclage wires at 5-cm intervals, as described by Duncan and associates.

Junctional Fractures

A junctional fracture is another type of C fracture, which can occur following treatment of a periprosthetic fracture at the distal femur, occurs between two implants at a site of stress concentration (ie, between the stems of the hip femoral implant and the knee femoral component, or between the hip stem and a fixation plate).

These fractures are very difficult to treat, given the very high stress concentrations at the junction, and often they require extensive surgeries to correct. Nonsurgical treatment has a high chance of nonunion or malunion with the component migrating into varus.

Surgical options are very challenging and should be undertaken only by surgeons familiar with extensile approaches. One option is to use bridging strut grafts or plates with cerclage fixation proximally and distally. The disadvantage of this technique is that extramedullary fixation is often insufficient to control the forces at the fracture site. A second option is to use a total femur reconstruction in which the entire femur is substituted with a tumor-type prosthesis after removal of the femoral components from both ends of the femur. This is an extensive procedure because the knee must be converted to a semiconstrained total knee arthroplasty requiring a tibial component with an intramedullary stem.

Acetabular Fractures

Classification
Acetabular fractures are not reported with the same frequency as femoral

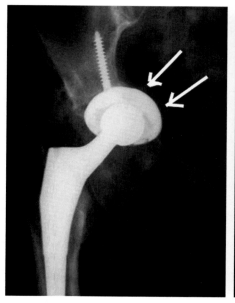

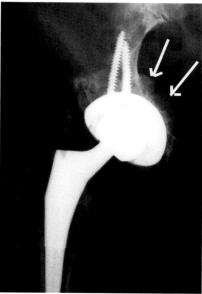

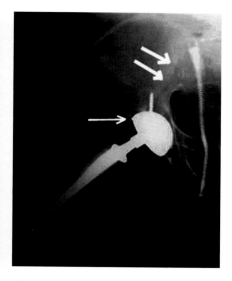

Figure 9 **A,** AP radiograph of an 80-year-old woman with a fracture of the medial wall and migration of the acetabular component in the early postoperative period (arrows). **B,** AP radiograph after removal of the smaller component and reaming up to a larger component, with medial bone grafting (arrows).

Figure 10 AP radiograph of a 75-year-old man who fell on his hip 6 years after hybrid THA shows a dome fracture (double arrows). The patient has had pain despite 3 months of protected weight bearing. The single arrow shows a developing zone 1 radiolucency.

fractures; thus, few classification strategies have been proposed. Fractures have been reported to occur on insertion, with trauma, and in patients with osteopenia. Typically these fractures are classified as one of two principal types: (1) those within the bony confines of the acetabulum; and (2) those adjacent to the bony acetabulum. Fractures of the acetabulum may be further divided into rim fractures (anterior, posterior, or inferior), medial wall fractures, vertical dome fractures, and transverse fractures.

Fractures that occur outside the acetabulum usually can be treated nonsurgically with protected weight bearing. These fractures are classified according to the anatomic portion of the pelvis affected. The most common site of fracture is the superior pubic ramus, and these usually heal with protected weight bearing over a 6-week period.

A high failure rate has been widely reported when fractures within the acetabulum are treated nonsurgically. In patients who report signifi-

cant symptoms after 3 months, loosening has likely occurred, and revision is needed if symptoms persist. Prior to the revision, the fracture pattern should be identified for effective surgical planning. A CT scan can be helpful in this situation, especially if the radiologist can vary the windows to suppress metal artifact.

Indications

Rim fractures usually occur during insertion of an uncemented socket, and unless the fracture encompasses more than 30% of the cup area, the addition of dome screws is sufficient if the fracture is recognized at the time of surgery. Surgeons should be alert when impacting press-fit cups in patients with osteopenic bone. If a fracture is seen, the cup should be removed and the fracture pattern assessed.

Medial wall fractures typically occur in patients with osteopenia (**Figure 9,** *A*). In patients with significant medial migration, surgery is usually required. If the acetabular rim is intact, revision often can be accom-

plished by removing the socket and reaming up to a larger-diameter socket that rests on the rim and is secured with dome screws, with particulate bone graft added into the defect (**Figure 9,** *B*). When the defects involve the anterior or posterior columns, an antiprotrusio cage should be used.

Dome fractures are a type of burst mechanism in which fractures originate in the dome of the acetabulum and propagate vertically into the ilium (**Figure 10**). These fractures are more commonly associated with trauma such as a fall or motor vehicle accident. As the fracture becomes displaced, the acetabular aperture is widened. These fractures can be treated with protected weight bearing initially, but if significant groin pain remains after 3 months, the patient should be assessed for signs of loosening (eg, increasing radiolucencies or migration of the socket).

In contrast to dome fractures, transverse fractures extend horizontally. If the transverse fracture extends through both the anterior and posterior columns, it is considered a pelvic discontinuity and should be managed surgically with plating of the posterior column, followed by reaming up to good rim interference and placing a press-fit cup with screw augmentation. The materials needed include a small fragment set, reconstruction plates, larger sockets, tools for disengaging the polyethylene liner, and bone graft.

Contraindications

These fractures need to be fixed once they are identified.

Alternative Treatments

Treatment is determined by when they are located. Some fractures may occur intraoperatively during implantation of an uncemented component or during removal of a well-fixed acetabular component during revision surgery. Others result from trauma, osteoporosis, or osteolysis. Treatment is determined by the stability of the acetabular component after the fracture.

Fractures that occur intraoperatively need immediate treatment. Those that occur secondary to trauma or osteopenia may be treated with non–weight-bearing status and observation. However, revision surgery is often necessary, and close follow-up is essential. Fractures that occur secondary to osteolysis usually require surgical treatment; careful analysis is necessary to determine the extent of bone loss and to identify or rule out pelvic discontinuity.

Technique

The equipment needed for surgical treatment of the patients includes larger uncemented sockets, dome screws, cancellous bone graft (fresh frozen or freeze dried), antiprotrusio cages, and all-polyethylene cups. The surgical approach should be either posterior or transtrochanteric in the event that a cage must be used.

EXPOSURE

The approach is selected when the fracture is identified. If a fracture occurs intraoperatively, then a more extensive exposure of the ilium, anterior and posterior columns, and the ischium is necessary. In some situations a trochanteric slide may be necessary to allow better access to the ilium for placement of a cage or a plate along the posterior wall. If the cup has migrated into the pelvis, consultation with a general surgeon is necessary because a retroperitoneal approach may be necessary to safely remove the component from the surrounding intrapelvic neurovascular structures.

The approach to a fracture that occurs postoperatively is determined by the type of defect. Some type of osteotomy may be necessary in this situation, depending on the bony defect present. The management of acetabular bony defects is described in chapters that address acetabular revision.

BONE PREPARATION

The type of fracture present will determine the type of bone preparation that is necessary. Rim fractures may be treated with multiple screws if the fracture encompasses less than 30% of the cup area. A cup with multiple screw holes is recommended. The extent of the fracture must be carefully assessed to determine if a plate or cage is also necessary.

Management of medial wall, dome, and transverse fractures depends on the extent of the fracture (**Figures 9** and **10**). With medial wall fractures, the integrity of the anterior and posterior columns needs to be assessed once the cup is removed. If these columns are intact, the surgeon can ream up in size until an interference fit is obtained. Often it is judicious to either ream by 1 mm or actually ream line to line and then use a cup that has multiple screw holes that can enhance fixation. The medial defect should be filled with particulate graft prior to cup insertion. If the an-

terior or posterior columns are involved, then an acetabular cage may be necessary. A more extensive exposure is required to visualize both the ilium and the ischium. In the presence of a dome or transverse fracture, treatment is determined by the bony defect. With dome fractures, plating of the ilium or posterior wall may be necessary. In general, these fractures can be managed with component revision using a larger uncemented socket and multiple screws. With transverse fractures, the stability of the cup needs to be assessed. If the cup is loose, the fixation screws should be removed and the extent of the fracture assessed. In general, a reconstruction plate along the posterior wall is required. The acetabulum should be reamed up to a good interference fit (do not underream by more than 1 mm), and a large cup with screws can be inserted in place.

Finally, in cases of fracture secondary to osteolysis, bone preparation is determined by the extent of the bone defect. Structural bone grafts may be necessary.

WOUND CLOSURE

The wound is closed in a standard fashion.

POSTOPERATIVE REGIMEN

In most cases, toe-touch weight bearing is advised for 6 weeks. The weight-bearing status will be increased gradually over the next 6 weeks, but the patient should be expected to ambulate with support for at least 3 months. The use of a hip abduction brace for 6 weeks also should be considered.

————————————■

Avoiding Pitfalls and Complications

Avoiding intraoperative fractures during a primary THA is essential because of the high rate of failure. Reaming must be done carefully, but overreaming of the anterior, posterior, or medial walls should be avoided. This may be difficult to determine when small incisions are used. The acetabulum should not be underreamed by more than 2 mm when inserting the component. If the prosthesis does not advance with each blow of the mallet, it is a warning sign for a potential fracture. The component should be removed, and the potential for soft-tissue impingement should be assessed. If the periphery of the acetabulum is free of soft tissue, then reaming either 1 mm or line to line should be considered. When treating patients with poor bone stock, underreaming by only 1 mm or line to line should be considered and adjunct screw fixation should be used.

If an intraoperative fracture occurs, the component should be removed and the extent of the fracture assessed. An intraoperative radiograph may be useful.

When treating postoperative fractures, the fracture must be carefully assessed with standard and Judet views. In most cases, CT also is needed to evaluate the extent of the fracture. It is important to confirm or rule out a pelvic discontinuity.

A thorough preoperative plan is necessary to address the most grave defects should they occur. Therefore, jumbo cups, pelvic reconstruction plates, cages, polyethylene cups, and structural allografts must be available during surgery.

——————■

References

Beals RK, Tower SS: Periprosthetic fracture of the femur: An analysis of 93 fractures. *Clin Orthop* 1996;327:238-246.

Berry DJ: Treatment of Vancouver B3 periprosthetic femur fractures with a fluted tapered stem. *Clin Orthop* 2003;417:224-231.

Callaghan JJ: Periprosthetic fractures of the acetabulum during and following total hip arthroplasty. *Instr Course Lect* 1998;47:231-235.

Garbuz DS, Masri BA, Duncan CP: Periprosthetic fracture of the femur: Principles of prevention and management. *Instr Course Lect* 1998;47:237-242.

Greidamus NV, Mitchell PA, Masri BA, et al: Principles of management and results of treating the fractured femur during and after total hip arthroplasty. *Instr Course Lect* 2003;52:309-322.

Jukkala-Partio K, Partio EK, Solovieva S, et al: Treatment of periprosthetic fractures in association with total hip arthroplasty: A retrospective comparison between revision stem and plate fixation. *Ann Chir Gynaecol* 1998;87:229-235.

Ko PS, Lam JJ, Tio MK, Lee OB, Ip FK: Distal fixation with Wagner revision stem in treating Vancouver type B2 periprosthetic femur fractures in geriatric patients. *J Arthroplasty* 2003;18:446-452.

Lewallen DG, Berry DJ: Periprosthetic fracture of the femur after total hip arthroplasty. *J Bone Joint Surg Am* 1997;79:1881-1890.

Logel KJ, Lachiewicz PF, Schmale GA, Kelley SS: Cortical strut allografts for the treatment of femoral fractures and deficiencies in revision total hip arthroplasty. *J South Orthop Assoc* 1999;8:163-172.

Peterson CA, Lewallen DG: Periprosthetic fracture of the acetabulum after total hip arthroplasty. *J Bone Joint Surg Am* 1998;78:1206-1213.

Sharkey PF, Hozack WJ, Callaghan JJ, et al: Acetabular fracture associated with cementless acetabular component insertion: A report of 13 cases. *J Arthroplasty* 1999;14:426-431.

Siegmeth A, Menth-Chiari W, Wozasek GE, Vecsei V: Periprosthetic femur shaft fractures: Indications and outcome in 51 patients. *Unfallchirurg* 1998;101:901-906.

Springer BD, Berry DJ, Lewallen DG: Treatment of periprosthetic femoral fractures following total hip arthroplasty with femoral component revision. *J Bone Joint Surg Am* 2003;85:156-162.

Tadross TS, Nanu AM, Buchanan MG, Checketts RG: Dall-Miles plating for periprosthetic B1 fractures of the femur. *J Arthroplasty* 2000;15:47- 51.

Wang JW, Wang CJ: Periprosthetic fracture of the femur after hip arthroplasty: The clinical outcome using cortical strut allografts. *J Orthop Surg* 2000;8:27-31.

Coding

CPT Codes		Corresponding ICD-9 Codes		
27132	Conversion of previous hip surgery to total hip arthroplasty, with or without autograft or allograft	808.0 808.8 820.22 996.4	808.41 820.20 821.00 996.77	808.49 820.21 821.01
27134	Revision of total hip arthroplasty; both components, with or without autograft or allograft	996.4	996.77	
27137	Revision of total hip arthroplasty; acetabular component only, with or without autograft or allograft	996.4	996.77	
27138	Revision of total hip arthroplasty; femoral component only, with or without allograft	996.4	996.77	
27215	Open treatment of iliac spine(s), tuberosity avulsion, or iliac wing fracture(s) (eg, pelvic fracture(s) which does not disrupt the pelvic ring), with internal fixation	808.41	808.49	
27226	Open treatment of posterior or anterior acetabular wall fracture, with internal fixation	808.0		
27227	Open treatment of acetabular fracture(s) involving anterior or posterior (one) column, or a fracture running transversely across the acetabulum, with internal fixation	808.0	808.49	
27245	Open treatment of intertrochanteric, peritrochanteric, or subtrochanteric femoral fracture; with intramedullary implant, with or without interlocking screws or cerclage	820.20	820.21	820.22
27248	Open treatment of greater trochanteric fracture, with or without internal or external fixation	820.20		

CPT copyright © 2004 by the American Medical Association. All Rights Reserved.

Chapter 35

Prophylaxis for Venous Thromboembolic Disease After Total Hip Arthroplasty

Clifford W. Colwell, Jr, MD

Indications

The 1986 Consensus Conference convened by the National Institutes of Health emphasized the unacceptable rates of venous thromboembolic disease (VTED), including proximal and distal deep vein thrombosis (DVT), pulmonary embolism (PE) and ultimately death, in orthopaedic surgery of the lower extremity without prophylaxis. In the intervening years, interest in use of prophylaxis has increased dramatically as the number of total hip arthroplasties (THAs) per year in the United States approximates 300,000. Moreover, the number of THAs, as well as the number of hip fractures, is predicted to increase over the next 20 years as the population ages.

The argument for prescribing thrombosis prophylaxis for all THA patients is based on the overall risk in this patient population for DVT and PE. THA patients treated with a placebo or as controls have a total DVT prevalence of 45% to 57% and a proximal DVT prevalence of 23% to 36% when examined by venography at 7 to 14 days. Prevalence of PE is less certain, but clinical studies have reported a range of 0.7% to 30% for total PEs and 0.1% to 0.4% for fatal PEs for control or placebo patients. Use of routine ventilation-perfusion lung scans in studies reported a prevalence of 7% to 11%, with high probability scans within 7 to 14 days after THA. Venography studies without prolonged out-of-hospital prophylaxis indicate that new evidence of DVT develops in up to 25% of patients within 4 to 5 weeks after hospital discharge, and intermediate or high probability lung scans are found in up to 6% of patients. Furthermore, the possibility of post-thrombosis syndrome remains in patients who experience a venous thromboembolic event. Such an event could mean a lifetime of treatment for these patients.

Some clinicians continue to rely on clinical signs and symptoms as the initial presentation of DVT or PE in THA patients. However, the accuracy of diagnosis by signs and symptoms is considered to be low. Results of objective testing indicate that many symptomatic patients are negative for venous thrombosis and that many asymptomatic patients are positive for venous thrombosis.

Withholding primary prophylaxis in favor of case findings, either by noninvasive screening techniques or serial techniques, has not demonstrated effectiveness as an alternative to primary prophylaxis. Many screening trials lack sensitivity, specificity and accuracy, particularly for calf thrombi and variable detection of proximal thrombi. Clinical trials and cohort studies indicate screening for proximal DVT with predischarge color duplex ultrasound is also ineffective. Consequently, primary prophylaxis continues to be recommended for all THA patients.

Contraindications

Providing prophylaxis may be more challenging in some patients, but no contraindications to prophylaxis are recognized for THA patients. Patients with a history of bleeding dyscrasias may be treated differently than the standard patient. Likewise, patients on long-term anticoagulant therapy for other reasons require a special protocol of prophylaxis. Special cases occasionally present themselves in which case consultation with another specialist may be needed to establish an appropriate prophylactic regimen.

Treatments and Results

Prophylactic treatment protocols and recommendations are available through evidence-based medicine published by the American College of

Table 1 Anticoagulation Agents, Dosage, and Administration

Agent	Dose	Administration
Warfarin	Adjusted INR 2.5 (range 2–3)	Oral once daily, starting preoperatively or postoperatively on same day as surgery
Enoxaparin	30 mg*	Subcutaneously every 12 hours, starting 12 to 24 hours postoperatively
Dalteparin	2,500 IU initially, then 5,000 IU	Subcutaneously once daily, starting 4 to 8 hours postoperatively†
Fondaparinux	2.5 mg	Subcutaneously once daily, starting 6 to 8 hours postoperatively‡

*A dose of 40 mg subcutaneously once daily may be used in THA patients for extended prophylaxis for 3 weeks after initial dosing of 7 to 10 days.
†May be started within 2 hours preoperatively at 2,500 IU
‡May be continued for 24 additional days in patients undergoing surgery for hip fracture

Table 2 Results of Major Randomized Trials

Agent	PE % (95% CI)	Proximal DVT % (95% CI)	Total VTED % (95% CI)
Placebo	1.5 (0.8–2.6)	26.6 (23–31)	54.8 (51–59)
Intermittent pneumatic compression	0.3 (0.01–1.4)	13.7 (11–17)	20.3 (17–24)
Warfarin	0.2 (0.02–0.6)	5.2 (4–6)	22.3 (20–24)
Unfractionated heparin	1.4 (0.9–2.0)	18.5 (16–21)	19.2 (26–32)
Low molecular weight heparins	0.4 (0.2–0.6)	4.9 (4–5)	15.4 (15–16)
Fondaparinux	0.3 (0.2–0.4)	1.2 (1–2)	4.7 (4–6)

Table 3 Incidence of Bleeding Events by Type of Anticoagulant Treatment

Agent	Major Event (%)	Minor Event (%)
Placebo	2.0%	3.0%
Unfractionated heparin	4.7%	9.1%
Warfarin	2.6%	5.7%
Enoxaparin	2.6%	9.9%
Dalteparin	3.4%	7.0%
Fondaparinux	0.3%	3.0%
Pneumatic compression	0	4.1%

Chest Physicians and updated every 2 years. These recommendations are based on available clinical trial results and are written with consensus from orthopaedic surgeons.

Pharmacologic Prophylaxis

Numerous anticoagulant-based prophylaxis regimens for THA have been studied. Meta-analysis has shown that low-dose unfractionated heparin or aspirin prophylaxis is more effective than no prophylaxis, but both are less effective than other prophylactic regimens in this high-risk THA patient group.

WARFARIN

Most orthopaedic surgeons in North America prescribe oral anticoagulation with adjusted-dose warfarin sodium. Adjusted-dose warfarin has the potential advantage of allowing continued prophylaxis after hospital discharge, provided the infrastructure is available to continue home therapy effectively and safely. Oral anticoagulation should be administered in a dose sufficient to prolong the international normalized ratio (INR) to a target of 2.5 (range 2 to 3) (**Table 1**). The half-life of warfarin is 36 to 42 hours and can be reversed with vitamin K. The

initial oral anticoagulant dose is administered either before surgery or as soon after surgery as possible. However, even with early initiation of oral anticoagulation therapy, the INR usually does not reach the target range until the third postoperative day. Use of warfarin in 13 studies of 1,828 patients revealed a 22% prevalence of total DVT (relative risk reduction [RRR], 59%) and a 5% prevalence of proximal DVT (RRR, 80%) (**Table 2**). The risk of symptomatic PE is between 0.16% and 0.40%, and the risk of fatal PE is 0.16%.

Warfarin has been compared with low molecular weight heparins (LMWHs) in a number of multicenter randomized trials in which venography was used as a surrogate outcome measure. In all of these studies, LMWH proved more effective than warfarin but were associated with higher bleeding rates.

The safety of warfarin prophylaxis requires that patients understand both the risks and the benefits of this medication. Clinical studies report a 2.6% prevalence of a major bleeding event, which is similar to placebo (**Table 3**). Many factors interact with warfarin as well, including medications, tobacco and alcohol use, foods, and changes in activity. Because many patients are discharged with warfarin prophylaxis, they must be advised about these interactions and must monitor themselves for any symptoms of overanticoagulation. Optimal use of warfarin requires consideration of the timeframe of its effects, use of INR for close monitoring of effect and interacting factors, patient education, and a systematic approach.

LOW MOLECULAR WEIGHT HEPARINS

LMWHs were approved for prophylactic use for THA in 1993 and have been adopted in practice by many clinicians. The most commonly used LMWHs in North America are enoxaparin given subcutaneously at a dose of 30 mg every 12 hours starting 12 to 24 hours after surgery and dalteparin, also given subcutaneously, started 4 to 6 hours after surgery at a dose of 2,500 IU, then continued once daily at a dose of 5,000 IU (**Table 1**). LMWHs have been studied extensively and are highly effective and generally safe. Twenty-six studies using LMWH prophylaxis on 6,216 THA patients showed a total DVT prevalence of 15% (RRR, 70%) and a proximal DVT prevalence of 5% (RRR, 78%), with a PE rate of 0.4%. (**Table 2**)

LMWHs are pharmacologically different from unfractionated heparin. LMWHs bind less to proteins and endothelial cells, resulting in (1) a more predictable dose response, (2) a dose-independent mechanism of clearance, and (3) a longer plasma half-life. With highly predictable pharmacokinetic properties and high bioavailability, LMWH can target factor Xa, while affecting factor IIa to a lesser extent (**Figure 1**), and are associated with a lower incidence of thrombocytopenia than unfractionated heparin. The half-life of LMWH is 4.5 hours, and its effects can be reversed by protamine sulfate. The propitious pharmacokinetics allows LMWH administration subcutaneously once or twice daily without

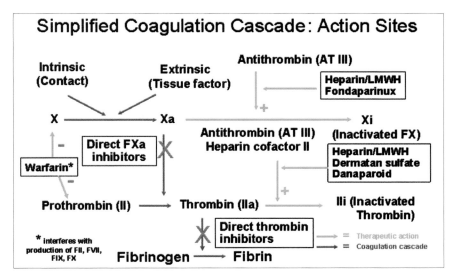

Figure 1 Simplified coagulation cascade with point of action of anticoagulation agents. (Courtesy of S.D. Berkowitz, MD, FACP.)

requisite monitoring of drug levels or activity.

However, the possibility of increased bleeding remains a concern with LMWH prophylaxis. Both increased bleeding and greater blood loss have been reported. The prevalence of major bleeding events in 5,412 patients is reported at 2.6%, a level not significantly different from placebo (**Table 3**).

PENTASACCHARIDES

Fondaparinux, a synthetic pentasaccharide that provides anticoagulation through inhibition of factor Xa (**Figure 1**), provides effective prophylaxis for DVT in a once daily subcutaneous fixed dose of 2.5 mg in THA and hip fracture surgery patients (**Table 1**). Pentasaccharide has a half-life of 18 hours with no known antidote. The reported total incidence of DVT in THA patients was 4.7% (RRR, 91%), with the incidence of proximal DVT of 1.2% (RRR, 95%) (**Table 2**). The reported rate of symptomatic VTED was 0.7% in THA. Major bleeding was reported at a rate of 0.3% in THA patients (**Table 3**). Clinical trials are in progress to compare the efficacy of earlier dosing versus first postoperative day dos-

ing, which may potentially decrease the bleeding rates in these patients.

Efficacy

Differences in efficacy among LMWH, pentasaccharide, and adjusted-dose warfarin prophylaxis are reported to be relatively small (**Table 2**). Pooled rates for major and minor bleeding events are presented in **Table 3**. In general, bleeding rates are comparable with placebo bleeding rates.

These data indicate that LMWH and pentasaccharide are more effective than warfarin in preventing asymptomatic and symptomatic in-hospital VTED. However, bleeding at the surgical site is increased in patients taking either LMWH or pentasaccharide compared with warfarin. The more rapid onset of anticoagulation activity with LMWH and pentasaccharide compared with warfarin accounts for the increase in bleeding.

Based on issues of cost, convenience, availability of an infrastructure to provide safe oral anticoagulation, potential bleeding and thrombosis risks, and duration of planned prophylaxis, the selection of LMWH, pentasaccharide, or warfarin prophylaxis is best made at the specific hospital level or, on occasion, at the individual patient level.

Nonpharmacologic Prophylaxis

MECHANICAL COMPRESSION

Prophylaxis via nonpharmacologic methods, including elastic stockings, intermittent pneumatic compression, plantar compression, and early ambulation has not proved to be effective as a single modality. These mechanical devices have a negligible effect on the proximal DVT rate. Additionally, with decreasing hospital stays for THA patients, the duration of prophylaxis is limited with these mechanical devices.

MULTIMODAL PROPHYLAXIS

The potential effect of combining nonpharmacologic methods and pharmacologic methods in multimodal prophylaxis has not been well studied. Although the use of layered modalities or multimodal prophylaxis is of considerable interest, no prospective randomized trials presently indicate that multimodal prophylaxis is more effective than single modality therapy.

REGIONAL ANESTHESIA

Hypotensive regional anesthesia (spinal or epidural) is associated with a significantly reduced incidence of postoperative DVT, in the absence or presence of other prophylaxis for THA. VTED prevalence after regional anesthesia, though reduced, remains substantial. Regional anesthesia alone has not been documented to match primary prophylaxis with other agents.

INFERIOR VENA CAVA FILTER

Inferior vena cava (IVC) filter placement has been suggested as a prophylaxis option for patients at extremely high risk for both postoperative VTED and bleeding. No randomized trials have reported using IVC filter prophylaxis alone or to add value to prophylaxis. In a treatment study using IVC filters, the incidence of PE (both symptomatic and asymptomatic) was significantly reduced in the short term. However, the IVC filter did not reduce mortality and revealed significantly more recurrent DVTs on follow-up. Thus, placement of a prophylactic IVC filter may reduce the immediate risk of postoperative PE in THA patients but will also increase the risk of future DVT. Prophylactic placement of an IVC filter should be relegated to patients who have failed previous adequate pharmacologic prophylaxis.

Length of Prophylaxis

Historically, prophylaxis has been continued during hospitalization of up to 14 days, but with the length of hospital stays now less than 5 days, the period of hospital prophylaxis may be inadequate. Screening for the presence of VTED is not recommended. Some studies suggest that the risk of DVT may persist for as long as 2 months after THA. A study continuing warfarin prophylaxis for 4 weeks after hospital discharge reported a 5.1% symptomatic confirmed DVT prevalence in the nontreated group and a 0.5% prevalence in the warfarin treated group. In an analysis of six THA studies in which LMWHs were used as extended prophylaxis versus placebo, the prevalence of DVT in the LMWH group was 7.9% (RRR, 41%), whereas in the placebo group it was 22.5%. The prevalence of proximal DVT was 11.2% in the placebo group and 3.0% in the LMWH group (RRR, 31%). Studies of extended LMWH use (up to 35 days) reported that prolonged LMWH prophylaxis is beneficial and significantly superior to conventional prophylaxis of 7 to 10 days, with a 50% reduction in DVT over placebo. Extended prophylaxis may be recommended in the future to reduce the number of thrombosis events after THA hospital discharge.

Cost Effectiveness

Cost effectiveness continues to be an elusive issue because of changing costs of prophylaxis agents, use of monitoring for oral anticoagulation, and use of extended prophylaxis. In a Canadian cost-effectiveness study, LMWHs were preferred over adjusted-dose warfarin. However, an analysis based on US health care costs found adjusted-dose warfarin to be more cost effective than LMWH. Other studies examining the cost of DVT after THA advocate prophylaxis as a cost-saving measure and indicate prevention of DVT is less expensive than treatment over the lifetime of the patient.

Genetics and Thrombosis

Areas of ongoing research include risk stratification with genetic markers. Genetic thrombophilia and hypofibrinolysis appear more frequently in patients who had PE after THA than in those who did not. Patients with activated protein C resistance appear to experience thromboembolic events more often than those without this resistance. Other genetic factors may be discovered that affect thrombosis formation, and testing for genetic factors may be done in the future.

Avoiding Pitfalls and Complications

Patients undergoing THA have been reported to be at greater risk for venous thrombosis and PE. Therefore, prophylaxis of THA patients is mandated for the prevention of thrombosis events, which cause venous sequelae and possible death. The American College of Chest Physicians recommends prophylaxis for THA for a minimum of 7 to 10 days and for 28 to 35 days after THA in high-risk patients. Choices are available as to the type of prophylaxis used, but in the practice of evidence-based medicine, the prophylaxis must be shown to be both effective and safe.

References

Freedman KB, Brookenthal KR, Fitzgerald RH Jr, et al: A meta-analysis of thromboembolic prophylaxis following elective total hip arthroplasty. *J Bone Joint Surg Am* 2000;82:929-938.

Geerts WH, Heit JA, Clagett GP, et al: Prevention of venous thromboembolism. *Chest* 2001; 119:132S-175S.

Mohr DN, Silverstein MD, Murtaugh PA, Harrison JM: Prophylactic agents for venous thrombosis in elective hip surgery: Meta-analysis of studies using venographic assessment. *Arch Intern Med* 1993; 153:2221-2228.

Prandoni P, Bruchi O, Sabbion P, et al: Prolonged thromboprophylaxis with oral anticoagulants after total hip arthroplasty: A prospective controlled randomized study. *Arch Intern Med* 2002; 162:1966-1971.

Prins MH, Hirsh J: A comparison of general anesthesia and regional anesthesia as a risk factor for deep vein thrombosis following hip surgery: A critical review. *Thromb Haemost* 1990;64:497-500.

Coding

CPT Codes	ICD-9 Codes		
CPT codes are based on procedures, and thrombosis prophylaxis does not fall into a diagnostic or procedural category unless thrombosis is suspected.	451.11 451.81 453.42	451.19 453.40	451.2 453.41

CPT copyright © 2004 by the American Medical Association. All Rights Reserved.

Femur

Chapter 36

Revision Total Hip Arthroplasty: Indications and Contraindications

Aaron G. Rosenberg, MD

■ Indications

The term "indications" carries a sense of certainty that is only rarely present in most surgical settings. Particularly in revision surgery, indications represents the end points of a complex decision-making process in which both surgeon and patient are involved.

The most common indications for revision total hip arthroplasty (THA) are pain or functional disability caused by diagnoses that may be corrected surgically. The symptoms must be related to an identified problem with the arthroplasty that is likely to be corrected by the revision, such as mechanical loosening, biomechanical abnormalities of the reconstruction, advanced bearing surface wear and its sequelae, recurrent dislocation, sepsis, and/or periprosthetic fracture.

The severity of the symptoms guides the decision-making process. The severity of pain usually can be quantified, but the patient also should be questioned about the frequency and the degree of disability the pain produces. In addition, a thorough understanding of the activities that cause and relieve the pain should be obtained.

Quantifying functional disability is more complex and functional problems are less often associated with reliable revision indications.

These problems include hip stiffness, recurrent dislocation, limb-length discrepancy, and persistent limp. Determining a patient's functional disability can be challenging but also is important in the decision to consider revision surgery.

Aseptic Loosening

The principal indication for revision THA in a patient with aseptic loosening is pain. The more frequent and intense the pain, the stronger the indication for revision, provided that the pain is likely to be improved by the revision. Pain associated with loosening usually occurs with weight bearing or hip motion and often is particularly intense when the patient stands from a resting position and begins to walk. Loose cups typically cause groin or buttock pain, whereas loose stems usually cause thigh pain, but these findings are not absolute. The patient must understand that all hip pain around a failed arthroplasty may not be relieved by reoperation.

Aseptic loosening can create functional disability related to pain or altered biomechanics of a failed implant, which may be an indication for revision THA. Hip biomechanics can be adversely affected when loose implants migrate, leading to poorer abductor function or limb shortening.

Bone loss associated with aseptic loosening also can be an indication for revision. Aseptic loosening often, but not always, causes bone loss as a result of mechanical bone erosion or particulate debris-induced (eg, metal, polyethylene, or cement) osteolysis. Bone loss associated with implant loosening tends to be progressive, but the rate at which the bone loss occurs varies. Grossly loose sockets tend to cause relatively rapid acetabular bone erosion, and stems with a rough surface finish that debond from the cement tend to cause rapid osteolysis. Conversely, bone loss usually is slow with loose uncemented stems. Regardless of the rate at which it occurs, bone loss may be an indication for revision, depending on the patient's specific circumstances.

Marked bone loss that predisposes to periprosthetic fracture also is a relatively strong indication for revision THA. Finally, if anticipated further bone loss will negatively affect the quality of a future reconstruction, revision THA is more strongly indicated.

Bearing Surface Wear and Periprosthetic Osteolysis

Osteolysis associated with well-fixed components usually is caused by particulate debris from the bearing surface, a process that often is not (but occasionally is) associated with hip pain. Patients with pain in this circumstance typically report pain in the groin, most likely the result of particulate debris-induced synovitis, iliopsoas tendinitis from particulate debris, or periprosthetic fracture through osteolytic lesions.

Radiographically evident bearing surface wear may or may not be associated with osteolysis. The indications for revision THA for wear in the absence of osteolysis are (1) pain secondary to particulate synovitis, (2) wear through or fracture of the polyethylene bearing surface, and (3) impending wear through or fracture of the polyethylene bearing surface.

The indications for reoperation for bearing surface wear and osteolysis are based on symptom severity, rate of progression, and location of osteolytic lesions. A more detailed discussion of reoperation for osteolysis is provided in chapter 42.

Other Indications

Indications for revision related to other complications of THA, including infection, dislocation, heterotopic bone formation, and periprosthetic fracture are discussed in separate chapters in the book.

■ Contraindications

Revision THA usually is not indicated unless a specific problem is identified that can be solved with reoperation. Revision THA also is contraindicated if the medical or orthopaedic risks of the surgery outweigh the potential benefits. A detailed discussion of risks and benefits occurs later in this chapter.

For a patient whose symptoms are clearly amenable to activity modification or in whom revision is not ideal because of age, comorbidities, or other specific anatomic factors, nonsurgical treatment may be appropriate. An obvious example is a young patient who has a well-fixed, functioning arthroplasty who must limit only the most vigorous of athletic activities. For some patients with few or no symptoms after activity modification, a nonsurgical approach is more reasonable than revision THA given the potential difficulty in revising components that are already well fixed and the relatively small benefit afforded by surgery.

■ Alternative Treatments

The main alternative to revision THA is ongoing observation of the primary THA. Oral analgesics and gait aids can reduce pain and improve function in some patients sufficiently to avoid reoperation. Nonsurgical treatment of a failing arthroplasty should not be considered if further bone loss, functional disability, and reduced likelihood of successful reoperation are potential sequelae.

■ Decision Making in Revision Total Hip Arthroplasty

Medical decision making requires consideration of the potential risks and benefits of a particular intervention and subsequent comparisons with other potential courses of action. A simple risk-benefit ratio can be considered by evaluating the sum of all potential medical and surgical risks faced by the patient. Medical risks may be best determined by the patient's internist (ie, who is likely to be familiar with the physiologic burden imposed on the patient by revision surgery). In some cases, however, the surgeon must describe these burdens so that the internist can accurately assess the medical risks involved. The general and specific surgical risks are then added to the medical risks, accounting for the specific anatomic features of the pathology, as well as the skills of the surgical team.

The presence of substantial comorbidities may preclude surgical intervention in all but the most incapacitated of patients. Certainly the risks of perioperative mortality following surgical intervention must be carefully weighed against the expected functional improvement and pain relief that can be expected with any type of surgical intervention.

An underlying assumption in most surgical decision making and one predicated on the relative unpredictability of surgical outcomes, particularly in the elective setting, is that nonsurgical treatment should be attempted first. Nonsurgical treatment may consist of assistive devices for ambulation, weight loss, systemic or local medications, and physical therapy and activity modification in an effort to make symptoms more tolerable.

Although the degree of functional disability, level of activity, and associated symptoms vary by patient and diagnosis, assessment of these factors can help in surgical decision making by determining whether revision THA has the potential to eliminate or minimize symptoms. In some settings, however, the symptoms, physical findings, and radiographic changes are severe enough that revision THA is indicated. In patients in whom revision is indicated for problems that are not currently causing symptoms (eg, progressive osteolysis or accelerated polyethylene wear), it is important to explain to the patient why surgical treatment is recommended, even though it will not relieve symptoms or improve function and carries substantial potential risks and complications.

All interventions must be evaluated in the context of the patient's overall health and personal expectations.

■ References

Abernathy CM, Hamm RM: *Surgical Intuition: What It Is and How to Get It.* Philadelphia, PA, Hanley & Belfus, 1995.

Baron J: *Thinking and Deciding,* ed 3. Cambridge, United Kingdom, Cambridge University Press, 2000.

Brown TE, Larson B, Shen F, Moskal JT: Thigh pain after cementless total hip arthroplasty: Evaluation and management. *J Am Acad Orthop Surg* 2002;10:385-392.

Eddy DM: *Clinical Decision Making: From Theory to Practice: A Collection of Essays From the Journal of the American Medical Association.* Sudbury, MA, Jones & Bartlett, 1996.

Fehring TK, Rosenberg AG: Primary total hip arthroplasty: Indications and contraindications, in Callahan JC, Rosenberg AG, Rubash HE (eds): *The Adult Hip.* Philadelphia, PA, Lippincott-Raven, 1997, pp 893-898.

Hastie R, Dawes RM: *Rational Choice in An Uncertain World: The Psychology of Judgment and Decision Making.* Thousand Oaks, CA, Sage Publications, 2001.

Mahomed NN, Barrett JA, Katz JN, et al: Rates and outcomes of primary and revision total hip replacement in the United States Medicare population. *J Bone Joint Surg Am* 2003;85:27-32.

Reigelman RK: *Minimizing Medical Mistakes: The Art of Medical Decision Making.* Boston, MA, Little Brown & Co, 1991.

Socket DL, Haynes RB, Guyatt GH, Tugwell PL: *Clinical Epidemiology: A Basic Science for Clinical Medicine.* Boston, MA, Little Brown & Co, 1991.

Sacket DL, Richardson WS, Rosenberg W, Haynes RB: *Evidence Based Medicine: How to Practice and Teach EBM.* New York, NY, Churchill Livingstone, 1997.

Schwartz S, Griffin T: *Medical Thinking: The Psychology of Medical Judgment and Decision Making.* New York, NY, Springer-Verlag, 1986.

Tversky A, Kahneman D: Judgments under uncertainty. *Heuristics Biases Science* 1974;185:1124-1131.

Wennberg J: Dealing with medical practice variation: A proposal for action. *Health Aff* 1984;3:6-9.

White RE: Evaluation of the painful total hip arthroplasty, in Callahan JC, Rosenberg AG, Rubash HE (eds): *The Adult Hip.* Philadelphia, PA, Lippincott-Raven, 1997, pp 1377-1386.

Chapter 37

Revision Total Hip Arthroplasty: Preoperative Planning

Jay R. Lieberman, MD
Daniel J. Berry, MD

Introduction

Preoperative planning is essential to the success of revision total hip arthroplasty (THA). These complex procedures require that the surgeon know what implants are in place, that the proper extraction instruments will be available if the implants will be removed, and that compatible matching trial and actual implants will be available for use. Preoperative planning helps the surgeon evaluate patterns of bone loss, anticipate the need for special implants or bone grafts, and consider whether alternative implants and materials might be needed at surgery as a result of intraoperative findings. Perhaps most importantly, good preoperative planning involves a mental rehearsal of the proposed surgery by the surgeon; this can help the surgeon move more efficiently once the procedure begins. The following outline lists important considerations that may be included in preoperative planning for revision THA. The worksheet that follows may be considered one way to preoperatively organize surgical needs.

1. Ensure the patient has had an adequate medical evaluation.
    Does the patient's medical status allow a major reconstructive procedure?
    Is the patient on warfarin on a chronic basis?
    Has the warfarin been stopped and is the INR normal now?
    Does the patient have a history of DVT or pulmonary embolism?

2. Understand the mechanism(s) by which the previous hip arthroplasty has failed.
    Will you be able to correct the problem that led to failure of the previous hip arthroplasty?

3. Determine if the arthroplasty is infected.
    Are the ESR and CRP normal? If not, has the hip joint been aspirated?
    What are the results of hip aspiration?

4. Understand what implants are in place and determine their design and size.
    Have you reviewed the previous operative reports?
    Do you have copies of the implant labels that were placed in the medical record at the patient's previous surgeries?

5. Make sure adequate, good-quality radiographs are available.
    Do you have radiographs that show enough of the femur?
    Are any special radiographs (Judet views) or scans (CT) needed?

6. Template the hip radiographs.
    Do you know the magnification of the hip radiographs?
    What type of socket do you plan to place? What socket diameter?
    What type of femoral component do you plan to place? What stem diameter? What stem length?

7. Ensure optimal perioperative systemic and local delivery antibiotics are available.
    Do you have optimal antibiotics for systemic perioperative coverage based on the patient's allergies or any previous infections?
    Do you have antibiotic-loaded cement if needed?

8. Consider which implants you plan to remove and which you plan to retain; determine what compatible implants may be needed.

 Do you have compatible liners if the metal socket will be retained?

 Will you cement a different liner into a retained metal socket?

 Do you have compatible femoral head sizes to match the socket if the socket and femoral component will be retained?

 Do you have compatible modular heads and trial heads to match the femur if it will be retained?

9. Consider the operative approach you will use.

 What exposure will help you best remove the implant and cement?

 What exposure will you need to place new implants?

 What exposure will optimize hip stability?

 Will an osteotomy be required? Do you have the wires or cables available to repair the osteotomy site?

10. Consider what special instruments are needed for implant or cement removal.

 Do you need special curved gouges to remove an uncemented socket?

 Do you have hand instruments for cement removal available?

 Do you need special power instruments? Metal-cutting instruments? Trephines? High-speed burrs? Ultrasonic cement removal instruments?

 Do you need company/implant-specific extraction devices for the acetabular PE?

 The acetabular screws? The acetabular component? The femoral component?

11. Consider what your options will be in the event your first choice of implants will not work at surgery.

 What are your first and second alternative choices for acetabular reconstruction?

 What are your first and second alternative choices for femoral reconstruction?

12. Consider what your options will be in the event of intraoperative complications.

 Do you have implants to manage unexpected bone fracture?

13. Evaluate bone graft needs.

 Do you anticipate needing acetabular bone grafts? Particulate? Bulk?

 Do you anticipate needing femoral bone grafts? Strut grafts? Particulate grafts? Large segment grafts?

 Do you have all potential necessary bone grafts readily available?

14. Evaluate the need for internal fixation devices.

 Is there evidence of pelvic discontinuity?

 Do you need pelvic reconstruction plates for pelvic discontinuity?

 Do you need screws to fix a bulk acetabular graft?

 Do you need cables or wires for femoral cerclage?

 Do you need femoral plates?

 Do you need special trochanteric fixation devices? Claws? Hook plates? Wire mesh?

15. Consider how you will manage intraoperative hip instability if it is present.

 Do you need extra-large diameter femoral heads and matching extra-large inside diameter acetabular liners?

 Do you need constrained acetabular components?

16. Consider blood replacement needs.

 Would intraoperative blood salvage be of value?

17. Will a postoperative abductor brace be necessary?

18. What type of DVT prophylaxis will be used and what will be the duration?

19. Consider the patient's postoperative needs.

 Do you need to arrange an ICU bed?

 Do you need social services for postdischarge planning?

■ **Revision Total Hip Arthroplasty Checklist**

1. Patient Name _____   2. Patient ID Number _____

3. Sex: M F   4. Date of Birth _____   5. Date of Planned Procedure _____

6. Primary Diagnosis (Original THA) _____

7. Secondary Diagnosis (Planned Procedure)

8. Procedure

       Acetabulum _____

       Femur _____

9. Components in place

       Acetabulum (Type/Company) _____

       Femur (Type/Company) _____

10. Acetabulum Revision: _____ Yes   _____ No

       If No

       Polyethylene liner exchange   Option 1 _____

                                            Type/Company _____

                                            Option 2 _____

                                            Type/Company _____

       If Yes

       Procedure

       Implant Selection   Option 1 _____

                               Type/Company _____

                               Option 2 _____

                               Type/Company _____

                               Option 3 _____

                               Type/Company _____

       Bone grafts   Morcellized _____ Yes   _____ No

                      Structural   _____ Yes   _____ No

                      Structural graft options:

                            Distal femur _____ Yes   _____ No

                            Femoral head _____ Yes   _____ No

                            Other _____

       Cage   _____ Yes   _____ No

                      Type/Company _____

       Cemented Cup   _____ Yes   _____ No

                      Type/Company _____

11. Femoral Revision: _____ Yes   _____ No

        If No

        Femoral head exchange   Type/Company _____

        If Yes

        Procedure

        Implant Selection   Option 1 _____

                                  Type/Company _____

                                  Option 2 _____

                                  Type/Company _____

                                  Option 3 _____

                                  Type/Company _____

        Cemented implant? _____ Yes   _____ No

                                  Option 1 _____

                                  Type/Company _____

                                  Option 2 _____

                                  Type/Company _____

        Bone graft   Morcellized   _____ Yes   _____ No

                                  Femoral Strut   _____ Yes   _____ No

                                  Proximal Femur   _____ Yes   _____ No

                                  Other   _____ Yes   _____ No

12. Special Equipment

                                  High-speed burrs _____ Yes   _____ No

                                  Ultrasound   _____ Yes   _____ No

                                  Type/Company _____

                                  Cables   _____ Yes   _____ No

                                  Type/Company _____

                                  Abduction Brace   _____ Yes   _____ No

                                  Cell Saver   _____ Yes   _____ No

                                  Other _____

                                  Other _____

Chapter 38

Revision Total Hip Arthroplasty: Surgical Approaches

Clive P. Duncan, MD, MSc, FRCSC
Jonathan R. Howell, MD, FRCSC
Bassam A. Masri, MD, FRCSC

Introduction

Successful reconstruction of the adult hip requires adequate exposure of the patient's anatomy, existing implants, and bony deficits while protecting vital neurovascular structures and minimizing the degree of unnecessary dissection, bone devascularization, and bone destruction. To achieve these objectives, the surgeon should be familiar with different surgical approaches to the adult hip. Each approach offers specific advantages and disadvantages that can be matched to the patient's needs and the requirements of the re-

construction. This chapter describes both the factors influencing the surgeon's choice of approach and the various surgical approaches and their strengths and weaknesses, emphasizing some of the more specialized techniques required for complex reconstruction. Specific indications for which each approach is particularly well suited are also described.

Factors Influencing Surgical Approach

Table 1 outlines the factors influencing the choice of approach. Any number of different approaches might be suitable, but the final choice depends on which factors the surgeon feels are most important in each case.

Patient Anatomy and Bony Deficits

Exposure of the bony anatomy is the key to a satisfactory reconstruction. For uncomplicated reconstructions the surgeon may choose any of the commonly used approaches that afford safe and adequate exposure for primary total hip arthroplasty (THA). However, anatomic anomalies have a major influence on the choice of approach.

Anatomy may have been altered by previous operations. For example, patients undergoing conversion of a previous hip fusion may have abnormal bone masses around the acetabulum that might disorient the surgeon. Heterotopic ossification may also hinder exposure, and varus remodeling of the femur may make exposure of the medullary canal difficult without an osteotomy. Patients with a previous diagnosis of developmental dysplasia of the hip (DDH) may require revision of the acetabular placement and bone augmentation if the location of the acetabulum was not established during the initial reconstruction.

Meticulous preoperative planning is the key to avoiding potential pitfalls. Alterations in the patient's anatomy may limit the choice of surgical approach in several ways. First, the approach chosen may limit the surgery that can be performed, and the patient's anatomy may require surgery beyond those limits. For example, the structural bone grafting required to reconstruct the acetabulum of a patient with Crowe III or IV DDH requires extensive exposure of the superolateral wall of the acetabulum and the pelvis. A transgluteal approach limits the degree of proximal dissection that can be safely performed, and this potentially compromises the surgical results. However, the posterior approach al-

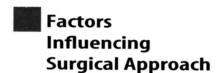

Table 1 Factors Influencing the Surgeon's Choice of Surgical Approach

Patient's anatomy, including contractures, presence of heterotopic bone, etc

Bone defects

Design and fixation of existing components

Position of existing components

Previous surgical approaches

Complications of previous surgery

Surgeon training and experience

Patient's ability to comply with postoperative restrictions

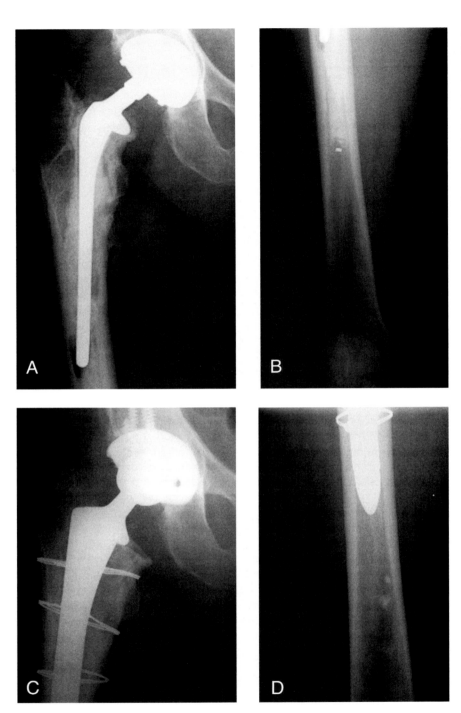

Figure 1 Preoperative AP radiographs of a failed cemented femoral stem **(A)** with a long column of well-fixed distal cement **(B)**. Attempted proximal removal of this column of cement risks inadvertent injury to the femur. **C** and **D**, Postoperative AP radiographs of the same patient. The cement was easily removed using an ETO, and the hip was reconstructed using an extensively porous-coated uncemented stem.

quired when the center of rotation is restored to its correct level.

Second, a patient's anatomy and degree of bone loss may predispose to complications with some surgical approaches. These complications may be avoided by using an alternative approach. For example, lysis affecting the trochanteric region may lead to such extensive bone loss that trochanteric osteotomy or trochanteric slide should be avoided because, although they provide excellent hip joint exposure, they also lead to predictable problems with reattachment of the trochanter.

In some patients with a high risk of postoperative dislocation because of neuromuscular imbalance, poor compliance, or a grossly deficient abductor mechanism, the anterolateral approach coupled with a constrained socket design may be preferred to the posterolateral approach, all other factors being equal.

Component Design, Fixation, and Orientation

Design and fixation features of the components to be removed often influence the choice of surgical exposure, especially on the femoral side. In the patient with a loose cemented stem, several factors to be considered include fixation of cement to the host bone, the need for complete cement removal, and the intended reconstruction method. A loosely bonded column of cement is easily removed from above and has little influence on the choice of surgical approach. However, rigidly fixed cement may be extremely difficult to remove, particularly if a long column of distal cement exists because a cement plug was not used during the initial operation. Attempted removal of well-fixed distal cement will risk inadvertent injury to the femoral cortex because of the difficulties in achieving adequate visualization of the distal canal and the tendency for instruments to wander from the line of the femoral canal. The risks of femoral perforation can be reduced

lows access to the pelvic sidewall through careful elevation of the glu-

teal muscles and also allows mobilization of the glutei, which is often re-

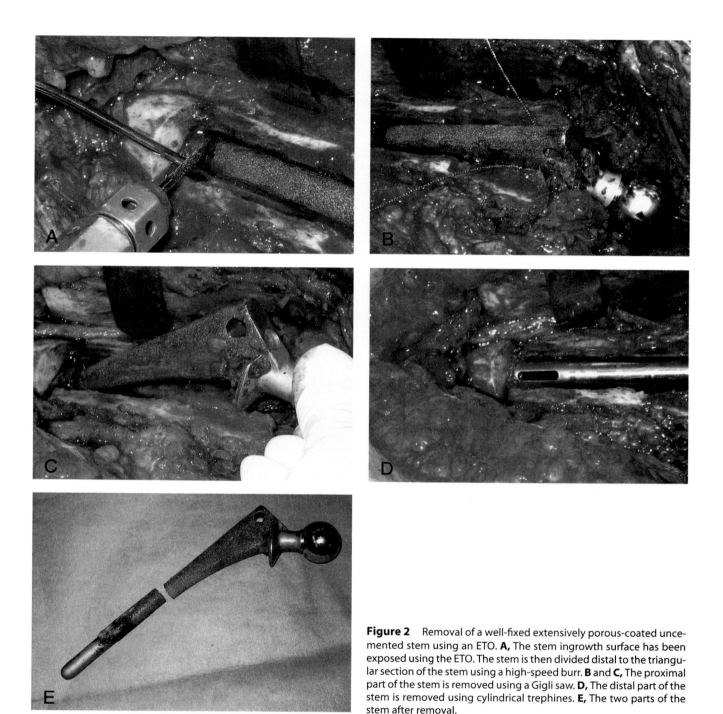

Figure 2 Removal of a well-fixed extensively porous-coated uncemented stem using an ETO. **A,** The stem ingrowth surface has been exposed using the ETO. The stem is then divided distal to the triangular section of the stem using a high-speed burr. **B** and **C,** The proximal part of the stem is removed using a Gigli saw. **D,** The distal part of the stem is removed using cylindrical trephines. **E,** The two parts of the stem after removal.

through selection of the surgical approach; in these circumstances, the extended trochanteric osteotomy (ETO) provides a safe route for distal cement removal (**Figure 1**).

Removal of a well-ingrown uncemented stem requires surgical ac-

cess to the ingrowth surface. The surgeon should be familiar with the stem design because it usually influences surgical approach and extraction techniques. Access to the ingrowth surface from the proximal femoral surface may be restricted by the presence of a

collar or by the proximal geometry of the stem. In such circumstances, attempted removal of the stem from above may cause significant injury to the proximal femur. For proximally coated designs, an ETO performed to or just beyond the distal extent of the

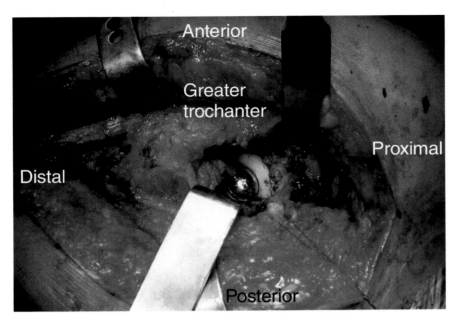

Figure 3 A posterior approach has been made to this left hip. At the primary surgery, the acetabular component was malpositioned in marked retroversion; therefore, revision of this component is required to ensure that the hip is stable postoperatively.

coating allows good access to the ingrowth surface. Fixation of the revision stem can be achieved by using the intact femur distal to the ETO. For extensively coated stems, access to the distal ingrowth surface from above is limited by the metaphyseal flare of the prosthesis. In these patients, an ETO can be performed to a point just beyond the junction of the cylindrical and triangular segments of the stem, with the stem sectioned at the junction. This allows removal of the proximal part of the stem using Gigli saws, flexible osteotomes, and high-speed burrs. The distal stem can be cored with cylindrical trephines (**Figure 2**).

Fixation of the acetabular component generally has less influence on the surgical approach because circumferential exposure of the cup is usually achievable using any common surgical approach. However, when removing hardware (such as reconstruction cages or plates) that requires access to specific regions (such as the pelvis side wall or the posterior column), the need for access influences the choice of approach. Similarly, the presence of pelvic discontinuity and the location of severe bone loss around the acetabulum modifies the choice of surgical exposure. The presence of large amounts of intrapelvic cement in an infected hip may require a retroperitoneal approach for cement removal, and a similar approach may be required for intrapelvic components if protecting the iliac vessels is necessary.

The orientation of existing components sometimes influences the choice of surgical approach, particularly if one of the components is to be retained. For example, in planning to retain a well-fixed uncemented shell that has been placed in minimal anteversion, the posterior approach should be avoided because it might produce postoperative instability. However, component position should be a relatively minor consideration. If there is any doubt about postoperative stability, the component should be revised to improve its orientation (**Figure 3**).

Previous Surgical Approaches

Multiple parallel incisions are unsightly and risk wound necrosis; thus, previous incisions should be used, if possible. Using existing incisions usually does not restrict the surgical approach because the skin is sufficiently mobile to accommodate multiple approaches though the same incision. Part (if not all) of a previous incision often can be used, the incision being modified at either end of the wound.

Deep dissection routes used in previous surgeries should be considered. If possible, the previous operative note should be studied to determine whether the capsule and surrounding tendons were repaired at the last operation. It is generally a good practice to limit the number of joint restraints damaged through surgical access, so if repair was not made or if repair has failed, it may be advantageous to use the same approach and allow virgin tissues to remain intact. For example, if a previous transgluteal repair has avulsed, use of the same route of access to the joint should be considered to avoid causing further damage. However, if this approach does not adequately expose the anatomy, the previous approach should not become the overriding factor.

Complications of Previous Surgery

Complications occurring since the original operation sometimes influence the surgeon's choice of future procedures. For example, nonunion of the trochanter after trochanteric osteotomy can provide excellent exposure of the hip and thus provide a useful access route. However, the surgeon should ensure that disturbing a stable fibrous nonunion will not prevent subsequent reattachment of the trochanteric fragment with a reliable expectation of bony union (**Figure 4**). Without such certainty, it is best to leave the trochanter undisturbed.

Instability is a common indication for revision surgery and its direc-

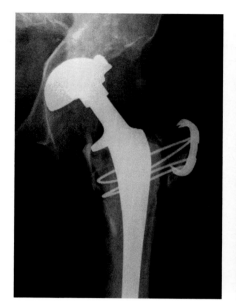

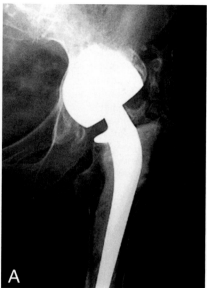

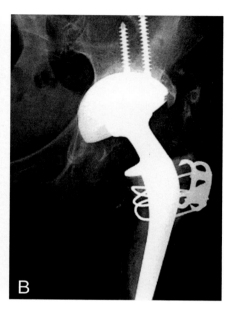

Figure 4 This acetabular component requires revision because of polyethylene wear. The previous trochanteric osteotomy has healed through fibrous union and could be used to access the hip joint for the revision. However, the shoulder of exposed cement underneath the trochanteric fragment means that problems with further trochanteric union could be expected using this approach. The surgery was performed through a transgluteal approach, and the fibrous union was left undisturbed.

Figure 5 **A,** Heterotopic ossification surrounding the right hip made exposure through the posterior approach extremely difficult. Use of a trochanteric slide allowed the femur and its retained component to be retracted, and good exposure was achieved. **B,** Postoperative radiograph showing repair of the trochanteric slide using a cable grip system.

tion will influence the choice of surgical approach. A detailed history combined with physical examination under anesthesia should determine the direction of instability and indicate whether there has been disruption of the anterior or posterior soft-tissue envelope. It can then be decided which part of the envelope to compromise through the approach and which soft tissues should be preserved.

Heterotopic ossification severely limits the pliability of the soft tissues surrounding the hip joint and thus may dictate the choice of approach. **Figure 5,** *A* is the preoperative radiograph of a patient requiring revision of the acetabular component with retention of the femoral stem. In this case, the posterior approach was used, and the tissue anterior to the hip was mobilized to create a pocket into which

the femoral neck could be placed while the surgeon worked on the cup. However, the presence of heterotopic ossification and dense scarring anteriorly made this impossible, and the approach was changed to a trochanteric slide (**Figure 5,** *B*), which gave excellent exposure.

When planning surgery for periprosthetic fractures, the surgeon should consider how the fracture's presence influences the surgical approach. A direct lateral approach usually suffices for patients requiring simple fixation with plates or strut allografts. If stem revision is required, the fracture may provide a route to the femoral canal for cement removal and reaming. In these patients, the vastus slide approach is ideal because it allows simultaneous exposure of the hip joint and the femoral shaft and permits easier dislocation of the proximal femoral fragment in the operated femur than does the posterolateral approach. Once the femur has been provisionally fixed, this approach makes it easy to prepare the femur for the revision sur-

gery and potentially reduce the risk of postoperative instability.

If the proximal femur is to be bivalved and reassembled around the new femoral component because of severe proximal bone loss, an ETO (or a sagittal bivalve) approach provides excellent exposure of the acetabulum and remaining distal femoral canal. Alternatively, a trochanteric slide can be used and the grossly deficient proximal femur simply excised.

━━━━━━━■

Classification of Surgical Approaches

A classification system can be useful when deciding which surgical approach to use. No universally accepted system exists, but the classification system presented in **Table 2** divides approaches into two main categories, standard and specialized, and further classifies the standard approaches de-

Table 2 Classification of Surgical Approaches

Category	Direction of Approach	Examples
Standard	Anterior	Smith-Petersen
	Anterolateral	Watson-Jones
	Transgluteal	Hardinge Omega Vastus slide
	Transtrochanteric	Trochanteric osteotomy Trochanteric slide
	Posterolateral	Kocher-Langenbeck Moore
	Medial	Ludloff
Specialized	Femoral osteotomies	ETO Vascularized scaphoid window Controlled perforations
	Extensive acetabular	Ilioinguinal Extended iliofemoral Combined approaches Triradiate
	Retroperitoneal	Modified ilioinguinal

Table 3 Anterior Approach: Strengths, Weaknesses, and Indications

Strengths	Weaknesses	Indications in Adult Reconstruction
Exposure of the anterior column	Poor exposure of the posterior column and the posterior wall	Pelvic fractures
Exposure of the medial wall of the acetabulum		Pelvic osteotomies
Patient position ideal for hip fusion	Extensive stripping of the abductors	Primary THA
		Hemiarthroplasty
		Intra-articular fusions
		Pelvic tumors
		Septic arthritis
		Synovial biopsy

pending on the direction of the deep dissection. An approach is deemed to be anterior if the dissection passes completely anterior to the gluteus medius muscle (eg, the Smith-Petersen approach). An anterolateral approach goes deep to the hip abductor muscles without going through them (such as in the Watson-Jones approach). A transgluteal approach goes through the hip abductor muscles either par-tially or entirely (examples include the Hardinge, Omega, and vastus slide approaches). Transtrochanteric approaches are characterized by os-teotomy limited to the greater tro-chanter. The dissection in posterolat-eral approaches passes behind the greater trochanter and gluteus medius. Ludloff's medial approach is included so the table of surgical approaches is complete, but it is not discussed fur-ther because it is seldom useful for adult hip reconstruction.

The specialized approaches rep-resent a diverse group of techniques usually reserved for specific indica-tions. This group includes osteoto-mies of the femur used to gain access to the hip joint and limited osteoto-mies used to access local areas of the femoral canal. The acetabular expo-sures are extensive dissections most commonly used for the surgical treat-ment of acetabular fractures. They are sometimes used for tumor resection and reconstruction or extremely diffi-cult acetabular revisions.

Standard Approaches

Anterior Approach

The anterior approach of Smith-Petersen, sometimes referred to as the iliofemoral approach, is performed through an internervous plane, super-ficially passing between the tensor fas-cia lata muscle laterally (superior glu-teal nerve) and the sartorius muscle medially (femoral nerve). The deep dissection passes medial to the gluteus medius (superior gluteal nerve) and lateral to the rectus femoris (femoral nerve). Structures at risk include the lateral femoral cutaneous nerve, which passes through the sartorius fascia approximately 3 cm below the anterior superior iliac spine, and the ascending branch of the lateral cir-cumflex femoral artery.

The indications for this ap-proach and its strengths and weakness are summarized in **Table 3**. The ante-rior approach provides good exposure of the anterior column and the medial wall of the acetabulum, but exposure of the posterior column and femur is limited. Femoral exposure can be improved using specialized equip-ment, including an operating table that places the hip in hyperextension, but the acetabular exposure is not sufficient to allow complex reconstruction of the posterior wall. In addition, the anterior acetabular exposure is achieved through extensive stripping of the abductors from the wall of the ilium, which can result in marked residual weakness and heterotopic ossification. As a result, this approach alone is rarely used for revision arthroplasty but may be combined with another approach when exposure of the anterior column of the pelvis is required. Because this approach is rarely used, and because in our experience this approach is almost never more advantageous than those described below, the anterior approach of Smith-Petersen is not described further.

Anterolateral Approach

The Watson-Jones approach passes anterior to the gluteus medius tendon beneath the tensor facia lata, which is retracted anteriorly. A retractor is passed around the inferior and medial borders of the gluteus medius and minimus muscles, and they are retracted laterally and superiorly to expose the fat pad overlying the anterior capsule of the hip joint. Exposure of the anterior capsule is facilitated through division of the vastus lateralis from the vastus ridge of the femur and retraction of this muscle inferiorly and laterally. Depending on the patient's anatomy and the intended procedure, the exposure may be further improved through partial division of the anterior fibers of the gluteus medius tendon, although the approach then becomes transgluteal. Our experience suggests that this approach is inferior to the Hardinge approach, and that its use offers no real advantages to the patient or the surgeon. We believe its role in revision THA is extremely limited.

Transgluteal Approaches

Several techniques are described for exposure of the hip through elevation of part or all of the gluteus medius muscle. McFarland and Osborne originally described detachment of the en-

Table 4 Transgluteal Approaches: Strengths, Weaknesses, and Indications

Strengths	Weaknesses	Indications in Adult Reconstruction
Circumferential exposure of the acetabulum	Not extensile	Primary THA
Need for trochanteric osteotomy avoided	Risk of abductor tendon avulsion, especially when the limb is lengthened	Simple revision THA
Posterior tissues remain intact	Risk of injury to superior gluteal nerve	Femoral neck fractures
Low dislocation rate	Increased rate of heterotopic ossification	Proximal femoral osteotomy
		Slipped capital femoral epiphysis

tire gluteus medius with posterior dislocation of the hip. This technique was later modified and popularized by Hardinge, who described elevation of the anterior half of the gluteus medius tendon and anterior dislocation of the hip while preserving the attachment of the muscle's thick posterior part to the greater trochanter.

These soft-tissue approaches avoid the problems associated with reattachment of a trochanteric osteotomy and preserve the posterior soft-tissue envelope, producing lower rates of dislocation compared with the posterior approach. The transgluteal approaches provide satisfactory exposure of the acetabulum for simple primary and revision THA, but proximal dissection is limited by the risk of injury to the inferior gluteal nerve and the subsequent loss of abductor function. Exposure of the posterior column can also be limited without the development of a separate subfascial plane passing posterior to the gluteus medius and minimus muscles and around the back of the femur. These approaches are further complicated by difficulties with tendon reattachment in patients with a lengthened limb, the inability to adjust abductor muscle tension through trochanteric advancement, and a higher rate of postoperative heterotopic ossification. The strengths and weaknesses of this approach, and some indications for it, are summarized in **Table 4**.

Many modifications of the transgluteal approach exist, including

Dall's anterior partial trochanteric osteotomy, in which a small flake of bone is taken with the attachment of the gluteus medius so that bony healing can occur to prevent postoperative abductor weakness. The patient may be placed in the supine or lateral position, depending on surgeon preference and training. A longitudinal skin incision is centered on the midline of the greater trochanter and is carried distally along the midline of the femur. The incision is curved posteriorly by 15° in the proximal arm to help access the proximal femur. The fascia lata is divided in line with the skin incision and retracted to expose the underlying trochanteric bursa, which is divided and swept aside.

The gluteus medius tendon is seen as a fan of muscle inserting into the superior aspect of the greater trochanter. The anterior one third to one half of the gluteus medius tendon is elevated from the anterior surface of the greater trochanter, carefully leaving a cuff of tendon attached to the trochanter for later repair. The most anterior aspect of the tendon remains attached to a portion of the vastus lateralis. The distal dissection continues by elevating a portion of the vastus lateralis from the medial aspect of the proximal femur. Alternatively, the tendon can be elevated with a thin flake of bone from the anterior trochanter to provide a cancellous surface for bony healing after reattachment. The split in the gluteus medius proximally is gently opened with retractors to ex-

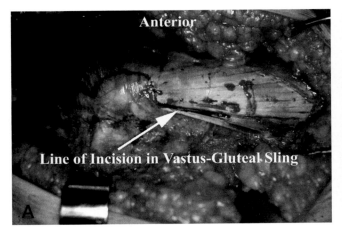

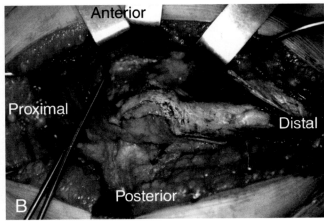

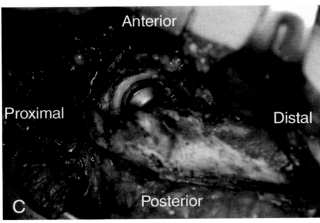

Figure 6 The vastus slide approach. **A,** The line of the incision in the vastus gluteal sling of this right hip (arrow) was marked intraoperatively. **B,** The vastus gluteal sling is elevated to expose the shaft of the femur. **C,** The limb is then externally rotated and the hip joint capsule opened anteriorly to expose the component.

pose the gluteus minimus tendon lying beneath. This is divided in line with its fibers, which lie longitudinally, and distally this cut is curved posteriorly toward the trochanter in line with the incision in the gluteus medius. The gluteal tendons are then elevated as a flap from the anterior aspect of the hip joint capsule, while the limb is placed in external rotation to help with capsule exposure. Wide exposure of the anterior capsule can be achieved using this approach, and the capsule is then either divided or excised to gain access to the hip joint.

Closure is achieved using bioabsorbable sutures in layers, starting with capsule repair, if the capsule was retained. The gluteus minimus tendon is repaired in a side-to-side manner, followed by reattachment of the gluteus medius tendon, either through repair of the tendon or reattachment of the bony flake, as discussed above.

In complex reconstructions, this approach can be modified to provide increased exposure of the femoral shaft through the vastus slide approach, originally described independently by Berman and Head (**Figure 6**). Using this technique, the proximal dissection is identical to that described above, but from the distal attachment of the gluteus medius the incision passes posteriorly just below the greater trochanter and then along the posterior border of the vastus lateralis, which is reflected anteriorly from the intermuscular septum, carefully ligating perforating vessels. This approach permits generous exposure and mobilization of the femur, but it also involves extensive stripping of soft tissue and does not allow the ad-

dition of a trochanteric osteotomy or a trochanteric slide.

The Omega approach described by Learmonth is similar to the vastus slide distally. In both procedures, the vastus lateralis is divided along its posterior border, and the muscle is reflected forward in continuity with the gluteus medius and minimus muscles. The difference between the Omega and vastus slide occurs proximally. In the Omega approach, the dissection passes behind the gluteus medius tendon, and the combined gluteus medius and minimus muscle mass is elevated forward with the superior gluteal nerve sandwiched between them (**Figure 7**).

Transtrochanteric Approaches

The classic trochanteric osteotomy provides excellent exposure of the ac-

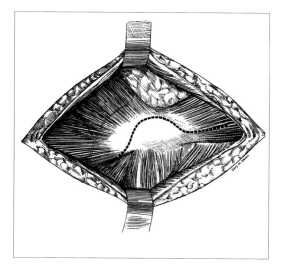

Figure 7 The Omega approach is similar to the vastus slide, except proximally, where the dissection is carried posterior to the gluteus medius tendon. The superior gluteal nerve is shown lying between the gluteus medius and gluteus minimus muscles and is protected as the muscles are mobilized anteriorly. (Reproduced with permission from Learmonth ID, Allen PE: The Omega lateral approach to the hip. *J Bone Joint Surg Br* 1996; 78:559-561.)

Table 5 Transtrochanteric Approaches: Strengths, Weakness, and Indications

Strengths	Weaknesses	Indications in Adult Reconstruction
Wide exposure of the acetabulum and femur Trochanteric advancement permitted	Risk of trochanteric nonunion and escape (can be reduced using trochanteric slide technique)	Complex primary THA Revision THA Femoral shortening (approach allows tensioning of the abductors)

etabulum and femur for complex reconstruction of the adult hip and also permits advancement and lateralization of the trochanter during reattachment (**Table 5**). This may improve soft-tissue tension around the hip and improve the function of the abductors through lengthening of the lever arm. The popularity of this approach for less complex reconstructions, for which other approaches provide very satisfactory exposure, has been limited by concerns over reattachment of the trochanteric fragment. This may also be a problem for revision surgeries, particularly if trochanteric bone loss erodes the bed for reattachment, thus predisposing to nonunion. The risks can be reduced by careful patient selection, thorough preoperative planning, and attention to detail during reattachment of the trochanter.

Two basic techniques of trochanteric osteotomy have been described, the intracapsular approach popularized by Charnley and the extracapsular technique advocated by Harris. Each may be performed with the patient in either supine or lateral position with the incision centered over the greater trochanter and curved posteriorly in the proximal limb.

Intrascapular Approach
With the intracapsular approach the fascia lata is divided in line with the skin incision, and then the anterior surface of the hip joint is located by release of the most distal insertion of the gluteus medius, which is then retracted superiorly and laterally. The proximal 2 to 3 cm of the vastus lateralis is elevated from the vastus ridge, and fatty tissue on the anterior surface of the capsule is cleared medially as far as the acetabular rim. The hip joint is then incised along the femoral neck, and an angled clamp is passed through

the incision and over the superior aspect of the femoral neck. This clamp is then pushed through the posterior superior aspect of the capsule and used to pass a Gigli saw to create the osteotomy, exiting at the level of the vastus ridge. Once the osteotomy is completed, the posterior capsule is carefully incised to allow retraction of the trochanter proximally. The piriformis muscle is often still attached to the trochanter and may be divided to facilitate retraction of this fragment.

The intracapsular technique thus leaves both abductors and the superior capsule attached to the trochanteric fragment. The attachment of the capsule may act as a static restraint and may limit excursion of the trochanter and the amount of limb lengthening that can be performed. It also potentially increases the rate of trochanteric nonunion. The extracapsular approach was developed in response to these limitations.

Extrascapular Approach
The extrascapular approach uses the plane between the gluteus minimus and the hip joint capsule. The key to the approach is locating the anterior edge of the gluteus minimus tendon. This is accomplished by passing the surgeon's index finger under the anterior border of the gluteus medius and directing the finger superiorly until the tendon edge is felt. A blunt retractor is passed between the gluteus minimus tendon and the capsule, and the posterior margin of the muscle is identified adjacent to the short external rotators. The sciatic nerve is palpated and protected throughout the procedure. Osteotomy is performed using an osteotome or an oscillating saw, beginning on the vastus ridge, which is exposed by elevating the vastus lateralis from its origin. The instrument is directed toward the blunt retractor lying between the minimus and the capsule, and the trochanteric fragment is reflected superiorly to expose the under-

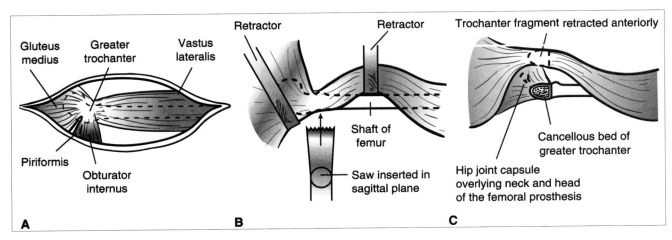

Figure 8 The trochanteric slide approach. **A,** The fascia lata is divided to expose the greater trochanter, with the gluteus medius proximally and the vastus lateralis distally. **B,** The vastus lateralis is reflected forward, distal to the vastus ridge, and proximally a retractor is placed underneath the glutei. This isolates the greater trochanter with its attached muscles. The osteotomy is then made in the sagittal plane from back to front, using an oscillating saw. Depending on the preoperative templating, the trochanteric fragment should be about 1 cm thick. **C,** The trochanteric fragment is retracted anteriorly, and the limb is externally rotated to expose the anterior surface of the hip joint capsule.

lying capsule, which is then incised or excised to gain access to the joint.

Trochanteric Slide

A major drawback to the trochanteric osteotomy is trochanteric nonunion, which may be a source of pain and may severely compromise abductor function. The trochanteric slide, an alternative approach originally described by Mercati and popularized by Glassman, reduces the risk of trochanteric nonunion and escape. The principle of this approach is to leave both the abductors and the vastus lateralis attached to the trochanteric fragment, which is then made to resemble a sesamoid bone within the vastus-gluteal muscle sling. The vastus lateralis and gluteal muscles pull in opposite directions, helping to prevent any superior migration of the trochanteric fragment, while their resultant force produces compression at the osteotomy site, thus theoretically promoting union. However, nonunions with trochanteric escapes have occurred with this approach.

The patient is placed in the lateral position, and a skin incision is made similar to that for a posterior approach to the hip. After division of the fascia lata, the posterior edge of the greater trochanter is defined along with the posterior edge of the gluteus medius proximally (**Figure 8**, *A*). The gluteus medius tendon is retracted anteriorly to expose the gluteus minimus tendon, and the interval between this tendon and the piriformis is located by blunt dissection. A periosteal elevator is passed anteriorly beneath the gluteus minimus muscle and then replaced by a cobra retractor. With the retractor in place, the insertion of the glutei into the superior aspect of the trochanter can be seen clearly (**Figure 8**, *B*). The posterior superior edge of the vastus lateralis is elevated distally from the intermuscular septum and reflected anteriorly. Attachment of the vastus lateralis to the vastus ridge remains intact.

Electrocautery is used to draw a line along the posterior aspect of the trochanter, starting just behind the insertion of the gluteal tendons and ending just behind the origin of the vastus lateralis from the gluteal ridge. An oscillating saw is used to create an osteotomy along this line, passing anteriorly, to elevate a fragment approximately 1 cm thick (depending on preoperative templating). This bony fragment is then retracted anteriorly while the limb is placed in external rotation to expose the anterior hip capsule (**Figure 8**, *C*).

Wide exposure of the anterior capsule is achieved by dividing the small amount of vastus lateralis that arises from the capsular surface. The capsule is then incised to gain access to the hip, which is dislocated anteriorly. This approach can also be performed after a posterolateral approach has been used if it is believed that dislocation is impossible without elevating the greater trochanter. The posterior soft tissue should then be repaired in a manner similar to that used with the posterolateral approach to the hip.

At the end of the procedure, the trochanter is easily replaced and usually is remarkably stable even before fixation is performed. Fixation of the trochanter can be performed using circumferential wires placed through the calcar or lesser trochanter or tucked distal to the lesser trochanter. This wiring technique may not be sufficient when trochanteric advancement is required so a trochanteric clamp device with cables may be needed.

Posterolateral Approaches

The deep dissection of the posterior approaches passes behind the greater trochanter. Several methods of exposure using this route have been described. The posterolateral, or Kocher-Langenbeck, approach is commonly used and provides easy, safe, and extensile exposure of the acetabulum, posterior pelvic column, and femur (**Table 6**). Traditionally, the posterolateral approach has been associated with a higher rate of postoperative dislocation, although this may be reduced through careful positioning of the components and meticulous repair of the posterior tissues. Because of the ease, safety, and extensile nature of this approach, we believe it is the single most useful approach for revision THA.

Descriptions of the approach vary. Most place the patient in the lateral position with the hip in extension and use a curved incision centered on the greater trochanter. The distal leg of the incision passes along the midline of the femur, while the proximal route is angled posteriorly at approximately a 30° angle to the long axis of the femur. The facia lata is divided in line with the skin incision to expose the trochanteric bursa, which is reflected posteriorly. The sciatic nerve is palpated and protected. By sweeping the bursa posteriorly, the short external rotators will become apparent, and lying superior to them is the posterior edge of gluteus medius. A retractor is passed around the edge of this muscle, and the muscle is retracted anteriorly to expose the underlying minimus tendon.

In a manner similar to that described for the trochanteric slide, a curved retractor is passed forward beneath the minimus tendon, thus isolating the short external rotators. The patient's limb is placed in internal rotation, and the piriformis, obturator internus, gemelli, and hip joint capsule are elevated from the bone as close to their insertion as possible.

Table 6 Posterior Approaches: Strengths, Weakness, and Indications

Strengths	Weaknesses	Indications in Adult Reconstruction
Wide exposure of the acetabulum, posterior pelvic column, and femur	Dislocation rate may be higher	Primary and complex primary THA, posterior pelvic column and femur
Abductors not violated		Revision THA
Mobilization of the abductors permitted when the limb is lengthened		Acetabular fractures and dislocations
Inadequate exposure may be combined with an ETO or an anterior approach		Septic arthritis

Maximum length on these structures may be achieved by maximally flexing the hip. After their origin is released, the hip is gradually extended to allow mobilization of these structures. The tendons are tagged with sutures for later repair and reflected posteriorly to protect the sciatic nerve. A T-shaped capsulotomy is performed, with the horizontal limb placed along the posterior edge of the greater trochanter and the vertical limb placed superiorly in line with the original direction of the piriformis tendon.

The quadratus femoris muscle is elevated at the point of insertion into the proximal femur and the branch of the medial femoral circumflex artery that runs deep to it is ligated. The hip may be dislocated by internal rotation and flexion of the adducted hip. Acetabular exposure is facilitated by anterior retraction of the proximal femur. If a monoblock stem remains in situ, an anterior pocket may be created by elevating the reflected head of rectus femoris muscle and adjacent soft tissue from the anterior aspect of the acetabulum. This allows safe anterior displacement and retraction of the femur. The anterior capsule may have to be released to achieve this retraction.

The importance of soft-tissue repair at the end of the procedure has become apparent in the last decade and has led to a reduction in dislocation rates after this approach. Occasionally, the limb is lengthened or the offset is increased to such a degree that closure of the capsule is not possible, but it should always be attempted. It is usually possible to repair the piriformis and obturator internus tendons, which provide a further restraint and help to prevent posterior dislocation.

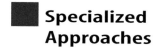

Specialized Approaches

Femoral Osteotomies

The ETO provides a useful route of access to the femoral canal. This approach extends the standard trochanteric osteotomy distally along the femoral diaphysis for a variable distance, depending on the indication for its use, and provides direct access to the endosteal surface of the femur. It can therefore greatly facilitate removal of an ingrown uncemented stem, a column of well-fixed cement, or a broken prosthesis. It may also be useful when there is varus remodeling of the femur around a loose prosthesis because revision using a straight stem may cause uncontrolled injury to the greater trochanter or a fracture of the femur.

Preoperative templating is vital in planning the ETO because its length is measured on the radiograph from the tip of the greater trochanter. Osteotomy length should be sufficient to provide access to the required extent of the component porous coating or to allow easy cement removal while retaining the length of intact femur required for subsequent reconstruction.

The approach is performed with the patient in the lateral position. Initially, a standard posterior approach is performed with dislocation of the hip joint posteriorly (**Figure 9**, *A*). The ETO is much easier to perform with the stem removed. Loose stems should be extracted first. The posterior approach extends distally along the posterior fascia overlying the vastus lateralis, which is then reflected anteriorly from the intermuscular septum, ligating perforating vessels as this is done. Reflection of a maximum of 1 cm of the vastus lateralis exposes the femoral. The osteotomy length planned during templating is then measured and marked (**Figure 9**, *B*). The limb is internally rotated approximately 45°, and the osteotomy is marked along the posterior surface of the femur. The ETO fragment should encompass approximately one third of the femoral circumference in the diaphysis and the entire greater trochanter proximally.

An oscillating saw is used to begin the cut in the sagittal plane, starting proximally and passing through both cortices of the femur. Caution is necessary when making the cut distal to the greater trochanter because this area of the osteotomy tends to be cut thin and can result in fracture. If the stem is well fixed in situ, the saw blade must be skived over the lateral surface of the stem to reach the anterior femoral cortex. If the shoulder of the existing prosthesis does not permit this technique, the anterior cortex can be divided by introducing an osteotomy through the muscle anteriorly. It is preferable to create a rounded tip at the distal end of the ETO to avoid any stress risers. This can be done several ways, such as using a burr or multiple drill holes. Once the distal end is completed, the trochanteric fragment is freed and is lifted and reflected anteri-orly, carefully preserving its soft-tissue attachments (**Figure 9**, *C* and *D*). The remaining proximal femur is freed from medial capsular attachments to allow mobilization of the femur posteriorly. This provides circumferential access to the acetabulum and direct access to the femoral canal for reconstruction. Femoral exposure provides direct access to the cement-bone interface and greatly facilitates cement and plug removal. Removing an ingrown uncemented stem may be done by passing a Gigli saw around the proximal end of the prosthesis and using it to divide the interface between the stem and the intact two thirds of the femoral circumference. If access to the interface cannot be achieved using a Gigli saw, then the femoral prosthesis may be sectioned below the metaphyseal flare and trephines used to remove the stem's distal portion.

To close the ETO, the limb is once again internally rotated and the trochanteric fragment brought back to its original position. It is often necessary to burr the inside of the trochanteric fragment, especially proximally, so that the newly implanted femoral stem does not prevent approximation of the osteotomy edges. The trochanteric fragment is held in place using circumferential wires or cables (**Figure 9**, *E* and *F*) passed from back to front to minimize the risk of injury to the sciatic nerve. A wire is placed just distal to the osteotomy site to prevent fracture during implantation of the prosthesis. If no fracture occurs, the wire may be removed.

In cases of varus remodeling of the proximal femur, it may be necessary to complete the osteotomy at the distal end of the ETO to allow straightening of the femur.

CONTROLLED PERFORATION TECHNIQUE

The metaphyseal region of the femur is usually easily visualized from above, and procedures such as proximal cement removal can be performed safely from the proximal femur. However, proximal removal of distal cement and cement plugs can be hazardous, particularly when revising a long-stemmed prosthesis or if there is a long column of cement extending beyond the anterior bow of the femur. Controlled perforations of the femur and limited osteotomies have been reported as alternatives to an ETO for stem and cement removal. These osteotomies may be used to control the position of instruments introduced into the femoral canal from above, permit additional light into the canal, remove debris from the canal, and introduce instruments from outside the femoral diaphysis, such as a punch inserted distal to a femoral stem. Perforations can be made at any point around the femoral circumference, but the lateral and anterior surfaces are the most accessible after reflection of the vastus lateralis. Circular perforations 7 to 9 mm in diameter are preferred to rectangular perforations because they reduce the risk of stress risers. It is advisable to leave at least two femoral diameters between adjacent holes to further reduce the risk of subsequent fracture.

SCAPHOID WINDOW

One drawback to use of controlled perforations is that access is often inadequate for the requirements of the procedure. More generous exposure is afforded by a femoral window, such as the scaphoid window osteotomy. These osteotomies provide wider access to the femoral canal and do not require mandatory detachment of the greater trochanter, an inherent feature of the ETO. It is important during preoperative planning to identify the window's level and length and to determine a bypass method to minimize the risk of periprosthetic fracture. The planned femoral component ideally should bypass the distal end of the window by at least two femoral diameters, but if this is not possible, then a strut allograft may be used to reinforce

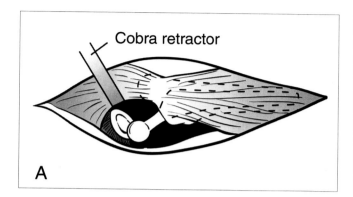

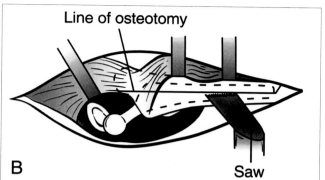

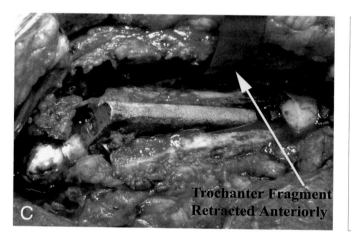

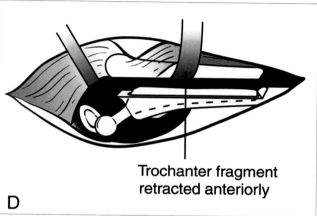

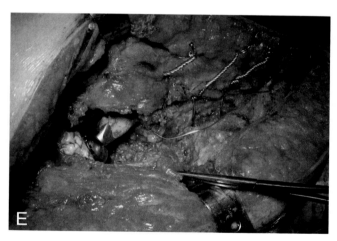

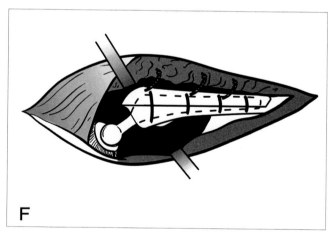

Figure 9   The ETO. **A,** A posterior approach is made to the hip, and the hip joint is dislocated posteriorly. A cemented stem may be removed prior to the osteotomy, but with a well-fixed uncemented stem the ETO can be performed with the stem in situ. **B,** The ETO includes the entire greater trochanter and the lateral third of the femoral shaft. The distal end is rounded to avoid creating a stress riser at that point. **C,** In this photograph, the ETO has been completed, and the trochanteric fragment has been retracted anteriorly (arrow) to expose the ingrowth surface of the uncemented stem. **D,** Illustration of the technique shown in C. **E,** This intraoperative photograph shows that following reconstruction of the hip, the trochanteric fragment is reduced and secured using cerclage wires or cables. **F,** Illustration of the technique shown in E.

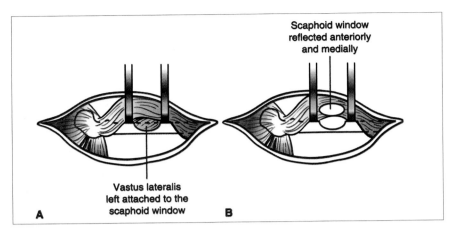

Figure 10 The scaphoid window. **A,** The femoral shaft is exposed above and below the proposed site for the scaphoid window, preserving the soft-tissue attachments of the osteotomy site. **B,** The osteotomy is made with a burr, osteotomes, or a saw, rounding the ends to avoid causing a stress riser. The window fragment is then reflected anteriorly and medially to expose the femoral canal.

the femur as long as there is no evidence of infection.

A standard approach to the hip joint may be used and extended distally along the femur to just beyond the expected level of the osteotomy. It is essential that the soft-tissue attachments of the osteotomy fragment be preserved so a limited exposure of the femoral cortex is performed above and below the level of the window, reflecting the vastus lateralis anteriorly and carefully ligating perforating vessels (**Figure 10**, A). Retractors are placed over the anterior femoral cortex at the proximal and distal ends of the window, and an oscillating saw is used to create the window's midsection, with the saw passing through both the lateral and medial cortices. The ends of the osteotomy should be rounded using a burr, osteotomes, or a saw. This completes the window, which is then elevated and reflected medially, carefully preserving its soft-tissue attachments (**Figure 10**, B). The window is replaced and secured using one or more cerclage wires at the end of the operation.

Extensive Acetabular Approaches

Although most acetabular reconstructions can be performed using one of the standard approaches, it is occa-

sionally necessary to obtain very wide exposure of the acetabulum and the pelvic columns. This need may arise with treatment of certain tumors, massive allografting of the acetabulum, or the treatment of pelvic discontinuity.

The ilioinguinal approach allows wide exposure of the anterior column of the pelvis and the medial wall of the pelvis and acetabulum as far proximally as the sacroiliac joint. Using this approach with release of the abductors from the pelvis may also provide access to the outer aspect of the ilium but at the risk of devitalizing bone fragments and causing heterotopic ossification. The ilioinguinal approach may also be combined with the posterior approach to provide access to both pelvic columns.

The extended iliofemoral approach can be used to visualize both the anterior and posterior columns of the pelvis and the outer surface of the ilium through complete release of the abductors from the wing of the ilium. The addition of a trochanteric osteotomy distally leads to near-circumferential exposure of the acetabulum but at the risk of serious postoperative abductor muscle dysfunction. Exposure of the inner aspect of the ilium can be achieved through elevation of

the iliopsoas, but this extension is usually best avoided because of the risk of devascularizing bone fragments. The triradiate approach provides an alternative to the extended iliofemoral and combined approaches when extensive exposure of both acetabular columns is required.

The triradiate approach provides an alternative to the extended iliofemoral and combined approaches when extensive exposure of both columns is required. This approach combines the posterolateral approach with the anterior dissection of the Smith-Petersen approach through use of a Y-shaped skin incision. Wide exposure is achieved either through trochanteric osteotomy or through detachment of the abductors from the greater trochanter. Full descriptions of these approaches can be found in the literature on acetabular fracture management.

The Retroperitoneal Approach

The retroperitoneal approach provides access to the pelvis. In adult hip reconstruction, it is most often used for the removal of cement and prostheses that have migrated medially and in patients with a risk of injury to pelvic viscera and neurovascular structures. Injuries to vascular structures, particularly the external iliac and femoral vessels, may be life threatening or pose risks to limb survival. Potential vascular injuries include blunt, sharp, thermal, and traction injuries. Blunt injuries may arise because of the careless placement of retractors, particularly with atherosclerotic vessels, which may become less pliable and predisposed to crush injury and occlusion. Sharp injuries may occur when making keyholes for cement or during placement of acetabular screws in uncemented reconstructions. Cement allowed to extrude medially may cause thermal injury to the vessels as it cures, and it is therefore essential that perforations of the medial wall be repaired before pressurizing cement in the acetabulum. With revision surgery, the vessels, particularly the external iliac vein, are most at risk during component removal, especially if there is medial migration of the existing components.

Several clinical and radiologic factors have been identified to warn of the possible risk of intrapelvic injuries during a revision procedure. Clinical indicators include a complaint of pelvic pain or mass, or the discovery of a pelvic mass, tenderness, or a bruit on examination. Indicators present on plain radiographs include marked medial migration of the components and previous medial extrusion of cement. The presence of any of these indicators requires further preoperative investigation, perhaps including vascular surgical consultation and angiography. Visceral structures can be studied through CT or MRI, and angiography allows investigation of often distorted vascular anatomy.

When preoperative investigations suggest that pelvic structures are at risk, the retroperitoneal approach should be considered for removal of an acetabular component. It is advisable that this part of the procedure be a joint effort between vascular and orthopaedic surgeons, with the vascular surgeon performing the abdominal part of the procedure.

———————————■

■ Conclusion

Surgical exposure is the keystone of complex reconstruction of the adult hip. Without proper exposure, bony anatomy and defects cannot be defined, existing implants cannot be safely removed, and reconstructive options are limited. No single surgical approach is suitable for all situations. Surgeons should be comfortable with several approaches so that the appropriate choice can be made for each patient. The surgeon must consider sometimes conflicting factors to determine the best approach. Although many of these deliberations will occur prior to the decision for surgery and during preoperative planning, the surgeon must consider intraoperative findings and be willing to modify the selected approach if necessary. Specialized techniques exist to enable the surgeon to modify the standard approaches and respond to the requirements of this demanding surgery.

———————————■

■ References

Blackley HR, Rorabeck CH: Extensile exposures for revision hip arthroplasty. *Clin Orthop* 2000;381:77-87.

Chen WM, McAuley JP, Engh CA Jr, Hopper RH Jr, Engh CA: Extended slide trochanteric osteotomy for revision total hip arthroplasty. *J Bone Joint Surg Am* 2000;82:1215-1219.

Glassman AH, Engh CA, Bobyn JD: A technique of extensile exposure for total hip arthroplasty. *J Arthroplasty* 1987;2:11-21.

Head WC, Mallory TH, Berklacich FM, et al: Extensile exposure of the hip for revision arthroplasty. *J Arthroplasty* 1988;2:265-273.

Kerry RM, Masri BA, Garbuz DS, Duncan CP: The vascularized scaphoid window for access to the femoral canal in revision total hip arthroplasty. *Instr Course Lect* 1999;48:9-11.

Learmonth ID, Allen PE: The Omega lateral approach to the hip. *J Bone Joint Surg Br* 1996;78:559-561.

Masterson EL, Masri BA, Duncan CP: Surgical approaches in revision hip replacement. *J Am Acad Orthop Surg* 1998;6:84-92.

Miner TM, Momberger NG, Chong D, Paprosky WL: The extended trochanteric osteotomy in revision hip arthroplasty. *J Arthroplasty* 2001;16:188-194.

Rorabeck CH, Partington PF: Retroperitoneal exposure in revision total hip arthroplasty. *Instr Course Lect* 1999;48:27-36.

Coding

CPT Codes		Corresponding ICD-9 Codes		
26990	Incision and drainage, pelvis or hip joint area; deep abscess or hematoma	682.5 711.45 730.05 998.1	682.6 711.95 924.01 998.5	711.15 726.5 958.3
26992	Incision, bone cortex, pelvis and/or hip joint (eg, osteomyelitis or bone abscess)	711.15 730.05 996.67	711.45 730.15 996.78	711.95 958.3 998.5
27030	Arthrotomy, hip, with drainage (eg, infection)	711.05 998.5	730.25	958.3
27033	Arthrotomy, hip, including exploration or removal of loose or foreign body	716.15 890.0	729.6 890.1	732.7
27036	Capsulectomy or capsulotomy, hip, with or without excision of heterotopic bone, with release of hip flexor muscles (ie, gluteus medius, gluteus minimus, tensor fascia latae, rectus femoris, sartorius, iliopsoas)	343.0 343.3 728.13	343.1 343.9 781.2	343.2 718.45 905.1
27052	Arthrotomy, with biopsy; hip joint	682.5		
27054	Arthrotomy with synovectomy, hip joint	714.0	719.25	
27087	Removal of foreign body, pelvis or hip; deep (subfascial or intramuscular)	729.6 996.67	890.0 996.78	890.1 998.4
27090	Removal of hip prosthesis; (separate procedure)	996.4	996.66	996.77
27091	Removal of hip prosthesis, complicated, including total hip prosthesis, methylmethacrylate with or without insertion of spacer	996.4	996.66	996.77
27125	Hemiarthroplasty, hip, partial (eg, femoral stem prosthesis, bipolar arthroplasty)	715.15 716.15 733.42	715.25 718.6 905.6	715.35 733.14
27130	Arthroplasty, acetabular and proximal femoral prosthetic replacement (total hip arthroplasty), with or without autograft or allograft	711.45 714.30 715.35 718.6 733.42	711.95 715.15 716.15 720.0 808.0	714.0 715.25 718.5 733.14 905.6
27132	Conversion of previous hip surgery to total hip arthroplasty, with or without autograft or allograft	715.15 718.2 733.14 996.4	715.25 718.5 733.42 996.66	715.35 718.6 905.6 996.77
27134	Revision of total hip arthroplasty; both components, with or without autograft or allograft	996.4	996.66	996.77
27137	Revision of total hip arthroplasty, acetabular component only, with or without autograft or allograft	996.4	996.66	996.77
27138	Revision of total hip arthroplasty, femoral component only, with or without allograft	996.4	996.66	996.77
27236	Open treatment of femoral fracture, proximal end, neck, internal fixation or prosthetic replacement	733.14 820.03 820.13	820.00 820.10 820.8	820.02 820.12 820.9

CPT copyright © 2004 by the American Medical Association. All Rights Reserved.

Chapter 39

Revision Total Hip Arthroplasty: Component Removal

Michael J. Archibeck, MD
Richard E. White Jr, MD

 ## Indications

The indications for removal of an acetabular component include loosening, chronic infection, worn polyethylene in a nonmodular component, instability resulting from a malpositioned component, and occasionally periacetabular osteolysis with a poor or damaged locking mechanism. Revising a cemented or nonmodular acetabular component at the time of femoral revision is controversial. Generally, retaining the component is warranted if the cement-bone and cement-prosthetic interfaces are well preserved, the polyethylene is not significantly worn, and the component is well positioned.

Femoral component revision is indicated in patients with loosening, chronic infection, a malpositioned (excessive anteversion or retroversion) component with instability, or a damaged femoral head on a nonmodular femoral component. It may also be necessary when adequate stability is not obtained at the time of acetabular revision. This can occur because of (1) inadequate neck length options, (2) inadequate femoral offset in the presence of osteolysis, which compromises fixation of the femoral component, or (3) in the case of distal osteolysis at risk for insufficiency fracture. The need to revise an early generation cemented or uncemented femoral component at the time of acetabular revision is controversial. Generally, retaining the component is warranted if the interfaces appear stable or ingrown and none of the above-mentioned indications is present.

 ## Contraindications

Absent the above-mentioned indications, removal of acetabular or femoral components should be avoided. The decision to retain one component during revision of the other can be a difficult one. Evidence supports the decision to retain femoral or acetabular components as long as the component is well fixed and appropriately positioned.

 ## Alternative Treatments

Failure of the polyethylene of a modular component does not always necessitate a complete acetabular revision. Such failure commonly occurs with polyethylene wear and retroacetabular osteolysis with a well-fixed uncemented acetabular shell. In these patients, removing the shell may leave a large defect that is not amenable to simple revision techniques. Polyethylene exchange with or without grafting of the osteolytic lesions may be a better option.

Most modern uncemented acetabular components are modular and allow for polyethylene exchange at the time of revision. This exchange requires identifying the design and obtaining appropriate polyethylene modular trial components and inserts. Polyethylene exchange may not be an option, however, in designs with poor or damaged locking mechanisms. Cementing a new polyethylene liner into a well-fixed metallic shell is mechanically sound and, done correctly, may exceed the strength of most modular capture mechanisms. Long-term durability of this construct is presently unknown.

This technique generally includes undersizing the liner to allow a 2- to 4-mm cement mantle between the shell and liner. Some controversy exists as to the need to score or texture the polyethylene and/or metallic shell. It is recommended that the inner surface of the metal shell be scored with a high-speed burr in components without holes. The polyethylene can be a pretextured, cemented design, or the back side can be scored with shallow troughs using a high-speed burr.

One alternative to femoral component removal is an isolated femoral

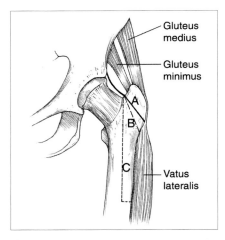

Figure 1 Trochanteric osteotomies can be a valuable tool in the atraumatic removal of femoral components or provide enhanced acetabular exposure in patients undergoing complex acetabular reconstruction. The standard trochanteric osteotomy (A), the trochanteric slide (B), and (most commonly) the ETO (C) can be used. (Reproduced from Archibeck MJ, Rosenberg AG, Berger RA, Silverton CD: Trochanteric osteotomy and fixation during total hip arthroplasty. *J Am Acad Orthop Surg* 2003;11:163-173.)

head exchange, which allows adjustments of femoral head length (adding to limb length and offset) and head size. This may provide acceptable stability for isolated acetabular revisions or revisions for instability with well-positioned components. Proximal femoral osteolysis that does not compromise component fixation can be treated without revision of the entire femoral component by addressing the articular surfaces (polyethylene and femoral head exchange) and grafting of the lesions.

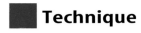

■ Technique

Exposure
Standard exposure techniques are used for component removal and are often dictated by the anticipated revision needs, ranging from polyethylene exchange to two-component revision with allograft reconstruction. Gener-

ally this includes either a modified direct lateral approach or, more commonly, a more extensile posterolateral approach. Additional exposure techniques may be required in difficult circumstances, such as acetabular protrusio in which dislocation is difficult, significant stiffness, or patients requiring extensile acetabular exposure (ie, allograft reconstruction and cage implantation). Use of trochanteric osteotomies such as a standard trochanteric osteotomy, a trochanteric slide, or an extended trochanteric osteotomy may be required (**Figure 1**).

The trochanteric slide can help provide access to the proximal femoral interfaces and additional acetabular exposure. This technique is preferred when a cemented revision femoral component is anticipated (cemented stem or impaction grafting). The extended trochanteric osteotomy (ETO) is an excellent technique for removal of well-fixed cemented or uncemented femoral components. However, this technique necessitates use of an uncemented revision stem with distal fixation.

Bone Preparation
At the time of revision, at least three sets of intraoperative cultures should be obtained before antibiotics are administered. Frozen sections and/or synovial fluid should also be evaluated by the pathologist. Femoral component removal is generally performed first because it enhances acetabular exposure for polyethylene exchange or acetabular component revision.

The ETO has become a valuable technique in revision total hip arthroplasty. It greatly facilitates the removal of well-fixed cemented or uncemented femoral components that are not easily removed through proximal exposure alone. This osteotomy also allows direct, in-line reaming of the diaphysis in varus remodeling of the proximal femur.

Preoperatively, this osteotomy is planned to be the longest length suffi-

cient to provide adequate component exposure and maintain at least 4 cm of isthmic diaphyseal cortex for revision component fixation. It should be at least 10 cm long, measured from the tip of the greater trochanter, and is generally performed through a posterolateral approach. The ETO can be completed before or after hip dislocation or after stem removal. It is easiest to perform after stem removal, because the anterior cut of the osteotomy can be made directly from the posterior exposure, but this is not always possible. The osteotomy extends down the posterior aspect of the femur along the linea aspera after exposure by partial elevation of the vastus lateralis and release of the gluteus maximus. Once appropriate length is obtained, the transverse portion of the osteotomy is performed, incorporating approximately one third of the circumference of the diaphysis. The distal-anterior extent of the osteotomy is initiated using a saw or high-speed burr. The desired proximal-anterior exit site is initiated as well. If the anterior limb of the osteotomy cannot be made directly, the anterior cortex is scored with an osteotome, or drill holes can be created to direct the controlled fracture to the desired exit point. With a series of broad curved osteotomes inserted posteriorly, the osteotomy is booked open on its anterior muscular hinge. After implantation of the revision femoral component, the trochanteric fragment can be contoured with a burr to accommodate the new stem. The fragment should be reapproximated to its posterior limb and secured with two to four cables or wires.

Prosthesis Removal
REMOVAL OF A CEMENTED FEMORAL STEM
Removal of a cemented femoral component generally begins with stem removal from within the cement mantle. This can be easily done with a loose stem or a stem with a smooth surface. Well-fixed textured stems or pre-

coated stems can be difficult to extract and may require special techniques such as an ETO. Sometimes the stem is easily removed but the cement mantle remains well-fixed. Although successfully cementing into a well-fixed mantle is possible, cement removal is generally preferable. An ETO is advisable for an inextractable stem or a well-fixed cement mantle because it allows direct access to the cement-bone interface for controlled removal without inadvertent canal penetration. Although hand tools (with or without a cortical window) can permit removal of cement, an ETO provides better visualization and direct access to all cement but the most distal, making fracture, retained cement, or cortical perforation less likely.

Once the ETO is complete, cement can be removed with hand tools until the stem is extractable. Remaining proximal cement can then be removed in piecemeal fashion with osteotomes or tools from the Moreland cemented revision trays (DePuy, Warsaw, IN). The distal cement and cement restrictor are generally removed using a drill and tap technique (**Figure 2**). The drill is centered in the distal plug and advanced in approximately 1 cm increments. A tap can be advanced into the predrilled hole in the cement (Segces, Zimmer, Warsaw, IN; Moreland) and back hammered to segmentally extract the plug. Reverse curettes can confirm complete cement removal. If retained distal cement is still a possibility, an intraoperative radiograph should be obtained prior to reaming. Ultrasonic tools can also be used for many of these tasks.

REMOVAL OF AN UNCEMENTED FEMORAL STEM

Removal of a loose uncemented stem can be relatively straightforward. Before extracting the loose component, any overhanging bone of the medial greater trochanter should be removed using a burr or hand tools to avoid trochanteric fracture during extrac-

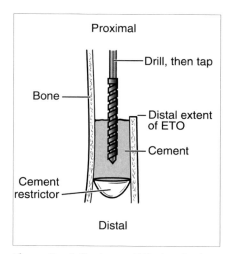

Figure 2 Following an ETO, the distal cement plug and cement restrictor are sequentially drilled and tapped, removing the cement in segments.

tion. Despite radiographic indications of loosening, stems with fibrous ingrowth occasionally can be difficult to remove. Instead of using excessive force, the surgeon should use the techniques described below.

The technique used to remove a well-fixed uncemented femoral component depends on the extent of the component's ingrowth surface. With a proximally coated femoral component, attempts can be made to disrupt the bone-prosthetic interface using thin flexible osteotomes inserted proximally and advanced distally. Stems with collars may require a high-speed, metal-cutting burr to remove the collar and thus provide access to the medial interface. Excessive force should be avoided when advancing the osteotomes distally because fracture can result if the osteotome is wedged between the stem and dense cortical bone. Once the interface is disrupted, standard extraction devices, such as a slap hammer attached to the proximal stem, can be used for stem extraction. Inability to adequately disrupt the interface may require additional exposure, such as that provided by a trochanteric slide or, more commonly, an ETO.

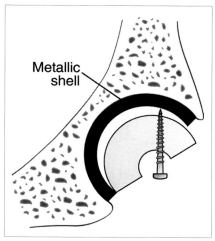

Figure 3 A helpful technique in removal of a modular polyethylene liner from its metal shell is to drill the polyethylene eccentrically and advance a screw into the polyethylene. When the screw engages the metal shell, it will pry out the liner.

Alternative techniques are required to remove extensively porous-coated uncemented stems. Paprosky and associates have described a technique that minimizes the chance of significant bone loss or fracture by incorporating the ETO. The ETO should extend distally to the cylindrical portion of the component. Once completed, flexible osteotomes or a Gigli saw are used to disrupt the bone-prosthetic interface proximal to the level of the osteotomy, and the stem is transected at or near the distal extent of the osteotomy with a high-speed, metal-cutting burr. The remaining cylindrical distal stem is then removed using a trephine of appropriate size. It is important to use the smallest trephine that fits over the stem. Using a trephine that is too large can leave a bridge of bone distally, making extraction difficult.

Isolated Polyethylene Exchange

The locking mechanism determines how easily a modular polyethylene liner is removed at the time of revision. The surgeon should be familiar with the locking mechanism's design

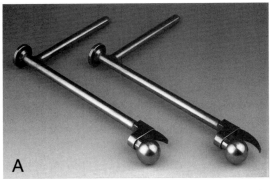

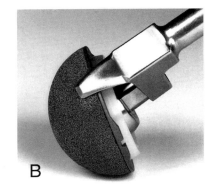

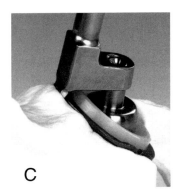

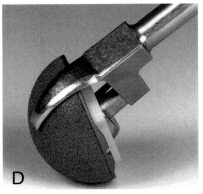

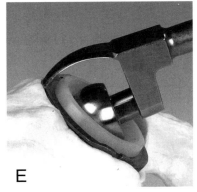

Figure 4 **A**, The Explant system consists of a short stout blade and a longer full-radiused blade for each diameter of shell. The short blade disrupts the exposed bone prosthetic interface by rotating the device (**B** and **C**), and then the longer blade disrupts the remainder of the interface (**D** and **E**). (Courtesy of Zimmer, Warsaw, IN.)

and the equipment needed for polyethylene removal. If the locking mechanism does not require disengagement of a locking ring or other special instruments, it can generally be removed by drilling into the polyethylene and inserting a screw (6.5 × 40 mm). Doing so will pry the polyethylene out as it advances and impinges on the underlying shell (**Figure 3**). With removal of the polyethylene, the locking mechanism (locking ring or wire) can be damaged, and replacement rings or wire should be available.

Removal of Cemented Acetabular Components

Removal of a well-fixed acetabular component, whether cemented or uncemented, first requires adequate circumferential exposure of the cement-bone or bone-prosthetic interface. This may require exposure techniques such as trochanteric osteotomies.

Removal of a well-fixed cemented acetabular component requires that the bone-cement interface be disrupted with minimal bone loss. The first step is to disrupt the prosthesis-cement interface, if possible, because this interface avoids inadvertent damage to adjacent bone. Disruption can be performed with curved osteotomes or gauges designed for this task (Moreland cemented revision set). The Explant system (Zimmer), which is described below in the section on uncemented acetabular component removal, can also be used with cemented components. Alternatively, the polyethylene can be reamed away with a standard acetabular reamer until only the cement mantle remains. A high-speed burr can also be used to section the polyethylene. Once the polyethylene is removed, hand tools (osteotomes and cement splitters) can be used to remove the cement in a piecemeal fashion. Ultrasonic tools have been used for these purposes as well.

Cement plugs are often present in the ilium, ischium, and pubis and must be identified and removed so they do not deflect the reamers when the bed is prepared for the uncemented revision component. Cement can occasionally "mushroom" through a small medial acetabular defect into the intrapelvic region. This cement does not need to be removed unless infection is present. A variation of the ilioinguinal approach can remove intrapelvic cement, and preoperative vascular and urologic imaging can identify structures at risk in these patients.

Removal of Uncemented Acetabular Components

Removal of a loose uncemented acetabular component is not difficult, but because failure of ingrowth into modern uncemented acetabular components is exceedingly rare, infection should be suspected. Polyethylene removal is the first step in revision of a well-fixed uncemented acetabular component. Once the polyethylene is removed, any screws present are also removed. Preoperative planning, such as anticipating the need for nonstandard screwdrivers, make this step simple and save valuable time in the operating room. Stripped screw heads can be removed using a metal-cutting burr. Broken screws that do not interfere with reaming can be left in situ. Broken screws that interfere with reaming can be removed using trephines in commonly available broken screw removal sets that extract the screw shank.

Removal of a well-fixed shell requires exposure of the bone-prosthetic interface circumferentially. A burr can be helpful in exposing this interface. Narrow curved osteotomes are available to disrupt the prosthesis-bone interface. Particular care should be exercised in preserving the posterior and superior bone because this bone is essential for fixation of the revision component. Sectioning a well-fixed shell and removing portions of the shell separately have been described elsewhere.

Although the techniques described above are useful, a new instrument set, the Explant (Zimmer), allows removal of a well-fixed shell with minimal bone loss (**Figure 4**). It contains a series of femoral heads (22, 26, and 32 mm) with a short robust starter blade and a thin full-radiused long blade at a fixed distance from the center of rotation. The head is inserted into the polyethylene or trial liner after screw removal. The blades, short followed by long, are then advanced circumferentially until the shell is loose. This tool set has greatly simplified the potentially difficult step of removing a well-fixed shell while minimizing bone loss (**Figures 5** and **6**).

Wound Closure

Once the revision components have been inserted, wound closure is dictated by the approach used.

Postoperative Regimen

Postoperative regimen is determined by the type of components and ap-

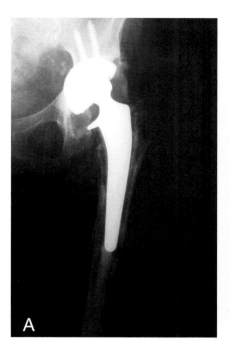 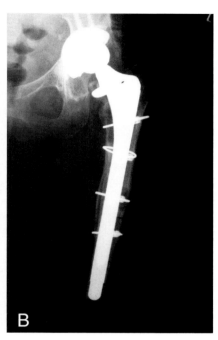

Figure 5 **A,** A loose cemented femoral component with some varus remodeling of the proximal femur and cement extruded well distal to the stem tip. **B,** An ETO facilitated distal cement removal and direct in-line diaphyseal reaming. An uncemented extensively coated revision femoral component was used to obtain distal scratch fit over at least 4 to 6 cm.

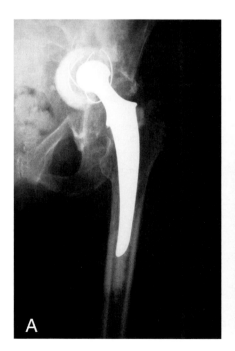 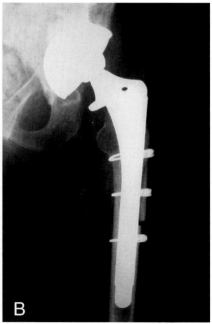

Figure 6 **A,** Patient with a loose acetabular component and a well-fixed distal cement column and nonmodular femoral component. **B,** At the time of acetabular revision, the retained femoral component did not allow adequate acetabular exposure. An ETO facilitated removal of cement and provided excellent acetabular exposure. The femur was again revised to an extensively coated component.

proach used. This generally includes limited weight bearing and no active abduction when a trochanteric osteotomy is performed.

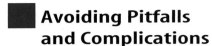 **Avoiding Pitfalls and Complications**

Adequate exposure, meticulous disruption of the fixation interfaces, and avoidance of excessive force minimize the risks of fracture, excessive bone loss, and retained cement.

References

Berger RA, Quigley LR, Jacobs JJ, et al: The fate of stable cemented acetabular components retained during revision of a femoral component of a total hip arthroplasty. *J Bone Joint Surg Am* 1999;81:1682-1691.

Haft GF, Heiner AD, Callaghan JJ, et al: Polyethylene liner cementation into fixed acetabular shells. *J Arthroplasty* 2002;17:167-170.

Paprosky WG, Weeden SH, Bowling JW Jr: Component removal in revision total hip arthroplasty. *Clin Orthop* 2001;393:181-193.

Paprosky WG, Martin EL: Removal of well-fixed femoral and acetabular components. *Am J Orthop* 2002;31:476-478.

Coding				
CPT Codes			**Corresponding ICD-9 Codes**	
27134	Revision of total hip arthroplasty; both components, with or without autograft or allograft		996.4	996.66
27137	Revision of total hip arthroplasty; acetabular component only, with or without autograft or allograft		996.4	996.66
27138	Revision of total hip arthroplasty; femoral component only, with or without allograft		996.4	996.66

CPT copyright © 2004 by the American Medical Association. All Rights Reserved.

Chapter 40

Acetabular Reconstruction: Overview and Strategy

William J. Hozack, MD

■ Introduction

Acetabular revision surgery is arguably the most complex procedure the adult hip reconstruction surgeon performs. Without a coordinated and organized overall strategy, significant problems can easily develop. This chapter provides an overview of a strategic approach to acetabular revision surgery and also describes specific aspects that can give the best chance of a good outcome.

From a surgical perspective, several factors are important to remember. First, more than one potential solution to the problem at hand should be ready; specifically, a "plan B" and "plan C" must be available if the original plan does not appear to be working well. Flexibility is also crucial; dogged persistence with the original plan is unwise if it becomes obvious that an alternative approach would produce a better result. Simplicity is important. Given the possibility of two different solutions to a specific problem, the alternative that is the easiest to execute should be selected.

The strategic plan to acetabular revision surgery can be conveniently divided into four basic areas: exposure, implant removal, assessing acetabular bone damage, and new implant selection.

■ Exposure

The surgical approach for acetabular revision is selected after review of a combination of factors, including surgeon training, experience, and preference. The technical details of a variety of different approaches are described in detail in chapter 38. Ultimately, the approach that allows the surgeon to follow the planned reconstruction with the least chance of complications and the greatest chance of achieving successful long-term clinical results is the best approach.

Multiple choices for surgical exposure are available in acetabular revision surgery. For example, for the patient whose radiograph is shown in **Figure 1**, an intrapelvic approach is appropriate for component removal. However, on closer examination of the situation, a less invasive alternative was used. In this case, the femoral component had a modular femoral head and neck attachment that could be disengaged from the component through a standard approach to the hip joint. The well-fixed femoral stem was easily removed after an extended osteotomy of the femur. Subsequently, the femoral head was extracted from its intrapelvic location. Thus, the options for surgical exposure must be fully understood, but the specific approach must be individualized.

■ Implant Removal

Preoperative Assessment

Knowledge of the fixation status of the acetabular component is helpful in planning implant removal. Radiographs can clearly identify either a loose or a well-fixed component with a high degree of reliability (**Figure 2**). A cemented acetabular component is assumed to be loose with migration of more than 5 mm (100% agreement between radiographic and intraoperative

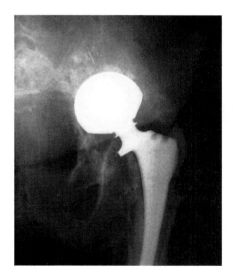

Figure 1 AP radiograph showing the intrapelvic location of hemiarthroplasty. Note that the modular femoral neck provides the surgeon with more than one option for exposure.

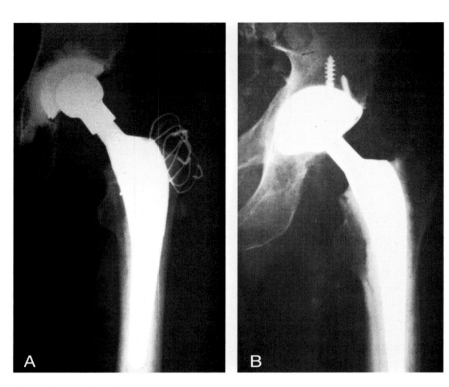

Figure 2 **A,** AP radiograph showing a well-fixed cemented acetabular component. Note the absence of radiolucent lines at the bone-cement interface. **B,** AP radiograph showing a well-fixed uncemented acetabular component.

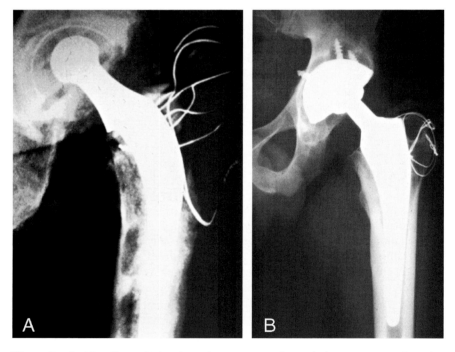

Figure 3 **A,** AP radiograph showing a loose cemented acetabular component. Note the presence of a radiolucent line comprising 100% of the bone-cement interface. **B,** AP radiograph showing a loose uncemented acetabular component. Note the presence of a radiolucent line comprising 100% of the prosthesis-bone interface.

findings) and if an area of radiolucency encompasses the entire bone-cement interface (94% agreement between radiographic and intraoperative findings) (**Figure 3,** *A*). An uncemented cup is considered loose for the same reasons, but the area of radiolucency is seen at the bone-prosthesis interface (**Figure 3,** *B* and **Figure 4**). A loose acetabular component must be removed, and a loose cup is usually relatively easy to extract. With a well-fixed prosthesis, however, several options must be considered before surgical extraction of the prosthesis.

Surgical Options
Cemented acetabular components must be removed in their entirety because they are not modular. Uncemented components are modular; therefore, they offer more options for component removal. With the latter, simple liner exchange can be an appropriate option if the shell is both well fixed and well positioned. In this situation, knowing how to remove the liner of a specific type of shell can simplify extraction. A generic technique of liner removal should be available as well. I drill a hole into the polyethylene liner in a peripheral location and then insert a screw into this drill hole. As the screw encounters the metal shell, the liner disengages.

Although loose shells can be achieved with relative ease, removing a well-fixed uncemented shell (eg, for infection or malposition) poses more of a challenge. Complete visualization of the periphery of the uncemented shell is necessary. I generally initiate the extraction process with a 2-mm burr, which disrupts the prosthesis-bone interface circumferentially at the cup periphery for a depth of 1 to 2 cm. I then use special curved osteotomes (**Figure 5**), which when used carefully, can remove even a fully ingrown socket. The prosthesis-bone interface must be completely disrupted before the uncemented shell can be extracted in order to minimize the damage to the underlying acetabular bony bed.

The residual integrity of the underlying acetabular bone stock is of paramount concern when extracting any acetabular component, especially a well-fixed uncemented shell (**Figure 6**). Pelvic discontinuities have been created during such attempts. Levering on bone during extraction should be avoided and, most importantly, patience is required. Additional specialized instrumentation is available to assist in these situations (chapter 39).

Assessing Acetabular Bone Damage

Preoperative assessment of bone damage is important for preoperative planning, but reassessment intraoperatively ultimately determines the choice of acetabular component and the need for bone graft. The AAOS and the Paprosky classification systems provide information helpful in surgical planning and prognosis (**Figures 7** and **8**).

Reconstruction of the acetabulum generally can be achieved with uncemented fixation (chapter 41), but occasionally this is not possible (ie, less than 5% of my revision cases). Cemented fixation is an option when contact between the uncemented shell and acetabular host bone comprises less than 50% of the surface area of the uncemented shell. A recent study reported a 78% failure rate for uncemented shells when structural bone graft was in contact with more than 50% of the shell. When treating severe bone stock deficiency with an antiprotrusio cage, a polyethylene liner is usually cemented directly into the cage. Finally, a cemented cup combined with the impaction-borne gravity technique has been used successfully by some surgeons.

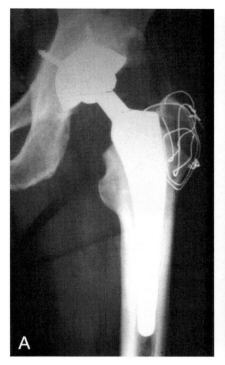
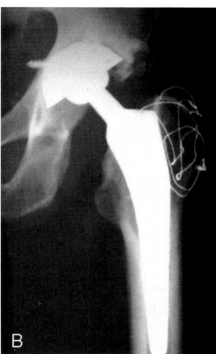

Figure 4 Early postoperative **(A)** and postoperative AP views obtained 2 years later **(B)** showing proximal and medial migration of an uncemented acetabular component, which is considered a definite sign of loosening.

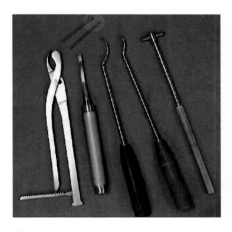

Figure 5 Special instruments used to extract both loose and well-fixed acetabular components. From left to right: cup extraction clamp, half-inch curved osteotome, long and short curve gouges, T-handle cup extractor.

The need for bone grafting depends on the degree of bone damage present after the acetabular component is removed. The primary reason for using bone graft is to restore bone

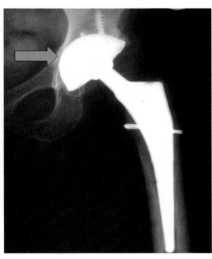

Figure 6 AP radiograph of an acetabular component requiring revision for malposition. Note the proximity of the shell to the medial wall of the pelvis (arrow). Careful extraction of this component is required to avoid creating a pelvic discontinuity.

stock in the event that future revision surgery is necessary. Bone graft is best used only as a supplement to missing bone stock, leaving the overall structural integrity of the acetabular reconstruction entirely dependent on the fixation of the acetabular component. In certain situations bone graft also may be needed for structural support. In these instances, the success and longevity of the reconstruction depends on the structural integrity of the bone graft. When bone graft is used in this fashion, the reconstruction is compromised because, ultimately, the bone graft will weaken mechanically and fail.

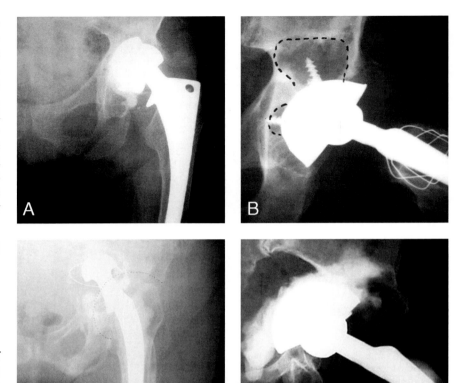

Figure 7 AAOS classification system of acetabular defects. **A,** Type I. Segmental deficiency in which the superolateral rim of the acetabulum is compromised. **B,** Type II. Cavitary deficiency in which the acetabular bed is damaged, but the rim is intact. **C,** Type III. Combined cavitary-segmental deficiency. **D,** Type IV. Pelvic discontinuity in which the structural integrity of the entire acetabulum is compromised, essentially a pelvic fracture.

New Implant Selection

In the chapters that follow, a variety of component choices are described. I prefer to achieve circumferential press-fit fixation using a hemispherical shell. I recognize that in patients with more severe defects, this is not possible. Expanded indications for uncemented fixation include placement of the shell in a high hip center, the use of bilobed or oblong shells, and the use of custom components. The advent of newer bone ingrowth surfaces on the acetabular components is promising and may increase use of uncemented shells in situations in which contact with host bone is severely compromised. The technical details of uncemented acetabular component insertion are described in chapter 41. Acetabular cage reconstruction is required only in special circumstances (chapter 44) and only infrequently.

Summary

A systematic approach to acetabular revision sets the stage for a successful reconstruction and a durable clinical result. The advice in this chapter reflects my experience and, therefore, my particular prejudices. What is written in the chapters to follow will expand on the groundwork laid in this chapter.

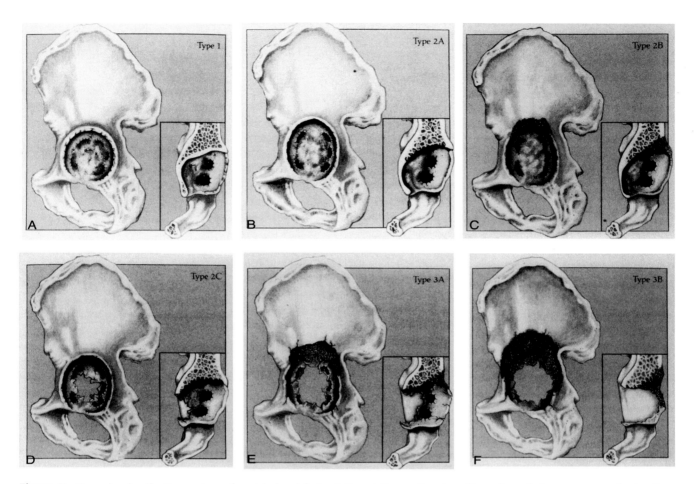

Figure 8 Paprosky classification system of acetabular defects. **A,** Type I. Supportive rim with no bone lysis or component migration. **B** through **D,** Type II. Distorted hemisphere with intact supportive columns and less than 2 cm of superomedial or lateral migration. **E,** Type IIIA. Superior migration greater than 2 cm and severe ischial lysis with Köhler's line intact. **F,** Type IIIB. Superior migration greater than 2 cm and severe ischial lysis with Köhler's line broken. (Reproduced with permission from Paprosky WG, Perona PG, Lawrence JM: Acetabular defect classification and surgical reconstruction in revision arthroplasty: A 6-year follow-up evaluation. *J Arthroplasty* 1994;9:33-44.)

References

D'Antonio JA, Capello WN, Borden LS, et al: Classification and management of acetabular abnormalities in total hip arthroplasty. *Clin Orthop* 1989;243:126-137.

Hodgkinson JP, Shelley P, Wroblewski BM: The correlation between the roentgenographic appearance and operative findings at the bone-cement junction of the socket in Charnley low friction arthroplasties. *Clin Orthop* 1988;228:105-109.

Paprosky W, Perona PG, Lawrence JM: Acetabular defect classification and surgical reconstruction in revision arthroplasty. *J Arthroplasty* 1994;9:33-44.

Chapter 41
Uncemented Acetabular Revision

John J. Callaghan, MD
Michael R. O'Rourke, MD
Steven S. Liu, MD
Wayne G. Paprosky, MD

 ## Indications

Uncemented acetabular components in revision total hip arthroplasty (THA) offer tremendous improvements in fixation over cemented components. Over the past 15 years, specific technical considerations in revision procedures have emerged as important factors in achieving long-term fixation and improved durability of uncemented acetabular components. These techniques are described in this chapter.

 ## Contraindications

Situations in which uncemented fixation is problematic are described below.

 ## Alternative Treatments

Alternative treatments include using cages or cement, with and without bone grafting. However, none of these methods works as well as uncemented fixation when adequate bone stock is available.

 ## Results

In our 10-year follow-up of cemented acetabular revisions, we reported revisions as a result of loosening and radiographic loosening in 13% and 33% of patients, respectively, compared with 0% and 2% of patients, respectively, with uncemented acetabular fixation. These results corroborate the experience of other investigators using uncemented acetabular revision THA.

 ## Technique

Preoperative Planning
The primary preoperative consideration when deciding whether to use uncemented acetabular components for revision THA, aside from septic loosening, is the amount of acetabular bone stock expected to be available for reconstruction. Patients are frequently asymptomatic for many years while loose acetabular components migrate and cause substantial bone loss or secure components develop extensive ballooning pelvic osteolysis, leading to massive acetabular bone loss. It is important to recognize that the bone loss present at surgery may be greater than that apparent on the preoperative radiographs. Oblique radiographs of the pelvis can be helpful in identifying both the extent of bone loss and the continuity of the posterior and anterior pelvic columns (**Figure 1**). CT is rarely helpful in this regard, however, because it principally assesses the relationship of the intrapelvic vessels to the remaining bone available at reconstruction.

Hip abductor function is another important preoperative consideration because constraint in the acetabular construct (or a larger femoral head size) may be needed if the abductors are deficient. The patient should be examined while lying on one side and actively elevating the limb. Preoperative identification of hip abductor insufficiency allows the surgeon to plan component options. Identifying cavitary and segmental defects in the acetabulum at this time can help ensure that cavitary-filling bone grafts or graft substitutes, as well as structural allografts, are available at surgery.

Classification Systems
The complexity of acetabular revision is currently based on the extent and location of bone loss at the time of surgery. Initially, however, the classification of acetabular bone loss was described as either contained (cavitary)

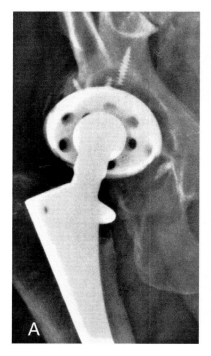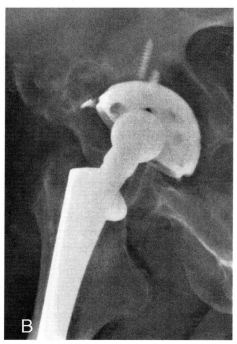

Figure 1 Obturator (**A**) and iliac (**B**) oblique pelvis radiographs demonstrate the extent of bone loss and fracture through the posterior column.

Table 1 Paprosky Classification of Acetabular Defects and Corresponding Preoperative/Intraoperative Characteristics

Type of Defect	Acetabular Rim	Walls and Domes	Columns	Bone Bed
I	Intact	Intact	Intact and supportive	> 50%; cancellous
II	Distorted	Distorted	Intact and supportive	> 50%; cancellous
III	Missing	Severely compromised	Nonsupportive	Membranous/sclerotic

or uncontained (segmented) defects. The use of these terms, along with recognition of pelvic continuity or discontinuity, provided a common vocabulary for surgeons performing revision THA. Over time, however, more formal classification systems have been devised.

The Paprosky classification system for uncemented acetabular fixation is based on the status of the acetabular rim, dome, columns, and contact area available for ingrowth at the time of revision (**Table 1**, **Figure 2**). This classification is based on the availability of supportive bone at the time of reconstruction.

Grafting patterns and methods of fixation differ, depending on the type of defect (**Table 2**). Type 1 acetabular bone defects exhibit minimal (if any) deformity. In cemented failures the only bone loss may be the cement-anchoring holes; thus, this bone can support an uncemented acetabular component. With type 2 defects,

the anterior and posterior columns are intact, but there is some destruction of the dome and medial wall of the acetabulum. In type 2A defects, there is superior bone loss from component migration or osteolysis but an intact acetabular rim so the defect is considered cavitary (contained). In type 2B defects, the superolateral rim is absent so the defect is considered segmental (uncontained). Type 2C defects demonstrate medial wall destruction. The key to the repair of type 2 defects is retention of the anterior and posterior columns to allow insertion of a stable uncemented acetabular component.

Type 3 defects demonstrate extensive superior migration of the acetabular component with more than 2 cm of superior bone loss and loss of the superolateral rim. In type 3A defects, the teardrop remains intact and therefore the medial wall remains intact. With type 3B defects, the acetabular component may migrate more than 2 cm, the teardrop is obliterated, and severe osteolysis of the ischium occurs (indicating posterior inferior wall and column deficiency). Type 3B defects may preclude use of an uncemented acetabular component; therefore, the preoperative radiographs should be scrutinized for these three signs.

To prepare the acetabulum for insertion of an uncemented component, whether for primary or revision THA, the surgeon must be correctly oriented to the acetabulum in the pelvis. Secure fixation of the pelvis in a reliable hip positioner is necessary to prevent the pelvis from rolling forward, which could cause the surgeon to inadvertently ream the posterior wall of the acetabulum and insert the acetabular component in a retroverted position (**Figure 3**). This can occur more frequently with the posterior approach to the hip. An inadequately secured pelvis rolls forward when the femur is retracted anteriorly to expose the acetabulum.

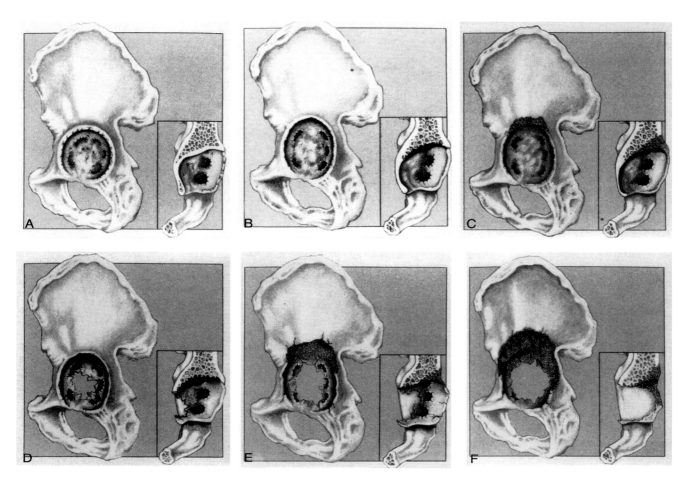

Figure 2 Paprosky classification system of acetabular defects. **A,** Type I. Supportive rim with no bone lysis or component migration. **B** through **D,** Type II. Distorted hemisphere with intact supportive columns and less than 2 cm of superomedial or lateral migration. **E,** Type IIIA. Superior migration greater than 2 cm and severe ischial lysis with Köhler's line intact. **F,** Type IIIB. Superior migration greater than 2 cm and severe ischial lysis with Köhler's line broken. (Reproduced with permission from Paprosky WG, Perona PG, Lawrence JM: Acetabular defect classification and surgical reconstruction in revision arthroplasty: A 6-year follow-up evaluation. *J Arthroplasty* 1994;9:33-44.)

Table 2 Grafting Patterns and Methods of Fixation by Acetabular Defect and Subtypes

Type of Defect	Grafting Patterns	Method of Fixation
1	Particulate graft	
2A	Particulate graft or femoral head allograft	Femoral head fixed inside acetabulum with 6.5-mm cancellous screws
2B	Number 7 femoral head allograft	Screws or plate outside the acetabulum
2C	Particulate graft or wafer-cut femoral head allograft	
3A	Number 7 distal femur or proximal tibia allograft	Screws or plate outside the acetabulum
3B	Proximal femur or acetabular "arc" graft	Plate

Exposure

Any approach to the hip can be used to expose the acetabulum, but the approach used must allow visualization of the ilium, pubis, and ischium to adequately assess the remaining bone available to support an uncemented acetabular component.

Bone Preparation

Sufficient skeletization of the proximal femur is necessary to allow mobilization of the femur and better visualization of the acetabulum. The status of the acetabular rim, anterior and posterior columns, and the medial wall also must be assessed. The acetabular rim may have remodeled around the loose

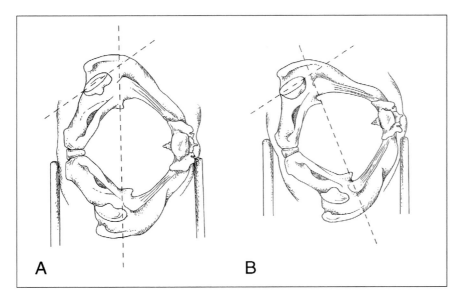

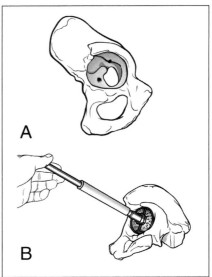

Figure 3 **A**, Correct positioning of the pelvis in a hip positioner with the patient in the lateral decubitus position. **B**, Forward tilt of the pelvis in a hip positioner gives the false impression of adequate anteversion of the acetabular component.

Figure 4 Model of a large cavitary defect. **A**, Opening of the defect to obtain contact with the native rim of the acetabulum. Stability is obtained by reaming between the anterior and posterior columns. **B**, Final reamer fits tightly between the anterior and posterior columns.

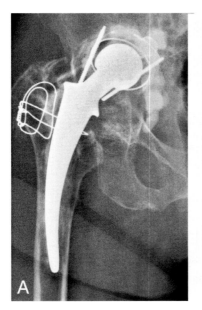

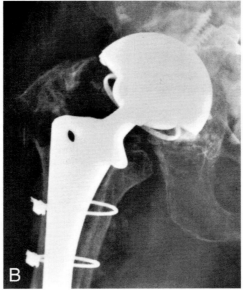

Figure 5 **A**, Large cavitary defect similar to the illustration shown in Figure 4. An uncemented component was stabilized by the intact anterior and posterior walls and columns. **B**, The medial defect was filled with impacted cancellous bone.

pect of the acetabulum generally is smaller than the superior inferior aspect. If the surgeon elects to widen the anteroposterior superior column support, the anterior column and rim should be selectively reamed, and the posterior column and posterior dome should be preserved. Similarly, to prepare the acetabulum for a larger-diameter component, the surgeon should avoid removing the medial wall, especially inferiorly and medially (ie, the teardrop region) because the medial wall supports the inferior medial aspect of the component, thus preventing postoperative horizontal movement or protrusio of the component.

Prosthesis Implantation
ACETABULAR PREPARATION FOR UNCEMENTED ACETABULAR FIXATION
All soft tissues surrounding the remaining acetabular rim should be resected before removing the acetabular component to save as much bone as possible at the time of component extraction. After component extraction, the amount of pelvic bone loss and the

component. A remodeled rim is usually inadequate for structural support so the opening of the acetabulum may need to be widened to achieve contact with the true acetabular rim and dome (**Figure 4**, *A*).

The anterior and posterior pelvic columns also must be assessed. Support of these columns is generally necessary to achieve stability with an uncemented acetabular component. At the time of revision THA, the anteroposterior as-

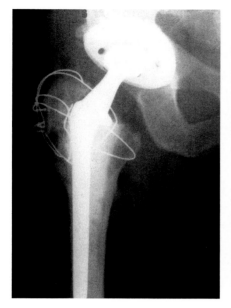
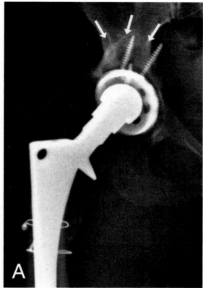
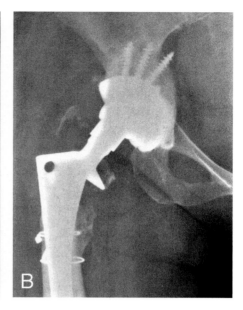

Figure 6 Typical acetabular cavitary defect allowing jumbo acetabular component insertion.

Figure 7 Preoperative (**A**) and postoperative (**B**) hip radiographs show a typical superior medial acetabular defect (arrows) that was treated with cancellous bone grafting and uncemented acetabular fixation.

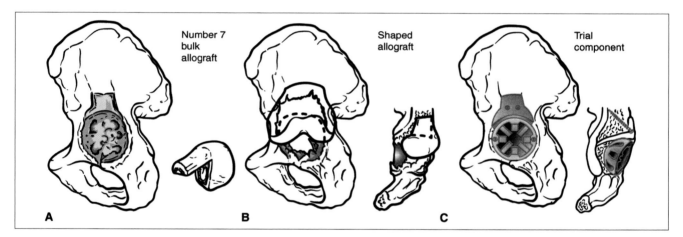

Figure 8 Preparation of distal femoral bulk allograft for the defect shown in Figure 7 (**A**), positioning of graft (**B**) and insertion of the trial component (**C**).

status of the true acetabular rim are assessed. This step may require removing the flimsy remodeled rim with enlarging reamers. The anterior and posterior columns should then be assessed for continuity and thickness. We assess any pelvic discontinuity for stability and the amount of posterior wall and column comminution present. We also assess the quality of ischium and superior aspect of the posterior column.

The goal of acetabular reaming should be to remove as little host bone as possible (**Figure 4**, *A*). Obtaining stability of the largest reamer used between the anterior and posterior columns permits use of uncemented acetabular components in all patients (**Figures 4**, *B* and **Figure 5**). In patients with only a contained cavitary defect, allograft cancellous bone or graft substitutes are impacted into the defect using reverse reamers, and

the components are impacted (**Figures 6** and **7**). The presence of massive ischial osteolysis on preoperative radiographs alerts the surgeon to the possibility of a posterior column defect that might prevent stability. If superior inferior stability is not obtained (typically a problem if more than 30% to 40% of the superior dome is absent), a Number 7 superior structural bone graft (**Figures 8** and **9**), superior metal augments (**Figure 10**),

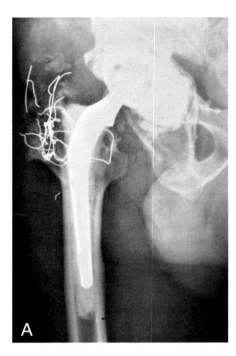

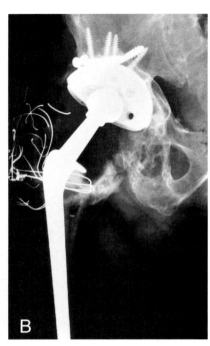

Figure 9 **A,** AP radiograph of a patient with a superior posterior acetabular wall and column defect that was treated with screw augmented posterior superior structural allograft. **B,** AP radiograph at 7 years follow-up.

or an oblong component (**Figure 11**) may be necessary.

If the anterior and posterior columns are intact superiorly and if the medial wall and superior dome have remodeled, the component can be placed in a high hip center (**Figures 12** and **13**). The advantage of the high hip center is that the component is placed on host bone. Disadvantages include the need to use a long femoral neck or calcar replacement component to obtain limb length and the fact that additional bone stock is not provided if another reconstruction is needed in the future (**Figure 14**).

Advantages of superior bone grafts include implant stability during the early postoperative period when bone ingrowth is occurring on those aspects of the acetabular component in contact with host bone and the preservation of bone stock if another procedure is required. Disadvantages include the potential for bone graft resorption during the injury-and-repair process and the lack of ingrowth in areas where the acetabular shell is in contact with graft bone. Bone grafts incorporate at the host-graft junction over time, but if structural or cancellous filler graft is used only partial incorporation of the graft bone itself occurs.

If the posterior column, especially in combination with the posterior superior dome, is absent or severely deficient, a posterior allograft with a posterior acetabular reconstruction plate is used (**Figure 15**). We currently use a partial acetabular allograft. This construct can be used only with an uncemented acetabular component if there is at least 50% to 60% host bone present (**Figure 10**). Superior posterior augments made of Trabecular Metal (Zimmer, Warsaw, IN) are beginning to be used in conjunction with acetabular components in patients with less than 50% to 60% host bone. It is too early to determine if these constructs provide durable results.

Uncemented acetabular components can provide stable reconstruc-

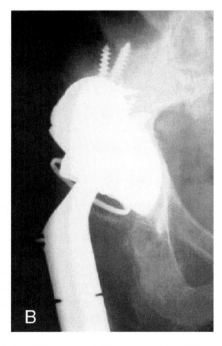

Figure 10 Posterior superior wall and dome defect (**A**) treated with Trabecular Metal (Zimmer) augments and Trabecular Metal component (**B**).

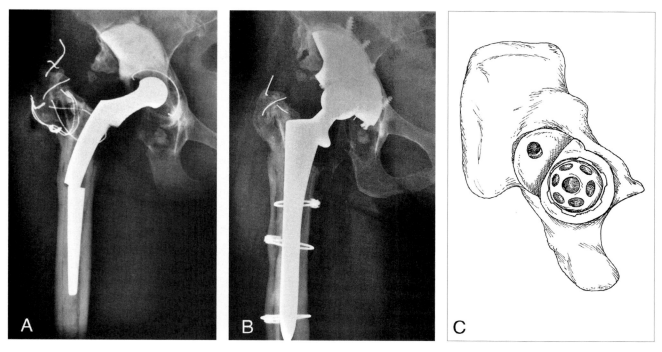

Figure 11 Preoperative **(A)** and postoperative **(B)** AP radiographs of a patient with a superior segmental defect that was treated with oblong component. **C,** Illustration shows component orientation.

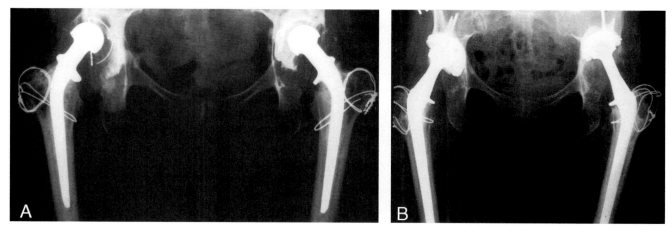

Figure 12 Bilateral AP hip radiograph shows superior segmental defects **(A)** treated with high hip center placement **(B)**. Note that long femoral neck or calcar replacements are needed to obtain appropriate limb length.

tions in many patients with pelvic discontinuity. If the posterior column is not severely osteoporotic and if the discontinuity has not created a markedly deficient or comminuted posterior wall, a posterior acetabular plate with bone grafting and an uncemented acetabular component can provide a stable, durable construct (**Figure 16**). In

patients with minimal column comminution and dense posterior column bone, we have obtained stable acetabular constructs using multiple bicortical screws through the shell above and below the discontinuity and bone grafting of the stable discontinuity while avoiding the dissection required for acetabular plating.

AUGMENTING UNCEMENTED ACETABULAR STABILITY
In primary THA, press-fitting the acetabular component (underreaming of the acetabular bone bed in relation to the outer diameter of the component) increases the stability of the uncemented acetabular construct. However, in revision THA, where ob-

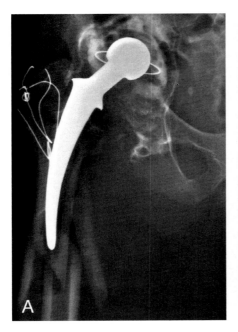
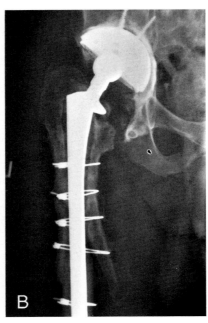

Figure 13 **A**, AP hip radiograph shows a large medial cavitary and segmental bone loss. The patient also has an acute periprosthetic femur fracture. **B**, AP radiograph obtained 6 years after revision of the acetabular and femoral components shows that remodeled bone around the migrated acetabular component made reconstruction without bone grafting possible.

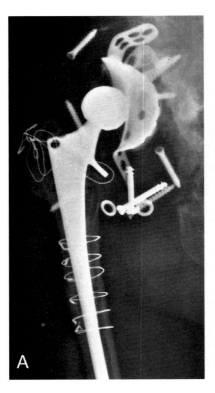
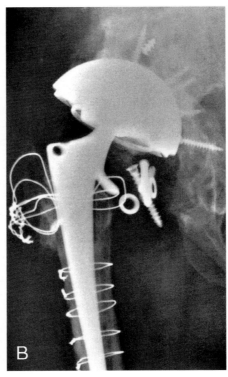

Figure 14 **A**, AP radiograph of a patient with failed acetabular cage with superior structural allograft. The separate structural allograft provided sufficient bone stock for reconstruction with an uncemented acetabular component with adjuvant screw fixation at revision (**B**).

taining contact with host bone is more challenging because of cavitary and segmental bone defects and the possibility of deficient structural bone, aggressive reaming and oversizing of components can result in greater bony deficiencies and fractures through the already thinned pelvic walls and columns. For this reason, the use of screws to augment fixation is preferable to excessive oversizing of the component in patients with the typical medial and superior defects present at the time of revision THA. Optimal screw purchase occurs in the posterior superior region of the pelvis, within or through the posterior column. Excellent screw purchase also can be obtained along the anterior superior column in larger patients. Peripheral screws also have been shown to provide excellent bone purchase in revision THA.

We have developed a technique for achieving component stability in typical revision THA in patients with a reasonable acetabular rim and an intact posterior superior dome and column. We place sequentially larger-sized reamers (as trial components) into the defect after obtaining anterior posterior stability (with the largest reamer) to determine the proper component size that allows medial wall contact with optimal stability. This reamer can be from 1 to 3 mm larger than the reamer used to obtain initial anteroposterior stability during the reaming process.

We then determine the orientation of the component in the acetabulum and place it in the proper lateral opening and anteversion, using the pubis and ischium as landmarks for anteversion and the superolateral rim as a landmark for the lateral opening. If the superolateral rim is absent, vertical placement of the cup must be avoided and superolateral and posterior uncovering of the component accepted. After impacting the component to a position of maximum medial and anteroposterior contact, we at-

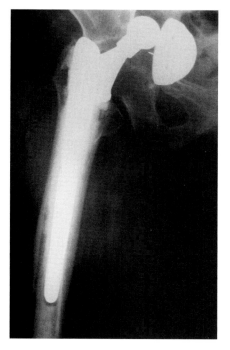

Figure 15 Medial wall and pelvic discontinuity treated by medial wall allograft, posterior plate and an uncemented acetabular component.

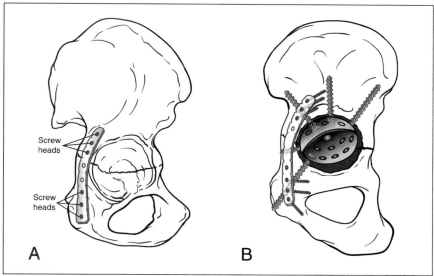

Figure 16 Illustration of posterior acetabular plating **(A)** and an uncemented acetabular component **(B)** using the dome screws to help secure the posterior column to the implant, superior and inferior to a pelvic discontinuity.

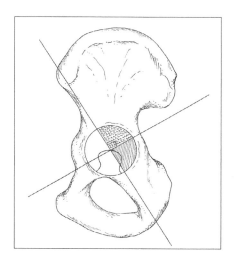

Figure 17 The quadrant system for safe screw placement is based on screws positioned posterior and superior to a line drawn between the anterosuperior iliac spine and the ischial tuberosity. The shaded areas are safe for screw placement and depict those areas with the strongest bone for screw placement.

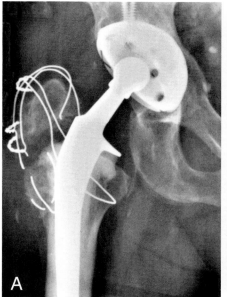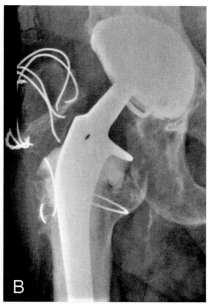

Figure 18 **A,** AP radiograph of a patient with a jumbo (68-mm) revision uncemented acetabular reconstruction using a 22-mm skirted modular head. **B,** The patient had recurrent hip dislocations requiring cementation of a constrained liner into the secure shell. Uncemented acetabular reconstruction permits this versatility.

tempt to use all available dome screw holes to obtain added stability of the acetabular construct. We generally attempt to use screw holes that are positioned posterior and superior to a line drawn between the anterosuperior iliac spine and the ischial tuberosity to avoid the iliac vessels and the obturator vessels, which are anterior and inferior to this line (**Figure 17**).

Wound Closure

Wound closure is routine. Drains are usually used.

Postoperative Regimen

Patients are kept on toe-touch or partial weight bearing for 6 to 12 weeks, depending on bone quality at the time of surgery.

———————————■

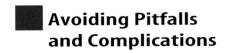

Avoiding Pitfalls and Complications

Hip instability following revision THA has been reported in up to 20% of patients. Use of modular components in the uncemented acetabular construct can help prevent or promote the insta-bility. Higher dislocation rates were reported in the mid 1990s because larger-diameter acetabular components were used in the uncemented acetabular revisions to span the deficient bone loss, and smaller diameter femoral heads were used to decrease polyethylene wear. The combination of large (< 60 mm) outer diameter acetabular components, smaller (≥ 28 mm) femoral heads, and skirted modular (22-mm) femoral heads had the highest rates of dislocation (**Figure 18**).

The use of extended lip liners and constrained acetabular liners (especially in patients with abductor muscle deficiencies) has decreased the prevalence of dislocation in revision THA. After placing the acetabular shell in the revision construct, trial liners should be used to assess stability, as should various femoral head sizes and liner inserts, to determine optimal stability. The use of larger femoral heads (especially with jumbo shells), along with extended lip liners or constrained inserts, should also be considered, but skirted modular heads should be avoided.

Using these techniques, uncemented acetabular reconstruction can be performed in almost all patients who require revision THA. Patients with loss of the posterior superior dome, posterior column, and posterior wall complex are the most problematic. A variety of femoral head sizes and different types of liners are necessary to ensure stability of the revision THA.

———————————■

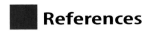

References

Behairy Y, Meldrum RD, Harris WH: Hybrid revision total hip arthroplasty: A 7-year follow-up study. *J Arthroplasty* 2001;16:829-837.

Buoncristiani AM, Dorr LD, Johnson C, Wan Z: Cementless revision of total hip arthroplasty using the anatomic porous replacement revision prosthesis. *J Arthroplasty* 1997;12:403-415.

Callaghan JJ, Kim YS, Pedersen DR, Brown TD: Acetabular preparation and insertion of cementless acetabular components. *Oper Tech Orthop* 1995;5:325-330.

Dewal H, Chen F, Su E, Di Cesare PE: Use of structural bone graft with cementless acetabular cups in total hip arthroplasty. *J Arthroplasty* 2003;18:23-28.

Garcia-Cimbrelo E: Porous-coated cementless acetabular cups in revision surgery: A 6- to 11-year follow-up study. *J Arthroplasty* 1999;14:397-406.

Gross AE: Revision arthroplasty of the acetabulum with restoration of bone stock. *Clin Orthop* 1999;369:198-207.

Heekin RD, Engh CA, Vinh T: Morselized allograft in acetabular reconstruction: A postmortem retrieval analysis. *Clin Orthop* 1995;319:184-190.

Hooten JP Jr, Engh CA, Heekin RD, Vinh TN: Structural bulk allografts in acetabular reconstruction: Analysis of two grafts retrieved at post-mortem. *J Bone Joint Surg Br* 1996;78:270-275.

Katz RP, Callaghan JJ, Sullivan PM, Johnston RC: Long-term results of revision total hip arthroplasty with improved cementing technique. *J Bone Joint Surg Br* 1997;79:322-326.

Leopold SS, Jacobs JJ, Rosenberg AG: Cancellous allograft in revision total hip arthroplasty: A clinical review. *Clin Orthop* 2000;371:86-97.

Leopold SS, Rosenberg AG, Bhatt RD, et al: Cementless acetabular revision: Evaluation at an average of 10.5 years. *Clin Orthop* 1999;369:179-186.

Patel JV, Masonis JL, Bourne RB, Rorabeck CH: The fate of cementless jumbo cups in revision hip arthroplasty. *J Arthroplasty* 2003;18:129-133.

Silverton CD, Rosenberg AG, Sheinkop MB, Kull LR, Galante JO: Revision total hip arthroplasty using a cementless acetabular component: Technique and results. *Semin Arthroplasty* 1995;6:109-117.

Sutherland CJ: Treatment of type II acetabular deficiencies in revision total hip arthroplasty without structural bone-graft. *J Arthroplasty* 1996;11:91-98.

Templeton JE, Callaghan JJ, Goetz DD, Sullivan PM, Johnston RC: Revision of a cemented acetabular component to a cementless acetabular component: A ten to fourteen-year follow-up study. *J Bone Joint Surg Am* 2001;83:1706-1711.

Udomkiat P, Wan Z, Dorr LD: Comparison of preoperative radiographs and intraoperative findings of fixation of hemispheric porous-coated sockets. *J Bone Joint Surg Am* 2001;83:1865-1970.

Whaley AL, Berry DJ, Harmsen WS: Extra-large uncemented hemispherical acetabular components for revision total hip arthroplasty. *J Bone Joint Surg Am* 2001;83:1352-1357.

Woodgate IG, Saleh KJ, Jaroszynski G, et al: Minor column structural acetabular allografts in revision hip arthroplasty. *Clin Orthop* 2000;371:75-85.

Coding

CPT Code		Corresponding ICD-9 Codes	
27137	Revision of total hip arthroplasty, acetabular component only, with or without autograft or allograft	996.4	996.66
27134	Revision of total hip arthroplasty; both components, with or without autograft or allograft (add this code if femoral component is also revised)	996.4	996.66
27134-52	Revision of total hip arthroplasty; both components, with or without autograft or allograft (add this code if the modular head is changed)	996.4	996.66

CPT copyright © 2004 by the American Medical Association. All Rights Reserved.

Chapter 42

Osteolysis-Polyethylene Liner Exchange

William J. Maloney, MD

 ## Indications

Osteolysis of the pelvis is a relatively common complication of cemented and uncemented acetabular components. With uncemented acetabular components, significant osteolysis can occur without implant loosening. With well-fixed uncemented components, the pathologic process does not necessarily affect the implant-bone interface. Thus, the surgeon must decide whether to remove a well-fixed socket or simply perform a polyethylene liner exchange. In general, the relative indications for a liner exchange include an osseointegrated socket, an available liner that fits into the existing shell or can be cemented in place, a well-positioned socket, and a shell that has a good clinical track record. Because these indications are merely guidelines, a surgeon may sometimes decide that it is in the patient's best long-term interest to perform a complete socket revision. These guidelines are described below.

Of critical and initial importance, the socket must be rigidly fixed to the pelvis if a liner exchange is to be performed. Radiographic evaluation to ascertain stability and ingrowth or ongrowth of uncemented sockets can be difficult. Thus, it is critically important to confirm intraoperatively that the socket is osseointegrated with the pelvis. Sockets with an ongrowth surface tend to fail catastrophically more often in the presence of osteolysis than do sockets with an ingrowth surface. Thus, sockets with an ongrowth surface (eg, a titanium plasma-spray) should be considered for socket revision, especially if the patient is young and active and has significant osteolysis. Revision of hydroxyapatite-coated sockets on macrotextured surfaces also should be strongly considered because these sockets are associated with a high intermediate-term loosening rate. Preoperative identification of the specific prosthesis is important to identify the type of fixation surface.

Dislocation is a relatively common complication after liner exchange. Preoperative assessment of variables such as component position, offset, and limb-length discrepancy will help the surgeon identify factors that may be correctable at surgery or may predispose the patient to dislocation following liner exchange. Careful trial reduction is necessary to assess hip stability following liner exchange. Use of offset, oblique, or elevated rim liners may enhance hip stability following liner exchange. In general, a larger femoral head should be used, if possible, when performing a polyethylene liner exchange to ensure stability. Stability also may be increased by using a slightly longer femoral neck. Use of a smaller femoral head or a head-neck combination that requires a skirted femoral head will decrease hip stability.

Surgical approach also may influence hip stability following liner exchange. In a recent study in which a direct lateral approach was used, no dislocations were reported in 24 hips 36 months after liner exchange. Similarly, repair of the posterior pseudocapsule after a posterior approach should improve hip stability. Postoperative bracing also should be considered. Patients who undergo liner exchange usually recover quickly and have relatively little pain; therefore, they may be more likely to violate precautions for dislocation. Malpositioned cups should be revised because of the higher dislocation rate after a revision procedure than after a primary procedure.

Damage to the metal shell and locking mechanism is another factor when considering liner exchange. If the locking mechanism is damaged or inadequate, either the socket should be revised or the liner should be cemented into the existing shell. Cementing a liner into an existing shell is a reliable way to provide liner stability. Biomechanical testing demonstrates that failure almost always occurs at the cement-liner interface, except in polished nontextured shells without screw holes, in which failure occurs at the cement interface. Texturing of smooth metal shells and polyethylene liners improves mechanical stability. In vitro testing has demonstrated that cementing of liners is as stable as most

Table 1 Results of Polyethylene Liner Exchange

Author(s) (Year)	Number of Hips	Implant Type	Mean Follow-up (Range)	Results Revision (%)	Dislocation (%)
Maloney, et al (1997)	35	Multiple*	3.3 years (2–5)	0%	NA
Boucher, et al (2003)	24	AML shell (DePuy, Warsaw, IN) S-ROM shell (Joint Medical Products, Stamford, CT)	56 months (24–108)	12%	25%
Griffin, et al (2004)	55	Multiple	30 months (9–51)	11%	18%

*Authors did not delineate types of acetabular components.
NA= Not available

commercially available locking mechanisms. The failure rate for cementing of liners is relatively low. It is important at the time of cementing a liner to fully seat the liner in the shell. A polyethylene liner that is 1 or 2 mm smaller than the diameter of the shell is generally advised to increase pressurization of the cement. Proud liners are at risk for impingement and loosening. Thus, it is not possible to significantly change the version of the socket by eccentric cementing without risking liner dissociation.

Contraindications

The contraindications for liner exchange include a loose socket, a socket with an ongrowth surface in the presence of a large osteolytic defect, a malpositioned socket, a badly damaged outer shell, and lack of availability of a liner. Ongrowth fixation surfaces are weaker in tension compared with three-dimensional ingrowth surfaces, and they are more susceptible to socket breakout in the presence of large osteolytic defects in the superior and lateral aspects of the acetabulum. Relative socket malposition, even if the hip did not dislocate after the index procedure, may be associated with an increased risk of postoperative dislocation following liner exchange. Preoperatively, a cross-table lateral view should be obtained to evaluate the version of the acetabular component. Depending on the results of the intraoperative trial reduction, complete socket revision should be considered for marginally positioned sockets.

Badly damaged shells also should be considered for revision because the polyethylene liner may be unstable, even if cemented in place. These contraindications are guidelines, and there may be cases where in the surgeon's judgment, liner exchange is indicated even if the conditions are suboptimal.

Results

Polyethylene liner exchange has been a reliable procedure for appropriately selected patients (**Table 1**). In most cases, osteolytic lesions tend to regress radiographically following liner exchange and bone grafting in the short to intermediate term. Component loosening is rare up to 10 years after isolated liner exchange. Quantitative evaluation of polyethylene wear and progression of lesion size indicates that liner exchange with removal of granulomatous tissue potentially decreases wear and slows the progression of osteolysis without subsequent component loosening. In one study, 10 hips were evaluated before and after component exchange. Prior to liner exchange, polyethylene wear rates averaged 0.36 ± 0.19 mm/year. At a mean of 6.2 years after liner exchange, wear rates were essentially cut in half (0.17 ± 0.11 mm/year). In addition, the growth rates of both the acetabular and femoral lesions decreased.

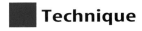

Technique

Exposure

Liner exchange, débridement of pelvic osteolytic lesions, and bone grafting of pelvic defects can be done from an anterolateral, direct lateral, or posterior approach to the hip joint. With a posterior approach, it is useful to take down the posterior pseudocapsule as a flap off of the posterior edge of the greater trochanter and repair it at the end of the surgery to enhance hip stability. Often, the femoral component is well fixed, and in some cases the femoral head is not modular. To move the femoral component out of the way of the socket, a complete capsulotomy is usually necessary.

With the posterior approach, the anterior capsule is released and the proximal femur partially skeletonized to allow mobilization of the femur. Release of the gluteus maximus tendon is sometimes necessary. A pocket can be created anteriorly to allow the femoral head and/or neck to be displaced from the acetabulum. This step allows visualization of the socket.

Bone Preparation

Following dislocation and exposure of the acetabulum, the polyethylene liner should be removed. In some patients, the locking mechanism is not easily disengaged. In these situations, the acetabular liner sometimes can be removed by drilling a hole in the liner using a 3.2-mm drill bit. Following that, a 6.5-mm cancellous screw can be inserted into the drill hole, which can dislodge most polyethylene liners. When using this technique, however, the surgeon has to ensure that the screw is not inserted into a screw hole in the socket and into the pelvis.

Following removal of the polyethylene liner, the remaining granulomatous tissue in the hip joint should be débrided and the periphery of the acetabular component clearly identified. Tissue may be sent for frozen sections to rule out infection. At this point, it is important to ensure that the socket is, in fact, osseointegrated. Once the rim of the acetabular component is exposed circumferentially and the screws in the socket are removed, socket stability can be tested. The socket can be grasped with Kocher retractors or by screwing the cup impaction device in place and then pulling on the component. If there is motion of the component, it should be revised. In addition, it is helpful to visualize the pseudopods of bone that have grown directly into the porous surface of the acetabular component. Once socket stability is confirmed, granulomatous tissue in the pelvis can be débrided. It is helpful to identify the access channel through which wear debris enters the pelvis; this is usually the easiest way to access osteolytic lesions. These lesions are preferably débrided through access channels around the periphery of the socket, but débridement also can be performed through screw holes. In some cases, a trapdoor can be made in the ilium, but care must be taken to avoid disrupting the pseudopods of bone that are stabilizing the cup. A variety

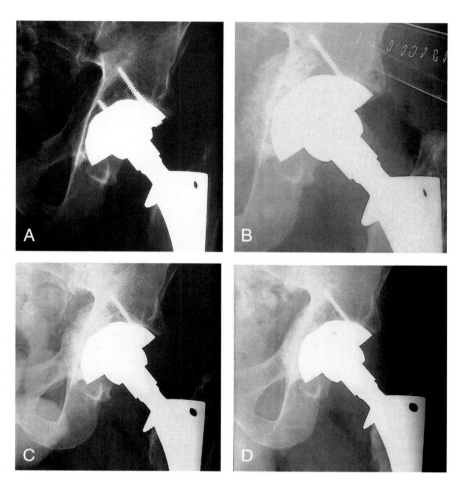

Figure 1 **A,** Preoperative radiograph demonstrating a well-fixed uncemented socket with retroacetabular osteolysis. Note the ballooning of the medial wall of the acetabulum. **B,** Immediate postoperative radiograph demonstrating graft material packed into the osteolytic defect through the dome hole of the acetabulum. **C,** Radiograph taken 3 months postoperatively demonstrating apparent graft incorporation. However, it is difficult to determine true graft incorporation on plain radiographs. **D,** Radiograph taken 1 year postoperatively demonstrating apparent radiographic healing of the osteolytic defect and incorporation of the graft.

of bone graft materials and bone graft substitutes have been used to fill osteolytic defects, but no one material is clearly superior. In addition, it is unclear whether bone graft and bone graft substitutes packed into osteolytic defects actually incorporate into the host bone (**Figure 1**). Radiographically, these lesions appear to heal in many patients; however, data are insufficient to suggest that actual incorporation into host bone occurs routinely.

Once the lesion has been grafted, a trial reduction should be performed.

At this time, an accurate assessment of hip stability is critical. Instability on the operating table is often equated with postoperative dislocation. Historically, femoral head size was often decreased to increase polyethylene thickness. The decision to use a smaller femoral head may increase the risk of postoperative dislocation after liner exchange. Therefore, the surgeon may want to consider using a larger head size and an enhanced polyethylene. Although no clinical data support the efficacy of this technique, the use of larger femoral heads clearly increases hip stability. A protrusio liner can be used with a large femoral head to increase the thickness of the polyethylene liner. Postoperative bracing for approximately 6 weeks also should be considered.

Prosthesis Implantation

If a liner is not available for a given metal shell or a locking mechanism is damaged but the shell is salvageable, a liner that seats fully into the acetabular shell can be cemented in place. If the inner aspect of the shell has no holes and is relatively smooth, a high-speed drill with a metal-cutting burr can be used to roughen the surface. This surface roughening may enhance the strength of the cement-metal bond. Some surgeons also use a high-speed burr to roughen the back of the liner to improve the bond between the polyethylene and cement. To cement the liner into the cup, dry the inner aspect of the cup and place the cement into the socket. Typically, a half pack of cement is adequate. Next, fully seat the polyethylene liner into the metal shell, remove the excess cement, and hold the liner in place until the cement hardens.

Wound Closure

Following placement of the acetabular liner, the hip is reduced and stability is assessed again. If a capsular flap was created at the time of exposure, standard wound closure is indicated.

Postoperative Regimen

Postoperatively, patients can be allowed to bear weight as tolerated, provided that the femoral component was not revised. Because one of the more common complications with isolated socket procedures (including liner exchanges) is postoperative instability, patients should be advised about the limits of range of motion in the postoperative period. Patients tend to recover quickly and often stop using assistive devices within 2 to 4 weeks, which may contribute to dislocation. therefore, patients should be encouraged to ambulate with support for 4 to 6 weeks. The use of a hip orthosis should be considered, particularly in patients in whom compliance with dislocation precautions is a concern.

Avoiding Pitfalls and Complications

Preoperative planning is an important part of approaching failed uncemented sockets secondary to polyethylene wear, with or without osteolysis. Both the position and specific type of acetabular component should be identified. Over the past 2 decades, subtle changes in component design have occurred, and some components are quite difficult to identify radiographically. With design changes, locking mechanisms have changed; thus, the appropriate acetabular liner should be available in the operating room if commercially available. The most reliable way to determine the specific acetabular component is to obtain the implant catalog numbers from the hospital records; however, this is not always possible. Obtaining this information preoperatively minimizes the risk of not having the appropriate liner available at the time of revision surgery. The type of femoral component in place needs to be identified, even if it is not going to be revised. Appropriate femoral heads need to be ordered.

The stability of the component must be thoroughly analyzed at the time of surgery. If there is motion of the acetabular component, it should be revised.

The trial reduction following liner exchange is also an important step in avoiding complications. If the hip is not stable on the operating table, steps should be taken to improve hip stability, and if these steps are unsuccessful the socket should be revised.

Finally, recognizing sockets with a poor track record and considering revision of those sockets may help to minimize failure secondary to aseptic loosening.

References

Boucher HR, Lynch C, Young AM, Engh CA Jr, Engh CA Sr: Dislocation after polyethylene liner exchange in total hip arthroplasty. *J Arthroplasty* 2003;18:654-657.

Griffin WL, Fehring TK, Mason JB, et al: Early morbidity of modular exchange for polyethylene wear and osteolysis. *J Arthroplasty* 2004;19(suppl):61-66.

O'Brien JJ, Burnett RS, McCalden RW, et al: Isolated liner exchange in revision total hip arthroplasty: Clinical results using the direct lateral surgical approach. *J Arthroplasty* 2004;19:414-423.

Haft GF, Anneliese DH, Callaghan JJ, et al: Polyethylene liner cementation into fixed acetabular shells. *J Arthroplasty* 2002;17:167-170.

Haft GF, Heiner AD, Dorr LD, Brown TD, Callaghan JJ: A biomechanical analysis of polyethylene liner cementation into a fixed metal acetabular shell. *J Bone Joint Surg Am* 2003;85:1100-1110.

LaPorte DM, Mont MA, Pierre-Jacques H, Peyton RS, Hungerford DS: Technique for acetabular liner revision in a nonmodular metal-backed component. *J Arthroplasty* 1998;13:348-350.

Maloney WJ, Herzwurm P, Paprosky W, Rubash HE, Engh CA: Treatment of pelvic osteolysis associated with stable acetabular components inserted without cement as part of a total hip replacement. *J Bone Joint Surg Am* 1997;79:1628-1634.

Maloney WJ, Paprosky W, Engh CA, Rubash H: Surgical treatment of pelvic osteolysis. *Clin Orthop* 2001;393:78-84.

Schmalzried TA, Fauble VA, Amstutz HC: The fate of pelvic osteolysis after reoperation. *Clin Orthop* 1998;350:128.

Terefenko KM, Sychterz CJ, Orishimo K, Engh CA Sr: Polyethylene liner exchange for excessive wear and osteolysis. *J Arthroplasty* 2002;17:798-804.

Coding

CPT Codes		Corresponding ICD-9 Codes	
27134	Revision of total hip arthroplasty; both components, with or without autograft or allograft	996.4	996.77
27137	Revision of total hip arthroplasty; acetabular component only, with or without autograft or allograft	996.4	996.77
Modifier 52	This modifier (Reduced Services) is usually used.		

CPT copyright © 2004 by the American Medical Association. All Rights Reserved.

Chapter 43
Acetabular Revision: Structural Grafts

Steven J. MacDonald, MD, FRCSC
Ramin Mehin, MD, FRCSC

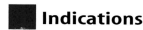

Indications

Adequate bone stock is critical in the success of any reconstructive technique in revision total hip arthroplasty (THA). In most patients, bone loss is rather minimal, either cavitary or small segmental bone loss. Deficiency in periacetabular bone is not uncommon, but massive loss of acetabular bone occurs less frequently.

Bulk structural allografts are indicated in acetabular reconstruction when host bone stock is insufficient to provide the support necessary for the implant. Host bone stock deficiencies are uncontained defects that cannot be treated solely with morcellized grafting, jumbo or oblong cups, or reconstruction rings. Specific indications regarding the use of bulk structural allografts in acetabular revision remain elusive. The evidence demonstrates that these revisions are associated with a much higher failure rate if a cup or reconstruction ring lacks adequate bony support.

Structural allografts can be anatomic or simulated. Anatomic structural allografts are anatomically representative of the deficient host bone stock (ie, a whole acetabular transplant allograft used in the reconstruction of a deficient acetabulum). Simulated structural allografts differ from their location in the reconstruction and are altered to augment the defi-

cient host bone stock (eg, a femoral head allograft used to restore deficient acetabular bone stock).

It should be emphasized that the use of structural allografts in revision acetabular THA is rare. In a review of 630 consecutive patients who underwent revision acetabular THA at our institution, structural allografts were required in only 35 procedures (5.5%), despite the fact that our institution is a referral center for patients undergoing complex revisions. Although structural allografts clearly are not commonly used, they are sometimes necessary in complex reconstructions.

Contraindications

The literature currently reports mixed midterm and long-term results for structural allografts. We believe they should be reserved for patients in whom other techniques cannot be used. Structural allografts should not be used in patients who need only a jumbo cup or a reconstruction ring with morcellized grafting. Newer techniques, such as the use of trabecular metal cups, may change the indications for structural grafts, although the techniques and their outcomes are not yet reflected in the literature.

Structural allografts are also contraindicated in the presence of active

infection. However, they can be a successful part of a second-stage reconstruction after treatment of infection.

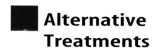

Alternative Treatments

Alternatives to structural allografting can be successful in most revision THA reconstructions. Small cavitary defects can be treated with morcellized grafting in deficient areas. Uncemented components are preferred even with moderate host bone stock loss. Most published series report that at least 50% of the uncemented acetabular component must be in contact with host bone stock to achieve long-term component fixation. Failure rates increase significantly when less than 50% host bone contact is present. A structural allograft can provide support but cannot substitute for adequate host bone contact. A bulk structural allograft clearly has no potential for bony ingrowth into an uncemented component. Posterior column fixation is critical to long-term component survival. Therefore, both the amount of available host bone contact and its location are critical. An uncemented component is an excellent alternative treatment when adequate host bone contact fixation can be achieved.

Reconstructive cages are an alternative to structural allografts when enough host bone contact is present. To achieve reproducible, long-lasting results with reconstruction cages, fixation to the ischium and ilium are required, as is maximum host bone contact with the columns, medial floor, and superior rim. Insufficient host bone stock will require bone stock restoration to achieve adequate fixation.

Impaction grafting techniques are another alternative to structural grafting in complex reconstructive procedures. Impaction grafting has been used for large acetabular defects and more routine segmental and cavitary defects. Impaction grafting is discussed in greater detail in chapter 45.

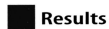

Results

Using structural allografts for reconstruction of acetabular bone loss is well documented in the literature. Some reports include patients with both primary and revision procedures, whereas others focus only on revisions. Several series are summarized in **Table 1**.

Grafts are reported to unite in most patients. However, several series describe significant acetabular component failures. Clearly, a structural graft can provide support to the acetabular reconstruction but cannot substitute for host bone fixation. All acetabular allografts undergo some degree of resorption and have no potential for bone ingrowth into uncemented components. Most reports conclude that when less than 50% of the acetabulum contains host bone, an alternative to the uncemented cup is required.

The results shown in **Table 1** demonstrate that several factors are critical to success when using structural allografts in acetabular revision reconstruction. Because many early series reported good short-term re-

sults but later described either graft failure or implant loosening, our review included only series with a mean 5-year follow-up. The duration of patient follow-up must be understood when reviewing study results.

Allograft type (eg, femoral head, distal femur, total acetabular allograft) and surgical technique are the most important criteria in successful procedures. Current thinking emphasizes aligning the graft trabecula with the host ilium trabecula and orienting fixation in an oblique fashion. Earlier reports essentially described bolting the allograft to the host ilium, with fixation generally perpendicular to the long axis of the limb. The earlier technique places the graft and its fixation at a biomechanical disadvantage, theoretically leading to higher graft failure rates.

The component selected for fixation must also be considered when reviewing the results. Earlier series described cemented cups. Because allografts undergo at least some degree of resorption, long-term failure of the cement-allograft interface might occur. A transition to uncemented fixation and its inherent limitations followed. Some series report on the outcomes with reconstructive cages.

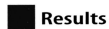

Technique

Exposure

Complete exposure of the acetabulum, including the anterior and posterior columns, medial floor, and superior dome and adjacent ilium, is mandatory in complex acetabular revisions requiring bulk structural allograft techniques. This exposure can be achieved with either posterolateral or modified direct lateral approaches. A trochanteric slide or extended trochanteric osteotomy may also be required in patients with severe acetabular protusio or with spe-

cific indications related to femoral component revision.

We performed a series of 35 reconstructions using the posterolateral approach in four procedures and a modified direct lateral approach in 31 reconstructions. Contrary to previous reports, we found that an extensile modified direct lateral approach provides excellent exposure and allows placement of both structural allografts and antiprotrusio cages. However, posterior column plating cannot be achieved with the direct lateral approach, and it is also technically very difficult to place screws into the ischium. We therefore prefer to place the ischial flange of the reconstruction ring into the body of the ischium rather than on its surface.

In patients with pelvic discontinuity, a modified direct lateral approach can be used in conjunction with a reconstruction ring. However, if the surgeon wishes to use an uncemented cup, or plate the posterior column, a posterolateral approach is preferred.

Bone Preparation

Both host bone and allograft bone must be prepared, and complete exposure of host bone is absolutely necessary before preparation of the acetabulum. The anterior and posterior columns must be well visualized with retractors placed over both columns and an inferior retractor placed at the inferior margin of the acetabulum. A systematic approach to component removal is essential and is detailed in chapter 39. It is essential to maximize the amount of host bone available for the reconstruction.

Direct visualization of the entire acetabular host bone stock is required. A Cobb elevator is used to remove the pseudomembrane that often develops between the host bone and the acetabular component or cement. All loose debris is removed, along with any well-fixed cement in the ischium or superior dome. Well-fixed cement

Table 1   Results of Structural Allografts in Acetabular Revision Total Hip Arthroplasty

Author(s) (Year)	Number of Reconstructions	Average Length of Follow-Up (Range)	Graft Source	Type of Component	Graft Union (%)	Component Loosening (%)	Comments
Jasty and Harris (1990)	29	5.9 years (4–9)	Femoral head	Cemented polyethylene cup	100%	32%	Update of an earlier series that had shown no early failures. Demonstrated the importance of midterm follow-up evaluations.
Paprosky, et al (1994)	87	5.7 years (3–9)	Femoral head or distal femur	Uncemented cup	100%	4%	All failures occurred in patients with less than 50% host bone contact.
Zehntner and Ganz (1994)	27	7.2 years (5–10)	Femoral head	Reinforcement roof ring	100%	20%	10-year survivorship of 79.6%, but 44% demonstrated migration of more than 2 mm. The component used in this series did not provide ischial fixation.
Garbuz, et al (1996)	33	7 years (5–11)	Acetabulum (whole or part)	Cemented polyethylene cup (14) Antiprotrusio cage (Burch-Schneider) (8) Uncemented cup (7) Bipolar (4)	76%	45%	The most successful reconstructive technique involved the antiprotrusio cage, which achieved ilial and ischial fixation.
Shinar and Harris (1997)	15	16.5 years (14–21)	Femoral head	Cemented polyethylene cup	100%	66%	The percentage of component coverage by the allograft did not influence the results, but a statistically significant increased failure rate in younger patients was demonstrated in a further update of an earlier series.
Gill, et al (2000)	37	7.1 years (5–13)	Femoral head	Antiprotrusio cage (Burch-Schneider) (30) Reinforcement roof ring (Muller ring) (7)	97%	10% (Definite or probable loosening)	All cases involved solid bulk allograft covering more than 50% of the socket. The success rate was high overall, with only 1 revision (because of sepsis).
Saleh, et al (2000)	13	10.5 years (5–16)	Acetabulum (whole or part)	Antiprotrusio cage (Burch-Schneider) (6) Reinforcement roof ring (Muller ring) (4)	92%	8%	Three resection arthroplasties (1 for graft resorption and 2 for recurrent dislocation) involved bulk allografts covering more than 50% of the socket.
DeWal, et al (2003)	13	6.8 years (2–10)	Femoral head or distal femur	Uncemented cup	100%	15%	Two loose cups not yet requiring revision. More than 80% of components had greater than 50% host bone coverage.

that is medial and adherent to soft tissue should be left in situ, with only the most superficial aspect of the cement removed with a high-speed burr if it blocks the reconstruction. It is both unsafe and unnecessary to remove all medial cement, particularly when it is past Köhler's line and adherent to underlying tissue. Once the entire ac-

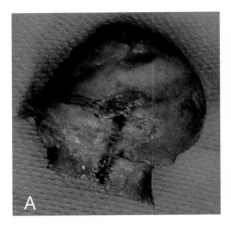 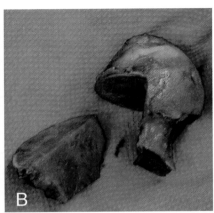

Figure 1 **A,** The femoral head allograft is cleared of all soft tissue and the numeral 7 is drawn on the graft. **B,** The medial portion of bone is removed, creating the classic number 7 femoral head allograft.

etabulum is exposed, the amount of host bone remaining for reconstruction is carefully assessed.

Acetabular reamers are placed at the true hip center, and gentle reaming is performed, taking care to avoid overly medializing with the reamers. After acetabular reaming is complete, a trial acetabular component can be placed to assess the extent of host bone contact present. When anterior and posterior column contact is sufficient, and host bone contact exceeds 50% but a significant host bone stock deficiency remains, a structural allograft can be used to restore bone stock in the location where the uncemented component will be placed. If less than 50% of host bone is present, an uncemented acetabular component will not provide adequate long-term fixation and a reconstruction ring should be used.

It is critical to assess posterior column support. In rare instances there is an isolated posterior column defect with an intact anterior column and superior dome. In this case, an uncemented acetabular component may not provide the desired results, even though the amount of host bone contact may be 50% or more. When fixation posteriorly is dependent on a structural graft, the posterior column should be reconstructed using a re-

construction ring, rather than an uncemented cup.

Allograft bone preparation depends on the type of structural graft chosen to restore the host bone stock loss. A femoral head or a distal femur can be used to create a "number 7" graft, or a whole acetabular allograft can be used in patients with severe acetabular deficiency. The surgical techniques involved in bone preparation are described in detail below.

We prefer a number 7 femoral head allograft when restoring bone stock deficiency of the superior dome of the acetabulum. Defects that occur from the 11 to 1 o'clock positions are ideal for femoral head allografts. We also prefer obtaining these allografts from male donors because the allograft material is generally large and strong. Greater host bone stock deficiencies involve more of the anterior and posterior column, and many femoral heads will not bridge that defect. Therefore, a distal femoral allograft is a better choice.

Prepare the femoral head allograft by removing all soft tissue from the graft itself. Draw the numeral 7 on the graft with a marking pen, orienting it to remove what would be the allograft's medial calcar section (**Figure 1**, *A*). Use an oscillating saw to remove the medial portion of the

bone, thus creating a classic number 7 femoral head allograft (**Figure 1**, *B*). This graft is then oriented in the host bone so that the angle of the number 7 locks into the superior rim of the acetabulum. The allograft is fixed by placing 6.5-mm partially threaded cancellous screws with washers through the long portion of the femoral head allograft into the host iliac bone (**Figure 2**). Screws should be placed superior enough to be well clear of the acetabular rim.

Some published reports indicate that it is important to align the allograft trabecula with host trabecula and to orient the screws in an oblique direction rather than a direction more perpendicular to the weight-bearing axis of the limb. The literature reports, however, that all techniques achieve 95% to 100% graft union, suggesting that nuances in allograft fixation probably do not influence long-term results. An oscillating saw is used to remove some of the overhanging femoral head, and a series of acetabular reamers is used to recreate a concentric host acetabulum (**Figure 3**).

Distal femoral allografts are used when more profound bone loss creates a defect greater than could be augmented with the femoral head alone. The technique for creating a number 7 graft using a distal femoral allograft is very similar to that for the femoral head allograft previously described.

Outline the number 7 on the allograft bone and remove the appropriate portion with an oscillating saw (**Figure 4**, *A*). Keystone the distal femoral allograft into the host acetabulum spanning the defect and lock the allograft's apex into the host acetabulum superior rim. The allograft is then fixed with 6.5-mm partially threaded cancellous screws with washers (**Figure 4**, *B*). Some excess allograft is removed with a saw while the remainder is removed with acetabular reamers as described above. The distal femoral allograft fills the void created by bone stock loss (**Figure 4**, *C*).

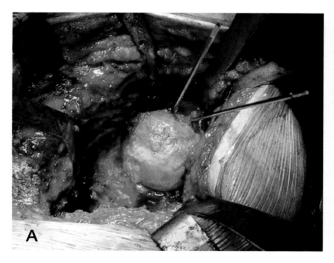
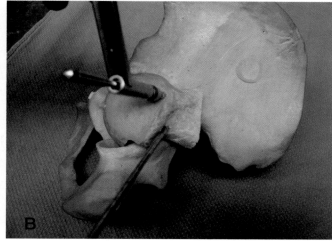

Figure 2   **A**, The femoral head allograft is hooked into the superior rim of the acetabulum and temporarily held in place with threaded pins or drill bits. **B**, A Sawbones (Pacific Research Laboratories, Vashon, WA) model representation.

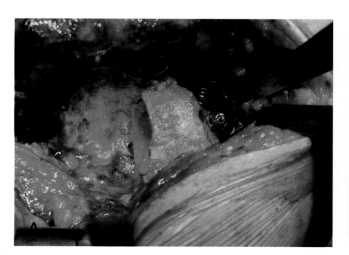
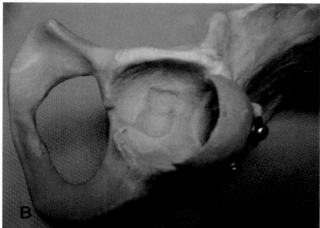

Figure 3   **A**, The femoral head allograft has been fixed to the host ilium with 5.5-mm cancellous screws, and a reamer has been used to recreate the acetabulum. **B**, A Sawbones model representation.

A whole acetabular transplant allograft, although rarely indicated in our experience, is used when there is massive circumferential host bone loss. Cut and shape the entire acetabular transplant allograft to allow placement into the host acetabulum (**Figure 5**). Cut the pubis, ischium, and iliac crest to reflect the host bone loss. Using a high-speed burr, create a trough on the backside of the graft to allow the graft to be locked into the bone remaining on the host acetabular rim. Impact the graft into position and

fix with 6.5-mm partially threaded cancellous screws with washers placed through the graft and into the host bone.

Prosthesis Implantation

After bone stock has been restored, an implant can be selected. The literature suggests that both uncemented sockets and antiprotrusio cages can be used if technical considerations are met. We do not recommend cementing polyethylene cups because of poor midterm and long-term results.

Newer implants, such as trabecular metal cups, may be indicated, but early results for these devices have not been published and therefore guidelines have not been established.

Uncemented acetabular components can be used successfully in conjunction with bulk structural allografts when there is sufficient host bone stock to allow ingrowth into the cup. This requires a minimum of 50% host bone stock with an intact posterior column. When less host bone stock is present, the implant of choice is the an-

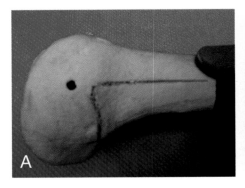
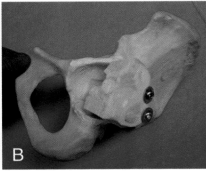
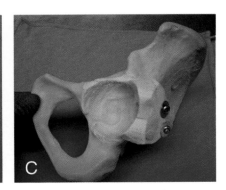

Figure 4　**A**, The numeral 7 is drawn on the distal femoral allograft. **B**, A Sawbones model representation of the distal femoral allograft fixed to host bone with 6.5-mm cancellous screws. **C**, An acetabular reamer removes excess allograft, and the deficient acetabular bone stock is restored in this Sawbones model representation.

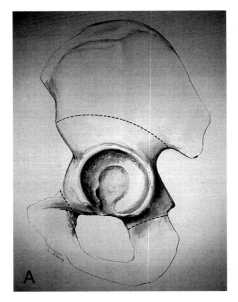
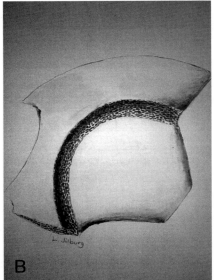
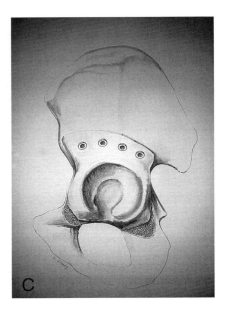

Figure 5　**A**, The whole acetabular transplant allograft is cut through the pubis, ischium, and ilium at locations determined by host bone stock loss. **B**, A trough is created on the undersurface of the acetabular allograft so that the graft can be locked into the host acetabulum. **C**, The acetabular allograft is fixed to the host bone with 6.5-mm cancellous screws. (Reproduced from Paprosky WG, Sekundiak TD: Total acetabular allografts. *Instr Course Lect* 1999;48:67-76.)

tiprotrusio cage. Good rim fit must be achievable when using an uncemented component, with the cup being stable between the anterior and posterior columns. Cups should be augmented with either peripheral or dome screw fixation. The principles of uncemented cup insertion in revision THA were detailed in an earlier chapter.

When using an antiprotrusio cage, it is critical to achieve fixation superiorly and inferiorly (ie, from the ilium to the ischium). Ischial fixation can be achieved by placing the ischial flange within the body of the ischium, or, conversely, using screw fixation. Once ischial fixation is achieved, screws are placed through the dome of the ring into either allograft or host bone. Finally, screws are placed through the superior flanges of the ring to achieve fixation to the ilium. A ring not fixed to host bone will be at increased risk of loosening over time as the allograft undergoes some degree of resorptive changes.

Postoperative Regimen

Patients requiring bulk structural allografts require postoperative care that is individualized to some degree. All patients should be maintained on postoperative intravenous antibiotic prophylaxis until all intraoperative cultures, including those from the allografts, are finalized. An increased risk of postoperative dislocation exists because of compromised soft tissues and deficient or absent abductors. Patients at increased risk for postoperative instability must be maintained on hip precautions for at least 3 months.

All patients require protected postoperative weight bearing, and toe-touch weight bearing is recommended for the first 6 weeks, followed by radiographic evaluation. Compliant patients can then begin graduated weight bearing, with 25% weight bearing for 3 weeks, followed by 50% weight bearing for 3 weeks. Noncompliant patients should be maintained on toe-touch weight bearing for 3 months.

Repeat radiographs are obtained 3 months postoperatively, and full weight bearing can begin if no concerns are raised on radiographic evaluation.

Avoiding Pitfalls and Complications

The use of bulk structural allograft reconstruction in complex acetabular revision is technically demanding. Adhering to technical principles minimizes some complications, but others are beyond the surgeon's control and arise because of the biologic processes involved with the use of structural allografts.

First, choosing appropriate allograft material is critical. Fresh frozen allograft and irradiated structural allograft constructs have both performed well in our experience, whereas freeze-dried allografts have not. We prefer using structurally strong, high-quality allografts, specifically whole acetabuli, distal femurs, and femoral heads. The femoral heads from male donors are often superior to those of osteopenic female donors.

To achieve long-term stability at the allograft-host bone junction, appropriate fixation and initial stability

at this interface are required. Both can be achieved by using large-fragment, 6.5-mm partially threaded cancellous screws and shaping the graft to the host bone to lock it into place. This procedure is described in greater detail earlier in this chapter. If stability of the construct cannot be achieved in the operating room, union will not occur and the graft will fail.

Some controversy exists regarding orientation of the graft to the host bone with respect to trabecular bone patterns and orientation of the screw fixation. Various techniques described in the literature almost uniformly achieve 95% to 100% union between the allograft and the host bone.

Most reported structural allograft construct failures do not occur because of nonunion. Rather, they occur because long-term fixation between the implant and the host-allograft acetabular construct fails. It is possible to minimize, although not eliminate, these failures. Cemented polyethylene acetabular components should be avoided when using large bulk structural allografts in acetabular revisions because these components have a higher failure rate than either uncemented cups or reconstruction rings.

Uncemented acetabular fixation can be successfully achieved by augmenting deficient bone stock with bulk structural allografts. Sufficient host bone stock is required to achieve long-term fixation, however. The literature suggests that a minimum of 50% host bone is necessary to achieve ingrowth into an uncemented socket. The posterior column also must be intact and able to support the uncemented component. Failure to adhere to the principles of uncemented cup fixation significantly increases failure rates.

When a structural allograft comprises more than 50% of the acetabu-

lum, a reconstructive cage provides the most predictable results. The cage must maximize host bone contact when possible. The cage must achieve inferior fixation into the ischium as well as superior fixation into the ilium, thus bridging the structural allograft. Reinforcement roof rings that do not allow ischial fixation have higher failure rates.

Certain complications arise that are representative of the biologic processes involved with the use of structural allografts. Most structural allografts uniformly undergo resorptive changes over time. The literature demonstrates that peripheral graft resorption ranging from 2 to 5 mm is not an uncommon occurrence. These resorptive changes naturally reduce support for the construct. Late failures occur when the selected component has not achieved adequate host bone stability.

Although the use of bulk structural allografts in acetabular revision is controversial, it remains a useful adjunct in treatment. Structural allografts unquestionably restore bone stock and have high rates of union. The ongoing challenge is achieving long-term component fixation. Applying the principles developed over the past 20 years using allografts in revision THA maximizes long-term success with this reconstructive technique. The use of structural allografts in complex acetabular revisions may diminish over time as new technologies develop, but their use will continue in massive acetabular defects requiring significant host bone stock restoration. When used appropriately, these allografts provide reproducible midterm results in these complex and challenging procedures.

■ References

DeWal H, Chen F, Su E, Di Cesare PE: Use of structural bone graft with cementless acetabular cups in total hip arthroplasty. *J Arthroplasty* 2003;18:23-28.

Garbuz D, Morsi E, Gross AE: Revision of the acetabular component of a total hip arthroplasty with a massive structural allograft. *J Bone Joint Surg Am* 1996;78:693-697.

Gill TJ, Sledge JB, Muller ME: The management of severe acetabular bone loss using structural allograft and acetabular reinforcement devices. *J Arthroplasty* 2000;15:1-7.

Gross AE, Duncan CP, Garbuz D, Mohamed EMZ: Revision arthroplasty of the acetabulum in association with loss of bone stock. *Instr Course Lect* 1999;48:57-66.

Jasty M, Harris WH: Salvage total hip reconstruction in patients with major acetabular bone deficiency using structural femoral head allografts. *J Bone Joint Surg Br* 1990;72:63-67.

Paprosky WG, Perona PG, Lawrence JM: Acetabular defect classification and surgical reconstruction in revision arthroplasty. *J Arthroplasty* 1994;9:33-44.

Paprosky WG, Sekundiak TD: Total acetabular allografts. *Instr Course Lect* 1999;48:67-76.

Saleh KJ, Jaroszynski G, Woodgate I, Saleh L, Gross AE: Revision total hip arthroplasty with the use of structural acetabular allograft and reconstruction ring. *J Arthroplasty* 2000;15:951-958.

Shinar AA, Harris WH: Bulk structural autogenous grafts and allografts for reconstruction of the acetabulum in total hip arthroplasty. *J Bone Joint Surg Am* 1997;79:159-168.

Zehntner MK, Ganz R: Midterm results (5.5-10 years) of acetabular allograft reconstruction with the acetabular reinforcement ring during total hip revision. *J Arthroplasty* 1994;9:469-479.

Coding					
CPT Codes				**Corresponding ICD-9 Codes**	
27134	Revision of total hip arthroplasty; both components, with or without autograft or allograft	996.4	996.66	996.77	
27137	Revision of total hip arthroplasty; acetabular component only, with or without autograft or allograft	996.4	996.66	996.77	

CPT copyright © 2004 by the American Medical Association. All Rights Reserved.

Chapter 44

Acetabular Revision: Cages and Rings

Allan E. Gross, MD, FRCSC
Stuart Goodman, MD, PhD

■ Indications

The goals of acetabular revision surgery are to restore anatomy and provide stable fixation for the new acetabular component. The quality of the existing bone stock is a key factor in surgical decision making. Protective rings help restore bone stock by providing a scaffold at the correct anatomic level to protect the graft while remodeling takes place and to provide a bed into which the cup is cemented.

Two types of rings can be used: (1) the roof reinforcement ring and (2) the antiprotrusio cage. The roof ring primarily protects the dome of the acetabulum and extends from the

ilium superiorly to the inferomedial aspect of the acetabulum (**Figure 1**). Use of the roof ring has decreased with the availability of better designs and larger sizes of uncemented acetabular components. The antiprotrusio cage is used for the reconstruction of much larger bone defects and extends from the ilium superiorly to the ischium inferiorly, spanning and protecting the entire acetabulum (**Figure 2**). This device can be used with morcellized or structural graft.

Rings and cages have certain advantages. They place the cup at the correct anatomic level and allow and protect morcellized or structural bone grafting. Cups are cemented into rings and cages, which allows for adjust-

ment of version independent of the ring and local delivery of antibiotics. Cement tends to penetrate the holes in the ring but only touches the surface of the impacted morcellized bone graft or the surface of structural graft; therefore, rings and cages are considered an uncemented reconstruction because the cement does not actually come into contact with host bone. Rings and cages can be used in irradiated bone and also allow for use of a constrained cup.

Cages and rings also have certain disadvantages. They can fracture or loosen early if not adequately supported by graft or host bone. Note that the rings and cages currently manufactured do not provide permanent bio-

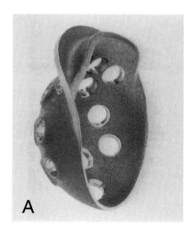
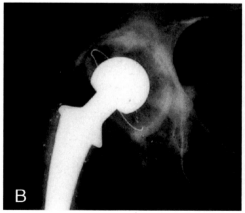
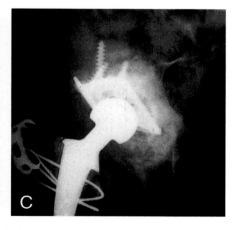

Figure 1 **A,** Roof reinforcement ring. **B,** Preoperative AP radiograph showing a loose acetabular component with contained bone defect. **C,** AP radiograph following reconstruction with morcellized allograft bone protected by a roof ring. Note that the roof ring is in contact with host bone superiorly and inferiorly.

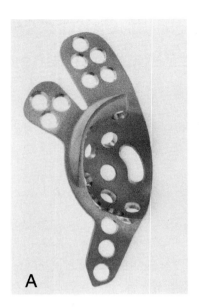
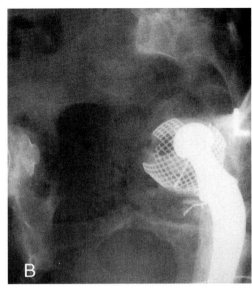
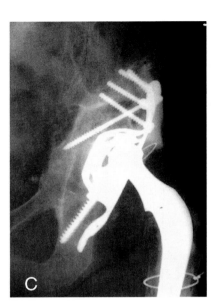

Figure 2   A, Antiprotrusio cage. **B,** Preoperative AP radiograph of a loose acetabular cemented cup with massive uncontained loss of bone stock. **C,** AP radiograph obtained 15 years postoperatively showing reconstruction with structural acetabular allograft protected by a cage.

logic fixation by bone ongrowth or ingrowth; thus, they can fail in the mid to long term. However, if failure occurs after the bone graft has remodeled and consolidated, revision with an uncemented component may be possible.

Bone stock deficiency can be defined as contained (cavitary) or uncontained (segmental). A contained defect is cavitary in that the acetabulum has expanded and weakened, but the columns are intact. A contained defect may be localized to only part of the acetabulum, or it may involve the entire acetabulum (ie, global defect). An uncontained defect is segmental in that there is full-thickness bone loss involving part of the acetabular rim and the adjacent anterior or posterior column. Uncontained defects may involve up to 50% or more of the acetabulum. With defects that involve less than 50% of the acetabulum, more surgical alternatives are available, and patients have a better prognosis. Most bone defects can be defined with radiographs. Specifically, Judet oblique views may be helpful to identify defects involving the columns. The final definition of the defect must be made

intraoperatively after removal of the old components.

Contained defects are usually treated with uncemented cups. Contact should be made with at least 50% bleeding host bone. If this is not possible, then morcellized allograft bone protected by a ring can be used. If the defect involves more than 50% of the acetabulum and contact with the inferomedial part of the host bone is possible, then a roof ring can be used. However, there is a fine line between using an uncemented cup and a roof ring. In some cases, additional reaming may increase contact with host bone, enough to use an uncemented cup. In contrast, when the contained defect affects the entire acetabulum and there is not enough contact with host bone (even with additional reaming and including the inferomedial host acetabulum), then a cage is necessary. A roof ring used under these circumstances will be sitting on morcellized bone inferomedially and eventually will toggle and become loose (**Figure 3**).

Some global contained defects are too large for jumbo (up to 90 mm in diameter) cups. Thus, the decision to

restore bone stock and use a cage is easily made. In other instances however, a large contained defect can be reamed enough so that it can accommodate a jumbo cup. In these circumstances the surgeon must decide whether to use a jumbo cup or restore bone stock and use a cage (**Figure 4**). The cage has a limited life span, but restoring bone stock at this time allows revision at the correct anatomic level the next time, potentially with an uncemented device. In a younger, higher demand patient, the cage may be a better choice. Morcellized allograft is typically used for contained defects, whereas structural grafts should be used only with uncontained (segmental) defects.

Uncontained defects that involve less than 50% of the acetabulum are usually superolateral and may extend anteriorly or posteriorly. These defects usually involve a weight-bearing area and can be managed by a high hip center, an oblong cup, or a structural graft that supports less than 50% of the cup. In these cases, the graft is relatively small and has a good prognosis (ie, cup and graft survival of 85% at 10 years) because it supports less

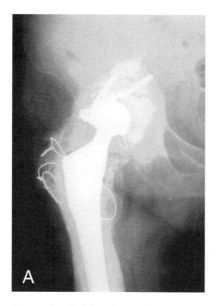
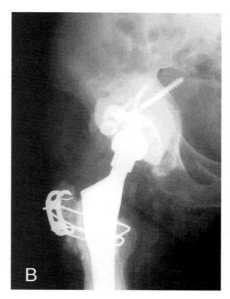
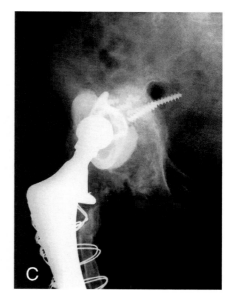

Figure 3   A, AP radiograph showing a loose cemented cup with contained bone defect. **B,** AP radiograph obtained after revision with morcellized allograft protected by a roof ring. Note that the ring is resting on the bone graft inferomedially. **C,** AP radiograph obtained 3 years postoperatively showing loosening as a result of failure to stabilize the ring by host bone inferomedially.

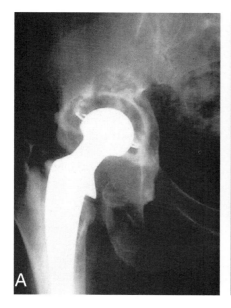
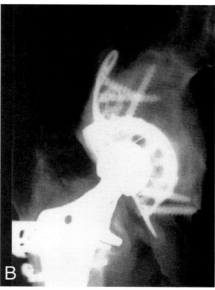

Figure 4   A, AP radiograph showing a loose acetabular component and a large contained bone defect. **B,** AP radiograph obtained 5 years postoperatively showing morcellized allograft bone protected by an antiprotrusio cage.

tive field on top of the structural graft where it meets the ilium to encourage union and remodeling.

Uncontained defects that involve more than 50% of the acetabulum are difficult to manage, and these patients have a guarded prognosis. The alternatives are a custom triflange cup or a large structural graft that replaces more than 50% of the acetabulum. We use a large structural graft (major column graft) and protect it with a cage.

Contraindications

There are no contraindications to the use of a cage or a ring.

Alternative Treatments

The use of trabecular metal has the potential to reduce the necessary amount of contact with host bone.

than 50% of the cup. The success of a structural graft in this situation is similar to that of a graft used to provide coverage for a cup in a primary THA done for congenital dislocation. This type of structural graft is called a shelf or minor column graft and is fixed by two 4.5-mm cancellous screws and used in conjunction with an uncemented cup. At some European centers, the graft is protected by a roof ring, but this has not been our practice. We place any morcellized autograft that is available in the opera-

Table 1 Results of Reconstruction With Cages or Rings

Author(s) (Year)	Number of Hips	Implant Type	Mean Patient Age (Range)	Mean Follow-up (Range)	Results
Kerboull, et al (2000)	53	Kerboull cage	57.7 years (24.8)	10 years (3 months–16 years)	90% success rate 3 loose cups
Gill, et al (2000)	63	Bürch-Schneider cage	63 years (41–83)	8.5 years (5–18)	90% success rate 5 repeat revisions
Perka and Ludwig (2001)	63	Bürch-Schneider cage	67.4 years (41–87)	5.45 years (3–10)	88% success rate with repeat revision or radiographic loosening as end point
Zehntner and Ganz (1994)	27	Roof reinforcement ring	72 years (52–87)	7.2 years (5.5–10)	80% survivorship at 10 years
Winter, et al (2001)	38	Bürch-Schneider cage	76 years (49–83)	7.3 years (4.2–9.4)	1 repeat revision for infection No loosening
Goodman, et al (2004)	61	Reconstruct ion ring, Bürch-Schneider cage	65 years (33–93)	4.6 years (2–17.8)	78% survivorship

Trabecular metal is a relatively new porous tantalum biomaterial that is being used as an acetabular shell in both primary and revision THA. Its porosity is similar to bone, and it may allow more effective bone ingrowth. It is feasible that this material will require less contact with bleeding host bone than conventional uncemented cups but medium- and long-term follow-up are needed. Another alternative is impaction grafting, a technique that involves cementing a cup onto a bed of impacted allograft bone. This technique is more accepted in Europe than in North America, and its advocates have reported excellent long-term results.

Uncontained defects involving less than 50% of the acetabulum can be managed by a high hip center, an oblong cup, or a minor column structural graft. Use of a high hip center requires reaming superiorly and medially to obtain cup coverage. Its advan-

tages are that it is technically easy, allows use of an uncemented cup, and rarely requires a bone graft. Disadvantages are that lengthening of the femur is necessary, bone stock is not restored, and the incidence of loosening on both the femoral and acetabular sides is higher. Excellent mid- to long-term results have been reported. The oblong or bilobed cup restores the cup to the correct level but does not restore bone stock. The midterm results have been good in some centers but not consistent.

Uncontained defects involving more than 50% of the acetabulum have fewer surgical solutions and a more guarded prognosis. The major column structural graft protected by a cage has already been described. An alternative is the custom triflange cup, but it is a complex procedure that does not restore bone stock. The clinical experience with this procedure is limited, but good midterm results have

been reported. This technique is described in more detail in chapter 47.

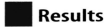

Results

Many reports support the use of protective rings and cages for revision arthroplasty of the acetabulum and have similar results (**Table 1**). The average follow-up is 5 to 10 years. For large contained and segmental defects, a cage rather than a roof ring must be used. Impacted morcellized allograft bone is used for contained defects, and structural allograft is used for large uncontained defects, especially those involving the dome and the posterior column. Large structural grafts should be fixed by screws and protected by a cage. In patients with an associated pelvic discontinuity, a posterior column plate should be considered in addition to the cage. Rings and cages must be firmly supported by graft or host bone. When following these principles, midterm (5 to 10 years) results should be at least 75% successful, with repeat revision rates of only 10% to 20%.

The results for contained and uncontained defects at our center have been reported separately. Morcellized bone protected by a roof ring was used for contained acetabular defects in 43 hips (average follow-up 5 years). Only one repeat revision was required, and four hips had asymptomatic loosening. A major column structural allograft was used in conjunction with a cage in eight patients who had an uncontained defect involving more than 50% of the acetabulum (average follow-up 7.5 years). Only one failure occurred as a result of infection. In a later study, we reported clinical and radiographic success in 10 hips in 13 (77%) patients (average follow-up 10.5 years).

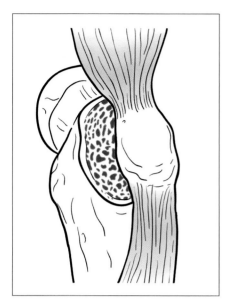

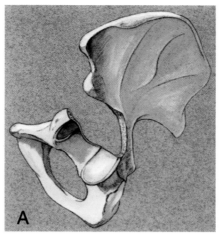

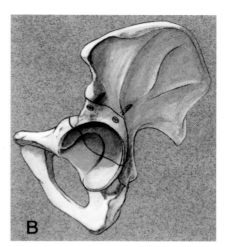

Figure 6 **A,** Segmental bone loss involving more than 50% of the acetabulum. **B,** The defect has been reconstructed with a structural acetabular allograft fixed by two cancellous screws. The graft will be protected by a cage.

Figure 5 The trochanteric slide. Note that the greater trochanter is maintained in a sling consisting of the gluteus medius and minimus proximally and the vastus lateralis distally.

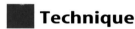 **Technique**

Exposure

A posterior or lateral (transgluteal) approach provides adequate exposure for insertion of a roof ring. Insertion of a cage, however, requires exposure of the ischium. We prefer a trochanteric osteotomy to expose the ischium, specifically the trochanteric slide because it has a lower incidence of trochanteric escape (**Figure 5**), but a posterior approach is adequate and can be converted to a trochanteric osteotomy if necessary. We use a trochanteric slide for all hips where a cage is used.

A trochanteric slide is performed through a straight lateral incision. After the fascia lata has been incised, the posterior border of the gluteus medius and minimus is identified and retracted anteriorly. The vastus lateralis is reflected off of the intermuscular septum 6 to 8 cm and reflected anteriorly 1 or 2 cm. We do not release the external rotators or posterior capsule. A trochanteric osteotomy is then performed using an oscillating saw, with

the osteotomy done posterior to anterior and exiting about 2 cm distal to the insertion of the vastus lateralis into the rough line (vastus ridge). To keep the posterior capsule and external rotators intact, we retain about 1 cm of bone posteriorly attached to the main femoral fragment. The main trochanteric fragment is retracted anteriorly, and a complete capsulectomy is done. The hip is dislocated anterolaterally but retracted posteriorly, and the trochanteric fragment is retracted anteriorly.

If additional exposure is required, a trochanteric slide can be converted to a transverse trochanteric osteotomy by releasing the vastus lateralis off of the trochanter so that the trochanter can be reflected superiorly. The ischium also can be exposed via an extended trochanteric osteotomy if a difficult femoral component removal is anticipated.

Bone Preparation

After the acetabular component and the membrane are removed, spherical reaming occurs. At this point, the surgeon must decide whether to use an uncemented cup, a roof ring, or a cage. A trial cup is inserted to determine whether at least 50% of the cup comes

into contact with bleeding host bone, particularly over the superior and posterior areas. With at least 50% coverage, an uncemented cup can be used. With less than 50% of the cup in contact with host acetabulum but sufficient bone superiorly and inferomedially, a roof ring can be used. If this is not possible, a cage is necessary. Most of this decision making is done preoperatively, but final confirmation occurs intraoperatively as described.

The nature of the defect dictates the type of bone graft used (cranial and posterior bone loss is most problematic). If the defect is uncontained and there is no more than 30% of cup coverage by host bone, then a structural graft is indicated. We prefer to use an acetabular allograft, but a male femoral head is also acceptable. We start with a whole acetabular allograft, gradually making it smaller and reshaping it to fit the defect. Radiographic matching of the pelvic allograft and the recipient is helpful but not necessary. The graft is fixed by two 6.5-mm cancellous screws inserted superiorly and posteriorly into the ilium (**Figure 6**). A finger placed in the sciatic notch protects the nerve. A cage is usually used with this large structural allograft. If a pelvic discontinuity has been demonstrated radiologically and intraoperatively, a posterior column plate should be considered along with the cage. The greater trochanter is then reattached with two 16-gauge cerclage wires.

With only 30% to 50% of cup coverage with host bone, a shelf (minor column) structural graft is used. This graft is fixed with two 4.5-mm cancellous screws and can be left unprotected, or it can be protected by a roof ring, depending on surgeon preference. The screws in the graft are directed in an oblique to vertical direction, and morcellized autograft or allograft is placed on top of the structural graft against the ilium to enhance union and remodeling. We prefer to use an uncemented cup, but some authors protect the graft by a roof ring. If there is any doubt as to whether the graft is supporting more or less than 50% of the cup, then a protective roof ring should be used. The diameter of the final reamer determines the outer diameter of the ring to be used. A structural graft may have to be reamed lightly, leaving the subchondral bone intact, to accommodate the outer diameter of the ring. When a structural graft is used, additional cavitary defects are filled with morcellized bone. The ring must be solidly supported by allograft or host bone. The optimal allograft bone for revision is deep frozen.

Prosthesis Implantation
ROOF RING

A roof ring must have host bone support both superoposteriorly and inferomedially (**Figure 7**, *A*); if not, a cage must be used. The outer diameter of the ring should correspond to that of the last reamer used. The ring is impacted into place and should feel solid before screws are inserted. The ring is then fixed by 6.5-mm fully threaded cancellous screws that are typically provided with the ring. The screws are inserted through the holes in the superior part of the ring, usually in a vertical to oblique direction and

should be anchored in host bone. At least three screws should be used (**Figure 7**, *B*). The cup is then cemented into the ring (**Figure 7**, *C*).

CAGE

A cage should be anchored onto the host ilium superiorly and ischium inferiorly. The ischium can be located by tracing down the posterior rim of the acetabulum. It is quite prominent as it extends out from the acetabular rim posteroinferiorly and can be cleared gently with an elevator for 1 or 2 cm for confirmation. The ligaments that come off of the ischium are encountered next, but caution is needed here because going beyond this point endangers the sciatic nerve.

A 3.2-mm hole is then drilled into the ischium at the point where the inferior flange of the cage is to be inserted. A depth gauge is inserted and should encounter bone for at least 2.5 to 3 cm (**Figure 8**). This also confirms the ischial anatomy. We prefer to slot the inferior flange into the ischium rather than on top so that the sciatic nerve does not have to be identified. If the flange is placed on top of the ischium and then fixed with screws, the nerve must be identified. The slot for the ischial flange is finished by drilling two more holes and connecting them with an osteotome. The muscle is cleared off of the ilium to create room for the superior flange(s).

Trial cages can be used, if available, to properly size the ring and determine whether the flanges need bending to make contact with host bone. The outer diameter of the cage should correspond to that of the last reamer used. The flanges should be bent in only one direction, or they will be weakened. Normally, the upper flanges have to be bent downward toward the ilium and the lower flange slightly upward to accommodate the shape of the ischium. The ischial flange is inserted first and then the cage is impacted, seating the superior flanges on the ilium (**Figure 9**). The

cage is then fixed with 6.5-mm fully threaded cancellous screws. One or two dome screws are inserted first to stabilize the cage superiorly. These screws may pass through structural graft on their way to host bone. The superior flanges are then fixed with three to five screws, and then one or two screws are inserted inferiorly through the cage into any available bone. These inferior screws are not absolutely necessary because the flange is slotted into the ischium.

POLYETHYLENE CUP

A polyethylene cup 2- or 3-mm smaller than the inner diameter of the ring is cemented into the ring or cage. Some cement penetrates the holes in the ring or cage and reaches the surface of the structural allograft or impacted allograft (**Figure 10**). The cup must be cemented in the correct anatomic position, regardless of the position of the cage or the ring. If indicated, a snap-in or constrained cup can be cemented into a ring.

Wound Closure

After the greater trochanter is wired, the fascia lata and subcutaneous tissue are closed with interrupted bioabsorbable sutures, and the skin is closed with staples.

Postoperative Regimen

Toe-touch weight bearing is maintained for 6 weeks followed by partial weight bearing (60 to 80 lb) for 6 weeks. Patients who cannot tolerate non–weight-bearing status can bear weight as tolerated. Intravenous antibiotics are administered for 5 days, and oral antibiotics are given for an additional 5 days. Gentle passive range-of-motion exercises are started at 2 to 3 days with no flexion beyond 70° and no adduction. Active abduction in the supine position is allowed at 6 weeks and against gravity at 12 weeks.

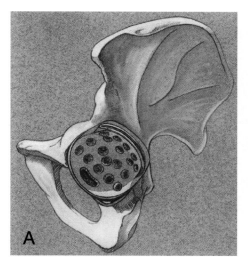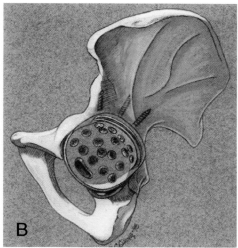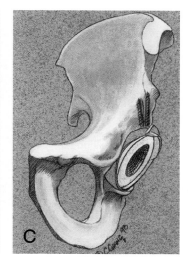

Figure 7 **A,** The roof ring is in contact with host bone superiorly and inferomedially. **B,** The ring is secured by at least three screws directed superiorly into the dome of the acetabulum. **C,** The cup is cemented into the ring. (© Copyright C. Chang, 1998.)

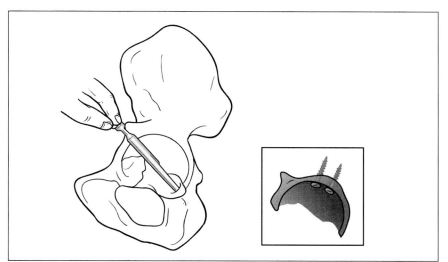

Figure 8 An osteotome creates a slot in the ischium for the inferior flange.

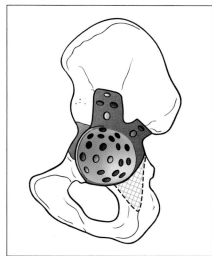

Figure 9 Placement of the cage with insertion of the inferior flange into the ischium and the superior flanges resting against the ilium. The cage is stabilized by screws into the dome, screws through the superior flanges into the ilium, and one or two screws into the inferior part of the cage adjacent to the inferior flange. The inferior flange is inserted into the ischium.

▪ Avoiding Pitfalls and Complications

We recently reviewed the records of 61 of our patients who required complex acetabular revision to evaluate complications associated with the cage. Of the 61 patients, 48 required a structural allograft and the rest morcellized allograft; average follow-up was 4.6 years. The complications we encountered were typical of those reported by other authors and representative of the problems of cages. In our series, none of the complications was associated with the use of structural or morcellized allograft bone, all of which healed uneventfully without radiographic evidence of resorption or fracture.

Twenty of the 61 patients had complications related to the use of the cage, but not all complications led to failure of the reconstruction. Six patients had sciatic nerve injuries, but all made significant partial or full recovery. In each case, the nerve injury occurred when the inferior flange was placed on top of the ischium rather than slotting it inside the ischium.

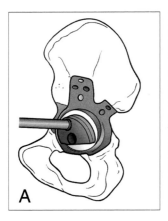
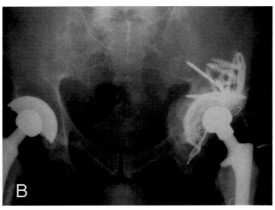

Figure 10 The cup is cemented to the cage with its position adjusted independent of the position of the cage.

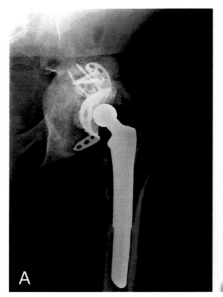
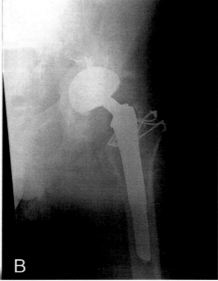

Figure 11 **A,** AP radiograph shows a loose cage several years after reconstruction with morcellized allograft bone. The graft has remodeled and restored bone stock. **B,** AP radiograph following a second revision with an uncemented cup at the correct anatomic level.

Placing the flange on top of the ischium puts it very close to the sciatic nerve, whereas slotting it inside the ischium keeps it well away from the nerve. In addition, when the flange is placed on top of the ischium, the cup is too lateralized. We now routinely slot the flange into the ischium.

Three rings had fractured flanges, one of which has been revised. This problem can be avoided by ensuring that the ring is solidly supported by host bone or bone graft. Seven hips dislocated, which can be avoided by orienting the cup independently of the position of the ring. Also in the multi-

ply operated hip with poor abductor function, a constrained cup can be cemented into the ring. Another preventive measure is use of a brace for 3 months following surgery. Three cups loosened requiring revision. We currently use a cup with cement spacers that have an outer diameter at least 2-mm smaller (excluding the spacers) than the inner diameter of the ring to enhance cement fixation.

Ten patients had a pelvic discontinuity associated with uncontained bone loss. A posterior column plate was not used. Of these 10 patients, three had rings that had loosened, and two had rings with fractured flanges. If a pelvic discontinuity can be demonstrated radiographically and intraoperatively, a cage should be used and it should be supplemented with a posterior column plate.

The most common complication related to the present generation of cages is loss of fixation. In our series, four cages lost fixation and required revision, and another three had fractured flanges, as described above. Loss of fixation occurs because this generation of cages does not achieve biologic fixation and really serves only as a buttress plate while the bone graft heals. If and when the metal fails, the bone graft may have incorporated enough to restore bone stock for an uncemented cup (**Figure 11**). Any motion between the cage or ring and host or grafted bone will eventually cause the cage or ring to loosen or fracture. In the future, cages and rings must be made of a material that achieves biologic fixation and provides a friendly environment for bone healing.

References

Garbuz D, Morsi E, Gross AE: Revision of the acetabular component of a total hip arthroplasty with a massive structural allograft. *J Bone Joint Surg Am* 1996;78:693-697.

Gill TJ, Sledge JB, Müller ME: The management of severe acetabular bone loss using structural allograft and acetabular reinforcement devices. *J Arthroplasty* 2000;15:1-7.

Goodman S, Saastomoinen H, Shasa N, Gross A: Complications of ilioischial reconstruction rings in revision total hip replacement. *J Arthroplasty* 2004;19:436-445.

Kerboull M, Hamadouche M, Kerboull L: The Kerboull acetabular reinforcement device in major acetabular reconstructions. *Clin Orthop* 2000;378:155-168.

Perka C, Ludwig R: Reconstruction of segmental defects during revision procedures of the acetabulum with the Bürch-Schneider anti-protrusio cage. *J Arthroplasty* 2001;16:568-574.

Saleh KJ, Jaroszynski G, Woodgate I, Saleh L, Gross AE: Revision total hip arthroplasty with the use of structural acetabular allograft and reconstruction ring: A case series with a 10-year average follow-up. *J Arthroplasty* 2000;15:951-958.

Winter E, Piert M, Volkmann R, et al: Allogeneic cancellous bone graft and a Bürch-Schneider ring for acetabular reconstruction in revision hip arthroplasty. *J Bone Joint Surg Am* 2001;83:862-867.

Woodgate IG, Saleh KJ, Jaroszynski G, et al: Minor column structural acetabular allografts in revision hip arthroplasty. *Clin Orthop* 2000;371:75-85.

Zehntner MK, Ganz R: Midterm results (5.5-10 years) of acetabular allograft reconstruction with the acetabular reinforcement ring during total hip revision. *J Arthroplasty* 1994;9:469-479.

Coding

CPT Codes		Corresponding ICD-9 Codes		
27130	Arthroplasty, acetabular and proximal femoral prosthetic replacement (total hip arthroplasty), with or without autograft or allograft	716.15 754.32 754.35 996.66	718.25 754.33 905.06 996.77	754.30 754.31 996.4
27132	Conversion of previous hip surgery to total hip arthroplasty, with or without autograft or allograft	716.15 754.32 754.35 996.66	718.25 754.33 905.06 996.77	754.30 754.31 996.4
27134	Revision of total hip arthroplasty; both components, with or without autograft or allograft	716.15 754.32 754.35 996.66	718.25 754.33 905.06 996.77	754.30 754.31 996.4
27137	Revision of total hip arthroplasty; acetabular component only, with or without autograft or allograft	716.15 754.32 754.35 996.66	718.25 754.33 905.06 996.77	754.30 754.31 996.4

CPT copyright © 2004 by the American Medical Association. All Rights Reserved.

Chapter 45

Acetabular Revision: Impaction Bone Grafting and Cement

Tom J.J.H. Slooff, MD, PhD
B. Willem Schreurs, MD, PhD
J.W.M. Gardeniers, MD, PhD

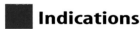 Indications

Acetabular bone impaction grafting is a hip reconstruction technique that is desirable from a biologic perspective. Based on the principle that bone stock loss should be restored by using tightly impacted, well-contained cancellous bone grafts, this method has been used since 1979, and long-term follow-up studies are now available.

Acetabular bone loss compromises the outcome in both primary and revision total hip arthroplasty (THA). Ideally, the surgeon should strive for reconstruction of this bone loss. The bone impaction grafting method, in combination with a cemented polyethylene cup, has been used for both complex primary and revision THA. This technique makes it possible to replace the bone stock loss and repair normal hip biomechanics and hip function with a standard implant. Although this technique works with all age groups, it is probably most beneficial for younger patients facing the possibility of future surgery.

Acetabular bone impaction grafting is suitable for both simple cavitary bone defects, as well as for extensive acetabular bone defects with loss of segmental structures such as the medial wall or the superolateral rim. In patients with acetabular wall or acetabular column defects, it is essential to use metal meshes to convert a combined segmental and cavitary defect into a contained defect. The impacted cancellous grafts adapt easily and closely to the irregularities of the host bone bed without gap formation. Even after tight impaction, the surface of the reconstructed bone bed is rough, and this facilitates cement interdigitation. Bone cement is pressurized to optimize cement extrusions into the graft, thus improving initial cup stability after the cup is inserted.

The incorporation process of these impacted morcellized bone grafts was studied both in animal experiments and in human biopsy specimens, with animal studies demonstrating almost complete incorporation of these grafts. To determine if this also occurs in humans, 24 acetabular bone biopsy specimens from 20 patients (21 hips) were examined. Biopsy specimens were obtained 3 months to 15 years after acetabular reconstruction in both complex primary and revision THA. Histology showed rapid revascularization of the graft, followed by osteoblast resorption and woven bone formation on graft remnants. New bone formation also occurred on fibrin accumulations or in the fibrous stroma that had invaded the graft. A mixture of graft, new bone, and fibrin was completely remodeled into a new trabecular structure with normal lamellar bone and remnants of graft material. In some patients, localized small areas of nonincorporated bone graft surrounded by fibrous tissue remained, regardless of the length of follow-up.

Acetabular bone impaction grafting is a demanding technique, especially with more extensive acetabular defects. Surgically related factors have a major effect on the outcome of revision procedures. We therefore strongly recommend that use of this technique be considered with relatively simple defects. Bone impaction grafting in simple cavitary defects is technically easy and reproducible, and favorable long-term results can be expected. Ongoing experience and familiarity with the technique's essentials permits more extensive defects to be successfully reconstructed.

Contraindications

Reconstruction using bone impaction grafting can be performed in a patient with septic loosening once the infection is treated. Bone impaction graft-

Table 1   Results of Acetabular Impaction Bone Grafting in Acetabular Revisions

Author(s) (Year)	Number of Hips	Implant Type	Mean Patient Age (Range)	Mean Follow-up (Range)	Results (End Point Cup Survival)
Schreurs, et al (2003)	35	Cemented polyethylene cups	57 years (31–73)	7.5 years (3–14)	85%, any reason 90%, aseptic loosening
Schreurs, et al (2004)	62	Cemented polyethylene cups	59 years (23–82)	16.5 years (15–20)	79%, any reason 84%, aseptic loosening
Schreurs, et al (2004; in press)	42	Cemented polyethylene cups	37 years (20–49)	17.5 years (15–23)	80%, any reason 91%, aseptic loosening

ing after treatment of infection is performed in a two-stage procedure. Stabilizing the fracture first is mandatory for acetabular revisions with pelvic dissociation. Bridging pelvic dissociation with thin metal mesh will fail; this fixation method is not adequate fracture treatment. Bone impaction grafting will fail in a high percentage of patients with bone stock loss or in patients whose hips have failed as a result of radiation therapy to the pelvis. Dead pelvic bone is not a suitable host bone bed for cancellous bone ingrowth, and the infection rate is also unacceptably high. Good results from bone impaction grafting cannot be obtained without basic knowledge of acetabular cementation techniques.

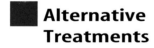

Alternative Treatments

Many options exist for acetabular revision. For example, cement-only reconstruction may be indicated in elderly patients with a limited life expectancy. Many different techniques and implants for uncemented reconstructions are also available. Impacted bone grafts have been described in combination with metal shells, recon-

struction rings, and uncemented cups. Although we have no experience with these alternative methods, adverse outcomes have been experienced as a result of seemingly small modifications of the original bone impaction grafting technique.

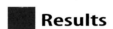

Results

Table 1 presents the outcomes for acetabular bone impaction grafting reconstruction presented in a 10- to 15-year follow-up study. Recently, the study was updated to include results at 15- to 20-year follow-up. Between 1979 and 1986, 62 acetabular reconstructions were performed in 58 consecutive patients with failed hip prostheses. One patient was lost to follow-up at review. The indications for revision hip surgery were aseptic loosening (57) and septic loosening (4). Defects were classified as cavitary (38) and combined cavitary-segmental (23, 10 central defects and 13 peripheral wall defects).

The Kaplan-Meier survivorship rate for cups with end point revisions (regardless of reason) was 79% at 15-year follow-up (95% CI, 67% to 91%). Excluding two revisions performed for

septic loosening at 3 years and 6 years, the Kaplan-Meier survivorship rate for end point aseptic loosening was 84% at 15 years (95% CI, 73% to 95%). Most patients appeared stable radiologically and none demonstrated radiologic loosening at the time of review (**Figure 1**). However, during follow-up, three patients with radiologic loosening died, but these patients had not undergone revision because their complaints were mild. At review, seven patients with acetabular reconstructions showed stable radiolucent lines in one or two zones.

We concluded from this long-term follow-up that the bone impaction grafting technique is a safe, adequate method of reconstruction of acetabular bone defects encountered in revision surgery for failed acetabular implants.

Patients with rheumatoid arthritis and an acetabular revision may also benefit from this procedure. Revision of a failed cup in patients with rheumatoid arthritis is very difficult because bone quality is so poor. Uncemented cup revisions in patients with rheumatoid arthritis demonstrate very high failure rates at midterm follow-up. Current literature indicates that the best results are obtained with simple recementation or bone impaction grafting with a cemented cup.

In a series of 28 patients with rheumatoid arthritis who underwent 35 consecutive acetabular revisions using bone impaction grafting and a cemented cup, acetabular bone stock defects were classified according to the AAOS system as cavitary (11) or combined segmental/cavitary (24). No patient was lost to follow-up, but 5 patients (6 hips) had died by the time of review. Patients were reviewed at a minimum follow-up of 3 years (range, 3 to 14 years), with average follow-up of 7.5 years. At an average follow-up of 7 years, 6 months, repeat revisions were performed in 6 patients (6 hips). Using the Kaplan-Meier analysis tool for this technique, and excluding sep-

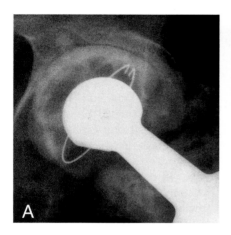
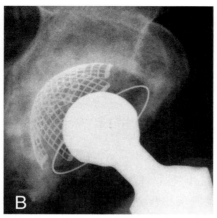
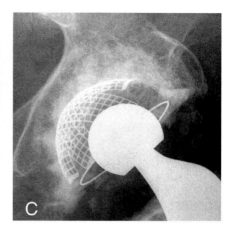

Figure 1 **A**, Preoperative AP radiograph of a pelvis showing a failed cemented cup that had been inserted for secondary osteoarthritis after an acetabular fracture in a 53-year-old man. **B**, A revision of both components was performed one month later, using acetabular bone impaction grafting and two femoral heads. Metal mesh was used on top of the bone graft. Metal mesh is no longer used on top of bone grafts and is the only modification of the technique in our 25 years of experience. **C**, Radiograph obtained 20 years after the reconstruction demonstrates no signs of acetabular loosening. The cup is stable with a radiologic incorporation of the grafts. The patient had two femoral revisions during 20 years of follow-up.

tic loosenings, at a follow-up of 8 years, the survival rate for aseptic loosening was 90% (95% CI, 80% to 100%).

Technique

Exposure

We generally use the posterolateral approach in which the patient is in a lateral position to perform acetabular bone impaction grafting, but other approaches can also be used. Extensive exposure of the acetabulum is mandatory. Trochanteric osteotomy is seldom necessary when using the posterolateral exposure. Identification of major anatomic landmarks is essential because normal anatomy may have been disturbed by previous surgeries and resultant scar tissue. These landmarks are the tip of the greater trochanter, the lesser trochanter, the tendinous part of the gluteus maximus, the lower border of the gluteus medius and minimus, and the sciatic nerve. Fluid for Gram stain may be aspirated from the hip. Femoral fractures can be prevented by performing a release of the proximal femur before dislocating the hip.

Wide exposure of the acetabulum is essential. All scar tissue is removed, and a circumferential capsulotomy is performed. The tendon of the iliopsoas muscle is released, if necessary. The failed implant can now be visualized and removed while preserving as much bone stock as possible. Biopsy specimens of the interface are obtained for bacterial cultures and intraoperative frozen sections. Systemic antibiotics are administered after all cultures are obtained. The interface membrane and bone cement remnants, if appropriate, are then thoroughly removed from the acetabulum using sharp spoons and curettes.

Bone Preparation

Meticulous inspection of the entire acetabulum is necessary to identify all bone stock defects (**Figure 2**). The transverse ligament, nearly always present, can be used as a landmark. A retractor beneath this ligament facilitates reconstruction. A trial cup is positioned against the ligament in the optimal and desired position, making it easy to detect the extent of any existing superolateral rim defect. Defects of both the medial wall and the rim should be reconstructed with flexible

stainless steel mesh (Acetabular X-Change mesh, Stryker-Howmedica, Newbury, England).

The mesh is adapted to the defects and trimmed to size using special scissors, clamps, and pliers. Peripheral rim mesh is placed on the outer side of the pelvic bone (**Figure 3**). The overlying muscles (abductors) can be elevated from the pelvic bone with only limited risk of neurovascular damage. The peripheral mesh should be fixed to the pelvic bone using at

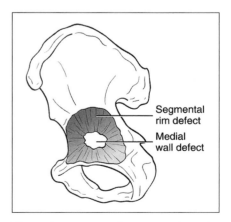

Figure 2 Diagram of a segmental rim defect and medial wall defect after removal of the failed acetabular component and the fibrous interface.

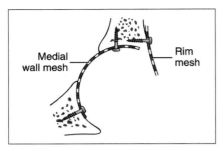

Figure 3 Flexible stainless-steel mesh is used to close the segmental defects. The rim mesh at the peripheral segmental defect should be fixed with at least three small screws to secure rigidity. The medial wall mesh may be fixed with screws, although this is not always necessary.

least three screws. Self-drilling and self-tapping screws are recommended because they are easier to use. Holding the trial cup in place during this part of the procedure helps determine the correct orientation of the mesh. The screws should be perpendicular to the pelvic bone to optimize the grip.

Medial wall mesh (if needed) is also trimmed to the proper size. To prevent fractures during the impaction process, it is recommended that a mesh be placed on the medial wall, especially if it is weak but intact. Vigorous impaction should not be diminished because the surgeon fears a medial wall fracture. Instead, the medial wall should be reinforced. Screw fixation is not always needed for medial wall mesh if perfect, stable fit of the mesh is obtained.

After the segmental defects are closed, the acetabulum is contained, and the reconstruction with bone grafts can begin once the host bone is prepared. Sclerotic areas in the acetabulum should be penetrated using multiple small but superficial drill holes (about 2-mm diameter). The drill holes create better surface contact between the donor bone bed and the graft and improve the possibilities for graft revascularization. The acetabulum can be cleaned just before impaction using pulsatile lavage.

Bone Graft Preparation

The ideal bone chips for acetabular bone impaction grafting are pure, cancellous, fresh frozen bone chips with a diameter of 0.7 to 1.0 cm. Our long-term experience is entirely based on use of fresh frozen trabecular bone chips produced by hand with a rongeur. However, this is a tedious, time-consuming part of the procedure, and it is tempting to use a bone mill. Although commercial bone mills can be used, most mills produce chips that are not optimal for the acetabulum (2 to 6 mm). A bone mill that produces 7- to 10-mm chips is now available (Noviomagus Bone Mill, Spierings Medical Technique, Nijmegen, The Netherlands).

All soft tissue and cartilage must be removed from the femoral head before milling because their presence will reduce the stability of the reconstruction and hamper the incorporation. Our only experience is with fresh frozen trabecular bone grafts made from femoral head allografts. However, it may be necessary to use a combination of trabecular and cortical bone or radiated bone, because experience with freeze-dried bone and bone impaction grafting is limited.

Bone Graft Impaction and Prosthesis Implantation

After lavage of the host bone, the contained acetabulum is packed tightly with bone chips. If necessary, small irregular cavities are filled and impacted using the small impactors. Then the entire cavitary defect is reconstructed layer by layer (**Figure 4**). The grafts are impacted using the specially designed acetabular impactors (Acetabular X-Change, Stryker-Howmedica) and a hammer. The graft layer should be at least 5-mm thick; otherwise, cement intrusion through the thin bone layer will hamper bone graft incorporation. During impaction the most caudal part of the new bone bed at the level of the transverse ligament should be reconstructed. The last im-

pactor used is oversized (2 to 4 mm) relative to the planned cup diameter to obtain a sufficient cement layer. During preparation of the antibiotic-loaded bone cement (Surgical Simplex, Stryker-Howmedica), pressure on the reconstructed acetabulum is maintained with the impactor last in use. Bone cement is pressurized after insertion by using a seal, just as in a primary cemented THA (**Figure 5**, A). The cup is then inserted and pressure is maintained until the cement is polymerized (**Figure 5**, B).

Wound Closure

After reduction of the hip joint, the surgical area should be inspected for bleeding vessels. All bone graft remnants and cement particles should be meticulously removed by intensive pressure lavage. A suction drain should remain in the hip joint area. If possible, we try to reconstruct the posterior capsule and the external rotators. Meticulous closure of the fascia, the subcutaneous layer, and the skin is essential.

Postoperative Regimen

We used to require 6 weeks of bed rest for patients with acetabular reconstruction. Currently, however, our protocol requires 2 days of bed rest followed by mobilization on two crutches, with touch toe weight bearing for the first 6 weeks. We establish both clinical and radiologic control of recovery. Patients then spend 6 weeks on crutches with 50% weight bearing. Patients are permitted to bear full weight at 12 weeks.

The only exceptions to this postoperative protocol are for patients whose medial walls were not adequately reconstructed and whose reconstruction may thus tend to migrate medially when they start weight bearing and for patients with extensive reconstructions.

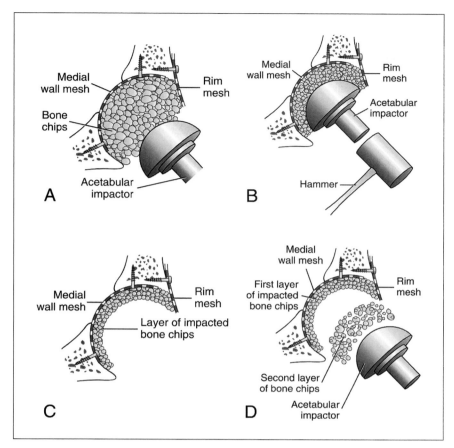

Figure 4 **A**, Fresh frozen morcellized bone chips with a size of 7 to 10 mm are recommended for acetabular reconstruction. Metal impactors in several diameters are used. **B**, The bone chips are tightly compressed using a hammer. **C**, After the first impaction, the layer is inspected. This layer sticks to the surrounding bone after the impactor is removed. **D**, A second layer of chips is impacted on the first layer, and the entire defect is reconstructed layer by layer.

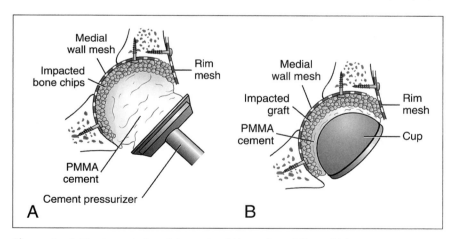

Figure 5 **A**, The impacted graft layer should be at least 0.5-cm thick to prevent cement penetration through the graft. Bone cement is introduced in a relatively viscous state and is pressurized to force bone cement into the graft. **B**, Illustration of cup placement with a reconstruction of the cup at the anatomic level.

Avoiding Pitfalls and Complications

Although bone mills are an option for producing the chips needed for reconstruction, there are several possible pitfalls. First, if using a mill and producing chips from fresh frozen femoral heads, the head should be cleaned of all soft tissue and cartilage. Cartilage particles remaining in the femoral head, if milled and included in the morcellized bone, will hamper the reconstruction's mechanical behavior. Human biopsy specimens demonstrate that these particles will never incorporate and will remain as pieces of cartilage within the reconstructed bone.

Second, most commercial bone mills produce bone chip particles between 2 and 5 mm. These sizes can be used on the femoral side because the dimensions of the grafts are limited by the diameter of the femoral canal. On the acetabular side, however, it is essential to use bone chips with a diameter of 7 to 10 mm. Smaller chips will produce acetabular reconstructions with less initial stability.

The bone impaction technique is also important. We use an impaction technique with specially designed impactors and a solid hammer. Bone impaction grafting using compression on an acetabular reamer rotating in the reverse direction to impact the graft will result in strongly reduced cup stability. It has been demonstrated in an experimental setting that the initial cup migration is two to three times higher when this modification of the original technique is used, especially when reverse reaming is combined with "slurry grafts" (1 to 3 mm).

■ References

Donk van der S, Buma P, Slooff TJJH, Gardeniers JWM, Schreurs BW: The incorporation process of impacted morsellized bone graft in cemented acetabular reconstruction: A study based on 24 human biopsies. *Clin Orthop* 2001;396:31-41.

Schreurs BW, Bolder SBT, Gardeniers JWM, et al: Acetabular revision with impacted morselized bone grafting and cemented cup: A 15 to 20 year follow-up of 62 revision arthroplasties. *J Bone Joint Surg Br* 2004;86:492-497.

Schreurs BW, Thien TM, de Waal Malefijt MC, et al: Acetabular revision with impacted morsellized cancellous bone graft and a cemented cup in patients with rheumatoid arthritis. *J Bone Joint Surg Am* 2003;85:647-652.

Schreurs BW, Slooff TJ, Gardeniers JWM, Buma P: Acetabular reconstruction with bone impaction grafting and a cemented cup: 20 years' experience. *Clin Orthop* 2001;393:202-215.

Slooff TJJH, Huiskes R, van Horn J, Lemmens AJ: Bone grafting in total hip replacement for acetabular protrusion. *Acta Orthop Scand* 1984;55:593-596.

Coding

CPT Codes		Corresponding ICD-9 Codes		
27130	Arthroplasty, acetabular and proximal femoral prosthetic replacement (total hip arthroplasty), with or without autograft or allograft	718.65	996.4	996.77
27132	Conversion of previous hip surgery to total hip arthroplasty, with or without autograft or allograft	718.65	996.4	996.77
27134	Revision of total hip arthroplasty; both components, with or without autograft or allograft	718.65	996.4	996.77
27137	Revision of total hip arthroplasty; acetabular component only, with or without autograft or allograft	718.65	996.4	996.77

CPT copyright © 2004 by the American Medical Association. All Rights Reserved.

Chapter 46
Acetabular Revision: Oblong Cups

Michael J. Christie, MD
David K. DeBoer, MD
J. Craig Morrison, MD

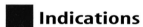 **Indications**

Acetabular reconstruction in the presence of significant bone loss is a reconstructive challenge. Reconstructive techniques can be classified into two major categories: defect matching and defect bridging. Defect-matching techniques achieve stability on host bone by shaping the defect to match the implant or by using bone grafts to fill the defect and bring the bone to the implant. Structural allografts fitted intraoperatively to match large defects are a common treatment choice. The allograft fills the defect, allowing the defect to be matched to the implant's shape. Long-term graft incorporation is unpredictable, however, and structural allografts without adjunctive fixation with a cage-type device will fail.

The most common defect-matching technique is reaming the acetabulum into a hemisphere. Many defects are small enough to be "reamed away." The acetabulum is then reconstructed with a large-diameter, rim-fit hemispherical cup. In patients with significant deficiency, reaming up to match the defect would result in significant bone loss to the anterior and/or posterior columns of the acetabulum. Despite these limitations, hemispherical cups in revision acetabuloplasty have outcomes approaching those of primary surgery

and should be used if bone loss is minimal.

Another defect-matching, non-hemispherical solution is the oblong cup. It is designed to achieve mechanical stability on host bone and thereby avoid the use of structural allograft while also restoring the normal anatomic hip center and creating better hip biomechanics to improve functional outcome. The cup is porous coated for uncemented fixation with adjunctive dome and rim screw fixation.

Loosening of a failed acetabular component is often accompanied by superior migration and an acetabular rim defect. The oblong cavity created by this migration inspired the design of the oblong cup. Although the shape of the cup is unique and better matched to the defect, the principles used to achieve support and initial stability are identical to those in revisions using hemispherical cups.

The primary indication for use of an oblong cup is an isolated superior rim defect (AAOS type I) too large to be easily converted into an oversized hemisphere (**Figure 1**). Although conversion of smaller rim defects into hemispheres is the most common method used for revision and has excellent long-term results, converting larger defects into hemispheres requires sacrificing a great

deal of host bone. In the most extreme instances, this results in reaming away the anterior and/or posterior columns. The oblong cup better matches the existing bone defect, limiting the amount of bone to be removed to that necessary to match the more symmetrically shaped bilobular prosthesis. Analysis of the bone sacrifice required to implant an oblong cup versus a jumbo cup in a superiorly deficient acetabulum indicates that bone retention is considerably higher with the oblong cup (**Table 1**).

The oblong cup is also indicated in circumstances in which the rim defect is accompanied by contained cavitary defects (AAOS type III). In these defects, it is necessary to ensure that the oblong cup rests on a supporting rim of acetabular bone sufficient to withstand weight-bearing loads. Rim and dome screws can be used as adjunctive fixation; however, to ensure cup stability and fixation, a supporting rim of bone is an absolute necessity.

Indications for use of the cup can also include superior rim defects with medial wall deficiency but only if the cup can be adequately supported by the acetabular rim. In patients with discontinuity, the oblong cup can be used only where the discontinuity can be stabilized with plates and adequate acetabular rim bone remains for implant support.

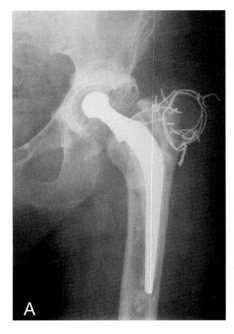
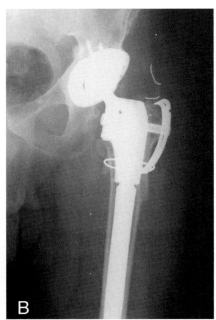

Figure 1   Radiographs of a failed THA with a superior defect preoperatively **(A)** and 3 years after reconstruction with an oblong cup **(B)**.

Table 1   Comparison of Bone Loss Required in Placement of an Oblong Cup Versus a Jumbo Hemispherical Cup for a Superiorly Deficient Acetabulum in Revision THA

Oblong Cup Versus Jumbo Hemispherical Cup	Mean Bone Saved (mm)			Volume difference		Joint Center Difference (mm)
	Anterior	Posterior	Medial	mL	%	
E-15*	8.65	8.65	8.65	35.1	30.7	7.5
E-25**	8.78	8.8	12.6	64.95	42.6	12.5

*15 mm of elongation
**25 mm of elongation

The oblong cup may occasionally be indicated in primary total hip arthroplasty (THA). For example, when a superior acetabular defect is present and there is insufficient femoral bone stock for autograft, an oblong cup may offer an ideal solution for a patient who has had an acetabular fracture with concurrent femoral head osteonecrosis. Patients who have developmental dysplasia of the hip with a Crowe III acetabulum may also be good candidates for this prosthesis because they exhibit superior acetabular bone deficiency in combination with poor femoral head bone quality, making autograft a less attractive option.

Contraindications

Although the oblong cup works well in the above-noted situations, it has performed poorly in several situations, and alternative means of reconstruction are recommended. These include situations in which Köhler's line is disrupted, there is evidence of pelvic discontinuity not amenable to stabilization with a plate, or when the previous reconstruction involved use of structural allograft and revision would require supporting the oblong cup on this allograft. In these situations, a custom-designed flanged component that attains stability through bony contact with the ilium, ischium, and pubis is our choice for more reliable and stable fixation.

Alternative Treatments

The goals of acetabular reconstruction are to achieve implant stability on host bone, restore the anatomic hip center, and preserve the native bone stock. Three reconstructive methods are available if the defect is too large to be reconstructed using a hemispherical device: using an oblong cup; placing a smaller hemispherical cup into the defect (the "high hip center" technique); and filling the defect with allograft or a mechanical bone substitute. Of the three methods, the oblong cup is best able to simultaneously achieve all three acetabular reconstruction goals (**Table 2**). It attains stability on host bone with a minimum of bone loss while maintaining or restoring the hip center to its native position.

Numerous studies have identified a high rate of loosening when acetabular components lack sufficient native bone contact and are instead supported primarily by bone grafts. In a series of 44 patients (46 hips) in which superior defects were revised by placing the acetabular component at least 35 mm above the interteardrop line (the so-called "high hip center" technique), only one patient (one hip) required revision for loosening and another was pending revision at a mean 10-year follow-up. Although the hip center's postoperative location (mean, 43 mm proximal to the inter-teardrop line) was virtually unchanged compared with its preoperative location (44.5 mm proximal), the prevalence of a positive Trendelenburg sign was reduced from a preoperative 98% to 44% at the most recent follow-up. The authors concluded that high placement of the acetabular cup does not adversely affect abductor function.

Despite satisfactory short-term results with bulk structural allograft, long-term survival of the reconstruction is poor. In another series of 62 patients (70 hips) treated with structural allograft and a cemented acetabular component at a mean follow-up of 16.5 years, there were several mechanical failures (10 of 15 hips) despite initial union of all grafts. Components supported by graft over more than 50% of the contact area had a significantly higher rate of loosening than components supported by host bone.

Mechanical bone substitutes, such as Trabecular Metal (Implex, Cedar Knolls, NJ; Zimmer, Warsaw, IN), offer a promising alternative to allograft for filling acetabular defects. The potential advantages of this material include its inherent permanent structural integrity and the high potential for bone ingrowth at the interface due to the friction generated by the terminal ends of the structural members. Potential disadvantages include the complexity of intraoperatively shaping the material to match the defect and the possibility of altering the material's frictional qualities during this shaping, thereby decreasing the potential for bone ingrowth. Early data are encouraging.

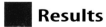

Results

The few published results for the oblong cup indicate that careful patient selection yields good outcomes (**Table**

Table 2 Comparison of Treatment Options for Reconstruction of Superior Defects in Complex THA

Revision Goal	Oblong Cup	Allograft	High Hip Center
Stability on host bone	Yes	No	Yes
Restoration of hip center	Yes	Yes	No
Preservation/addition of bone stock	Yes	Yes	Yes

Table 3 Results of Oblong Cups

Author(s) (Year)	Number of Hips	Implant Type	Mean Patient Age (Range)	Mean Follow-up (Range)	Results
DeBoer and Christie (1998)	15 revision 3 primary	oblong cup	65 years (41–82)	4.5 years (3.4–6.9)	0 revisions 0 loose
Chen, et al (2000)	37 revision	oblong cup	61.7 years (34–84)	3.4 years (2–5.5)	2 revisions 9 loose
Berry, et al (2000)	38 revision	oblong cup	60.5 years (35–88)	3 years (2–5)	1 revision 0 loose

3). Berry and associates reported a series of 38 revision THAs followed for a mean of 3 years during which one patient (one hip) underwent revision for loosening. The oblong cup in this hip rested on less than 50% structural allograft from a previous revision. All other patients were stable at latest follow-up, and Harris hip scores improved significantly. The hip center was brought to a more normal position in all patients without the need for allograft.

Chen and associates reported on 34 patients (37 hips) who underwent revision using an oblong cup and were followed for a mean of 41 months. Two patients (two hips) underwent revision for loosening. Seven additional cups were considered loose or probably loose, and 8 of 9 hips demonstrated a disrupted Köhler's line (a Paprosky type IIIB defect) on preoperative radiograph, indicating significant medial wall bone loss. All patients had improvement in vertical position of the hip center.

We reviewed the results of our first 50 patients (23 women, 27 men) who received the oblong cup as part of either a primary or revision THA. All surgeries were performed by the two senior authors and involved placement of an off-the-shelf oblong cup prosthesis in either the 15 or 25 mm of elongation (E-15 or E-25 configuration, respectively). At the most recent review, 11 patients were deceased, and 6 were considered lost to follow-up, leaving 33 patients (33 hips) available for review. Mean follow-up was 6.6 years (range, 3 to 12 years). Twenty-four arthroplasties were primary surgeries, and 26 were revision surgeries. Surgeries were performed on the right side in 35 patients and on the left side in 15 patients.

Two patients (two hips, or 6%) in this series (both revision THAs) have been revised again because of loosening. The first patient underwent a second revision 10 years postoperatively because of buttock and groin pain with all weight-bearing activities and pro-

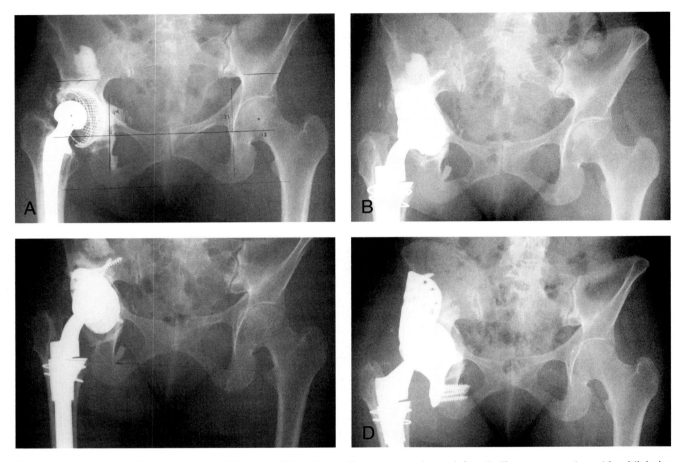

Figure 2   **A,** A 61-year-old woman has a failed right THA with significant superior bone defect. **B,** The reconstruction with a bilobular prosthesis initiallyappeared stable. **C,** However, 10.5 years after the revision there was evidence of migration and loosening. **D,** The patient then underwent re-revision to a custom flanged acetabular component and exchange of the modular stem without removal of the well-fixed proximally coated sleeve on the femoral side.

gressive loosening and superomedial migration of the component. Comorbidities included history of stroke, cervical fusion, and pulmonary embolus following previous THA. The patient had four previous arthroplasty procedures. The revision THA included placement of a custom-designed, flanged component and stem exchange without removal of the well-fixed, proximally coated sleeve of the modular femoral component (**Figure 2**). Two years later, the patient continues to ambulate with a significant limp and has good pain relief and excellent range of motion. Another patient with the underlying diagnosis of rheumatoid arthritis and three previous THAs had a second revision at approximately 9 years post-

operatively because of osteolysis and loosening (**Figure 3**). This re-revision arthroplasty also included placement of a custom flanged component as well as femoral head ball exchange.

No other hips are considered loose or are pending revision. Criteria for evaluating osseointegration include absence of progressive radiolucent lines, migration, or broken screws. Radiographic review of 31 patients (31 unrevised hips) with minimum follow-up indicates that the cup remains stable at midterm, with 5 patients (5 hips) demonstrating small nonprogressive radiolucent lines and 5 patients (5 hips) demonstrating polyethylene wear but no migration or progressive radiolucency.

Three patients (three hips) have had additional surgery for placement of new polyethylene liners, with one hip implant exchanged for a constrained insert at 4 months because of recurrent dislocation, and two hips demonstrating excessive polyethylene wear, both at approximately 9 years postoperatively.

The oblong cup allows the hip center to be returned to a more anatomic location without sacrificing host bone at revision. We analyzed hip center correction with the oblong cup. Vertical migration of the prosthetic hip center in 14 patients (14 hips) with a superior defect was compared to the native contralateral hip center preoperatively and postoperatively.

The average preoperative vertical migration of the hip center was 45.7 mm (range, 25 to 72 mm) above the interteardrop line. This compared to an average 18.8 mm (range, 13 to 25 mm) for the native contralateral hip. Postoperatively, the reconstructed hip center improved to 20.7 mm (range, 14 to 31 mm) above the interteardrop line. Horizontal migration of the hip center was also evaluated and found to be near anatomic after reconstruction. The average postoperative difference between the reconstructed hip center and the native hip center was 5.2 mm.

This series included 24 patients (24 hips) implanted with the oblong cup as part of a primary THA. Three patients died prior to achieving minimum follow-up, and 2 patients were lost to follow-up, leaving 19 patients to be followed for a mean of 5 years (range, 3 to 8 years). Patient age was an average 59 years at time of primary THA (range, 23 to 85 years). The indications for implantation were developmental dysplasia of the hip (7 patients), posttraumatic arthritis (8 patients), osteoarthritis (4 patients), osteonecrosis of the femoral head (2 patients), postpolio syndrome (2 patients), and septic arthritis (1 patient).

At latest follow-up, all patients reported improvement in hip pain and function. Eight patients walked without a limp, five had a slight limp, four had a moderate or severe limp, and two were nonambulatory for reasons unrelated to the surgery. Fourteen patients report no pain, and five patients rate their pain as slight. No patient has moderate or severe pain.

Nonprogressive radiolucent lines were present in two of these patients (11%) with minimum 3-year radiographic follow-up. Two patients (two hips) had polyethylene wear at latest follow-up, both less than 2 mm, with neither demonstrating signs of osteolysis. One patient had heterotopic ossification.

Complications include two dislocations, one treated successfully

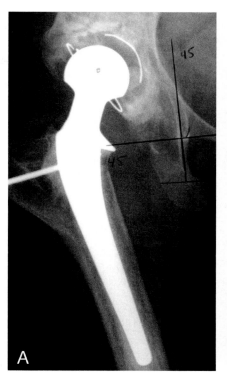
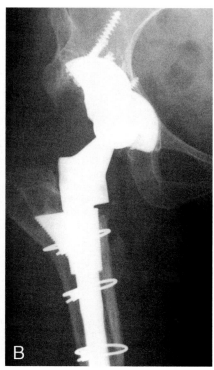

Figure 3 **A,** AP radiograph obtained 11 years after primary THA with cemented components shows osteolysis and component loosening. **B,** Nine years later, the hip demonstrates polyethylene wear but no loosening.

with closed reduction and the other converted to a constrained liner at 4 months postoperatively. In another patient, a sciatic nerve palsy developed secondary to limb lengthening. No cup has been removed or revised or is pending revision.

———————■

■ **Technique**

As with all revision surgery, careful preoperative planning is necessary. Templates are used first to determine the diameter of the inferior hemisphere. Once the inferior hemisphere size is selected to match the anatomic acetabular diameter, the amount of elongation (15 or 25 mm) that best matches the defect is selected. Both anteroposterior diameter and elongation can be confirmed at surgery using the trial implants.

The oblong cup has a bilobular shape created by two overlapping hemispheres. The diameter of the inferior hemisphere determines the minor diameter of the cup, and the amount of projection of the upper hemisphere beyond the lower hemisphere (either 15 or 25 mm) determines the cup's major diameter (**Figure 4**). The cup face of the 15 mm oblong cup (E-15) is adducted 15° in neutral version. The oblong cup with 25 mm of elongation (E-25) adducts the face of the inferior hemisphere 20° and adds 15° of anteversion. It is important to note that the two hemispheres are coplanar, that is, the two hemispherical portions of the cup are created on a single axis. Although the surgical instruments are designed to reproducibly machine the bone to match the more complicated shape of the implant, the reaming of the upper hemisphere must be done in matching planes (adduction and anteversion) of

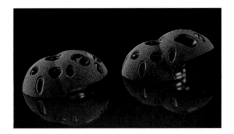

Figure 4 The Oblong Cup acetabular component shown in the E-15 configuration, with 15 mm of elongation, 15° of adduction and neutral version (left), and the E-25 configuration, with 25 mm of elongation, 20° of adduction and 15° anteversion (right). (Courtesy of DePuy Orthopaedics, Inc, Warsaw, IN.)

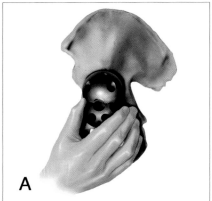

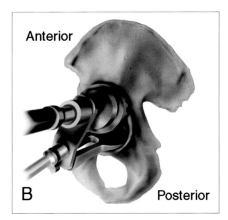

Figure 5 **A,** A trial Oblong Cup can help determine which extension, E-15 or E-25, is appropriate. **B,** The superior and inferior hemispheres must be coplanar, and the superior hemisphere must be reamed in a plane matching the final cup face angle. (Courtesy of DePuy Orthopaedics, Inc, Warsaw, IN.)

the lower hemisphere so that optimal rim contact can occur.

Bone Preparation

Once adequate exposure of the acetabulum is achieved, the anatomic acetabulum is reamed 1 mm under the designated minor diameter of the cup and no deeper than a hemisphere (the prosthesis is available in 3-mm increments from 51 to 60 mm). This is 2.5 mm less than the real diameter of the inferior hemisphere to maximize rim contact.

Prosthesis Implantation

The trial components are then used to confirm the amount of elongation necessary (**Figure 5**, *A*). Shaping the cavity for the superior hemisphere is done with a specialized reamer set to both the minor hemisphere diameter and the amount of needed elongation. The inferior portion of the reamer is seated into the prepared anatomic acetabulum. Anteversion and adduction are matched to the planned cup face angle. The upper cavity is then reamed by pistoning the specialized reamer into the defect. It is critical that the

upper cavity be created to match the plane of the ultimate position of the cup face (**Figure 5**, *B*). This allows interference fixation as the cup is impacted. The depth and accuracy of the reaming can be checked with the trial implant.

Cavitary defects are then filled with morcellized bone graft, and the implant is attached to the impaction handle and impacted. Dome and rim screws can then be placed for adjunctive fixation. At least one dome screw should be placed before a trial reduction of the femoral head is performed. Because of the unusual shape of the implant, a clumsy trial reduction can shift the cup, and a dome screw reduces the likelihood that this will occur. A full range of highly cross-linked polyethylene liners in a variety of inner diameters is available, including constrained inserts, lateral offset inserts, and raised lip inserts.

Postoperative Regimen

Postoperative treatment and restrictions are essentially the same as with

any revision acetabular procedure with uncemented fixation.

———————————————————■

■ Avoiding Pitfalls and Complications

The most common pitfall is extending the oblong cup beyond its limits. The component attains fixation on the rim of the acetabulum, and the shape allows it to reach the rim of superior defects, but the remaining host bony rim must be adequate for cup fixation and load bearing.

The most common intraoperative pitfall is failure to ream the cavity for the upper lobe of the oblong cup in a plane identical to that of the planned plane of the cup face. The cup will not fit properly if the two cavities are not coplanar. As with any uncemented hemispherical cup, accuracy of reaming is necessary to achieve stable fixation.

———————————————————■

References

Berry DJ, Sutherland CJ, Trousdale RT, et al: Bilobed oblong porous coated acetabular components in revision total hip arthroplasty. *Clin Orthop* 2000;371:154-160.

Bozic KJ, Freiberg AA, Harris WH: The high hip center. *Clin Orthop* 2004;420:101-105.

Chen WM, Engh CA Jr, Hopper RH Jr, McAuley JP, Engh CA: Acetabular revision with use of a bilobed component inserted without cement in patients who have acetabular bone-stock deficiency. *J Bone Joint Surg Am* 2000;82:197-206.

Christie MJ, Barrington SA, Brinson MF, Ruhling ME, DeBoer DK: Bridging massive acetabular defects with the Triflange Cup: 2- to 9-year results. *Clin Orthop* 2001;393:216-227.

Dearborn JT, Harris WH: High placement of an acetabular component inserted without cement in a revision total hip arthroplasty: Results after a mean of ten years. *J Bone Joint Surg Am* 1999;81:469-480.

DeBoer DK, Christie MJ: Reconstruction of the deficient acetabulum with an oblong prosthesis: Three- to seven-year results. *J Arthroplasty* 1998;13:674-680.

Padgett DE, Kull L, Rosenberg A, Sumner DR, Galante JO: Revision of the acetabular component without cement after total hip arthroplasty: Three to six-year follow-up. *J Bone Joint Surg Am* 1993;75:663-673.

Pagnano W, Hanssen AD, Lewallen DG, Shaughnessy WJ: The effect of superior placement of the acetabular component on the rate of loosening after total hip arthroplasty. *J Bone Joint Surg Am* 1996;78:1004-1014.

Shinar AA, Harris WH: Bulk structural autogenous grafts and allografts for reconstruction of the acetabulum in total hip arthroplasty: Sixteen-year-average follow-up. *J Bone Joint Surg Am* 1997;79:159-168.

Coding

CPT Codes		Corresponding ICD-9 Codes	
27134	Revision of total hip arthroplasty; both components, with or without autograft or allograft	996.4	996.66 996.77
27137	Revision of total hip arthroplasty; acetabular component only, with or without autograft or allograft	996.4	996.66 996.77
Modifier-22	Unusual procedural service		
Modifier-52	Reduced service		

CPT copyright ©2004 by the American Medical Association. All Rights Reserved.

Chapter 47
Acetabular Revision: Triflange Cups

Michael J. Christie, MD
David K. DeBoer, MD
J. Craig Morrison, MD

Indications

Stable fixation on host bone is the chief underlying principle of successful acetabular revision. Most often, this is accomplished by reaming the acetabulum to fit a larger hemisphere. The acetabular defect is reamed away until stable fixation can be achieved on the acetabular rim. With severe bone loss, however, it is impossible to reshape the defect to match the component; the loss is simply too great to achieve stability on the acetabular rim. In these instances, a device that bypasses the defect to achieve stability on pelvic bone beyond the acetabulum is required.

These defects generally are classified as AAOS type III or IV or Paprosky type IIIA or IIIB. With these defects, major structural allografts or antiprotrusio cages are often considered to salvage the reconstruction. Standard radiographic views of the pelvis, augmented by other views (pelvic Judet, inlet/outlet), alert the surgeon to defect size or the presence of pelvic discontinuity. We use CT and computerized three-dimensional CT reconstructions to help determine whether a custom triflange cup can be used and whether creating a plastic hemipelvic model is warranted. Studies confirm that our experience with three-dimensional models is accurate.

Using the model, the surgeon can confirm the location and quality of remaining bone. Using operating room instruments and hemispheric trial implants, the surgeon can perform a trial reconstruction and determine whether a rim-fit (defect-matching) reconstruction will be adequate.

The triflange cup is a custom-designed, porous- and/or hydroxyapatite-coated flanged device made from solid titanium. As an alternative to the antiprotrusio cage, the triflange cup is rigid, biologically fixed, modular, and can be matched to an individual pelvis and defect for excellent fit. Since 1992, we have used the triflange cup in patients with severe acetabular bone loss that exceeds the limits of hemispheric components, specifically in AAOS type III (combined deficiency) or type IV (pelvic discontinuity) bone defects. Combined segmental and cavitary defects are often present when osteolysis is the underlying source of the bone loss. These defects will be increasingly common as more total hip arthroplasties (THAs) approach long-term follow-up (**Figure 1**).

Pelvic discontinuity, defined as a defect across the anterior and posterior columns with total separation of the superior from the inferior acetabulum, represents a formidable challenge. This condition is not simply a larger, more complicated acetabular defect; rather, it more closely resembles a fracture nonunion because the rate of osteogenesis is often low or zero, being outweighed by bone resorption. Successful treatment of fracture nonunion (ie, creation of conditions that will encourage union) demands rigid fixation to stabilize the bony fragments. Pelvic reconstruction rings and antiprotrusio cages are, by design, flexible to allow intraoperative modification and therefore cannot provide the rigid fixation that pelvic discontinuity requires. Broken plates and screws on postoperative radiographs are not uncommon in these patients. The solid titanium flanges of the triflange cup, approximately 5- to 7-mm thick, provide the rigid fixation that pelvic discontinuity demands.

Contraindications

The proven reliability and long-term success of hemispheric components in revision THA have made these devices the treatment of choice for less complex defects. The triflange cup is an excellent option for patients with severe acetabular bone loss, but its relative cost and design complexity render it unsuitable when a simpler method of reconstruction will suffice.

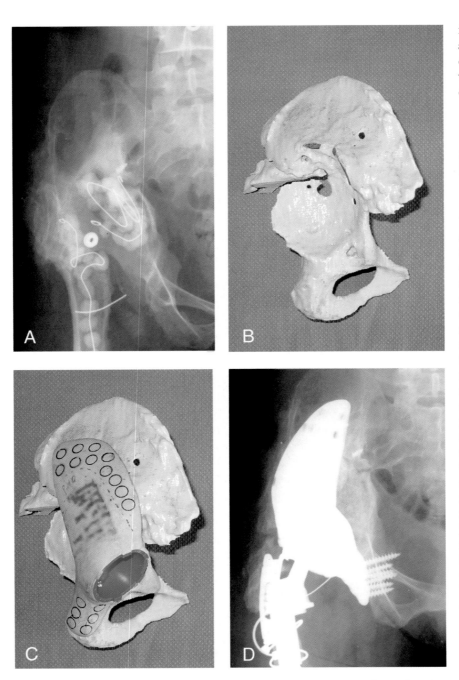

Figure 1   **A,** Preoperative AP radiograph of a 37-year-old woman 21 years after undergoing primary THA for developmental dysplasia of the hip. She presented following resection after failed revision THA with a jumbo hemispheric prosthesis. Revision with an antiprotrusio cage was abandoned intraoperatively because of its inability to fit to the remaining host bone. **B,** A one-to-one model of the patient's hemipelvis, showing the severity of the bone loss. **C,** The model with the clay prototype in place. **D,** Postoperative AP radiograph of the patient 6 months after revision with a triflange cup.

fection always should be considered and subsequently ruled out as a cause of pain. Careful attention to this tenet will increase the likelihood of success of the revision THA.

————————■

■ Alternative Treatments

To achieve long-term stability, use of structural allograft or metal augments to supplement deficient host bone requires that these augments attain sufficient osteointegration with the acetabular bone. Relying on structural allograft alone to achieve stability ultimately dooms a reconstruction to failure. Allografts may or may not heal to the host bone; therefore, they run the risk of long-term failure as a result of resorption or mechanical failure. The addition of an antiprotrusio cage improves the chances of success, but because the cage is an off-the-shelf device and essentially unchanged since its introduction in 1974, it must accommodate a wide range of deformities. This necessarily results in a relatively poor fit between cage and host bone. To improve fit, the cage must be made of relatively thin, malleable metal so that the flanges can be bent and twisted intraoperatively to maximize contact with remaining bone. This flexibility precludes the application of any type of coating to enhance biologic fixation. This inherent flexibility also increases the likelihood that the construct may move or bend as it bears load, contributing to the potential for fatigue failure of the flanges and screws.

The chief alternate treatment to the triflange cup is the antiprotrusio cage, chiefly used in combination with structural allograft. Both short-term and midterm results of this combination have been generally favorable, but as patients are followed long term, increasing numbers of failures have been reported. As described previ-

Orthopaedic contraindications are few. There must be enough remaining pelvic bone so that appropri- ate screw fixation of the component flanges can be obtained. As in all patients who require revision THA, inously, the utility of these devices is limited because of certain inherent design features, specifically the lack of inherent structural strength and ingrowth surfaces, which probably contribute most to their ultimate failure.

Trabecular Metal (Zimmer, Warsaw, IN) augments, metal augments of porous tantalum, show promise with their potential for bone ingrowth and use in filling bony defects. Success beyond the initial term is not known, however, because of lack of published data with this technique. Finally, there is interest in using a cage within an uncemented cup to obtain stable fixation. However, no long-term data have been reported.

Table 1 Results of the Triflange Cup in Acetabular Revision

Author(s) Year	Number of Hips	Implant Type	Mean Patient Age (Range)	Mean Follow-up (Range)	Results
Joshi, et al (2002)	27	Triflange cup	68 years (55–77)	39.5 months (25–56)	No mechanical failures
Dennis (2003)	24	Triflange cup	68 years (44–82)	48 months (24–78)	1 revision for loosening 2 additional radiographic failures (patients refuse additional surgery)
Christie, et al (2001)	67	Triflange cup	59 years (29–87)	53 months (24–107)	No mechanical failures

Results

We have inserted more than 150 triflange cups since 1992 and have removed none. In a retrospective review of the radiographic and clinical results in 21 patients (19 women, 2 men) at mean follow-up of 10 years (range, 8 to 12 years), 10 patients had combined defects and 11 had pelvic discontinuity, according to the AAOS classification system. The mean patient age was 54 years (range, 34 to 73 years) at the time of surgery.

At the time of the last follow-up, 12 of 21 hips (57%) showed radiographic evidence of bony remodeling of the medial wall. Three hips demonstrated small, nonprogressive radiolucent lines. No hip showed loosening, migration, or broken screws. Clinically, Harris hip scores improved from a preoperative mean of 33 (range, 16 to 68) to a postoperative mean of 73 (range, 46 to 100) (**Table 1**). Long-term follow-up of a larger group of patients will be required to determine the success of this technique, particularly in patients with pelvic discontinuity.

Technique

Component Design

Because the triflange cup is a custom device, component design must be finalized preoperatively. This changes the work of surgical planning from intraoperative fabrication (as is done with antiprotrusio cages and structural allografts) to preoperative fabrication. The component is designed to accept standard, snap-in acetabular liners, which allows for some intraoperative modification. The choices include ultra-high molecular weight polyethylene, alternative bearings such as metal-on-metal and constrained liners.

Design begins with obtaining a CT scan of the patient's hemipelvis, which is used to construct a one-to-one hemipelvic model using stereolithography (**Figure 2**, *A*). The surgeon, in consultation with the design engineer, uses the model to select flange size and orientation and to identify thin, fragile bone along the remaining acetabular rim, which will be removed at the time of insertion. This incompetent bone is marked and removed from the model (**Figure 2**, *B*). The sterilized model can be referenced during surgery to help the surgeon in removing this bone. Next, the surgeon

sketches the general size and orientation of the flanges on the model. The engineer then uses these markings to create a clay prototype of the component.

The flanges are designed to facilitate initial fixation through intimate contact with host bone. The iliac flange should achieve fit on the two planes of the ilium delineated by the gluteal ridge and target its screw holes at the most inferior structural iliac bone. The ischial flange normally has three to seven screw holes and is designed to rest primarily on the posterior surface of the ischial tuberosity when inserted through a posterior approach. The pubic flange is generally the smallest and does not contain screw holes.

Using the clay prototype, the surgeon can select the optimal placement of the head center and orientation of the cup. The location of the head center is chosen based on patient-specific considerations, including limb-length discrepancy, planned retention or revision of the femoral component, length of the contralateral leg, and cup size. Generally, the location of the vertical head center is established by first approximating the anatomic position of the head center using the superior aspect of the obtu-

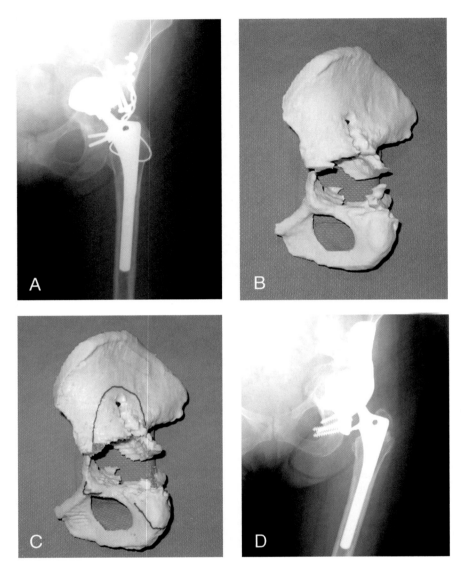

Figure 2 **A**, Preoperative AP hip radiograph of a 54-year-old woman 3 years following revision THA with acetabular structural allograft and 13 years after primary THA for osteonecrosis secondary to failed internal fixation of a femoral neck fracture. The acetabular defect is classified as AAOS type IV (pelvic discontinuity) or Paprosky type IIIB. **B**, An unmarked hemipelvis model showing the bony deficiency. A pelvic discontinuity is visible in this model. **C**, The same hemipelvis model after the flanges have been sketched on and thin, incompetent bone removed (marked). **D**, Postoperative AP hip radiograph 2 years after reconstruction with a triflange cup.

the plane of the iliac wing and the obturator foramen as references. Throughout the design process, a standard, full pelvic Sawbones (Pacific Research Laboratories, Vashon, WA) model is used as a reference.

Exposure

Although the size of a triflange cup may suggest that implantation will be difficult, the exposure necessary for implantation is no greater or more complicated than that required for placement of an antiprotrusio cage or structural allograft. A standard posterior approach is typically used; however, an extended trochanteric osteotomy may be used, when necessary, to facilitate femoral component revision.

The sciatic nerve must be identified and traced from the greater sciatic notch to beyond the ischium so that the ischial flange can be placed without injuring the nerve. The ischial flange intimately fits on the "sciatic" surface of the ischium. Because this contact is crucial for ultimate implant stability, the nerve must be mobilized enough that the flange can be placed without risk of traction or compression injury (**Figure 3**). This is usually easily accomplished. If surgical planes are confused, or if the nerve is densely scarred from previous surgery, meticulous dissection is required. The surgeon can identify an area in the nerve that is not densely scarred (either deep to the gluteus maximus insertion or directly over the ischium), and follow it proximally. Occasionally an external neurolysis is necessary to free the nerve. If scarring is severe, mobilization of the sciatic nerve can take an hour or more.

The gluteus medius and minimus are then elevated off the ilium to allow placement of the iliac flange. Sufficient elevation must be achieved to allow the iliac flange to slide under the muscle. When the femoral component is retained, it is necessary to obtain additional elevation of the soft tis-

rator foramen as a reference point. The remaining bone of the anterior and posterior columns is used to determine the head center in the coronal plane, whereas the flange geometry and cup face diameter guide the position of the head center in the sagittal plane.

The orientation of the cup face is determined by specifying the abduction and anteversion angles of the cup. The abduction angle generally is targeted at 35° to 40° from horizontal and is established using the plane of the obturator foramen as a reference. The anteversion angle is established using

sue anterior on the iliac wing. Care must be taken to avoid traction injury to the superior gluteal nerve. If the femoral component is retained, the femoral head is displaced anteriorly into the space created between the abductor muscles and the ilium. A small pocket is created anterior to the pubis for the pubic flange. After referencing the model, the surgeon palpates the location of the pubic flange with the patient in the lateral decubitus position (usually straight down toward the table). An elevator is used to create the small pocket necessary to accommodate the small flange.

Prosthesis Implantation

The gas-sterilized pelvic model is referenced, and the thin, fragile bone identified preoperatively is removed to match the model. The engineer has marked the model in red to indicate where bone has been removed; the surgeon identified this bone during the design process. Prosthesis implantation begins with insertion of the iliac flange, which is facilitated by translating the leg proximally, with some flexion and abduction, to relax the hip abductors. The iliac flange can then be slid under the gluteus minimus along the iliac wing. It is important to avoid undue traction on the gluteus medius to prevent superior gluteal nerve injury. The pubic flange is then rotated into position as the hip is extended. The ischial flange is then pushed down into position. The knee is flexed and the hip extended to relax the posterior soft tissues. Great care is taken to avoid placing the ischial flange on top of the sciatic nerve. Releasing the soft tissue at the inferior corner of the posterior inferior acetabulum often mobilizes the soft tissue. Using an elevator and sharp dissection, the soft tissue, including a portion of the hamstring origin, is elevated from the bone of the ischium. With the posterior soft tissue relaxed, the nerve and accompanying soft tissue are swept posteriorly as the flange is placed. Screws are

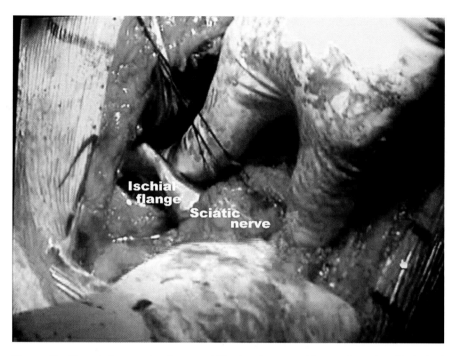

Figure 3   The sciatic nerve has been mobilized and retracted for cup insertion. The ischial flange sits intimately on ischial bone with the nerve overlying.

first fixed in the ischial flange where the bone is poorest and osteolysis common, and then in the ilium.

All ischial screws are placed before any iliac screws are added. The combined fixation of these screws is necessary to reduce the possibility of the flange being pulled away from the ischium, particularly if pelvic discontinuity is present. With severe osteolysis, the ischium can be filled with bone cement before screw placement to improve purchase. The iliac screws (usually four to five) are placed last. The iliac bone is usually better and screw purchase excellent. It is important to avoid undue traction on the superior gluteal nerve when placing the iliac screws. When screws are proximal on the iliac flange, drilling and insertion occur directly through the gluteus medius and minimus.

In patients with pelvic discontinuity, the iliac screws will pull the flange down into intimate contact with host bone, which will reduce the discontinuity and rotate the inferior

half of the hemipelvis into correct orientation relative to the superior half.

Wound Closure

After the procedure is completed, wound closure is done in the routine manner.

Postoperative Regimen

Postoperatively, patients are restricted to partial weight bearing for 6 weeks with use of a walker or crutches for ambulation.

Avoiding Pitfalls and Complications

The subset of patients who require reconstruction with a device such as the triflange cup, by definition, often have a variety of other difficult reconstructive issues such as severe femoral bone loss with weak or absent abductors or preexisting nerve compromise.

In our experience with triflange cups, subsequent dislocation rates are higher than that of our revision THA population as a whole. We have, however, noted a general trend toward less frequent dislocation in patients who have had surgery more recently. Of the 95 hips (93 patients) who had a triflange cup inserted before 2000 as either a primary or revision THA, 20 (21%) had at least one dislocation. For patients whose surgery occurred since 2000, the dislocation rate is 7% (4 of 57 hips). We speculate that a variety of factors have contributed to this decrease. Chiefly, constrained liners are now placed with much greater frequency at the index procedure. Also, our expertise with designing components, especially in determining head center and cup orientation, has improved. Accurate and anatomic placement of the cup face and head center is crucial to the ultimate stability of the implant.

Although implantation of the device is relatively straightforward, seating the component on host bone occasionally can be difficult. This difficulty can occur for a number of reasons, but all are easily remedied reasons. First, the surgeon must ensure that the incompetent rim bone planned for removal preoperatively has been removed. Careful referencing of the sterilized model helps in this process. Second, application of excessive cancellous bone graft as back fill can prevent the component from seating appropriately; removing the extra graft should facilitate proper seating. Third, in patients with pelvic discontinuity, the cup will not appear to be intimately seated until the iliac screws (after first inserting the ischial screws) are inserted and are used to pull the superior and inferior halves of the hemipelvis together.

Sciatic nerve palsy was a complication in early surgeries. Partial sciatic nerve injury occurred in five of the first 78 reconstructions we performed. All of these patients, however, have shown significant or complete recovery. Two nerves were injured intraoperatively, one during dissection of a densely scarred nerve and one while using a bipolar electrocautery near the nerve. Three others were injured as a result of acute hematomas that formed postoperatively. These injuries were promptly decompressed, and nerve function was restored. No nerve injuries have occurred because of the size or placement of the ischial flange, and no nerve palsies have occurred since 1998.

More careful monitoring of anticoagulation therapy has reduced the incidence of postoperative hematoma. Injury during dissection is avoided by identifying the nerve distally, beyond the involvement of the scar, and then carefully dissecting proximally. Occasionally the nerve cannot be clearly freed from dense scar, particularly with acetabular fractures that have undergone previous surgery. In these situations, the nerve must be made mobile enough to allow placement of the ischial flange without undue traction while avoiding more proximal dissection that could result in nerve injury.

Acknowledgment

The authors would like to thank Martha Brinson, MSN, for her assistance in preparation of the manuscript.

References

Christie MJ, Barrington SA, Brinson MF, Ruhling ME, DeBoer DK: Bridging massive acetabular defects with the triflange cup: 2- to 9-year results. *Clin Orthop* 2001:216-227.

D'Antonio JA, Capello WN, Borden LS, et al: Classification and management of acetabular abnormalities in total hip arthroplasty. *Clin Orthop* 1989:126-137.

Dennis DA: Management of massive acetabular defects in revision total hip arthroplasty. *J Arthroplasty* 2003;18:121-125.

Garbuz D, Morsi E, Gross AE: Revision of the acetabular component of a total hip arthroplasty with a massive structural allograft: Study with a minimum five-year follow-up. *J Bone Joint Surg Am* 1996;78:693-697.

Gill TJ, Sledge JB, Muller ME: The management of severe acetabular bone loss using structural allograft and acetabular reinforcement devices. *J Arthroplasty* 2000;15:1-7.

Hooten JP Jr, Engh CA Jr, Engh CA: Failure of structural acetabular allografts in cementless revision hip arthroplasty. *J Bone Joint Surg Br* 1994;76:419-422.

Jasty M, Harris WH: Salvage total hip reconstruction in patients with major acetabular bone deficiency using structural femoral head allografts. *J Bone Joint Surg Br* 1990;72:63-67.

Joshi AB, Lee J, Christensen C: Results for a custom acetabular component for acetabular deficiency. *J Arthroplasty* 2002;17:643-648.

Marsh D: Concepts of fracture union, delayed union, and nonunion. *Clin Orthop* 1998:S22-S30.

Pollock FH, Whiteside LA: The fate of massive allografts in total hip acetabular revision surgery. *J Arthroplasty* 1992;7:271-276.

Robertson DD, Sutherland CJ, Lopes T, Yuan J: Preoperative description of severe acetabular defects caused by failed total hip replacement. *J Comput Assist Tomogr* 1998;22:444-449.

Saleh KJ, Jaroszynski G, Woodgate I, Saleh L, Gross A: Revision total hip arthroplasty with the use of structural acetabular allograft and reconstruction ring: A case series with a 10-year average follow-up. *J Arthroplasty* 2000;15:951-958.

Shinar AA, Harris WH: Bulk structural autogenous grafts and allografts for reconstruction of the acetabulum in total hip arthroplasty: Sixteen-year-average follow-up. *J Bone Joint Surg Am* 1997;79:159-168.

Coding

CPT Codes		Corresponding ICD-9 Codes		
27134	Revision of total hip arthroplasty; both components, with or without autograft or allograft	733.81 996.77	996.4	996.66
27137	Revision of total hip arthroplasty; acetabular component only, with or without autograft or allograft	733.81 996.77	996.4	996.66
Modifier 22	Unusual procedural service			

CPT copyright © 2004 by the American Medical Association. All Rights Reserved.

Indications

Pelvic discontinuity is the loss of structural continuity between the superior and inferior portions of the pelvis. It occurs predominantly through deficient acetabular bone around a failed acetabular component, but it also can be produced iatrogenically during component removal or revision component insertion or as a pathologic fracture through abnormal bone (as occurs, for example, in radiation necrosis).

Pelvic discontinuity is of great clinical significance because attempts at standard hemispheric cup insertion in the presence of pelvic discontinuity are prone to failure. Pelvic discontinuity traditionally has been viewed as a single classification group, despite the fact that requirements for successful treatment differ significantly, depending on the amount of associated bone loss. The significance of bone deficiency in the treatment of pelvic discontinuity has been clearly illustrated in the literature: treatment is determined by the extent of acetabular bone loss.

The absence of pelvic continuity must be specifically addressed in any hip reconstruction procedure, with particular attention directed to the need for both acetabular component stability and stability of the pelvis.

 ## Contraindications

Major reconstructive surgery is contraindicated in patients with systemic health concerns, no local bone potential for healing or providing component stability, and local or systemic sepsis.

 ## Alternative Treatments

Many surgical options have been described to treat pelvic discontinuity. Standard cemented and uncemented acetabular components, with or without adjunctive screw and/or plate fixation, reinforcement rings or cages, and custom uncemented components have been used, often with allograft augmentation.

 ## Results

Many reports exist on small numbers of patients, usually subgroups of larger acetabular revision series. Although no true comparison studies are available, overall results reveal some trends. Pelvic discontinuity is a major negative prognostic factor, particularly with standard acetabular components, regardless of whether cement is used (**Table 1**).

The major challenge is to achieve both stabilization of the pelvis and stable fixation of the contained acetabular construct. Some procedures do not work well, specifically uncemented acetabular fixation with simple screw augmentation, cemented cup fixation without grafting (even with plate stabilization), and uncemented hemispheric cups with extensive grafting (with or without plates or cages). However, success can be achieved if a few simple principles are followed.

If the discontinuity occurs in the presence of good acetabular bone stock that would ordinarily support an uncemented cup, posterior column plating followed by uncemented cup fixation is appropriate. If there is less than 50% contact between host bone and a hemispheric cup, uncemented fixation is not indicated. In these complex situations, the fracture requires stabilization, and acetabular reconstruction is necessary to produce a stable acetabular component. Structural allografts alone cannot be expected to provide long-term stability to either cemented or uncemented acetabular components. However, acetabular reconstruction cages can provide both fixation to the pelvis and much more predictable stability of the acetabular component (**Figure 1**).

The custom triflange cup is a novel, more physiologic option de-

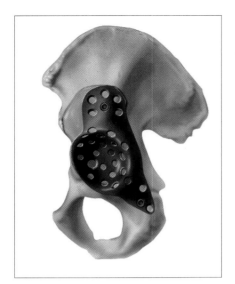

Figure 1 Typical acetabular reconstruction cage.

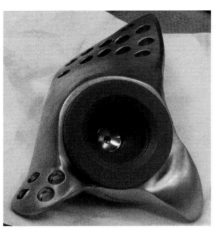

Figure 2 A custom triflange cup is created from a CT scan of the patient and is based on the available bone stock.

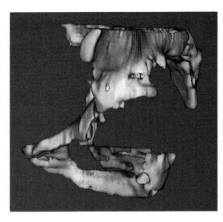

Figure 3 Three-dimensional CT reconstruction of acetabular deficiency. Note the superior bone loss and posterior wall deficiency.

scribed in chapter 47 (**Figure 2**) that has the potential to provide stability of the pelvic discontinuity, promote osseointegration of the construct to the surrounding bone, and eliminate the need for structural grafting and intraoperative contouring of cages.

■ Technique

The technique varies by patient, depending on the characteristics of the discontinuity and the surrounding bone deficiency. Successful treatment addresses both facets of this complex problem.

Preoperative Planning
Preoperative planning is essential. Pelvic discontinuity is often evident on plain radiographs; specifically, AP, lateral, and oblique pelvic views reveal clear displacement or rotation of the inferior pelvis. However, radiographs markedly underestimate the amount of acetabular bone damage that results from loosening or lysis. CT reconstruction techniques (**Figure 3**) can be very helpful in predicting pelvic integrity in that they provide an accurate

Table 1 Acetabular Revisions Treated With Cages or Triflange Cup

Author(s) (Year)	Number of Hips	Implant Type	Mean Patient Age (Range)	Mean Follow-up (Range)	Results
Berry, et al (1999)	24	Varied	61 years (38–80)	3 years (0.2–7)	17 hips, successful
Christie, et al (2001)	39 of 78 discontinuity	Custom triflange	59 years (28–87)	53 months (24–107)	2 hips, incomplete union; no iliac loosening
Garbuz, et al (1996)	32 type III or IV	Varied	60 years (32–85)	7 years (5–11)	18 hips, successful 7 hips, clinical failure, graft okay 8 hips, clinical and graft failure
Stiehl, et al (2000)	10 of 17 discontinuity	Bulk allograft	67.5 years (N/A)	N/A	3 hips revised for infection 2 hips revised for loosening 1 hip revised for dislocation

N/A = Not applicable

view of the extent of structural deficiency of the periacetabular bone.

Pelvic discontinuity can be inadvertently produced during component removal, bone preparation of the deficient acetabulum, and insertion of revision sockets. The presence of pelvic discontinuity should be assessed in all patients undergoing acetabular revision by directly visualizing the acetabulum and stressing the superior and inferior pelvis manually.

Exposure
The surgical approach used depends on the requirements of the reconstruction technique. Most surgeons prefer the posterior approach because it pro-

vides ease of extensile exposure and femoral osteotomy. In patients with discontinuity, I prefer to expose the sciatic nerve because it provides direct visualization. This approach also protects the nerve during the critical ischial exposure and fixation necessary for posterior column plating and screw insertion through the ischial flange of cages or triflange cups.

An extensive exposure is absolutely essential for placement of a posterior column plate, reconstruction cage, or triflange cup. The ischium needs to be completely exposed. In addition, the abductor muscles need to be gently elevated off of the ilium. The superior gluteal nerve is usually located 5 cm above the superior aspect of the normal acetabulum.

Trochanteric osteotomy can facilitate exposure of the acetabulum and prevent injury to the superior gluteal nerve. I prefer the extended trochanteric slide for predictability of fixation and flexibility for trochanteric advancement or displacement to optimize stability.

Bone Preparation

Fractures must be stabilized so they can heal, and local conditions must favor healing. Specifically, the fracture must be curetted and bleeding bone exposed. The acetabulum must be meticulously cleaned of granulation tissue, fibrous tissue, and debris to produce a biologically active interface to promote graft healing and ingrowth into an uncemented socket. The discontinuity site may be grafted with either morcellized allograft bone or autograft bone, if it is available.

Prosthesis Implantation

For patients with minimal acetabular deficiency (more than 50% of the cup in contact with viable host bone), posterior column plating is indicated to stabilize the fracture, followed by uncemented cup insertion with screw augmentation.

For patients with more significant bone loss (less than 50% of host

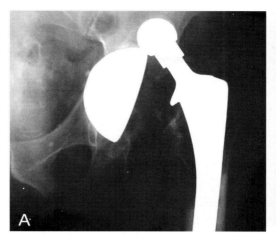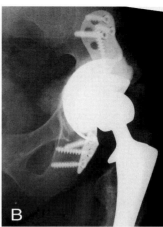

Figure 4 **A,** AP radiograph after attempted uncemented fixation demonstrates migration of the acetabular component. Intraoperatively, loss of integrity of the pelvic column and a pelvic discontinuity were found. This combination prohibited the use of posterior column plate/hemispheric cup reconstruction. **B,** The patient underwent revision to address the deficiency and fracture; a reconstruction cage with allograft augmentation was used.

bone in contact with the cup), the principles of acetabular revision must be followed to optimize component stability. For acetabular bone deficiencies that require structural grafting, the graft must be protected with a reconstruction cage, and a cemented cup is placed within the cage. Cages can simultaneously bridge the defect and provide pelvic stability by iliac and ischial screw fixation through the superior and inferior flanges. If it appears that bone loss will preclude obtaining stability with a cage alone, then posterior column plating also is required.

When combining posterior column plating and cage reconstruction, an integral part of fixation is optimal contouring of the implant to the underlying bone. The plate should be applied along the posterior column in such a way that it will not impede subsequent placement of the cage. The specifics of structural grafting and the use of cages and rings are discussed in chapter 44. The complicating issue in pelvic discontinuity is the need to reduce and stabilize the pelvis and ensure that the construct does not displace or distract the fracture (**Figure 4**).

The triflange cup provides several unique benefits in reconstructive procedures. After preoperative imaging of the pelvis with CT, a three-dimensional model of the deficiency is produced. The surgeon can use this model of the acetabulum to select flange size and orientation, and a patient-specific implant is produced from titanium alloy. The implant is thus already anatomically suited to the patient. Because the contouring required with off-the-shelf cages is avoided, the implant can be made much thicker and can be porous and hydroxyapatite-coated in an attempt to obtain osseointegration. A more detailed discussion of the use of the triflange cup is presented in chapter 47.

The cup center is selected and appropriate anteversion produced. The socket accepts standard, angled, and constrained polyethylene inserts. The technique includes insertion of the iliac flange first, relaxing the abductors with proximal displacement and some flexion of the femur. The inferior flanges are then inserted as the hip is extended. The ischial screws are inserted, then the iliac flange is opposed and screws inserted, which re-

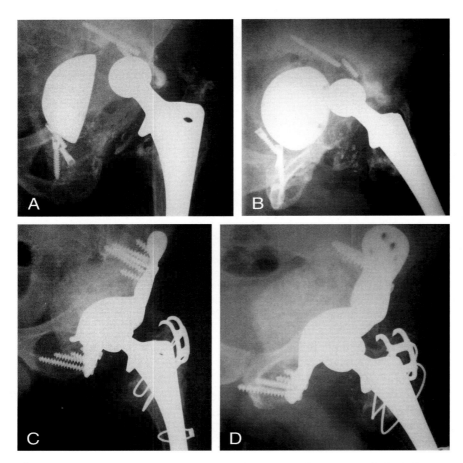

Figure 5 AP (**A**) and oblique (**B**) radiographs of a patient with severe acetabular deficiency. The cup has migrated into the pelvis, which often suggests the presence of a pelvic discontinuity. Postoperative AP (**C**) and oblique (**D**) radiographs demonstrating custom triflange reconstruction. Note the screw fixation in ilium and ischium.

duces the discontinuity. The appropriate liner is then inserted (**Figure 5**).

Wound Closure
I recommend following standard hip revision protocols for wound closure.

Postoperative Regimen
The interval of protected weight bearing, the need for bracing, and the duration of brace wear depend on the severity of the discontinuity and the specific needs of each patient, such as the use of femoral osteotomy, the apparent stability of the construct, and osteotomy. Because these procedures require extensive soft-tissue dissection, the use of a hip abduction brace may be useful.

■ Avoiding Pitfalls and Complications

Complex acetabular revision surgery is prone to frequent and serious complications. Careful preoperative planning is necessary to ensure that all necessary equipment is available for patients undergoing complex revisions. Avoiding aggressive component removal, insertion, and forceful retraction are good preventive measures as well. Ultimately, these measures will reduce the number of patients with unrecognized pelvic discontinuity.

Infection, neurovascular injury, and hip instability often occur with revision procedures. Preoperative screening for sepsis reduces the number of patients with unrecognized low-grade infections, and standard preoperative antibiotic regimens minimize infection risk. Major pelvic surgery requiring screw or plate augmentation always has an inherent risk of vascular injury; therefore, it is necessary to avoid screw placement in high-risk zones. The sciatic nerve is particularly at risk in patients requiring exposure and fixation to the ischium or significant limb lengthening. I recommend sciatic nerve exposure and direct visualization to minimize direct or tension injury. Postoperative hematomas can compromise sciatic nerve function; simple decompression is recommended for improvement.

Instability is common in complex hip revisions for many reasons, including the loss of stability during exposure, preoperative abductor insufficiency, and difficulty optimizing acetabular orientation in the presence of severe deficiencies and complex cage constructs. With superior deficiencies and cages, there is a natural tendency for the acetabulum to be vertical and of inadequate anteversion. Use of a metal-backed cup cemented into a cage can permit subsequent changes in orientation or degree of constraint of the liner. In the presence of inadequate muscle tension, advancement of the trochanter or the use of constrained liners should be considered.

Complications such as nonunion and loss of fixation depend on bone quality, but these complications also should be reduced by meticulously following the principles of fracture fixation. The use of uncemented hemispheric cups in the absence of good host bone, the use of large segment grafts without cage support, and the use of cemented cups alone are associated with generally disappointing results.

References

Berry DJ: Identification and management of pelvic discontinuity. *Orthopedics* 2001;9:881-882.

Berry DJ, Lewallen DG, Hanssen AD, Cabanela ME: Pelvic discontinuity in revision total hip arthroplasty. *J Bone Joint Surg Am* 1999;81:1692-1702.

Chen WM, McAuley JP, Engh CA Jr, Hopper R, Engh CA Sr: Extended slide trochanteric osteotomy for revision total hip arthroplasty. *J Bone Joint Surg Am* 2000;82:1215-1219.

Christie MJ, Barrington SA, Brinson MF, Ruhling ME, DeBoer DK: Bridging massive acetabular defects with the triflange cup: 2- to 9- year results. *Clin Orthop* 2001;393:216-227.

D'Antonio JA, Capello WN, Borden LS, et al: Classification and management of acetabular abnormalities in total hip arthroplasty. *Clin Orthop* 1989;243:126-137.

Garbuz D, Morsi E, Gross AE: Revision of the acetabular component of a total hip arthroplasty with a massive structural allograft: Study with a minimum five-year follow-up. *J Bone Joint Surg Am* 1996;78:693-697.

Stiehl JB, Saluia R, Dienet T: Reconstruction of major column defects and pelvic discontinuity in revision total hip arthroplasty. *J Arthroplasty* 2000;15:849-857.

Coding

CPT Codes		Corresponding ICD-9 Codes		
27132	Conversion of previous hip surgery to total hip arthroplasty, with or without autograft or allograft	733.82 996.66	808.0 996.77	996.4
27134	Revision of total hip arthroplasty; both components, with or without autograft or allograft	733.82 996.66	808.0 996.77	996.4
27137	Revision of total hip arthroplasty; acetabular component only, with or without autograft or allograft	996.4	996.66	996.77
27227	Open treatment of acetabular fracture(s) involving anterior or posterior (one) column, or a fracture running transversely across the acetabulum, with internal fixation	808.0		
27228	Open treatment of acetabular fracture(s) involving anterior and posterior (two) columns, includes T-fracture and both column fracture with complete articular detachment, or single column or transverse fracture with associated acetabular wall fracture, with internal fixation	808.0		

Chapter 49

Femoral Revision: Overview and Strategy

Harry E. Rubash, MD
David Manning, MD

 Introduction

Failure of total hip arthroplasty (THA) is a complex, multifactorial process. Sepsis, dislocation, and failure of prosthetic fixation are frequent causes of early failure. Late failure routinely is linked to the limits of prosthetic biomaterials and the biologic response to their degradation products. Cellular responses to wear products (polyethylene, metal, cement, and ceramic) ultimately can lead to osteolysis and failure of a previously well-functioning arthroplasty. In many cases, the process of failure is silent. Without regular, stringent, clinical and radiographic postoperative review of patients, early detection of failure is impossible. In the unmonitored patient, the revision surgeon may be faced with difficult clinical scenarios with only compromised options for restoring the arthroplasty. This chapter describes revision of the femoral side of THA and the management of compromised soft tissues and bone stock.

 Bone Loss

Revision surgery is technically demanding and associated with decreased survivorship and increases in surgical time, blood loss, risk of dislocation, and rates of infection and other complications. This array of undesirables is primarily linked to compromise of host soft tissue and bone stock. Scarred tissues and compromised abductors result in poor wound healing, a limp, and hip instability. Fixation of the revision femoral component is compromised not only by the obvious bony deficiencies but also by the biologic shortcomings of the violated medullary spaces. As the demand for revision surgery has increased, investigations into the management of these problems have resulted in many different classification schemes of femoral bony defects. The aim of these classifications is to enhance understanding and guide the treatment of these problems. However, no consensus on classification or treatment exists.

Femoral bone loss in revision THA has been presented in many ways (**Table 1**). All of these measures use preoperative radiographs as the sole instrument for assessing the severity of bone loss anticipated at the time of revision. It is clear from related studies that attempts at classification may be inherently flawed because radiographs often understate the true severity of disease. Bony deficiencies undetected by routine radiographs should be expected intraoperatively. In difficult cases, CT scans are a useful adjunct to routine radiographs. Nevertheless, radiographs are easily obtainable and commonly used as the basis to evaluate bone stock in most cases.

Bone stock classifications may be quite complicated and cumbersome for routine clinical use, whereas others are far too simple to be clinically useful. Most present a single perspective and have poor inter- and intraobserver reliability. Only the Gross classification system was developed using research principles derived from multiattribute utility theory and consensus group techniques (**Table 1**). However, it also has shortcomings. The surgeon is not always easily led from classification to reconstruction option. This classification system also groups ectatic femurs with cases of simple cancellous bone loss because both have intact cortical tubes. The reconstruction challenges in these two situations are different.

We use a slight modification of the Paprosky classification for preoperative assessment of bone loss for the purpose of guiding reconstruction. This classification, like many others, is predominantly applicable to reconstructions other than standard cement techniques: (1) type I: proximal bone can fully support the prosthesis (proximal is at the level of lesser trochanter); (2) type II: proximal bone can only partially support the prosthesis; (3) type III: proximal bone cannot support the prosthesis but the isthmus is intact; and (4) type IV: type III with-

Table 1 Classification Systems of Femoral Bone Loss

System	Type I	Type II	Type III	Type IV	Type V
AAOS*	Segmental: Involves supporting cortical shell	Cavitary: From contained lesion—Ectasia	Combined	Malalignment	Femoral stenosis
Paprosky	No significant bone loss	A: Calcar nonsupportive B: Anterolateral deficient C: Posteromedial deficient	Circumferential loss to proximal diaphysis	N/A	N/A
Gross	No significant bone loss	Contained loss, Cortical sleeve intact	Noncircumferential loss or proximal circumferential loss < 5 cm	Circumferential loss > 5 cm	Periprosthetic fracture with proximal circumferential loss
Engh	Mild: Neck and isthmus intact	Moderate: Neck damaged but isthmus intact	Severe: Neck and isthmus damaged	N/A	N/A
Pak†	Head and neck	Proximal quarter	Second quarter	Third quarter	Distal quarter

*Segmental and cavitary are each subclassified by location: Level I (proximal to inferior border of lesser trochanter); Level II (inferior lesser trochanter to 10 cm distal); Level III (distal to level II).
†Classification designed to identify location of stable fixation of femoral component regardless of type of bone loss.
N/A= Not applicable.

Table 2 Results of Cemented Femoral Revision

Author	Number of Hips	Cement Type	Mean Follow-up (Range)	Rate of Radiographic Loosening (%)	Revision Rate for Loosening (%)	Survivorship (%)
Pellici	99	First generation	97 months (60-130)	21%	13%	81% (8 years)
Kavanaugh	210	First generation	54 months (24-126)	44%	3%	91% (4.5 years)
Kershaw	276	Unknown	75 months (30-144)	10%	5%	95% (5 years) 77% (10 years)
Rubash	43	Second generation	74 months (60-111)	11%	2%	93% (6 years)
Engelbrecht	138	Second generation	89 months (36-186)	31%	8%	91% (7.4 years)

out an intact isthmus or ectasia (defined as a canal diameter of > 22 mm).

As in most classification systems, the greater trochanter is not included because of its unique soft-tissue relationship. In each case, the continuity of the abductor mechanism is carefully considered. Trochanteric osteotomy, extended osteotomy, and soft-tissue slide in continuity with the vastus lateralis are all used routinely.

This view of bone stock will be used throughout the chapter as we discuss individual reconstruction techniques.

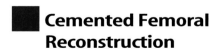

Cemented Femoral Reconstruction

The first significant experience in revision THA was with cemented techniques. So-called first-generation cement techniques were applied in which an unrestricted femoral canal was finger packed with high-porosity cement. This technique allowed for filling of cancellous defects with cement and managing cortical defects with graft and/or mesh. The initial short-term results of cemented femur revision tended to be poor, with reoperation required for mechanical failure, infection, symptomatic loosening, and poor function in a high percentage of patients. In one series more than 20% of patients eventually required resection arthroplasty, and the mortality rate was reported as 3%.

A summary of five different series is presented in **Table 2**. The radiographic loosening rate of revision femoral stems in these series is alarming. Mechanical failure is correlated with radiographic loosening, and increased failure rates are expected with longer-term follow-up of these patients.

Research on cement techniques in primary THA eventually led to improved methods, including canal restriction, canal irrigation, hemostasis with epinephrine sponges, cement pressurization, porosity reduction, and stem centralization. Optimal thickness of the cement mantle was determined to be 2 to 4 mm. When some of these techniques were applied to the revision setting in combination with improved metallurgy, the results naturally improved.

In 1994 Estok and Harris reported on 43 hips in 41 patients at an average follow-up of 11.7 years. The cement technique used at this time included canal restriction and irrigation and cement pressurization. Only four femoral components (10.5%) required revision for aseptic loosening at a mean duration of 99 months. Four additional hips (10.5%) had radiographic evidence of definite femoral component loosening at an average of 119 months. Kaplan-Meier survivorship with revision of the femoral component as the end point was 90% at 11.7 years. Among the hips that were not revised, the average Harris hip score was 81. The observation that 79% of femoral components were well fixed at 11.7 years was attributed to improved metallurgy and cement techniques. However, these results were not as favorable as the Mulroy and Harris report of an overall prevalence of loosening in primary arthroplasty using the same tech-

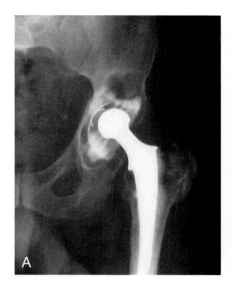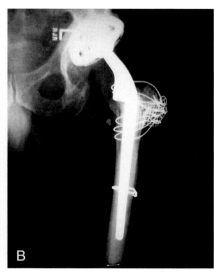

Figure 1 **A,** AP pelvis radiograph depicting failed cemented THA. **B,** AP hip radiograph 7 years after hybrid reconstruction with a cemented, calcar-replacing, long-stem femoral component. There is no evidence of mechanical loosening.

niques of only 3%, at a mean follow-up of 11 years.

In 1996, McLaughlin and Harris reported on cemented femoral revision surgery in a more challenging group of patients. Forty-eight hips in 44 patients with major bone loss in the region of the medial aspect of the femoral neck, significant limb shortening, or a high hip center were managed with a calcar-replacing femoral component cemented with second-generation techniques. A total of 38 hips were followed for an average of 10.8 years. The authors reported an overall mechanical failure rate of 29%, with 18% of patients requiring revision for aseptic loosening (**Figure 1**). They also cited a high prevalence of C2 cement mantles in this group associated with the availability of a single (large) medullary stem size. Thus, the prosthesis frequently came in contact with the femoral cortex, perforating the mantle. Despite the authors' explanation for their results, this report illustrates the difficulties of performing revision femoral surgery with cement techniques (**Figure 2**).

Long-term studies using more versatile femoral component designs

and fourth-generation cement techniques have not been reported to this point. Thus, we infrequently use cement techniques in revision femoral surgery. More durable options are available for most patients. The technique is occasionally used in revising primary cemented arthroplasties in low-demand patients with medical comorbidities.

———————————■

■ Tap Out Tap In

A modification of a revision cemented primary stem is the "tap out tap in" technique. This technique involves removing a cemented stem from an intact cement mantle. Surgical exposure during isolated revision of the acetabulum is often improved by using this technique. The intact femoral cement mantle is reused as the original stem is returned with minimal additional cement. The technique is based on the concept that polymethylmethacrylate functions as a grout and not an adhesive and with the knowledge that new methylmethacrylate can bond to the old methylmethacry-

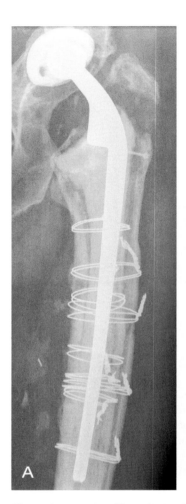
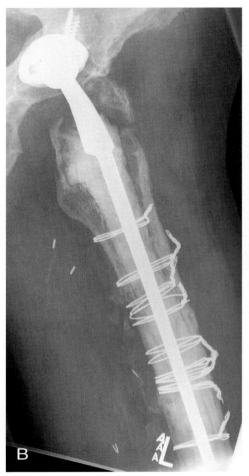
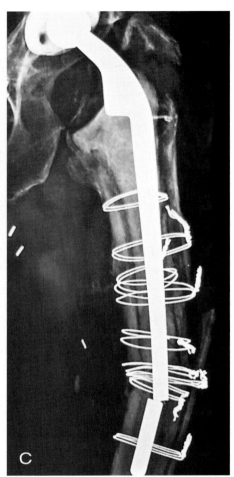

Figure 2 AP **(A)** and lateral **(B)** radiographs of a loosened, cemented, long calcar-replacing, revision femoral arthroplasty. Note the near-circumferential radiolucent lines and greater trochanteric fracture, nonunion, and escape. **C,** The patient went on to fracture the stem.

late. As such, polished tapered stems are ideal components for this technique.

In 1996, a retrospective review was published of all patients who underwent removal and reinsertion of cemented Muller and Aufranc-Turner femoral components during isolated acetabular revision. All components were reinserted into the original, intact cement mantle. Forty-two hips were followed for an average of 67 months (range, 2 to 10 years). At most recent follow-up, the cement mantle remained serviceable for an average of 191 months. Only two femoral components were radiographically loose by Harris criteria, both of which had

asymptomatic cement mantle fractures. No stems were revised for loosening. The study design included in vitro testing of eight cadaver hips, none of which showed any increase in rotational micromotion following removal and reinsertion. The authors concluded that this technique aids in isolated acetabular revision surgery without compromising femoral component stability and survivorship.

We routinely use this technique to facilitate acetabular exposure in the setting of isolated acetabular revision (**Figure 3**). However, we prefer femoral components that have an acceptable track record and design features similar to those in the original report.

In general, our criteria for applying the "tap out tap in" technique include the following: (1) intact cement mantle; (2) component with a good track record; (3) tapered geometry; (4) straight or continuously curved lateral border; (5) low stem surface roughness; and (6) absence of precoated cement.

It is unclear whether components with roughened surfaces or precoated surfaces should be inserted with this technique. Stems with a precoat or a surface roughness greater than 40 Ra may bond with cement and not truly function as a wedge fixed with grout. It is unknown whether "tap out tap in" techniques with such

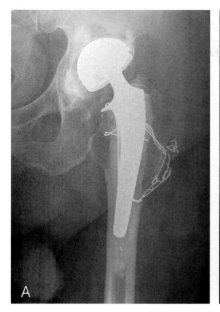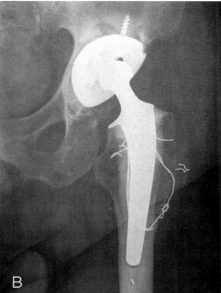

Figure 3 **A,** AP hip radiograph showing failed cemented metal-backed acetabulum with well-fixed cemented CAD stem 17 years after primary arthroplasty. **B,** AP hip radiograph 6 months after uncemented acetabular revision with "tap out tap in" procedure on the femur.

stems could be successful, or if they result in early femoral loosening with associated cement abrasion and osteolysis. Also, femoral components with differing geometry, such as proximal fins designed to promote rotational stability, may not be ideal candidates for this technique. Removal may not be possible without incurring significant damage to the cement mantle.

In performing this technique, the lateral shoulder of cement must be cleared prior to extraction to avoid fracturing the cement mantle. The mantle is carefully inspected and dried prior to replacing the stem. A disposable, sterile light source may be used to aid inspection of the mantle. Mantle fractures are not tolerated. The stem is replaced with a thin coating of cement in the liquid phase. The high monomer content in liquid cement improves the prosthesis-cement interface by reacting with the established mantle.

A natural extrapolation of this technique is cemented revision femoral arthroplasty in the situation of a "debonded" primary cemented femur.

Again, the cement mantle must be intact, the cement-bone interface must be intact, and the femoral component must have an acceptable track record and appropriate design features. Although there are no reported data in this setting, recementing a "debonded" stem may be appropriate in certain situations.

━━━━━━━ ■

■ Extensively Coated Uncemented Implants

Favorable short-term reports of uncemented femoral revision by Engh and others began to appear in the literature at the same time as the disappointing midterm reports of cemented femoral revision. Interest in extensively porous-coated femoral components for revision surgery thus increased. In most later reports, the results have been good. However, these should be interpreted as design specific. Enthusiasm for the technique

does not provide blanket endorsement of all porous-coated stems.

The technique is generally flexible and reasonably applied in many settings. One specific reason for the interest in extensively porous-coated femoral revision is the ease in which proximal femoral bone loss is managed by distal bypass fixation. This method achieves immediate axial and rotational prosthetic stability based on machining the available distal host bone to the specific dimensions of the implant.

Long-term stability that occurs with bony integration into the prosthetic surface is highly dependent on bone quality, the surface porosity of the component, and immediate construct rigidity. Viable host bone incorporates best into surface pores of approximately 250 µm. The importance of immediate implant stability is highlighted by the finding that micromotion greater than 50 µm inhibits bony ingrowth into prosthetic surfaces despite optimal surface porosity.

Paprosky and associates reported midterm follow-up on 297 patients who underwent femoral revision arthroplasty with the Anatomic Medullary Locking (AML) femoral component (DePuy, Warsaw, IN). The AML is extensively porous-coated cobalt chrome with a surface porosity of 150 to 350 µm. The radiographic mechanical failure rate was reported as 2.4% at 8.3 years. Survivorship was 98% at 8 years. All mechanically unstable reconstructions had been performed in Paprosky type III femurs (**Table 1**). The diameter of stems used in the seven failed reconstructions was not reported nor was there any attempt to assess the quality of fixation. However, it is clear from this study that early mechanical failure is associated with radiographically undersized femoral stems. Less than 75% canal fill was radiographically documented in the seven failed cases, whereas canal fill in the remaining 290 patients averaged more than 88%. As previously re-

Table 3   Midterm Results of Extensively Porous-Coated Uncemented Femoral Components in Revision Surgery

Author	Number of Hips	Mean Follow-up (Range)	Type of Implant	Radiographic Loosening	Repeat Revision for Mechanical Failure	Survivorship
Paprosky	297	8.3 years (5-13)	AML	2.4%	1.6%	98% (8 years)
Engh*	26	13.3 years	AML	15%	4%	89% (10 years)
Engh	127	53 months (24-72)	AML	4%	2%	97% (4.4 years)

*All patients had extensive bone loss prior to revision to at least 10 cm below the lesser trochanter.

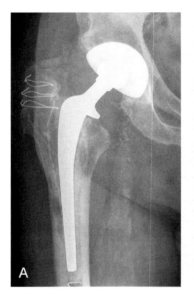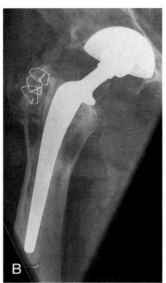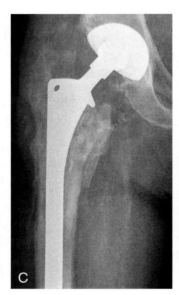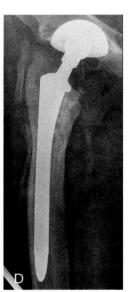

Figure 4   AP **(A)** and lateral **(B)** radiographs showing failed debonded cemented femoral component. AP **(C)** and lateral **(D)** radiographs after uncemented femoral reconstruction with an extensively porous-coated femoral component.

ported by Engh in the setting of primary THA with the AML stem, undersized stems do not provide the construct rigidity necessary for bony ingrowth.

Thigh pain in patients with mechanically loose stems was correlated with straight components that achieved immediate rigidity via three-point fixation. Repeat revision with curved canal-filling stems resulted in good short-term results and radiographically stable implants.

Other peer reviewed reports of extensively coated stems in the revision setting demonstrate radiographic

mechanical failure rates of up to 11%. **Table 3** summarizes some midterm results of uncemented femoral fixation in revision surgery.

Proximal stress shielding of the femur occurs in many settings, including cemented femoral arthroplasty. Yet it remains the major concern associated with extensively coated stems in both primary and revision settings. Several factors appear to be responsible for the phenomenon. Extensive coating, canal filling, stem diameter greater than 13.5 mm, distal fixation, and patient age all play a role. Together these factors result in a situa-

tion in which load is transmitted from the femur to a stiff implant fixed at the isthmus and ultimately to the pelvis and axial skeleton. Wolff's law dictates that the unloaded proximal femoral bone undergoes atrophy. Recently, McAuley and Engh have quantified the change in proximal femoral density associated with extensively coated stems via DEXA analysis. The change is noted to be greatest in patients with lower starting bone density, but the severity of stress shielding is not correlated with outcome. We frequently use extensively porous-coated femoral components in revision surgery.

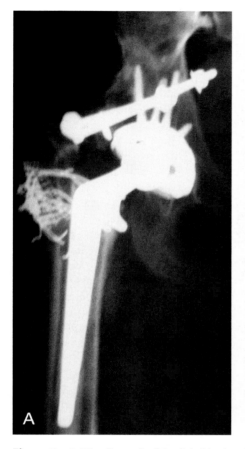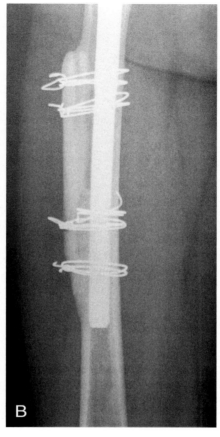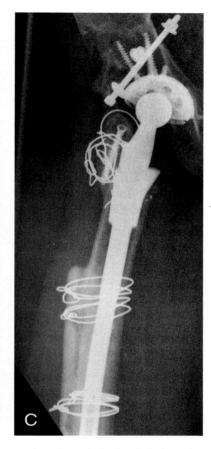

Figure 5 **A,** AP radiograph of the right hip showing a failed femoral component in complex reconstruction of acetabular dysplasia. Note the distal cement mantle fracture. AP **(B)** and lateral **(C)** radiographs of the right femoral revision arthroplasty with a modular femoral component composed of a proximal ingrowth collar and fluted stem.

When the principles of mandatory intraoperative stability and maximal canal fill are maintained, reliable results are routinely achieved with this technique. We accept no less than 4 to 5 cm of canal fill. This provides excellent stability and a large surface for ingrowth potential (**Figure 4**).

The flexibility to ignore proximal femoral deficiencies with regard to long-term fixation makes this technique suitable to almost any revision situation. However, distally ingrown stems that are not proximally supported are at risk for fracture. Smaller diameter stems (13.5 mm and less) are at highest risk for fracture. We consider an ectatic femoral diaphysis to be a second contraindication for this technique. Not only is the immediate

fixation often compromised but also a significant bone-prosthesis modulus mismatch exists. This situation may result in component instability, unacceptable thigh pain, and a potential stress riser at the prosthesis tip. Thus, in what we consider type III (no proximal bone support but isthmus intact) or type IV femurs (ectatic isthmus greater than 22 mm), different reconstruction options are considered.

■━━━━━━━━■

Modular Uncemented Implants

There are two types of modular uncemented femoral implants. One type de-

pends primarily on the metaphysis for biologic fixation, whereas the other relies primarily on the diaphysis. In general, the results of both types, when used in modular uncemented femoral revision, are equivalent to the midterm results of extensively coated uncemented femoral revisions, although patient selection criteria, and hence severity of bone loss, vary in different series. Modularity was originally introduced to provide a flexible solution to the metaphyseal-diaphyseal mismatch frequently encountered in femoral revisions. Independent sizing of both metaphyseal and diaphyseal regions maximizes component contact in both areas. Additional concerns with nonmodular prostheses in the revision setting include proper restoration of kine-

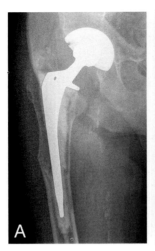
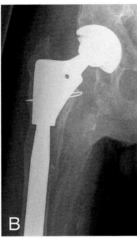
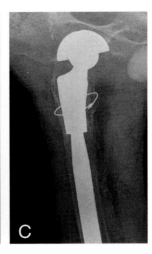

Figure 6 AP (**A**) radiograph of a failed cemented femoral component with a cement mantle fracture and bony remodeling. AP (**B**) and lateral (**C**) radiographs after uncemented femoral revision with a modular extensively porous-coated femoral component.

matics (ie, offset, anteversion, limb length, and muscle tensioning), proximal bone stress shielding, thigh pain, and difficulty in removal. Consideration of all of these issues has led to an increase in the popularity of modular components for femoral revisions.

One of the most commonly used modular uncemented femoral stems is the S-ROM prosthesis (DePuy, Warsaw, IN) (**Figure 5**). Since its introduction in 1984, more than 100,000 of these stems have been implanted. The variable sizing of stems (in length and diameter), proximal sleeves, neck lengths, and head sizes allows a total of 8,364 possible combinations to provide maximum proximal femoral bone contact with optimum version, length, and stability. Although the S-ROM was designed to rely on metaphyseal fit for axial stability and diaphyseal fit for rotational control, increased stem length and diameter can provide greater diaphyseal axial stability in patients with proximal bony deficiencies. The versatility of the S-ROM has allowed it to be used in conjunction with allograft prosthetic composites and structural allografts, and it can be used following extended trochanteric osteotomies.

Cameron and other authors have reported results with the S-ROM sys-

tem in femoral revisions, with radiographic mechanical failure rates of up to 8% and repeat revision rates for mechanical failure of up to 3%.

There is growing concern over the risk of mechanical loosening in proximal, metaphyseal-filling, modular, uncemented femoral revisions when proximal bone deficiencies prevent adequate formation of hoop stresses. Such is the case in femurs with significant metaphyseal destruction and/or following extended trochanteric osteotomy. In Cameron's midterm results, the only mechanical failures were reported in patients with marked proximal bone loss despite the use of long-stemmed S-ROM components. Chandler and associates reported that 44% of their revisions required proximal structural allografts due to major bone loss, and the overall mechanical rate of loosening was 10%.

Proximal loading provided by such stems appears to reduce the incidence of proximal stress shielding. Bono and associates reported only a 6% incidence of stress shielding in 63 hips using the S-ROM prosthesis with an average follow-up of 5.9 years. This is a dramatic decrease compared with the 33% incidence of stress shielding reported by Engh and associates in a

series of extensively coated implants for femoral revision. Along with the decrease in stress shielding, there has also been evidence of proximal bony ingrowth. Christie and associates reported an 81.4% incidence of spot welds at the sleeve-bone interface and a 45% incidence of metaphyseal-diaphyseal junction cortical hypertrophy.

Thigh pain also appears to be diminished with reliance on proximal fixation for stability, reducing the need for large-diameter stems to fill expanded canals. Rates vary from 4% to 12%, with most patients reporting that their thigh pain does not interfere with daily activities. In contrast, Krishnamurthy and associates reported a 31% incidence of thigh pain, and Engh and associates noted a 14% incidence of activity-limiting thigh pain with extensively coated revision stems.

A number of manufacturers have introduced newer modular uncemented femoral revision systems to address the concern of inadequate proximal fixation (**Figure 6**). Some of these systems provide surgeons with different distal fixation options including extensively porous-coated segments and fluted tapered grit-blasted distal segments. The fluted tapered grit-blasted titanium stems are designed to allow bone ongrowth. These stems are modular successors to the Wagner revision stems commonly used in Europe in the last decade.

Modularity has theoretical disadvantages, including failure at the modular junction and the potential for increased wear debris. Fracture of several different designs of modular distally fixed implants at the modular junction have been reported, typically in the setting of poor proximal bone support. Manufacturers are striving to provide stronger modular implants, but the materials' strength limitations in these designs must be recognized. To date, no modular junction failures have been reported in any of the revision series with the S-ROM implant,

Table 4 Short-Term Results of Femoral Reconstruction With APC Reconstruction

Author	Number of Hips	Mean Follow-up (Range)	Revision for Mechanical Failure (%)	Nonunion at Junction (%)	Trochanteric Escape (%)	Survivorship
Chandler	30	22 months (2-46 months)	10%	26%	10%	90% at 22 months
Head	25	28 months (21-40 months)	12%	12%	N/A	88% at 28 months
Masri	44	5.1 years (2-8.3 years)	10%	10%	25%	N/A
Gross	168	4.8 years (0.5-11.5 years)	4%	4%	25%	89% at 4.8 years

N/A = Not available

which typically has good proximal bone support. Although Bobyn and associates demonstrated in laboratory testing that particulate debris can be generated with modular femoral components, it is likely to be minimal compared with that generated at the polyethylene articulation. So far, little evidence of increased osteolysis associated with these systems exists. Several authors have failed to measure modular junction titanium debris in hip aspiration fluid or repeat revision tissue samples. The published results are encouraging, but longer follow-up study is needed on these early to mid-term results.

We frequently use modular uncemented systems in femoral revisions. We enjoy the flexibility of independently sizing each metaphysis and diaphysis to maximize prosthetic contact. Our choice between the two types of modular systems is based predominantly on the condition of the proximal bone. We sometimes use proximally fixed modular implants when the metaphyseal bone can maintain the proximal hoop stresses necessary for proximal stability. However, we find that the proximal bone stock often is deficient. In this situation, fixation within the diaphysis is preferable. When we believe that the reconstruction will not be supported proxi-

mal to the modular junction, we routinely opt for diaphyseal fixation with a nonmodular prosthesis, a megaprosthesis, or an allograft prosthetic composite (APC).

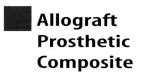

Allograft Prosthetic Composite

Severe circumferential femoral bone loss of greater than 5 cm in length often makes conventional revision techniques difficult or impossible, especially if obtaining adequate distal bypass fixation is not possible. It is in this setting that APC techniques are most helpful. APC reconstructions may be performed in several fundamentally different ways (chapter 57).

Short-term results of femoral reconstruction with APC have been encouraging (**Table 4**), specifically with predominantly compromised patients (principally Paprosky type III and IV) that are similar to Engh's series of patients managed with 10-inch AML reconstruction (**Table 3**).

Blackley and associates reported long-term follow-up (9 to 15 years) in 60 consecutive patients revised with proximal femoral APC. The average

graft was 15 cm in length (range, 10 to 22 cm). All femoral defects were circumferential and measured 8 to 22 cm in length from the greater trochanter. The defects in this series were graded using the AAOS classification as combined defects in level II or III (**Table 1**). This roughly converts to Paprosky type III or IV. In this extremely difficult patient population, only three hips failed because of aseptic loosening. Another three patients required revision for graft-host nonunion. All other failures were related to sepsis or dislocation. The Kaplan-Meier survivorship was 90% at 5 years and 86% at 10 years. The values are reported at the 95% confidence limit.

Despite the good results reported by Blackley and associates, they do not perform APC reconstruction of the proximal femur frequently. In most cases, simpler reconstruction options with equally good or better outcomes can be used. We typically reserve this technique for Paprosky type IV femurs in which extensive proximal bone loss is accompanied by isthmic bone that does not support bypass fixation.

APC reconstruction is associated with a significant complication rate. Dislocation is linked predominantly to management of the abductors. If the greater trochanter is present at the

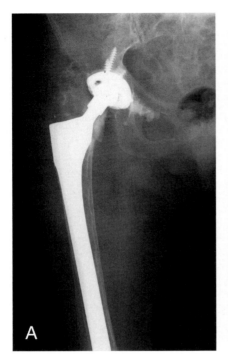
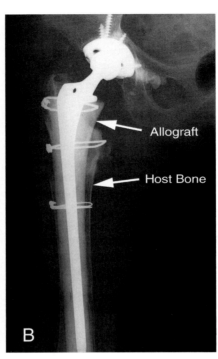

Figure 7 **A,** AP radiograph of a failed THA with massive proximal bone loss. **B,** Reconstruction with proximal femoral allograft fitted inside host femur with the intussusception method.

Table 5 Results of Impacted Cancellous Allografts and Cement for Revision THA

Author	Number of Hips	Mean Follow-up (Range)	Revision for Mechanical Failure	Fracture	Survivorship
Gie	56	30 months (18-49 months)	0	4	N/A
Ullmark	57	64 months (47-84 months)	4%	8 (4 intraoperative, 4 postoperative)	89% at 64 months
Leopold	29	63 months (minimum 4 years)	4%	6 (all intraoperative)	92% at 6 years
Lind*	87	3.6 years (1-7 years)	3.5%	2	96% at 3.6 years†

N/A = not available

*Exchange impaction grafting

†Greater than 20% clinical failure rate at 7 years

time of revision, then union to the allograft is attempted. Nonunion and trochanteric escape can result in global hip instability. Soft-tissue repair with allograft abductor tendon is at-tempted when the greater trochanter is severely compromised, and use of a constrained acetabular liner is always considered when performing this procedure. APC reconstruction also has a higher infection rate (up to 20% of patients) than revision surgery in general. In fact, even Blackley and associates reported that five patients required a second revision because of sepsis. Graft fracture and failure of the reconstruction have also been reported. Concerns about graft source and the potential for transmission of viral and prion diseases have recently been reported in the lay press.

APC reconstruction of the proximal femur is a technically challenging procedure with risk of significant potential complications. The technique is not frequently performed but can be indispensable when reconstructing the Paprosky type IV femur (**Figure 7**).

Impaction Grafting

Femoral impaction grafting used to restore bone stock in revision surgery is an adaptation of a previously described technique for primary acetabular protrusio. This technique was first developed in 1985 in which cancellous allograft and prosthesis reconstruction without cement were used to treat serious loss of femoral bone stock in one patient. Slooff modified the acetabular technique to include cement later in 1985, and in 1991, Simon similarly modified the femoral technique. The first early clinical results were reported by Gie and associates in 1993 and are summarized in **Table 5**.

The technique, as described by Gie and associates, requires complete removal of granuloma and the remnants of primary arthroplasty. The restricted canal is then filled, starting distally, with unwashed, cancellous allograft bone chips no larger than 5 mm in size. Specialized femoral phantom components with a central cannula for suction are used to force (ie, impact) the graft firmly against the femoral

Table 6 Results of Femoral Reconstruction Using Megaprostheses

Author	Number of Patients/Hips	Mean Follow-up	Indication	Stem Fixation	Abductor Repair	Articulation	Rate of Dislocation	Survivorship
Ilyas	13 of 15	6.7 years	Tumor	Uncemented	Suture	Bipolar	20%	N/A
Bickels	57 of 57	6.5 years	Tumor	Cemented and uncemented	Complex	Bipolar and unipolar	1.7%	N/A
Haentjens	16 of 19	5 years	Revision	Cemented	N/A	Total	22%	N/A
Malkani	32 of 49	11 years	Revision	Cemented	Suture	Total	30%	64% at 12 years

N/A = Not available

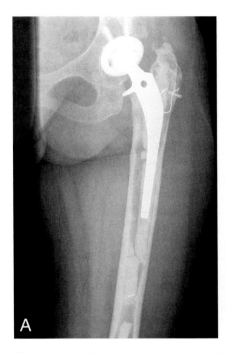
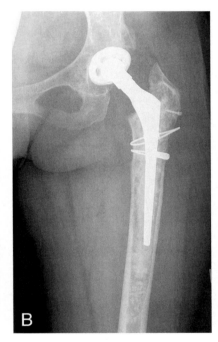
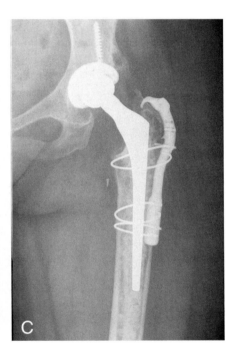

Figure 8   **A,** AP radiograph depicting a failed 10-year-old cemented femoral component in a 30-year-old woman whose original diagnosis was dysplasia. **B** and **C,** Sequential AP hip radiographs after revision with impaction grafting. A greater trochanter fracture in association with severe polyethylene wear necessitated acetabular revision and fixation of the fracture. The revision femoral component has remained stable.

cortex to create a "neocortex." The canal is dried, and then cement is pressurized into the neocortex in a fourth-generation fashion. Finally, a femoral component smaller than the phantom component is inserted, creating an adequate mantle thickness.

This technique is time consuming and demanding but extraordinarily flexible. Large and small metaphyseal defects are easily filled with cancellous graft. Large segmental bone deficien-

cies may be reconstructed by containing the defect with mesh and/or structural graft prior to impacting cancellous chips. The universal applications, promising midterm results, and the concept of restoring bone stock have resulted in great excitement about this technique, despite the technical demands.

More recently, high complication rates associated with this technique have been reported, including

perioperative and late femoral fracture rates as high as 24%. Late follow-up has also raised concern over symptomatic subsidence of the femoral component. In their report, Meding and associates described an average subsidence of approximately 10 mm. Complications reported in early series may now be reduced with refinements in both patient selection and surgical technique as the technology has matured.

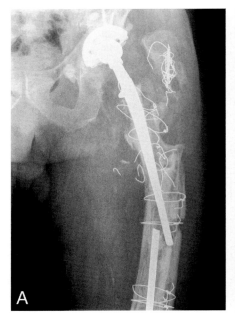

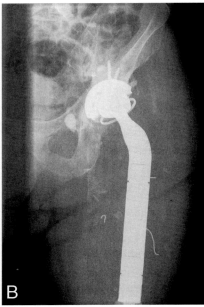

Figure 9 **A,** AP hip radiograph shows a failed cemented femoral revision in an elderly, low-demand patient. Note the component fracture and greater trochanter fracture with escape. **B,** AP hip radiograph shows reconstruction with a femoral megaprosthesis cemented distally into remaining host femur. Note that the liner has been exchanged to a constrained liner. The patient walks with a cane and a moderate limp.

Retrieval and histologic assessments of the impacted bone graft confirm that this technique can restore bone stock. Ullmark and Obrant reported on 31 biopsies performed in 21 femurs between 1 and 48 months after reconstruction using impaction grafting. At 3 to 4 months, fibrous tissue with neovascularization and pluripotential cells had reached 3 mm within the graft. At 8 to 11 months, the fibrous tissue extended to 7 mm. At the same time osteoid and living bone had progressed 3 to 5 mm from the cortex. In some cases new osteoid penetrated the entire thickness of the graft. At 48 months, the proximal graft was a composite of living bone, living bone on dead bone, and fibrous tissue that extended to the cement layer. At the midstem and distally, no dead bone or fibrous tissue was identified. In partial contact with the cement mantle was a thin neocortex with trabeculae projecting toward the cortex. The intracortex space was filled with hematopoietic marrow.

We prefer techniques other than impaction grafting in most patients. The technical complexity and rate of complications exceed those of other options, without the benefit of improved results. However, because bone stock can be enhanced with impaction grafting, we will perform it in some younger patients who have severe bone compromise (**Figure 8**). The ideal candidate has a capacious femur (> 22 mm in diameter) in which adequate initial fixation is not possible with uncemented devices. In this situation, impaction grafting may restore bone stock needed in future revisions and provide reliable intermediate survivorship.

———▬

■ Megaprosthesis

Use of a megaprosthesis in femoral reconstruction is a viable option for managing severe circumferential prox-

imal femoral bone stock deficiencies. Experience with this technique predominantly has been limited to femoral reconstruction after tumor resection. However, it has been expanded to include reconstruction of failed arthroplasty when structural bone loss is similar to that encountered after tumor resection (**Table 6**). Indications for this technique and its capacity to manage bone deficiency are similar to APC reconstruction of the proximal femur. Most surgeons rarely use megaprostheses because they do not restore bone stock or provide for reattachment of the remaining proximal femoral or trochanteric bone as readily as APCs. However, megaprosthesis reconstruction is a simpler, faster surgical alternative compared to APC reconstruction.

However, like APC reconstruction of the proximal femur, the principal complication associated with megaprostheses is the high rate of dislocation. The predominant reason for this problem is the loss of abductor function from either iatrogenic muscle injury, lysis-related trochanter loss, or resection along with tumor. The literature reports dislocation rates as high as 30%. To date, Bickels and associates' 1.7% dislocation rate is the lowest reported in the literature. The low rate of dislocation in their series has been attributed to an elaborate technique of abductor restoration, including Dacron tape capsulorrhaphy and extensive tenodesis of the iliopsoas, gluteus medius, gluteus maximus, and vastus lateralis.

The largest series to date of megaprosthesis use for proximal femur reconstruction in the setting of severe bone loss after failed arthroplasty was reported by the Mayo Clinic. Investigators retrospectively reported on 49 patients with 50 revision THAs involving proximal femoral replacements. Of these, 33 THAs were available to study. The 1985 early follow-up by Sim reported a high rate of failure and dislocation. Longer-term follow-up in 1995 by Malkani and associates reported

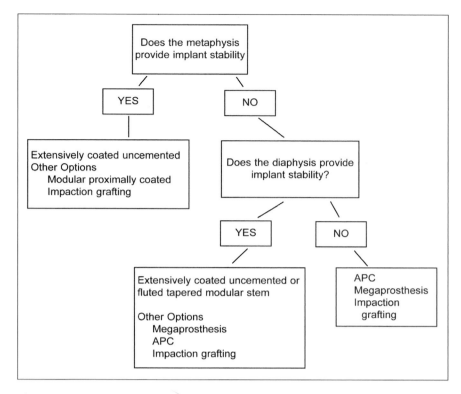

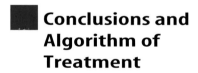

Figure 10   Reconstruction algorithm.

similarly high rates of dislocation and mechanical failure.

The results of this technique for severe bone loss after failed arthroplasty generally appear to be inferior to those of APC reconstruction with similar complications. We do not frequently use megaprostheses as a primary option. Our indication for using a megaprosthesis as our primary option is severe bone loss in an extremely low-demand older patient. We routinely combat the dislocation problem by using a unipolar or bipolar prosthe-sis when possible or implanting a constrained liner when acetabular reconstruction is performed concurrently (**Figure 9**).

━━━━━━━━━━ ■

■ Conclusions and Algorithm of Treatment

Revision reconstruction of the femur ranges from the relatively straightfor-ward to the incredibly complex. The magnitude of difficulty depends primarily on the bone quantity and quality at the time of revision. Preoperative assessment of bone loss based on plain radiographs is frequently misleading. Each patient must be considered individually, and the unexpected must be planned for accordingly. Flexibility in planning allows for flexibility in the operating room. Thus, the ultimate reconstruction method should be based on the intra-operative assessment of femoral bone stock.

We have adopted an algorithmic approach to managing femoral bone loss. This algorithm helps guide our choice for the optimal reconstruction technique and is based on our interpretation of the literature and our specific capabilities. The most flexible and frequently used reconstruction technique we use is distal bypass fixation with either a modular or solid extensively porous-coated implant. We will occasionally perform cemented, APC, or megaprosthesis reconstruction when deemed appropriate (**Figure 10**).

Finally, the integrity of the soft tissues is critically important when managing bone loss and failed prostheses. Reports of all revision techniques include increased rates of dislocation, limp, wound problems, and infection. Special attention to the abductor mechanism, skin, and other soft tissues may decrease the incidence of these complications and ultimately improve patient outcomes.

━━━━━━━━━━ ■

■ References

Bickels J, Meller I, Henshaw RM, Malawer MM: Reconstruction of hip stability after proximal and total femur resections. *Clin Orthop* 2000;375:218-230.

Blackley HRL, Davis AM, Hutchinson CR, Gross AE: Proximal femoral allografts for reconstruction of bone stock in revision arthroplasty of the hip. *J Bone Joint Surg Am* 2001;83:346-354.

Bobyn JD, Tanzer M, Krygier JJ, Dujovne AR, Brooks CE: Concerns with modularity in total hip arthroplasty. *Clin Orthop* 1994;298:27-36.

Bono JV, McCarthy JC, Lee J, Carangelo RJ, Turner RH: Fixation with a modular stem in revision total hip arthroplasty. *Instr Course Lect* 2000;49:131-139.

Cameron HU: The long-term success of modular proximal fixation stems in revision total hip arthroplasty. *J Arthroplasty* 2002;17:138-141.

Chandler HP, Ayers DK, Tan RC, Anderson LC, Varma AK: Revision total hip replacement using the S-ROM femoral component. *Clin Orthop* 1995;319:130-140.

Christie MJ, DeBoer DK, Tingstad EM, et al: Clinical experience with a modular noncemented femoral component in revision total hip arthroplasty. *J Arthroplasty* 2000;15:840-848.

Engh CA Jr, Christi SJ, Young AM, et al: Interobserver and intraobserver variability in radiographic assessment of osteolysis. *J Arthroplasty* 2002;17:752-759.

Engh CA Jr, Ellis TJ, Koralewicz LM, McAuley JP, Engh CA: Extensively porous-coated femoral revision for severe femoral bone loss (minimum ten year follow-up). *J Arthroplasty* 2002;17:955-960.

Estok DM II, Harris WH: Long-term results of cemented femoral revision surgery using second-generation techniques: An average 11.7-year follow-up evaluation. *Clin Orthop* 1994;299:190-202.

Gie GA, Linder L, Ling RS, et al: Impacted cancellous allografts and cement for revision total hip arthroplasty. *J Bone Joint Surg Br* 1993;75:14-21.

Krishnamurthy AB, MacDonald SJ, Paprosky WG: 5 to 13 year follow-up study on cementless femoral components in revision surgery. *J Arthroplasty* 1997;12:839-847.

Malkani AL, Settecerri JJ, Sim FH, Chao EYS, Wallrichs SL: Long term results of proximal femoral replacement for non-neoplastic disorders. *J Bone Joint Surg Br* 1995;77:351-356.

McLaughlin JR, Harris WH: Revision of the femoral component of a total hip arthroplasty with the calcar-replacement femoral component: Results after a mean of 10.8 years postoperatively. *J Bone Joint Surg Am* 1996;78:331-339.

Meding JB, Ritter MA, Keating EM, Faris PM: Impaction bone grafting before insertion of a femoral stem with cement in revision total hip arthroplasty: A minimum two-year follow-up study. *J Bone Joint Surg Am* 1997;79:1834-1840.

Nabors ED, Liebelt R, Mattingly DA, Bierbaum BE: Removal and reinsertion of cemented femoral components during acetabular revision. *J Arthroplasty* 1996;11:146-152.

Saleh KJ, Holtzman J, Gafni A, et al: Reliability and intraoperative validity of preoperative assessment of standardized plain radiographs in predicting bone loss at revision hip surgery. *J Bone Joint Surg Am* 2001;83:1040-1046.

Ullmark G, Obrant KJ: Histology of impacted bone-graft incorporation. *J Arthroplasty* 2002;17:150-157.

Chapter 50

Femoral Revision: Component Removal

Charles L. Nelson, MD

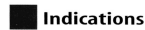
Indications

Indications for revision total hip arthroplasty (THA) include infection, symptomatic mechanical loosening, component malposition, hip instability, significant polyethylene damage or wear, periprosthetic fractures, and implant fracture or failure of modular connections.

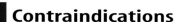
Contraindications

Contraindications to revision THA and component removal include medical illness or severe comorbidities whose risk precludes major surgery. In the absence of infection or malposition, it is generally preferable to leave a well-fixed femoral component in place, particularly if modularity allows appropriate restoration of limb length and soft-tissue tension.

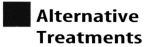
Alternative Treatments

Alternative treatments to revision THA depend on the specific indication for surgery. For deep infection, alternatives include irrigation and débridement with retention of components and/or treatment with chronic suppressive antibiotics. Hip instability may be managed with bracing. Alternatives to femoral revision for periprosthetic femur fractures include conservative management for isolated trochanteric fractures and open reduction with internal fixation for fractures with a well-fixed femoral component. Aseptic loosening or osteolysis are quality of life issues; possible alternatives include sufficient analgesia, activity limitations, and physical therapy. Adjunctive ambulatory aids should always be considered, including canes, crutches, walkers, or wheelchairs.

Technique

Every successful surgery—whether primary or revision—is preceded by careful preoperative planning. Imaging should include radiographic AP and lateral views of the femur and an AP view of the pelvis. Every attempt should be made to identify the existing components and their mode of fixation. The most reliable way to identify components is to obtain copies of the implant stickers from prior surgical procedures, usually found in the progress note section of the hospital chart or hospital orthopaedic operating room logbook. Many surgeons indicate in the operative report which prosthetic device was implanted, and some previous surgeons can be contacted directly. When these methods are not successful, an experienced orthopaedic surgeon or an industry representative may be able to identify components based on radiographic criteria. Identifying the components may decrease morbidity, the extent of surgery, and surgical time. Implant-specific extraction devices can be ordered preoperatively. Revision of a well-fixed modular implant can be avoided by ordering appropriate modular parts.

Once the implant and mode of fixation have been identified, appropriate instrumentation can be ordered. The surgeon preparing for a revision hip procedure should be aware of all available options. Various hand tool sets exist in both cemented and uncemented versions; these generally have variations of the same type of instruments (**Figure 1**). Examples include, but are not limited to, the Moreland Hand Tool Set (DePuy, Warsaw, IN); the Zimmer Manual Hip Revision Set (Zimmer, Warsaw, IN); and the Gray Revision Instrument System (Stryker-Howmedica-Osteonics, Allendale, NJ). These instruments permit removal of cement at the bone-cement interface. Because areas of cement interdigitation are visualized, the surgeon can be confident that all cement has been removed.

A number of high-speed burrs are available that greatly facilitate

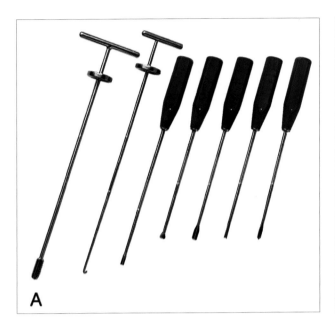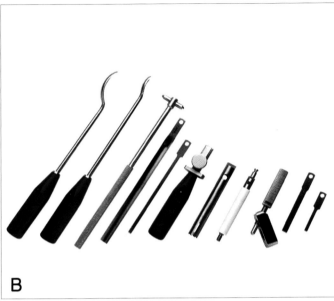

Figure 1 **A,** Examples of manual cement removal instruments. **B,** Examples of manual implant extraction instruments. (Courtesy of DePuy and Johnson & Johnson, Warsaw, IN.)

component and cement extraction. Examples include the Midas Rex (Medtronic, Minneapolis, MN); the Ultrapower (Linvatec, Largo, FL); the Anspach (Forth Medical, Berkshire, England); and the Stryker TPS (Stryker-Howmedica-Osteonics).

Motorized hand instruments are also available and allow rapid, controlled impact as well as visualization facilitated by fluorescent light sources. Some surgeons achieve more rapid cement removal with hand tools, but motorized devices are an alternative. I am aware of only one motorized osteotome set currently being manufactured, the AcuDriver (Exactech, Gainesville, FL). Ultrasound devices for cement removal can also be quite useful. Examples include O.S.C.A.R. (Orthosonics, Upper Montclair, NJ) and the Ultradrive (Biomet, Warsaw, IN). Ultrasonic devices are particularly useful because they are less likely to penetrate bone when creating a hole through the distal cement plug. Unlike hand tools, ultrasonic devices may blur the bone-cement margins, so I recommend using reverse curettes

following use of ultrasonic tools to ensure that all cement has been removed.

The surgical approach is the surgeon's preference. The most common approaches are the posterolateral and direct lateral (modified Hardinge). The posterolateral approach offers better exposure of the posterior acetabular wall and column. The greater trochanteric osteotomy (GTO) and the extended trochanteric osteotomy (ETO) can provide increasing amounts of exposure, greatly facilitating component extraction while decreasing the risk of femoral perforation. GTO allows enhanced acetabular exposure and improved abductor tensioning but only a limited increase in femoral exposure. GTO can be complicated by nonunion, fibrous-union, proximal migration, and abductor weakness with associated abductor lurch.

ETO offers several advantages. It provides greater exposure for femoral implant removal, allows correction of deformity, especially varus-remodeled femurs, has predictable healing, and

allows abductor advancement and neutral reaming of the femoral canal with decreased chance of cortical perforation. Extensively porous-coated uncemented stems that are osteointegrated require an ETO for safe removal. Most cemented components may be extracted from the cement mantle without an ETO. However, there are certain prostheses in which the anterior-posterior diameter is wider in the midsection, thus occasionally necessitating an ETO. This approach can also be used when the cement mantle extends beyond the anterior bow of the femur, for difficult textured stem-cement interfaces, or if varus or valgus remodeling has occurred.

Disadvantages of an ETO are the need for cerclage fixation, hardware-related pain, and (rarely) nonunion with abductor weakness secondary to proximal migration. For a planned cemented femoral revision, with or without impaction grafting, concerns about potential cement extrusion from the osteotomy site make ETO less optimal.

Cemented Stems

Extraction of cemented stems can be divided into two phases: disimpaction of the stem from the cement mantle and removal of cement. Cemented stems are either highly polished or matte finished or roughened with or without polymethylmethacrylate precoating. The surgeon must clear away any bone or cement from the medial aspect of the greater trochanter that may overhang the shoulder of the prosthesis. The path for implant disimpaction must be clear to avoid inadvertent greater trochanteric fracture. Use of a high-speed burr allows removal of overhanging bone and cement without introduction of an osteotome. Use of osteotomes is discouraged because they occupy space and may lead to trochanteric fracture through increased hoop stresses.

Removal of the femoral component is made more difficult with marked subsidence. A medial collar may often be overgrown by bone after subsidence and this area must be cleared before disimpaction. Subsidence may compromise attachment of universal extraction devices to the trunion. Once the trajectory of the prosthesis is clear, an implant-specific femoral extraction device or universal device may be applied. When using a universal device on components with nonlipped tapers, it may be necessary to notch the undersurface of the neck with a metal-cutting diamond wheel to allow the extraction device to firmly grasp the prosthesis. Most highly polished and textured stems can be removed with three to five firm but controlled disimpaction blows. If these blows do not free the prosthesis, the cement-prosthesis interface may be disrupted with a pencil-tipped burr or thin flexible osteotomes. However, because of the risk of fracture with the use of osteotomes, I prefer use of an ETO in more difficult extractions. Once the prosthesis-cement interface has been disrupted, the surgeon can begin retrograde disimpaction.

Cement removal can be a formidable task. If a good bone-cement interface exists it may be possible to cement a revision prosthesis into an existing cement mantle. To do so, the existing cement mantle would need to be modified with burrs or ultrasonic tools to allow space for the new prosthesis and texturing of the existing cement to allow increased cement-to-cement bonding. The criteria for the cement-within-cement technique include an absence of infection and an undisturbed bone-cement interface in the middle and distal portions. When loose, the cement mantle may be removed en masse by threading a tap into the cement mantle and disimpacting it in retrograde fashion. An ultrasound device may also be used to gain purchase on a loose cement mantle and allow removal. This is a rare situation; usually the cement must be removed in pieces. The surgeon's arsenal includes hand tools, burrs, drills, and ultrasonic devices. Metaphyseal cement mantles can often be thick and may be debulked with a high-speed burr. Hand tools in the form of splitters, "T" and "V" osteotomes, reverse hooks, and pituitary rongeurs are then used to methodically and patiently break and remove metaphyseal and diaphyseal cement.

Motorized osteotomes are another alternative. A fluorescent headlight greatly facilitates removal of cement in the diaphysis, where visualization is poor. Removal of a well-fixed distal cement plug requires creation of a central hole in the plug with a burr drill or ultrasonic device. The surgeon should progressively enlarge this hole and use reverse hooks to drive the cement fragment proximally. Placement of space-occupying objects prior to creation of a central hole may lead to femoral fracture. If the distal cement plug expands past the isthmus of the femur, an ETO or cortical window may be necessary for safe extraction. In most instances, an ETO allows more rapid cement removal with de-

creased risk of perforation. This advantage must be weighed against the ETO risks previously discussed.

Uncemented Stems

Uncemented stems are either proximally or extensively porous-coated and undersized rather than canal-filling. These specifications affect extraction. Removal of a loose, proximally coated, undersized stem is a much easier undertaking than the converse, removal of a well-fixed, extensively porous-coated, canal-filling stem. As in cemented-stem extraction, any overhanging bone from the greater trochanter must be removed to clear the trajectory of the prosthetic shoulder. At this point, if the stem has been determined to be radiographically loose, a proximal extraction device can be attached. Three to five firm, controlled disimpaction blows should be administered. If the stem proves to be well-fixed, then the surgeon must disrupt the bone-prosthesis interface or the fibrous tissue-prosthesis interface. Fibrous ingrowth may require thin, flat, "U-shaped" osteotomes. Caution must be used with osteotomes because they are space-occupying devices and can easily fracture the femur. The surgeon should not hesitate to perform an ETO if resistance is encountered.

A pencil-tip burr can be used to divide the anterior, posterior, and lateral interfaces. The medial interface may be blocked by a collar. In these cases, a metal-cutting burr may be used to divide the collar and gain access to the medial aspect. Before using a metal-cutting device, the patient's bone and soft tissues should be isolated with sponges or plastic drapes to minimize the spread of metal debris. When using burrs, be sure to stay along the prosthesis at all times and not perforate the cortices of the femur. Once the interface has been divided, the surgeon may again attempt to disimpact the prosthesis. If this is unsuccessful after three to five blows, the surgeon should reassess the situation.

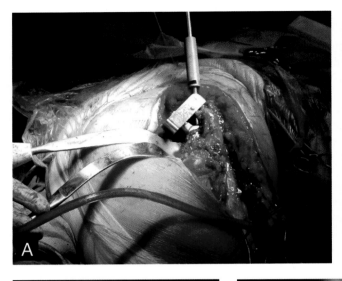

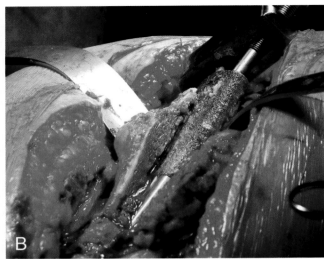

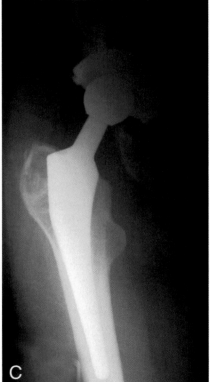

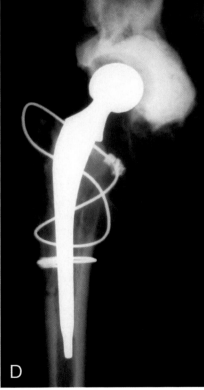

Figure 2 **A**, Intraoperative photograph with universal femoral extraction device attached to femoral trunion. **B**, Intraoperative photograph following ETO. **C**, Preoperative radiograph of infected THA demonstrating well-fixed uncemented femoral component. **D**, Postoperative radiograph following removal of femoral and acetabular components and placement of an articulated antibiotic-loaded spacer. Note that an ETO was necessary to facilitate removal of the well-fixed femoral component.

Even if the distal aspect of the stem is not coated in some fashion, there may be bone ongrowth distally and measures used on a fully porous-coated stem must be applied.

An ETO is useful in facilitating removal of both proximally and extensively porous-coated stems (**Figure 2**). The distal margin of the osteotomy is determined after preoperative templating. The goal with an extensively porous-coated component is to create an osteotomy sufficiently distal to facilitate prosthetic removal and allow correction of varus remodeling, but proximal enough to maintain 4 to 6 cm of isthmic bone to allow reliable fixation. The distal aspect of the osteotomy should be located just distal to the site where the stem becomes cylindrical, thereby allowing the distal portion of the stem to be removed using trephines, if necessary. When removing proximally coated stems, an

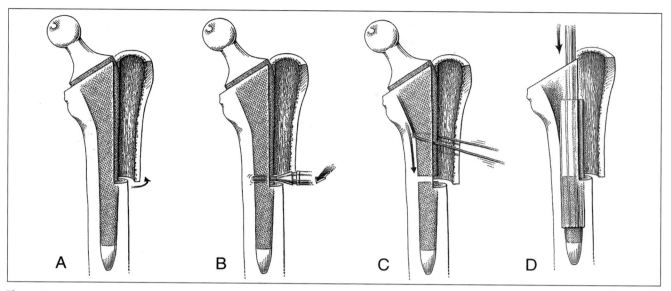

Figure 3 **A,** Access to an extensively porous-coated stem with an extended greater trochanteric osteotomy. **B,** Dividing the implant below the metaphyseal flare with a high-speed, metal-cutting instrument. **C,** A Gigli saw is used to cut the medial bone-ingrown areas of the proximal stem. **D,** A trephine is used to cut the distal stem free of the diaphysis. (Reproduced with permission from the Mayo Foundation, Rochester, MN.)

osteotomy just distal to the coating will usually suffice.

The ETO technique has been described in the literature. I prefer to use an oscillating saw to cut the femur posteriorly, just anterior to the linea aspera. A pencil-tip burr is used to make the distal cut, with rounded corners, across one third of the femoral diameter. The burr is also used to section the anterior femur a distance of 1 to 2 cm. A ½-inch osteotome can then be used proximally and distally along the anterior femoral cortex and under the vastus lateralis to create stress risers at the desired location. At this point, two wide osteotomes are placed posteriorly and levered gently to allow a controlled break at the anterior aspect of the osteotomy. An ETO is usually necessary in extensively porous-coated, bone-ingrown stems (**Figure 3**). Several burrs, trephines, diamond cutting wheels, and Gigli saws should be available because rapid dulling occurs when cutting cortical bone and metal. Flat, oscillating saws can divide the bone-prosthesis interface anteriorly and posteriorly. Several Gigli saws will be necessary to divide the medial interface from the

calcar to the cylindrical aspect of the stem. The surgeon may then attach a proximal disimpaction device and apply three to five blows. If unsuccessful, the stem must be cut with metal-cutting burrs. The distal cylindrical aspect of the stem may then be removed using motorized trephines. Choose a trephine size slightly larger than the stem diameter to avoid as much bone loss as possible. Several trephines may be necessary. If a curved stem is being removed, the osteotomy needs to be sufficiently distal to allow a straight pathway below the bow of the stem. Copious irrigation is necessary to avoid thermal damage from motorized trephines.

Fractured Stems

Fractured stems can be removed using a combination of techniques. A distal angled drill hole, cortical window, or an ETO are almost always used to remove the distal aspect of the fractured stem. The simplest technique involves drilling a hole at a 45° angle through bone near the proximal aspect of the distal stem segment. A carbide punch is then driven into the stem at a 45° angle and the stem pushed proximally.

The carbide punch is placed more distally on the stem through the same drill hole, and force is applied to drive the stem more proximally. This process is repeated until the stem can be removed from above. Alternatively, an ETO allows placement of a trephine over the distal stem as described for the removal of the distal segment of an extensively coated stem.

—————◼

Avoiding Pitfalls and Complications

Femur fracture is a dreaded complication in explanting femoral stems and is best avoided by using the techniques described above and avoiding use of space-occupying osteotomes between the prosthesis and cement or host bone. Generous release of soft tissue around the femur allows less forceful femoral rotation and decreases the risk of spiral fractures in the setting of osteopenic bone. In most cases, patience and nonforceful extraction will help avoid fractures.

—————◼

References

Aribindi R, Paprosky WG, Nourbash P, Kronick J, Barba M: Extended proximal femoral osteotomy. *Instr Course Lect* 1999;48:19-26.

Berry DJ: Removal of cementless stems. *Instr Course Lect* 2003;52:331-336.

Glassman AH: The removal of cementless total hip femoral components. *Instr Course Lect* 2002;51:93-101.

Glassman AH, Engh CA: The removal of porous coated femoral hip stems. *Clin Orthop* 1992;285:164-180.

Hozack WJ: Removal of components and cement, in Callaghan JJ, Rosenberg AG, Rubash HE (eds): *The Adult Hip*. Philadelphia, PA, Lippincott Williams & Wilkins, 1998, pp 1387-1412.

Lieberman JR, Moeckel BH, Evans BG, Salvati EA, Ranawat CS: Cement-within-cement revision hip arthroplasty. *J Bone Joint Surg Br* 1993;75:869-871.

Paprosky WG, Weeden SH, Bowling JW Jr: Component removal in revision total hip arthroplasty. *Clin Orthop* 2001;393:181-193.

Coding

CPT Codes		Corresponding ICD-9 Codes		
27091	Removal of hip prosthesis; complicated, including total hip prosthesis, methylmethacrylate with or without insertion of spacer	996.4	996.66	996.77
27132	Conversion of previous hip surgery to total hip arthroplasty, with or without autograft or allograft	996.4	996.66	996.77
27134	Revision of total hip arthroplasty; both components, with or without autograft or allograft	996.4	996.66	996.77
27138	Revision of total hip arthroplasty; femoral component only, with or without allograft	996.4	996.66	996.77

Chapter 51
Femoral Revision: Cemented Stems

Dennis K. Collis, MD
Brian A. Jewett, MD

◼ Indications

The indications for revision hip surgery are intolerable pain and/or progressive bone loss. In most patients, we believe that another cemented femoral component can be used in revision of a loose femoral component. The three interrelated criteria a surgeon should use in choosing to use cement in femoral revision are the patient's age, the amount of bone loss, and the anatomy of the existing residual bone. If considerable cortical loss is present, structural allografting (chapter 58) and/or allograft composite replacement (chapter 57) may be necessary. However, a cemented stem may be used with either of these bone grafting methods. If the intramedullary bone loss is significant, morcellized impaction techniques may be valuable to replace the loss. Thus, the use of a cemented femoral component for revision has a wide spectrum of indications.

The ideal candidate for revision of a cemented stem with another cemented stem is a patient who does not require intramedullary or extramedullary grafting. It is helpful if some cancellous bone remains in the upper metaphyseal region. However, this procedure can be used when there is some segmental loss of the cortical bone. If the entire upper third of the femur is shiny cortical bone, it is im-

portant that the upper diaphysis be prepared for some bone interdigitation. The adequacy of cancellous bone is determined at the time of surgery; it cannot always be predicted by radiographs because cancellous bone can be found in parts of the upper metaphyseal region, such as in the lesser trochanter. When the previous stem has been 13 to 14 cm long, a stem that is 4 to 5 cm longer will incorporate the use of primary bone distally. If the remaining intramedullary canal is very wide, some surgeons consider the use of an extensively porous-coated uncemented stem to be contraindicated (**Figure 1**). Angular deformities of the residual bone stock can be accommodated more easily with a cemented stem than with an uncemented stem.

The patient's age should be used in judging whether to use a cemented femoral component. We believe that most patients with moderate residual bone stock are candidates for a revision using a cemented femoral component based on our results using this technique over the last 30 years. In patients older than age 75 years, more bone loss can be accepted before a grafting technique is used. In patients in their 50s, cemented stem revision is less commonly used, and in patients younger than 50 years, unless there is significant bone stock loss or unusual anatomy is present, uncemented revi-

sion may be the best choice. Cemented stem revision should be considered for patients of any age when remaining bone stock allows adequate cement technique and the bone stock is deficient or deformed enough that standard uncemented techniques are not likely to produce a good result.

◼ Contraindications

The most significant contraindication to using a cemented stem is a patient younger than age 50 years with a normal life expectancy and a bony anatomy that would allow use of an uncemented stem with an expected successful result. The other major contraindication is a patient in whom the bone stock is so deficient that a cemented stem will not provide adequate secure fixation. Such deficient bone stock, however, may be supplemented by the use of impaction grafting techniques (chapter 56). It is neither expected nor essential that a cemented stem be recemented into primary bone stock with the classic interdigitation grouting techniques proposed by Charnley.

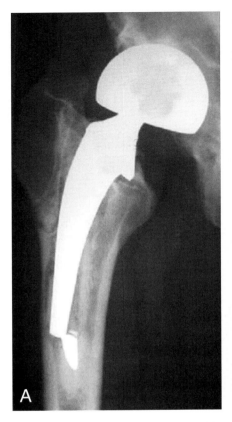

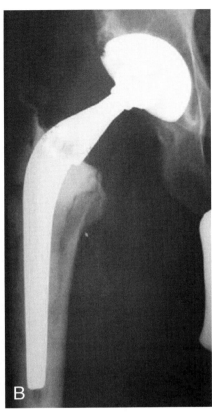

Figure 1 A 6-foot tall, 220-lb, 45-year-old man with a failed cemented bipolar arthroplasty with a wide canal and anatomy that indicated a cemented standard stem length revision. **A,** Preoperative AP radiograph shows the fractured loose stem. **B,** Postoperative AP radiograph shows the cemented arthroplasty.

Alternative Treatments

The alternate treatments to using only cemented stems in revision are the use of composite allograft, strut allograft, or impaction grafting and the use of an uncemented stem revision if the bone quality is sufficient to provide a good result. Both modular and nonmodular proximally and extensively porous-coated stems may be alternatives depending on the residual bone. Uncemented devices should be considered when revising failed uncemented stems where prior surgery used aggressive canal reaming, which leaves no cancellous bone in the upper half of the femur.

Results

Cemented femoral components in revision total hip arthroplasty (THA) have been reported to give unsatisfactory results at early and midterm follow-up of patients operated on in the 1970s. Since that time, better cementing techniques and availability of numerous revision components have been reported to give better results. Cemented revisions done in the 1980s and 1990s illustrate the potential of achieving a long-standing successful revision THA (**Table 1** and **Figures 2** and **3**). From 1980 to 2000, Collis inserted 274 cemented femoral components; 90 in the 1980s and the other 184 in the 1990s (**Table 1**). Only 5 of the 184 stems inserted in the 1990s were longer than 210 mm, and antibi-

otics were used less than 30% of the time. By 2004, 6 of the stems inserted in the 1980s and 13 of the stems inserted in the 1990s were revised for loosening. In addition, 6 of the 274 stems required prosthetic removal for late deep infections. Six of the 19 re-revised stems were revised after 10 years of clinical success. Radiographs of the remaining stems showed no unequivocal loosening and no major lysis.

Technique

Exposure

The patient is placed in a lateral decubitus position on the table with the torso secured by a beanbag or hip positioners. Previous incisions about the hip should be noted and marked, but the skin incision is typically a straight, direct lateral incision. Depending on the difficulty expected with the removal of the failed implant, the trochanter may or may not be osteotomized. Frequently, an anterolateral or posterior approach without trochanteric osteotomy can be readily performed. Because it is best to have as much continuity of the primary femur as possible so that a new stem can be cemented, an extended trochanteric osteotomy (ETO) is contraindicated. If the surgeon anticipates that removing a large distal cement plug will be difficult, an anterior cortical window would be preferred over the ETO to maintain an intact cylinder of femur proximally. The entire hip capsule is removed so that the proximal femur is well mobilized and the medullary canal can be readily accessed. Pins are placed in the ilium, a mark is placed on the lateral shaft, and the distance between the two is measured for future limb-length assessment.

Prosthesis and Cement Removal

Once the proximal femur is fully accessed, any cement lateral to the

Table 1 Results of Femoral Revision Using Cemented Stems

Author(s) (Year)	Number of Hips	Implant Type	Mean Patient Age (Range)	Mean Follow-up (Range)	Average Rating	Femoral Component Revisions for Aseptic Loosening
Jewett and Collis* (1980s)	90	Iowa, Harris, and others	66.5 years (28–83)	7.1 years (1–21)	Iowa hip score = 88	6
Jewett and Collis* (1990s)	184	Iowa, Heritage, and others	70.6 years (40–88)	3.2 years (1–14)	Iowa hip score = 89	11
Schmale, et al (2000)	56	Centraligh, Precoat, Iowa Precoat, and others	68 years (40–87)	4 years (2–8)	Harris hip score = 79	9
Gramkow, et al (2001)	84	Lubinus ster (Stanmore, UK)	69 years (30–88)	11.4 years (7.9–15)	Harris hip score = 91 (Maximum; average not reported)	10
Hultmark, et al (2000)	109	Charnley, Spectron, Brunswick, and others	65 years (42–80)	8.7 years (0.5–14.5)	Harris hip score = 74	13
Crawford, et al (2000)	74	Custom modular femoral component (Charnley with modifications)	66 years (34–84)	5.7 years (1–12)	Not reported	3
Haydon, et al (2004)	97	Biomet, HNR, Harris Design 2, and others	68 years (39–86)	10.3 years (5–23.2)	Harris hip score = 71	9

*Personal database of Dennis K. Collis, unpublished.

shoulder of the implant is to be removed so that the failed stem and any surrounding attached cement can be readily removed without damage to the femur. Residual cement that has adhered to the bone is best removed with hand chisels and osteotomes, taking care to avoid perforating the femur. If there is no infection, it is not essential to remove all cement, but it is necessary to ensure that the canal is open enough to permit a revision stem that is often longer than its predecessor. Reverse cup curettes, available in cement removal instrument sets from several manufacturers, are valuable to remove not only residual diaphyseal cement but also the membrane that is usually present at the bone-cement interface (**Figure 4**). Removal of a retained distal cement plug can be facil-

itated by an ultrasonic plug puller device with an attached slap hammer. Alternatively, a thin blade curette may be passed between the bone and the cement and the plug removed with a slap hammer attachment. A canal light that extends down into the canal and provides good visualization of the diaphyseal region of the femur and any distal cement can be helpful. The distal cement plug also can be removed by drilling through the center of it with an 8-mm cement drill, and once the surgeon is sure that he or she is within the confines of that distal cement plug, the cement can be removed with conical cement taps. An alternative to these devices is to place an anterior window to expose the plug and remove it with hand instruments. We rarely use the high-speed burrs in the

diaphysis when approaching the femur from the proximal end because of the risk of perforation.

Bone Preparation

After removal of the prosthesis, cement, and distal plug, the bone is prepared for the new prosthesis by roughening the sclerotic surfaces, if this can be done without cortical penetration, even using the light touch of a high-speed burr to make the surfaces irregular. Also, small osteotomes can be used to make irregularities in the metaphyseal region, and it is often helpful to clean out new areas for cement interdigitation into the bone of the greater and lesser trochanters. If new primary bone is being used in the upper diaphysis, endosteal bone should not be aggressively reamed or curetted.

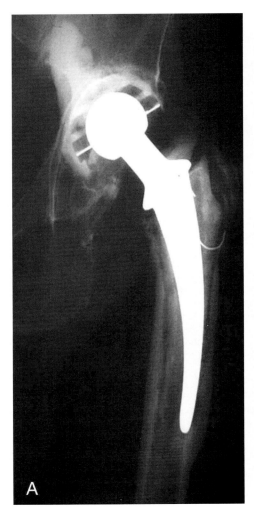
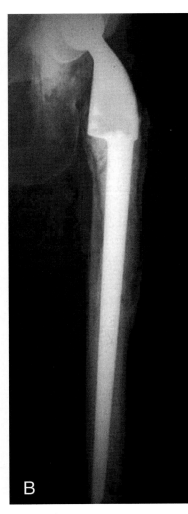

Once the canal has been prepared and the prosthesis has been selected, the distal canal needs to be plugged. In most instances, a standard polyethylene cement plug can be used to plug the mid- to distal diaphysis. Occasionally, leaving the old cement plug in place is advisable if proximal bone stock is reasonable without too much lysis. If the stem is going to extend into the lower metaphyseal region where the femur flares, another method of canal plugging must be used. Usually a separate batch of cement is injected with a long cement gun and allowed to harden after ensuring that it is distal to where the tip of the prosthesis will be located.

Prosthesis Implantation

Once the canal is prepared and plugged as described above, it should be prepared with pulsatile lavage and carefully dried with a gauze or sponge packing that has a dilute epinephrine solution to decrease bleeding. The packing is left in place until the cement is ready to be inserted. Just before cement insertion, the packing is removed, and new dry packing is placed to further dry the canal. If there is a voluminous canal or a long prosthesis, two separate batches of two packs of cement, each with two separate cement delivery guns, need to be mixed. Very rarely are more than four packages of cement necessary for good canal filling. The cement is either mixed under vacuum or centrifuged and inserted with a gun that allows retrograde insertion relatively late in the mixing stage. The cement should be doughy and not stick to the surgeon's gloves. The canal is filled completely, the cement column is pressurized, and then the prosthesis is introduced carefully into the appropriate alignment position and inserted to the proper level as determined from trial reductions. The prosthesis must be held very still in the cement bed and not allowed to either rotate or subside until the ce-

Figure 2 **A,** Preoperative AP view of the hip in a 53-year-old man with 12 previous hip surgeries. Three were THAs resulting in marked proximal bone loss. **B,** AP view of the same hip treated with a calcar replacement prosthesis with a cemented stem 11 years after surgery. The patient was still doing well with this revision when he died 12 years postoperatively.

Prosthesis Selection

Once the canal has been prepared, a new prosthesis must be selected. Preoperatively, it is important to have templated a number of different components and have them available (**Figure 5**). It is especially important to have prosthetic components with extended neck lengths available. Use of extra-long modular heads with skirts should be avoided because they increase the neck diameter and can lead to impingement on the bone or acetabular component. Calcar replacement prostheses or extended neck

length prostheses can provide limb length and reduce the need for "skirted" extra-long modular neck lengths. Stem length selection is important. An important principle is that the stem length should exceed any defects or perforations in the femur by at least two diameters of the width of the femur. Most stem lengths in revision surgery using cement a second time are between 140 and 210 mm. Trial prostheses should be available so that the surgeon can obtain the appropriate length in order to achieve good stability.

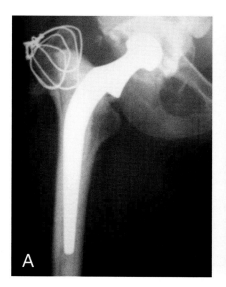
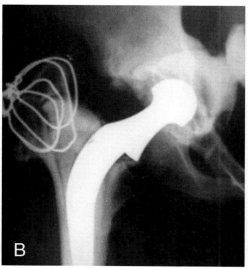
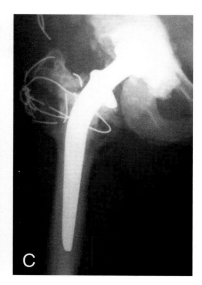

Figure 3   **A,** AP radiograph of a 20-year-old patient after undergoing an initial THA. **B,** AP radiograph obtained 5 years postoperatively shows obvious proximal loosening and prosthesis subsidence. **C,** Twenty years after the revision, the bone, cement, and prosthesis look good.

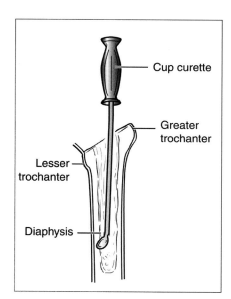

Figure 4   Removal of loose bone, membrane, and residual cement using reverse cutting (cup) curette. The shaded area represents membrane, bone, and cement.

ment is hardened over approximately a 15-minute period.

When the cement is fully hardened, trial heads are used to obtain the proper length and stability. As with any standard hip operation, the appropriate modular head is applied to a clean dry trunion. In revision surgery, we prefer to use a larger-diameter modular head, at least 32 mm. When the cup also has been exchanged, a 36- or 40-mm head size can be considered to optimize hip stability.

Wound Closure

Once the femoral head has been placed and the hip is reduced and stable, the leg is placed on a Mayo stand and the wound is closed in the standard fashion. If the trochanter has been osteotomized, two wires usually are placed through the lesser trochanter and then brought circumferentially around the trochanter and two wires are placed in the lateral cortex prior to cement insertion. If only soft tissue needs repair, standard closure is appropriate with drains placed deep in the wound.

Postoperative Regimen

In the recovery room the patient is placed in balanced suspension, with plans to ambulate the day after surgery using crutches. If there is any question about stability, a hip abduction brace can be used because dislocations are much more frequent after revision surgery. Routine protection includes 6 to 8 weeks on crutches and another 6 to 8 weeks on a cane, but unless unusual instability is present or extensive bone grafting done, the patient is walking at full weight bearing within 4 months. No particular extra physical therapy other than gait training is done until 3 to 4 months postoperatively when patients are started on abduction and extension leg raises. Permanent restrictions are the same as for a primary THA, no lifting of more than 40 lb or running or jumping. For patients with a multiply revised hip and soft tissues of questionable strength, a cane might be recommended for an extended period of time and, on rare occasions, permanently. Patients are checked routinely at 6 weeks, 3 months, 6 months, and yearly intervals and radiographs taken. Because revision surgery has been done, the usual criteria of radiolucencies at the bone-cement interface suggesting early failure are not valid (**Figure 4**). The surgeon must depend more on change in prosthetic position to diagnose stem loosening.

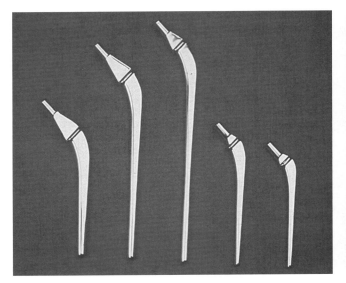

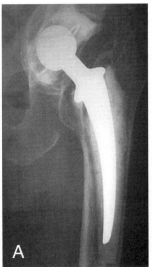

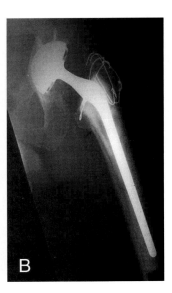

Figure 5 Examples of cemented revision stems with varying proximal offset and lengths so that the bone loss in the femoral head-neck region can be restored with the prosthetic device above the calcar.

Figure 6 **A,** AP radiograph of a 72-year-old patient with a loose cemented stem and a generous medullary canal. **B,** Following THA with a cemented stem and an adequate bone-cement interface, the result does not achieve the results of the primary cemented stem.

■ Avoiding Pitfalls and Complications

Numerous prosthetic components must be available so that alterations can be made intraoperatively. The best possible cementing technique must be used to ensure that the stem is securely set in the best mantle that can be obtained. If there is a femoral fracture during the operation, the fracture can be reduced and cabled, with either allograft bone plating or metal plating done before cementing the stem. However, if this step is necessary, the fracture must be well reduced to avoid cement extrusion through the fracture areas.

If there are defects in the femoral cortex, the assistant surgeon can control cement extrusion during insertion merely by holding his or her fingers over the defects. If the defects are quite large, cortical allografts may be needed to place over them. However,

allografts are usually best placed after the cement has been inserted. This allows close attachment of the allograft plates with surrounding cerclage wires directly to the bone so that cement is not extruded beneath them. Some authors have tried various methods of hoses and clamps and rubber dams. If there are segmental defects in the upper femur, it is important to ensure that there is not excessive cement extruding from them, and if cement is found to be extruded through either a cortical window or segmental area, it can be easily removed after the cement has cured.

Surgeons not familiar with cemented revision techniques are often concerned about cement hardening too early. It has been our experience that cement inserted in the 6- to 8-minute range, with the temperature in the operating room at 67° to 68°F, will allow careful insertion of the prosthesis with no early hardening. In less experienced hands, it might be prefer-

able to insert the stem a minute or so earlier. However, it is not advisable to be holding a fully inserted stem if the cement has not achieved a doughy consistency because it is difficult to maintain the stem in its proper position in a more liquid cement mantle. It is also helpful to have a bony anatomic positioning mark to confirm the insertion level selected in trial reduction. It is often possible to seat the small collar of the prosthesis on this bony landmark for further security (**Figure 6**).

Using cemented stems in revision surgery is a successful method of treatment; however, it should not be used in all instances. Extensively porous-coated stems should be used in young patients with good bone stock and small inside diameter femoral canals. However, in most patients older than age 65 years, cemented stem revision usually results in long-term success.

———————————————■

References

Collis DK: Revision total hip arthroplasty with cement. *Semin Arthroplasty* 1993;4:38-49.

Crawford SA, Siney PD, Wroblewski BM: Revision of failed total hip arthroplasty with a proximal femoral modular cemented stem. *J Bone Joint Surg Br* 2000;82:684-688.

Estok DM, Harris WH: Long-term results of cemented femoral revision surgery using second-generation techniques. *Clin Orthop* 1994;299:190.

Gramkow J, Jensen TH, Varmarken JE, Retpen JB: Long-term results after cemented revision of the femoral component in total hip arthroplasty. *J Arthroplasty* 2001;16:777-783.

Haydon CM, Mehin R, Burnett S, et al: Revision total hip arthroplasty with use of a cemented femoral component. *J Bone Joint Surg Am* 2004;86:1179-1185.

Hultmark P, Karrholm J, Stromberg C, et al: Cemented first-time revisions of the femoral component. *J Arthroplasty* 2000;15:551-561.

Marti RK, Schuller HM, Cesselarr PP, et al: Results of revision of hip arthroplasty with cement: A five to 14 year follow-up. *J Bone Joint Surg Am* 1990;72:346-354.

Mohler CG, Collis DK: Femoral revision: Cemented, in Steinberg ME, Garino JP (eds): *Revision Total Hip Arthroplasty*. Philadelphia, PA, Lippincott-Raven, 1999, pp 339-350.

Mulroy WF, Harris WH: Revision total hip arthroplasty with use of so-called second generation cementing techniques for aseptic loosening of the femoral component: A 15-year average follow-up study. *J Bone Joint Surg Am* 1996;78:325-330.

Pellicci PM, Wilson PD, Sledge CG, et al: Long-term results of revision total hip replacement: A follow-up report. *J Bone Joint Surg Am* 1985;67:513-516.

Schmale GA, Lachiewicz PF, Kelley SS: Early failure of revision total hip arthroplasty with cemented precoated femoral components. *J Arthroplasty* 2000;15:718-728.

Weber KL, Callaghan JJ, Goetz DD, Johnston RC: Revision of a failed cemented total hip prosthesis with insertion of an acetabular component without cement and a femoral component with cement. *J Bone Joint Surg Am* 1996;78:982.

Coding				
CPT Codes		**Corresponding ICD-9 Codes**		
27134	Revision of total hip arthroplasty; both components, with or without autograft or allograft	996.4	996.66	996.77
27138	Revision of total hip arthroplasty; femoral component only, with or without allograft	996.4	996.66	996.77

CPT copyright © 2004 by the American Medical Association. All Rights Reserved.

Chapter 52

Femoral Revision: Extensively Porous-Coated Stems

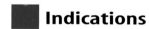

Wayne G. Paprosky, MD
Scott M. Sporer, MD, MS

Indications

Despite the overwhelming success and long-term reliability of total hip arthroplasty (THA), several situations necessitate the revision of a femoral component. The incidence of femoral revisions has not changed significantly; however, the absolute number of revisions continues to increase. The most frequent indications for femoral revision include aseptic loosening, recurrent instability from a malpositioned component, component fracture, delayed infection, and the need for improved acetabular exposure. Relative indications for femoral component removal include progressive distal femoral osteolysis or discretionary revision of a femoral component with a poor track record during acetabular revision.

A successful surgical result following femoral reconstruction requires the extraction of the previous component with as little bone loss as possible, the insertion of a new component with resistance against rotational and axial stresses, and a stable hip following reduction. The use of an extended trochanteric osteotomy (ETO) often is recommended to extract a well-fixed stem, to address a femur that has shown varus remodeling, or to facilitate removal of distal cement. This surgical technique al-

lows both preservation of bone stock and concentric reaming of the femur.

The type of femoral component used during reconstruction depends on the quality of remaining host bone. The Paprosky system of classifying femoral defects is helpful in preoperative planning and in assisting the surgeon with reconstructive options (**Figure 1**). Patients with type I bone have minimal metaphyseal bone loss; reconstruction can be done with a component that is similar to the one used in the index procedure. Successful results can be expected with a cemented, a proximally porous-coated, or an extensively coated stem (**Figure 2**). However, most femoral revisions have intact diaphyseal bone with compromise of the metaphyseal region (Paprosky type II) or involvement of the proximal diaphysis with more extensive metaphyseal bone loss (Paprosky type IIIA). In these patients, the metaphyseal region is not consistently supportive to provide stable component fixation. Extensively porous-coated stems, which rely on the intact diaphyseal bone rather than the deficient metaphyseal bone, are recommended in these situations (**Figures 3** and **4**). Patients with type IIIB bone have extensive metaphyseal bone loss and significant involvement of the diaphysis. In these patients, less than 5 cm of diaphyseal bone stock is available for implant fixation. A long-stemmed (8- or

10-inch) extensively porous-coated implant can still be used in this situation, particularly if the endosteal diameter is less than 19 mm. Patients with a type IIIB femur and an associated endosteal diameter greater than 19 mm have a higher incidence of subsidence and a decreased likelihood of achieving bone ingrowth. Alternative methods of reconstruction are recommended in this patient population, as well as in patients with type IV defects (**Figure 5**).

Contraindications

We consider other reimplantation methods in patients with Paprosky type IIIB and IV bone loss with femoral canals greater than 19 mm. In these situations, the large femoral components required for surgery are very stiff, and we are concerned about the risk of thigh pain and proximal stress shielding.

Alternative Treatments

Most patients in need of a femoral revision can be treated successfully with

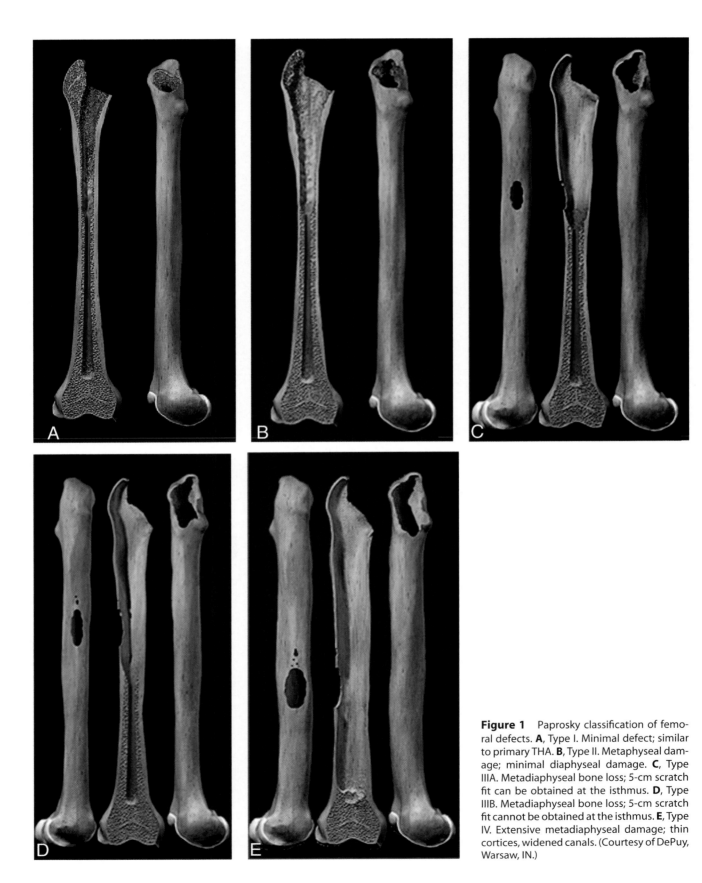

Figure 1 Paprosky classification of femoral defects. **A**, Type I. Minimal defect; similar to primary THA. **B**, Type II. Metaphyseal damage; minimal diaphyseal damage. **C**, Type IIIA. Metadiaphyseal bone loss; 5-cm scratch fit can be obtained at the isthmus. **D**, Type IIIB. Metadiaphyseal bone loss; 5-cm scratch fit cannot be obtained at the isthmus. **E**, Type IV. Extensive metadiaphyseal damage; thin cortices, widened canals. (Courtesy of DePuy, Warsaw, IN.)

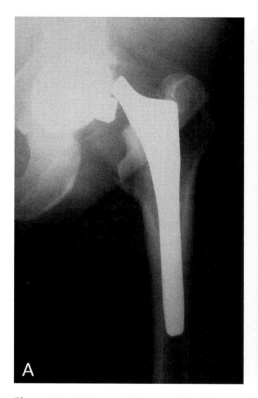

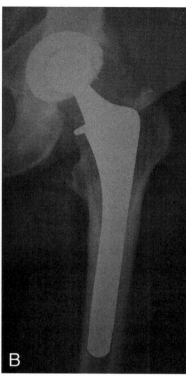

Figure 2 A 55-year-old man with a fracture of the neck of the femoral component. **A,** Preoperative radiograph of a type I femoral defect. **B,** Postoperative radiograph showing a 6-inch extensively coated stem.

either a 6- or 8-inch extensively porous-coated stem. Alternative options are considered in patients with a type IV defect, a type IIIB defect with an associated large endosteal diameter, and in a patient with a canal diameter too large to gain fixation with available extensively porous-coated stems. In these situations, patient age, medical comorbidities, and patient activity level are important considerations. Surgical options include the use of an allograft prosthetic composite (APC), impaction bone grafting, a modular tapered stem, or a cemented long-stemmed component. In general, the surgeon should attempt to restore bone stock with an APC or impaction bone grafting in a younger, healthier, more active patient. Impaction bone grafting requires a residual shell of cortical bone or a canal that can be constructed with metal mesh or allograft struts in the proximal aspect of the femur. A modular tapered stem can also provide excellent results in some patients with enlarged endosteal

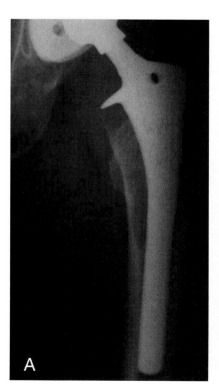

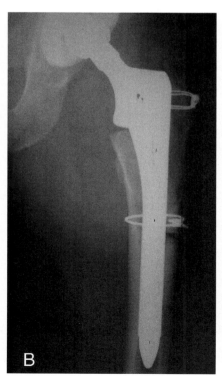

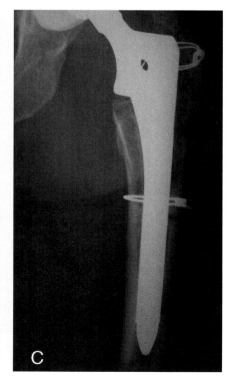

Figure 3 Preoperative **(A)**, postoperative **(B)**, and 8-year postoperative **(C)** radiographs of the extensively coated prosthesis in a 61-year-old patient with a loose cemented femoral component. Note the healed trochanteric osteotomy.

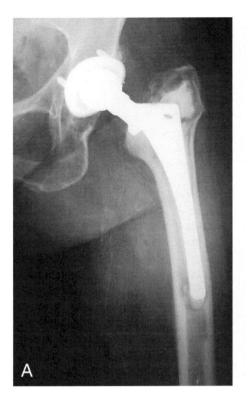
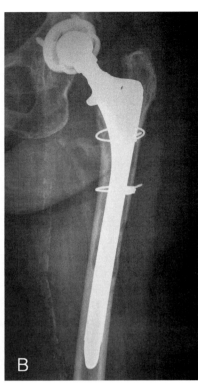

Figure 4 A 67-year-old woman with a loose femoral component. **A,** Preoperative radiograph of a type IIIA femoral defect. **B,** Postoperative radiograph showing an 8-inch bowed femoral component.

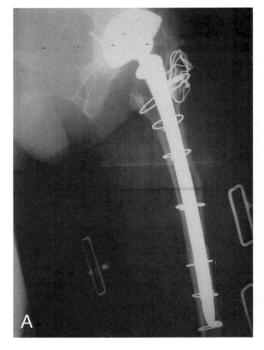
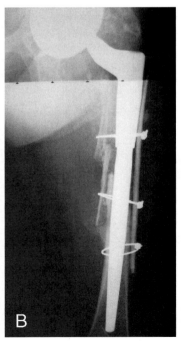

Figure 5 A 74-year-old man with a loose 10-inch extensively coated stem. Preoperative **(A)** and postoperative **(B)** AP radiographs showing a modular tapered revision femoral component.

diameters. The use of a cemented long-stemmed component or a tumor prosthesis is an attractive option for the low-demand patient in whom the surgeon strives to minimize blood loss and operative time.

Results

An extensively porous-coated stem used during femoral revision surgery has been shown to provide reliable and predictable long-term results. Most surgeons now consider an extensively porous-coated stem the standard implant during most femoral revision surgery. A series of 188 patients who had extensively porous-coated stems inserted at the time of revision had an overall mechanical failure rate of only 4.1% at 14-year follow-up. Extensive bone loss and a large endosteal canal were highly predictive of a poor outcome. Similarly, in another series of 204 patients evaluated at an average follow-up of 12.2 years, only 3.4% of patients required revision for loosening or progressive osteolysis. These results are superior to those reported for either a cemented or monoblock proximally porous-coated implant (**Table 1**).

Technique

Exposure
Similar to other surgical procedures, adequate preoperative planning is essential for a successful surgical outcome. If the femoral component appears to be well fixed and must be removed, if there is a long column of well-fixed cement, or if there is marked femoral varus remodeling, an extended greater trochanteric osteotomy provides strong advantages (**Figure 6**). It is imperative that an os-

Table 1   Results With Extensively Porous-Coated Revision Femoral Components

Author(s)/ Year	Number of Hips	Implant Type	Mean Patient Age (Range)	Mean Follow-up (Range)	Results
Weeden and Paprosky (2002)	170	AML & Solution (DePuy, Warsaw, IN)	61.2 years	14.2 years (11–16 years)	3.5% revision for aseptic femoral loosening 4.1% mechanical failure rate
Engh, et al (2004)	777	AML & Solution	N/A	20-year experience	Revision for any reason: 97.7% at 5 years 95.8% at 10 years 95.8% at 15 years Increased rate of revision with bone loss >10 cm below lesser trochanter
Moreland and Moreno (2001)	137	AML & Solution	63 years	9.3 years (5–16 years)	4% revision rate of aseptic femoral loosening 83% radiographic bone ingrowth
Krishnamurthy, et al (1997)	297	AML & Solution	59.6 years (24–86)	8.3 years (5–14 years)	1.7% femoral revision for aseptic loosening 2.4% mechanical failure rate
Moreland and Bernstein (1995)	175	AML & Solution	62.4 years	5 years (2–10 years)	96% component survival 98% survival for aseptic loosening 83% bone ingrowth
Lawrence, et al (1994)	83	AML & Solution	57 years (21–83)	9 years (5–13 years)	10% femoral re-revision 11% mechanical failure of femoral component

AML = Anatomic Medullary Locking

cillating saw, pencil-tip burr, several wide osteotomes, cerclage wires, and in selected cases, trephines, Gigli saws, and metal-cutting burrs be available in the operative suite.

The surgical approach in the revision setting may be directed by previous surgical incisions. In general, a posterior lateral approach is used to facilitate visualization of both the femur and the acetabulum. This approach allows extension both proximally and distally if needed. A lateral surgical skin incision is made in line with the femur based on the posterior third of the greater trochanter. The tensor fascia lata and the fascia of the gluteus maximus are then split in line with the surgical incision and retracted with a Charnley bow. The posterior pseudocapsule and the short external rotators are then elevated as a posteriorly based flap. A portion of the gluteus maximus insertion is then released to allow mobilization of the fe-

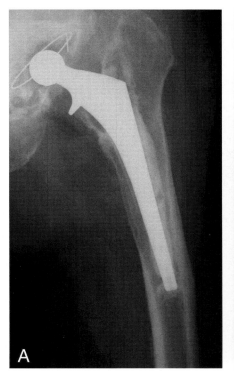
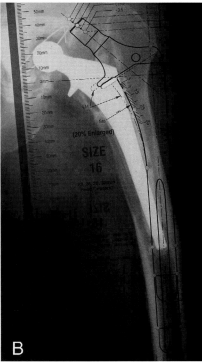

Figure 6   **A** and **B,** Femoral varus remodeling. An ETO is required to avoid lateral cortical perforation during femoral preparation.

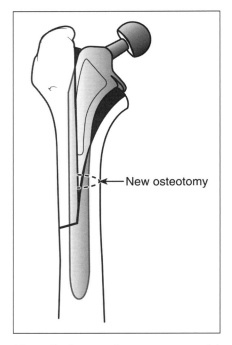

Figure 7 In cases of severe varus remodeling, an osteotomy of the remaining reduced bone can be required to provide good bone apposition. The osteotomy is usually made with a Gigli saw 1 or 2 cm above the most distal aspect of the lateral osteotomy.

mur. The femoral head is then dislocated, and the hip is placed in internal rotation with the knee flexed. The stability of the femoral component is then assessed. If the stem is grossly loose and the greater trochanter is not preventing extraction, the component is removed. However, if the trochanter prevents component removal or if the stem is well fixed, an in situ ETO is performed.

An ETO is initiated by identifying the posterior margin of the vastus lateralis. This muscle belly is mobilized anteriorly without stripping muscle from the anticipated osteotomy fragment. The length of the osteotomy is determined, and the distal extent of the osteotomy is marked. The femur is held in full extension and internally rotated. The saw is directed from posterolateral to anterolateral. Ideally, the osteotomy fragment should encompass the posterolateral third of the proximal femur and

should be oriented perpendicular to the anteversion of the hip. An oscillating saw is used to make the longitudinal arm of the osteotomy. Proximally, the saw is angled medially so that the entire greater trochanter is released with the osteotomy. The distal transverse limb of the osteotomy is made with the use of a pencil-tip burr, and the corners are rounded. This will minimize stress risers and will decrease the risk of propagating a fracture. Wide osteotomes are used to gently lever the osteotomy site from posterior to anterior. The greater trochanteric fragment is retracted with the attached abductors and vastus lateralis. Because the remaining blood supply and innervation to the vastus enter anteriorly, it is important to minimize dissection along the anterolateral limb of the osteotomy.

Once the osteotomy has been completed, the femoral component now can be adequately visualized and removed (chapter 50).

Bone Preparation
Preparation of the femoral canal can begin once the previous component has been successfully removed. It is imperative to concentrically ream the remaining diaphyseal bone. If the femur has undergone varus remodeling, an ETO helps to avoid perforation of the lateral cortex. The femoral canal is sequentially reamed until cortical resistance is encountered. Throughout reaming, the surgeon should be aware of the depth of the anticipated insertion of the new stem. A minimum of 5 cm of diaphyseal bone, "scratch fit," is required when using an extensively porous-coated stem. Alternative methods of reconstruction should be considered if this is not feasible.

The femoral canal is reamed sequentially with straight reamers until endosteal contact is encountered if a straight 6- or 8-inch extensively porous-coated prosthesis is chosen. The canal is underreamed by 0.5 mm compared to the diameter of the femoral

implant to provide axial and rotation implant stability. If the femoral bow is encountered and distal fixation with either an 8- or 10-inch stem is required, flexible reamers are used to sequentially ream the diaphysis. The femoral canal is initially underreamed by 0.5 mm, and an attempt is made to place the femoral component. If the final implant cannot be placed within 5 cm of the final position by hand, without impaction with a hammer, the canal is reamed line to line. Prior to placement of the implant, a cerclage wire placed distal to the osteotomy site is recommended to avoid inadvertent femoral fracture during component insertion.

A femoral trial component is placed, the hip can be reduced, and stable range of motion can be assessed. Provided that the hip is stable, the anticipated femoral component anteversion is marked. If an 8- or 10-inch bowed stem is used, the bow of the femur and the prosthesis, to some degree, control the ultimate amount of femoral anteversion. If the hip is not stable in this configuration, alternative methods of reconstruction such as a modular stem should be considered.

Prosthesis Implantation
The placement of an extensively porous-coated stem in the revision situation is similar to that used during primary THA. A hole gauge should be used to verify that the manufacturing process has resulted in the appropriate distal femoral diameter (eg, an 18-mm component should be able to pass through the 18.25-mm hole, not the 18-mm hole). If the component is slightly oversized, the femoral canal can be reamed an additional 0.5 mm to avoid femoral fracture. A series of gentle blows are used to seat the implant. The stem should advance with each strike with the mallet.

Wound Closure
Once the femoral component has been placed, the wound is closed in a rou-

tine manner. Two cables are used to secure the greater trochanter osteotomy fragment if an ETO was performed. The fragment can be advanced slightly distally and posteriorly to improve stability and avoid anterior greater trochanteric impingement with the pelvis in flexion and internal rotation. Bone grafting of the osteotomy site is not routinely performed. Our preference is to repair the posterior capsule and short external rotators to the posterior aspect of the gluteus medius. The gluteus maximus fascia and the iliotibial band are closed with interrupted sutures. If there is marked varus remodeling of the proximal femur that precludes gaining good apposition of the osteotomized bone and the medial bone, then the medial bone can be osteotomized (**Figure 7**).

Postoperative Regimen

Following a femoral revision, patients are treated with an abduction orthosis for 6 weeks postoperatively. During this time, partial weight bearing on the affected leg (30% of body weight) using a walker or crutch for ambulation is indicated. Patients are instructed to avoid active abduction for 6 weeks while the osteotomy site is healing. At the end of 6 weeks, they can use a cane and begin a strength training program.

Avoiding Pitfalls and Complications

Extensively porous-coated stems can provide reliable and predictable results if the appropriate indications are followed. A minimum of 5-cm "scratch fit" is required to provide immediate component stability. If this cannot be obtained, alternative methods of reconstruction should be considered. During preparation of the femur, it is imperative that the femur is reamed centrally and concentrically. An ETO allows direct access to the femoral canal with little associated morbidity in patients with retained cement, a well-fixed stem, or varus remodeling. An ETO helps minimize undersizing of the components, thereby providing intimate endosteal contact and reducing the likelihood of inadvertent cortical perforation.

If an 8- or 10-inch stem is planned, the magnitude of the anterior femoral bow must be assessed with appropriate preoperative templates. A curved stem should be used if templating indicates that a straight stem would cause anterior cortical perforation. If anterior cortical perforation occurs, the defect can be bypassed with a longer curved stem, or a protective anterior allograft strut can be placed.

A cerclage cable placed distal to the site of an ETO reduces the risk of distal fracture during insertion of an extensively coated stem. If an intraoperative fracture occurs, the stem can be removed, and distal cerclage cables should be placed around the femur extending beyond the extension of the fracture. The extensively coated stem can then be reinserted once the canal is reamed 0.5 mm larger than the prior ream. Alternatively, if a minimally displaced stable longitudinal fracture occurs and the stem fixation is good, the fracture can be treated with cerclage wires with the stem in situ.

References

Berry DJ, Harmsen WS, Ilstrup D, Lewallen DG, Cabenela M: Survivorship of uncemented proximally porous-coated femoral components. *Clin Orthop* 1995;319:168-177.

Engh CA Jr, Claus AM, Hopper RH Jr, Engh CA: Long-term results using the anatomic medullary locking hip prosthesis. *Clin Orthop* 2001;393:137-146.

Krishnamurthy AB , MacDonald SJ , Paprosky WG: 5- to 13-year follow-up study on cementless femoral components in revision surgery. *J Arthroplasty* 1997;12:839-847.

Lawrence JM, Engh CA, Macalino GE, Lauro GR: Outcome of revision hip arthroplasty done without cement. *J Bone Joint Surg Am* 1994;76:965-973.

Moreland JR, Bernstein ML: Femoral revision hip arthroplasty with uncemented, porous-coated stems. *Clin Orthop* 1995;319:141-150.

Moreland JR, Moreno MA: Cementless femoral revision arthroplasty of the hip: Minimum 5 years followup. *Clin Orthop* 2001;393:194-201.

Weeden SH, Paprosky WG: Minimal 11-year follow-up of extensively porous-coated stems in femoral revision total hip arthroplasty. *J Arthroplasty* 2002;17(suppl 1):134-137.

Younger TI, Bradford MS, Magnus RE, Paprosky WG: Extended proximal femoral osteotomy: A new technique for femoral revision arthroplasty. *J Arthroplasty* 1995;10:329-338.

Coding

CPT Codes		Corresponding ICD-9 Codes		
27130	Arthroplasty, acetabular and proximal femoral prosthetic replacement (total hip arthroplasty), with or without autograft or allograft	711.45 711.95 714.0 714.30 715.15	715.25 715.35 716.15 718.5 718.6	720.0 733.14 733.42 808.0 905.6
27132	Conversion of previous hip surgery to total hip arthroplasty, with or without autograft or allograft	715.15 715.25 715.35 718.2	718.5 718.6 733.14 733.42	905.6 996.4 996.66 996.77
27134	Revision of total hip arthroplasty; both components, with or without autograft or allograft	996.4	996.66	996.77
27138	Revision of total hip arthroplasty; femoral component only, with or without allograft	996.4	996.66	996.77

CPT copyright © 2004 by the American Medical Association. All Rights Reserved.

Chapter 53

Femoral Revision: Modular Proximally Porous-Coated Stems

David A. Mattingly, MD

 ## Indications

Use of modular proximally porous-coated stems in femoral revision total hip arthroplasty (THA) depends on the extent of femoral bone deformities and deficiencies after implant and cement removal. The success of modular femoral revision implants depends on distal diaphyseal stability (fit and fill) and adequate proximal bone to provide proximal rotational stability and ingrowth fixation. Modular proximally porous-coated stems work best when some degree of fixation to the proximal femur is possible, such as Paprosky type I, II, and IIIA defects (**Figure 1**). Modular proximally porous-coated stems can rarely be used effectively in Paprosky type IIIB and IV defects. Extensive metaphyseal bone loss usually requires a calcar replacement prosthesis, and stems longer than 200 mm usually are required for diaphyseal stability. Modular proximally porous-coated stems also may be used as an allograft prosthetic composite (APC) in Paprosky type IV defects.

Fit and fill of the proximal and distal femur are determined independently, permitting many different options for proximal size for each diameter stem. This unique modularity and stem flexibility permit use of this implant in femurs with multiple deformities, allowing intraoperative customization. Proximal sleeves are placed independent of the stem to allow for maximum contact with host bone in any degree of version, whereas the stem is placed in 10° to 25° of anteversion to maximize joint stability.

———■

 ## Contraindications

Modular proximally porous-coated stems are not indicated when proximal diaphyseal bone loss prevents adequate stability and fixation of the proximal sleeve (such as Paprosky type IIIB and IV defects). These stems should not be used in patients with severe proximal ectasia. Bone loss of more than 2 cm distal to the lesser trochanter does not provide adequate fixation of the proximal sleeve unless used as an APC.

Extended trochanteric osteotomy (ETO) is a relative contraindication for use of a modular proximally porous-coated stem. It should only be used in Dorr type A and B bone where there is excellent proximal bone stock and when an extremely tight diaphyseal fit and anatomic repair of the osteotomy fragment can be achieved. When these conditions were met, I have successfully used this stem in combination with an ETO in more than 30 patients.

———■

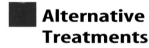 ## Alternative Treatments

Although modular proximally porous-coated stems can be used for most femoral revisions, other stems may be preferred in certain situations. Extensively porous-coated stems provide reliable fixation and results in Paprosky type IIIA and IIIB defects, where 4 to 5 cm of diaphyseal fixation is possible. These stems typically are preferred when an ETO is performed. The modular proximally porous-coated stem is useful in these situations only when reliable proximal sleeve contact and stability can be achieved.

For Paprosky type IV defects, a distally fixed, fluted tapered implant or impaction grafting should be considered. Modular proximally porous-coated stems are useful in this situation only if used as an APC (**Figure 2**).

———■

 ## Results

I began to use S-ROM modular proximally porous-coated stems for femoral revision in 1987. In clinical and radiographic reviews of my first 73 patients (75 hips) at an average follow-up of 10 years (range, 8 to 14 years), preoperative Harris hip scores and pain scores averaged 34 and 17, respectively, improving to 75 and 37, respec-

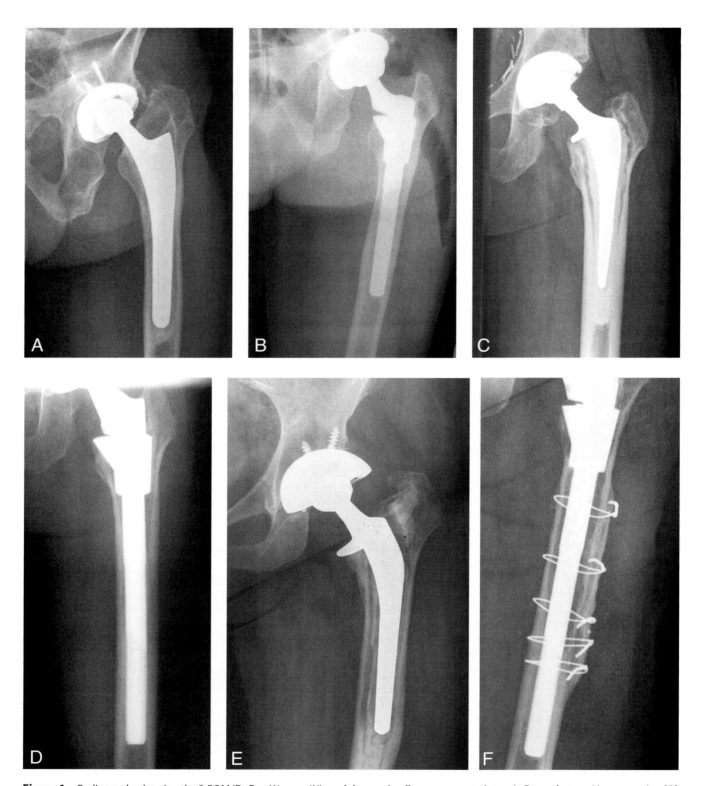

Figure 1   Radiographs showing the S-ROM (DuPuy, Warsaw, IN) modular proximally porous-coated stem in Paprosky type I (preoperative, [**A**] and postoperative [**B**]), type II (preoperative, [**C**] and postoperative [**D**]) and type III (preoperative, [**E**] and postoperative [**F**]) defects.

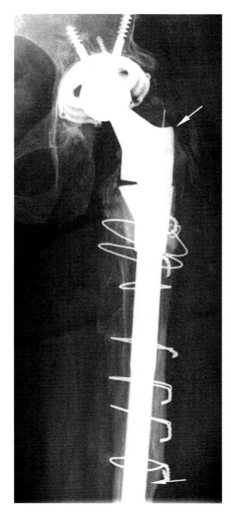

Figure 2 AP radiograph of a femur 5 years postoperatively shows cementing of an S-ROM sleeve (top arrow) into a proximal allograft. The bottom arrow shows healing at the allograft-host bone junction.

Table 1 Results of Modular Proximally Porous-Coated Stems

Author(s) (Year)	Number of Hips	Implant Type	Mean Patient Age (Range)	Mean Follow-up (Range)	Results
Mattingly and Bierbaum (2001)	75	S-ROM (DePuy)	59 years (44–83)	10 years (8–14)	No revisions for aseptic loosening 2 stems removed for sepsis Ingrown (94%), stable fibrous (3%), unstable fibrous (3%) No osteolysis distal to sleeve
Chandler, et al (1995)	52	S-ROM (DePuy)	60 years (NR)	3 years (2–5)	Greater trochanter bursitis and nonunion (38%) Minor nonpropagating fracture (25%) Dislocations (23%) Mechanical loosening (9%) No radiographic or histologic evidence of fretting at modular sleeve-stem junction or along stem Thigh pain (4%) directly related to stem diameters >17 mm Patient satisfaction (84%)
Christie, et al (2000)	129	Modular proximally porous-coated	NR	6.2 years (4–7)	Aseptic failure rate 2.9% 3 hips with osteolytic lesions < 5 mm No complications related to modularity
Christie, et al (1999)	175	S-ROM (DePuy)	59 years (22–93)	5.3 years (4–7.8), clinical 4.9 years (4–7.3) radiologic	Failed femoral component (0.6%), revised acetabular component (1%) Ingrowth (98%), stable fibrous (1%), unstable fibrous (0.6%) Periprosthetic osteolytic lesions (7%) No osteolytic lesions distal to the stem-sleeve junction

NR = Not reported

tively, at last follow-up. Only 4.5% of the patients reported activity-limiting thigh pain. No stems were revised for aseptic loosening. Two stems were removed from the same patient for sepsis. Radiographic review classified stem fixation as ingrown (94%), stable fibrous (3%), or unstable fibrous (3%). Both unstable fibrous stems were septic. No femur demonstrated osteolysis distal to the sleeve, although 16% demonstrated lysis proximal to the sleeve. Proximal femoral trabecular consolidation occurred in 82% of femurs, with no instances of proximal femoral stress shielding. Similarly satisfactory results using the S-ROM prosthesis for femoral revision also have been reported by other investigators (**Table 1**).

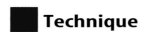

Technique

Exposure

Posterolateral and anterolateral approaches to the hip are preferred when using modular proximally porous-coated stems. Trochanteric osteotomy approaches (conventional, anterior trochanteric slide, and ETO) also may be used with adequate contact and stability of the proximal sleeve. These stems provide excellent stability and fixation when femoral cortical windows or diaphyseal osteotomy (transverse or oblique) are performed with a posterolateral or anterolateral approach. When femoral osteotomy or cortical windows are used, the inserted stem should bypass the most

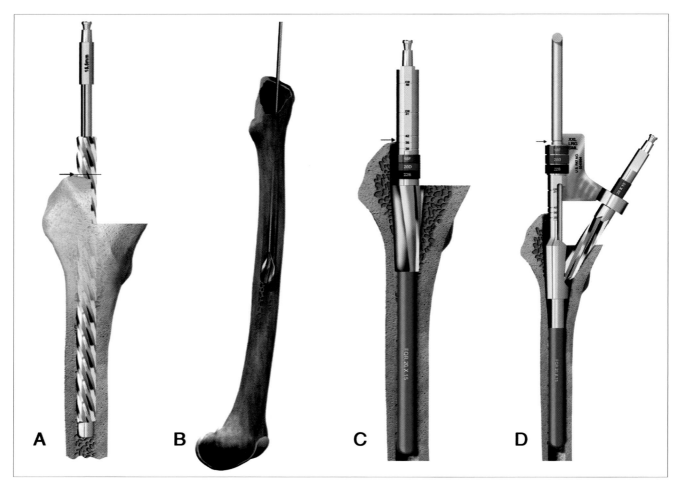

Figure 3   The three-step milling process demonstrating distal diaphyseal stem preparation with axial cylindrical (**A**) (step 1A) and flexible reamers (**B**) (step 1B); proximal bone preparation involves sequential conical reaming (**C**) (step 2) and calcar milling (**D**) (step 3) for the cone and triangle portions of the proximal sleeve. (Courtesy of DePuy and Johnson & Johnson.)

distal area of cortical weakness by 2 to 2.5 cortical diameters (5 to 7 cm).

Bone Preparation
After obtaining initial exposure, prophylactic 16-gauge cerclage wires are placed in those areas demonstrating femoral cortical deficiency on preoperative radiographs. This is done prior to removing the implant and cement to prevent or contain fractures resulting from this process. Adequate mobility and exposure of the femoral canal must be ensured before implant and cement removal. If necessary, complete capsulectomy or soft-tissue releases are performed to ensure proper access and visualization of the

femoral canal. Implant-specific extractors are recommended for femoral component removal. Femoral cement is removed by a combination of hand instruments, power burrs, and ultrasonic devices. All cement, membrane, and endosteal projections must be removed before bone preparation to prevent instrument deflection.

Femoral bone preparation for the S-ROM modular proximally porous-coated stem involves a three-step milling process. This not only entirely avoids broaching and reduces hoop stresses during instrumentation but also reduces the incidence of femoral fracture during revision THA. Distal diaphyseal preparation occurs first,

using axial cylindrical reamers (**Figure 3**, *A*) in a sequential process until firm diaphyseal cortical contact is obtained. This step is important in determining the proper stem diameter size for trialing and implantation. For Dorr type A and B bone, cylindrical reaming is performed to a diameter 0.5 mm greater than the minor stem diameter. In type C bone, reaming is performed to only the minor stem diameter. When long stems (greater than 200 mm) are selected, flexible reaming (**Figure 3**, *B*) of the distal femoral canal is recommended to avoid anterior cortical abutment, perforation, or fracture. With longer stems, flexible reaming is performed to either 1.0 mm greater (Dorr, type C bone) or 1.5 mm greater (Dorr, type A and B bone) than the minor stem diameter. This permits easier anteversion adjustments during stem placement and avoids distal perforations and fractures while allowing excellent three-point fixation of the stem.

Proximal bone preparation begins with sequential reaming using conical reamers (**Figure 3**, *C*) until firm anteroposterior endosteal cortical contact has been achieved. The size of the proximal cone for the final sleeve depends on the distal stem chosen. Three standard sizes and one oversized cone diameter may be used for each stem diameter. The stem version is selected independent of the trial sleeve.

Final bone preparation occurs with calcar miller reaming (**Figure 3**, *D*) to prepare the proximal femur to accommodate the calcar triangle portion of the final sleeve. The final triangle usually is placed in the proximal medial femur, often posteriorly into the lesser trochanter where bone deficiency exists because of femoral stem retroversion or lysis. The miller frame does not dictate stem placement. It can be placed in any degree of version to maximize contact with the remaining proximal host bone. The miller frame is lowered into the proximal femur until the miller cutter makes contact with the host cortical bone.

A trial sleeve is then inserted into the prepared proximal femur. The trial prosthesis is assembled by snapping the chosen neck onto the appropriate size distal stem. The trial prosthesis is introduced into the sleeve, and the trial neck can be adjusted in increments of 10° until desired version is obtained (**Figure 4**, *A*). Trial reduction can be performed with long, extra-long and double extra-long S-ROM distal stems. Trial assessments for motion, impingement, stability, offset, and limb length are then performed until a satisfactory construct is achieved. Differences in stem and

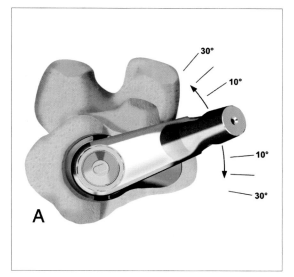

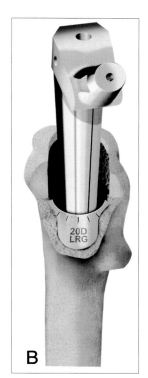

Figure 4   A, The trial neck can be adjusted in 10° increments until the desired anteversion and stability are obtained. **B,** Final stem version positioning by matching witness marks on the stem and sleeve at 20° increments. (Courtesy of DePuy and Johnson & Johnson.)

sleeve version are noted prior to removal of the trial prosthesis.

The final sleeve implant is then impacted into the proximal femur. Initially it is placed by hand until cortical contact is achieved. The stem is then rotated into its desired version by referencing witness marks on the medial stem against witness marks on the sleeve placed at intervals of 20° (**Figure 4**, *B*). The stem is then impacted. Alternatively, when placing long stems into altered femoral canals, the sleeve is initially placed as a "loose-fit" proximal to its final impaction site. The longer stem is then placed by hand past the anterior lateral bow of the femur until the desired anteversion is achieved. The stem is then impacted to within 5 mm of the sleeve and followed by final sleeve and stem seating to avoid canting of the sleeve that may dictate final stem position and to reduce stem malposition, distal fracture, and perforation.

Intraoperative AP and lateral radiographs of the femur are obtained when stems greater than 200 mm in

length are used to assess any unrecognized distal fractures, which can then easily be treated with cerclage wiring or cortical onlay grafts.

Wound Closure

Tight layered closure is performed over drains, followed by application of a dry, sterile compression dressing.

Postoperative Regimen

Postoperative rehabilitation is identical to that for primary THA if no fractures or osteotomy is present. Patients are immediately permitted 50% weight bearing with crutches, increasing to 100% weight bearing with crutches until 6 to 8 weeks postoperatively. Weight bearing as tolerated using a cane is encouraged until the patient can walk 0.5 miles without pain or a limp (usually 3 weeks). Progression of weight bearing and initiation of active abduction exercises are individually adjusted if femoral or trochanteric osteotomy, APC, or complex acetabular reconstruction is required.

——————■

Avoiding Pitfalls and Complication

Strict adherence to indications, surgical technique, and principles of revision THA is necessary to avoid complications. Modular proximally porous-coated stems work best when some fixation to the proximal femur is possible (such as Paprosky types I, II, and IIIA defects). These stems rarely can be used effectively in Paprosky type IIIB and IV defects. Alternative treatments described earlier in the chapter should be considered for these more severe deficiencies.

Surgical technique should focus on preventing further injury to the femoral canal. Surgeons should not hesitate to perform prophylactic wiring, extensile exposure, or osteotomy to contain or prevent fractures and perforations. Easy access to the femoral canal is necessary for proper implant removal, instrumentation, and implantation. Longer stems (greater than 200 mm) cannot be forced into the femoral canal. Although the S-ROM modular proximally porous-coated implant provides for distal stem flexibility, the femoral canal should generally be reamed 1 to 1.5 mm more than the minor stem diameter to avoid fractures and perforations. This step also permits safe placement of longer stems past the femoral diaphysis in the desired amount of anteversion.

In addition, the proximal sleeve does not dictate final stem position. This is easily achieved by placing the long stem femoral component by hand into the distal diaphysis before fully seating the proximal sleeve. The stem position must be determined prior to final sleeve placement.

———■

References

Bono JV, McCarthy JC, Lee J, Carangelo RJ, Turner RH: Fixation with a modular stem in revision total hip arthroplasty. *Instr Course Lect* 2000;49:131-139.

Cameron HU: The long-term success of modular proximal fixation stems in revision total hip arthroplasty. *J Arthroplasty* 2002;17:138-141.

Chandler HP, Ayres DK, Tan RC, Anderson LC, Varma AK: Revision total hip replacement using the S-ROM femoral component. *Clin Orthrop* 1995;319:130-140.

Christie MJ, DeBoer DK, Tingstad EM, et al: Clinical experience with a modular noncemented femoral component in revision total hip arthroplasty: 4 to 7 year results. *J Arthroplasty* 2000;15:840-848.

Christie MJ, DeBoer DK, Trick LW, et al: Primary total hip arthroplasty with use of the modular S-ROM prosthesis: Four to seven-year clinical and radiographic results. *J Bone Joint Surg Am* 1999;81:1707-1716.

D'Antonio J, McCarthy JC, Bargar WL, et al: Classification of femoral abnormalities in total hip arthroplasty. *Clin Orthop* 1993;296:133-139.

Dorr LD: Total hip replacement using the APR system. *Tech Orthop* 1986;1:23-34.

Paprosky WG, Lawrence J, Cameron H: Femoral defect classification: Clinical application. *Orthop Rev* 1990;19:9-16.

Coding

CPT Codes		Corresponding ICD-9 Codes		
27134	Revision of total hip arthroplasty; both components, with or without autograft or allograft	996.4	996.66	996.77
27138	Revision of total hip arthroplasty; femoral component only, with or without allograft	996.4	996.66	996.77
Modifier 22	Unusual procedural service			

CPT copyright © 2004 by the American Medical Association. All Rights Reserved.

Chapter 54
Femoral Revision: Calcar Replacement Stems

Adolph V. Lombardi, Jr, MD
Thomas H. Mallory, MD
Keith R. Berend, MD

Indications

The primary goal of revision total hip arthroplasty (THA) is to provide pain relief and maximize the patient's functional capacity. On the femoral side, this requires establishing a femoral construct that will provide long-term stable fixation. The femur in revision surgery is generally compromised by a combination of stress shielding and osteolysis. The quality of bone proximal to the calcar femora is frequently inadequate for prosthetic support, resulting in early failure of uncemented prosthetic components designed for proximal fit and fill. These prostheses tend to be longer versions of components used for primary uncemented fixation. The failure of such prostheses led to development of extensively porous-coated devices for distal fixation, which essentially ignores the proximal femur. The calcar replacement prosthesis, which has experienced a resurgence in popularity in recent years, is another approach to the compromised proximal femur.

Leinbach's early work used this head and neck prosthesis for the treatment of failed open reduction and internal fixation of peritrochanteric fractures, comminuted proximal femur fractures, and pathologic fractures. The device was further modified by Harris, but long-term results revealed 30% clinical or radiographic loosening and 21% dislocation. These devices, however, depended on polymethylmethacrylate for fixation.

The Mallory-Head uncemented calcar prosthesis (Biomet, Warsaw, IN) was developed in response to early and late failures with cemented revision THA. Titanium was chosen as the substrate metal for optimization of load transfer to bone. A circumferential coating of plasma spray effectuated an endosteal seal. To accommodate varying levels of bony deficiency, five calcar replacements are currently available in 34-, 45-, 55-, 65-, and 75-mm sizes (**Figure 1**).

Three modalities accomplish proximal loading. The primary method is direct platform loading of the calcar replacement prosthesis. The second technique uses the tapered geometry of the proximal third of the stem with its associated plasma spray osseointegration surface. The third process involves compressive forces applied to the trochanter via the trochanteric bolt with plate or claw (**Figure 2**). The calcar prosthesis, originally available as a monoblock device, is currently available in both monoblock and modular systems (**Figure 3**), the latter allowing for accommodation of proximal and distal mismatch via a variety of stem lengths and degrees of porous coating.

The calcar replacement prosthesis is our choice for all revision THAs and works particularly well for Paprosky type II and III femora. Paprosky type I femora can generally be treated with primary components, whereas Paprosky type II and III femora require revision prostheses. Paprosky type III femora also require supplemental bone grafting. Cortical strut allografts combined with the calcar prosthesis have consistently demonstrated excellent femoral bone reconstitution (**Figure 4**). Many manufacturers produce uncemented calcar-type femoral revision prostheses.

————————■

■ Contraindications

Some relative contraindications to the calcar prosthesis include total loss of the proximal femur, as in Paprosky type IIIB and type IV femora. Modular calcar devices should not be used because the modular junction would be at significant risk for fracture. One option is the monoblock calcar prosthesis combined with a proximal femoral allograft versus a proximal femoral replacement prosthesis. The late failure of proximal femoral allografts has raised increasing concern. Proximal femoral replacements are a viable op-

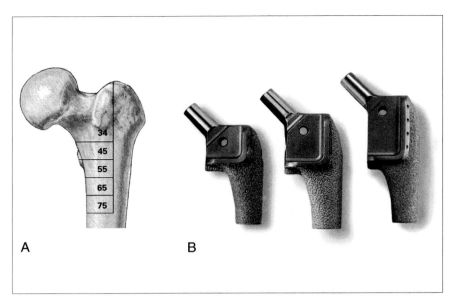

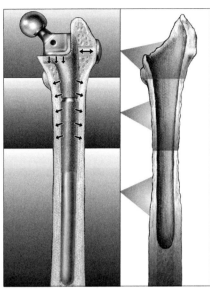

Figure 1 **A,** Bony deficiencies of the calcar region are addressed by various size options. (Joint Implant Surgeons, Inc, Columbus, OH.) **B,** The 34-, 45-, and 55-mm sizes are the most frequently used calcar replacements. (Courtesy of Biomet, Warsaw, IN.)

Figure 2 The calcar prosthesis is designed for proximal loading via three modalities: (1) Direct platform loading; (2) Tapered geometry of the proximal third of the stem to progressively offload; (3) Compression loading of the trochanter via the trochanteric plate and/or claw. Arrows indicate points of loading. (Copyright © Joint Implant Surgeons, Inc.)

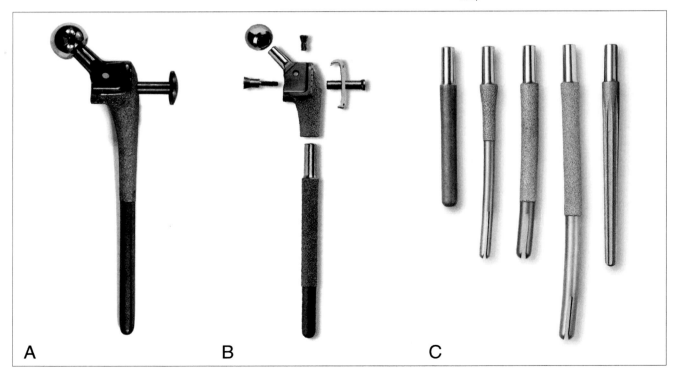

Figure 3 **A**, Mallory-Head calcar femoral component with bolt and plate (Biomet). **B**, Mallory-Head modular calcar femoral component with bolt and claw device for adjunctive reattachment, fixation, and stability of the greater trochanter. **C**, Multiple stem options are available with varying lengths and amounts of porous coating. (Courtesy of Biomet, Warsaw, IN.)

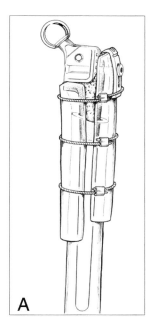
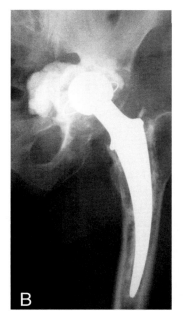
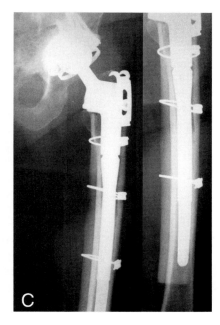
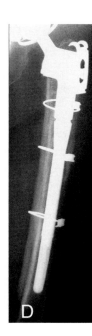

Figure 4 Reconstitution of the compromised femur. **A**, Cortical strut allografts in combination with the calcar prosthesis, cerclage cables, and the trochanter bolt (with claw or plate) present an extremely reliable construct for reconstitution of the compromised femur in revision THA. Preoperative (**B**), immediate postoperative (**C**), and 3-year follow-up (**D**) AP radiographs demonstrating the reconstitution of femoral bone stock via incorporation of the cortical strut allograft. (Copyright © Joint Implant Surgeons, Inc.)

tion in catastrophically damaged femora (**Figure 5**).

Another relative contraindication to using the calcar replacement prosthesis is very large patulous femora that require stem diameters greater than 20 mm. However, these femora recently have been approached using a tapered, splined (STS [splined, tapered, straight] modular stem, Biomet) stem combined with the modular calcar device. The splined stem has a significantly lower modulus of elasticity, thus resulting in less stress shielding. The excellent rotational stability of these stems is combined with the subsidence resistance of the calcar-loading prosthesis, a concept that evolved in an effort to capture the positive aspects of the Wagner SL prosthesis (Centerpulse Orthopaedics, Austin, TX) and to avoid the reported complication of subsidence.

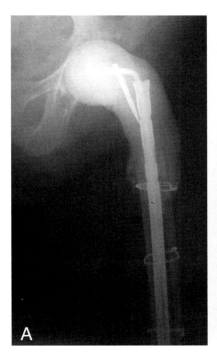
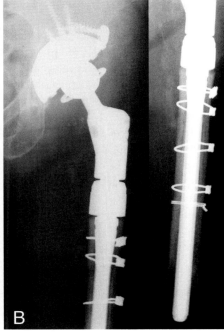

Figure 5 **A**, Preoperative AP radiograph demonstrating significant compromise of the proximal third of the femur with a prosthesis with antibiotic-loaded acrylic cement in place. **B**, Postoperative AP radiographs demonstrating reconstitution of the proximal femur using the Orthopaedic Salvage System (Biomet). (Copyright © Joint Implant Surgeons, Inc.)

■ Alternative Treatments

Reconstitution of the femur in revision THA has been attempted with many techniques. Cemented THA may be appropriate in Paprosky type I femora. However, when there is more extensive involvement of the femur, such as in Paprosky type II and III femora, cemented THA results have been less encouraging. This has led to a preference for uncemented fixation in both primary and revision THA. Several uncemented revision THA devices were designed as extensions of standard length components, but these generally resulted in continued postoperative pain secondary to aseptic loosening and associated subsidence.

The literature supports the concept of distal fixation. However, although these studies demonstrate that reliable distal fixation can be achieved, they also reveal that the disadvantage of this fixation is atrophy of the proximal femur. For the patulous femur, two techniques have been performed with varying degrees of success. The first procedure involves impaction grafting combined with a cemented, smooth, tapered prosthesis. Mixed results reveal complications including stem subsidence and periprosthetic femoral fracture distal to the prosthesis. The other technique uses splined stems that reconstitute the proximal femur at the expense of stem subsidence.

————————————■

■ Results

Table 1 and **Figure 6** illustrate the reported results of calcar replacement prostheses.

————————————■

■ Technique

Exposure

Any surgical technique begins with meticulous preoperative planning. Appropriate preoperative radiographs are mandatory, and reviewing serial radiographs can also be helpful. In revision THA of a cemented prosthesis, assessment of the cement mantle and its extent is critical. A careful review of the radiographs includes an assessment of the bone defect classification and the degree and location of osteolysis. This information determines the appropriate stem length. Furthermore, the degree of bone loss may dictate the requirements for particulate and structural allografting. The reconstructive armamentarium may include cables, wires, plates, and screws. Extracting the stem is easier if the surgeon is familiar with the existing implant. If a cemented stem is being removed, is it smooth? Precoated? Grit blasted? Has the prosthesis debonded from the cement mantle, or has the cement mantle debonded from the bone? If an uncemented device is being extracted, is it a fully porous-coated device or is the porous coating limited to the proximal third? Is the surface below the level of the porous coating smooth, or is it grit blasted? All of these conditions have a direct impact on the implant removal process.

The classic Charnley trochanteric approach is most appropriate for the patient presenting with nonunion of a previous trochanteric osteotomy. The trochanteric slide is appropriate for the patient presenting with significant lysis distal to the trochanter itself, thus rendering it difficult or impossible to perform an extended trochanteric osteotomy (ETO). The ETO, an approach that extends the osteotomy 6 to 12 cm distal to the trochanter, has gained wide acceptance. It facilitates the creation of a large lateral window that makes removal of the prosthesis and cement easier. This technique has been associated with a

lower incidence of trochanteric nonunion that is believed to be secondary to the increased surface area available for fixation and the ability to maintain a large soft-tissue sleeve with adequate blood supply. The posterolateral surgical approach is also a well-accepted approach for revision THA. Its main advantage is preservation of the abductor mechanism, although its main disadvantage is an increased incidence of dislocation. Furthermore, its close proximity to the sciatic nerve may predispose the patient to the risk of nerve injury.

We prefer the anterolateral approach (**Figure 7**). We try to incorporate into the new skin incision at least a portion of the previous skin incision. The landmarks for this incision involve the anterior superior iliac spine, the iliac crest, and the tip of the greater trochanter and the lateral aspect of the femur. The proximal and distal lengths of the incision depend on the required extent of reconstruction of the acetabulum and femur, respectively. The proximal portion of the average incision begins 4 cm proximal to the trochanter, bisecting the iliac wing, extending distally across the tip of the greater trochanter, and continuing along the lateral shaft of the femur. Incision of the fascia exposes the lateral aspect of the femur. The vastus lateralis is elevated from the posterolateral aspect of the femur just anterior to the linea aspera and reflected anteriorly. It is released proximally from the anterior aspect of the femur in continuity with the anterior third of the gluteus medius and minimus, in a fashion we previously described as the abductor muscle split. The procedure splits the anterior third of the gluteus medius and gluteus minimus along the line of the muscle fibers, followed by flexion, external rotation, and adduction maneuvers to facilitate dislocation. The anteromedial aspect of the femur is visualized by elevating the muscle sleeve. In the presence of a modular stem, the femoral head and neck unit is removed

Table 1 Results of Femoral Revision With Calcar Replacement Stems

Author(s)/Year	Number of Hips	Implant Type	Mean Patient Age (Range)	Mean Follow-up (Range)	Harris/Mayo Hip Score	Results
Cemented						
Harris and Allen (1981)	15	Harris Calcar	57 years (32–74)	2 years	82 (Harris)	1 (5.5%) stem revision for malposition
McLaughlin and Harris (1996)	38	Howmedica	55 years (20–73)	10.8 years (5.8–16.6)	84 (Harris)	7 (18%) revisions for aseptic loosening 4 radiographically loose but not revised 1 (2.6%) extensive proximal femoral lysis
Clarke, et al (1999)	52	Osteonics	73.5 years (23–90)	3.2 years (1.8–6.1)	55.2 (Mayo)	1 (1.9%) stem revision for sepsis
Uncemented						
Head, et al (1994)	177	Mallory-Head Calcar	Not reported	3 years (2–5.8)	85 (Harris)	2 (1.1%) revised for aseptic loosening 2 (1.1%) revised for subsidence 2 (1.1%) revised for thigh pain
Lombardi, et al (1997)	264	Mallory-Head Calcar	64 years	5 years (3–10)	Not reported	
	325	Mallory-Head Calcar with strut graft	59 years	5 years (3–10)		Not reported
Mallory, et al (1999)	351	Mallory-Head Calcar	62.6 years (39–88)	5.9 years (5–9)	79 (Harris)	21 (6%) revised for aseptic loosening
Head, et al (2000)	304	Mallory-Head Calcar	Not reported	Minimum 10 years	84 (Harris)	96% survivorship at 10 years 3 (0.7%) revised for aseptic loosening 3 (0.7%) revised for recurrent dislocation 2 (0.5%) revised for sepsis 2 (0.5%) thigh pain
Shilling, et al (2000)	34	Mallory-Head Calcar	67 years	3.8 years (2–5)	79 (Harris)	2 (5.9%) revised for aseptic loosening
	30	Mallory-Head Modular Calcar	66 years	3.0 years (2–5)	89 (Harris)	None revised for aseptic loosening 1 (3.3%) revised for prosthetic fracture
Emerson, et al (2001)	111	Mallory-Head Calcar	63 years (27–94)	4.4 years (0.5–9.5)	N/A	1 (0.9%) revised for sepsis
Head, et al (2001)	1,179	Mallory-Head Calcar (758 1-piece; 209 1-piece hydroxyapatite; 129 short 170-mm; 83 modular)	63 years (18–89)	6.2 years (up to 13.9)	N/A	95.2% stem survivorship at 13 years 17 (1.4%) revised for sepsis 9 (0.8%) revised for aseptic loosening 7 (0.6%) revised for recurrent dislocation 6 (0.5%) revised for end of stem pain (strut only) 1 (0.1%) revised for periprosthetic fracture

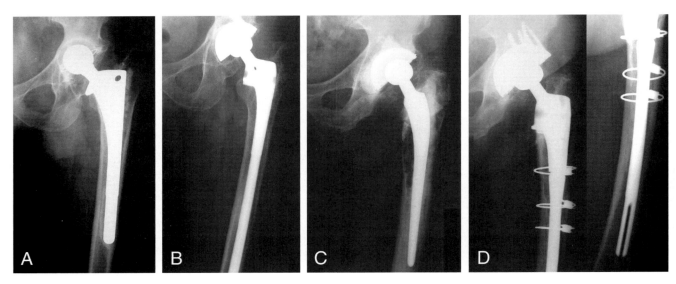

Figure 6 **A**, Preoperative radiograph demonstrating failed THA. **B**, AP radiograph obtained at 6.5-year follow-up after uncemented calcar replacement demonstrates a well-fixed component and maintenance of femoral bone stock. **C**, Preoperative AP radiograph of a different patient demonstrating failed THA. **D**, AP radiographs obtained at 4-year follow-up after uncemented calcar replacement demonstrate a well-fixed component and restoration of femoral bone stock. (Copyright © Joint Implant Surgeons, Inc.)

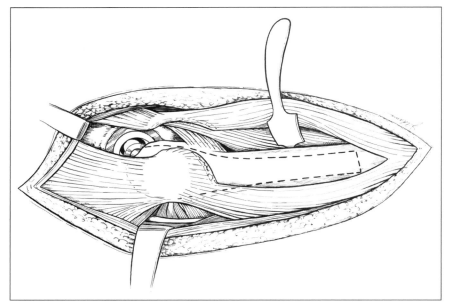

Figure 7 The anterolateral approach allows for direct visualization of the femur. It extends as far distally and proximally as required and can be further enhanced with an ETO. (Copyright © Joint Implant Surgeons, Inc.)

to allow release of the scarred capsule from the posterior aspect of the neck.

Bone Preparation

At this point, the integrity of the proximal femur is assessed. Generally, bone absent to the level of the lesser trochanter requires a 34-mm calcar prosthesis. If the bone deficiency extends to the distal third of the lesser trochanter, a 45-mm calcar replacement is generally the right choice. A deficiency distal to the calcar may require a 55- to 75-mm calcar replacement (**Figure 1**, *A*). The calcar template is applied to the lateral aspect of the femur, and a resection parallel to the long axis of the trochanter and perpendicular to the long axis of the femur is outlined and performed. This procedure affords an opportunity to débride the proximal femur and therefore assists in component removal. The trochanteric fossa is then débrided.

Whether or not to proceed with an ETO depends on the complexity of the revision. Positive indications include a cemented precoat or grit-blasted prosthesis with evidence of satisfactory distal fixation, an intact and well-fixed distal cement mantle with a debonded and loose femoral component, and an extensively porous-coated stem. An oscillating saw is used anteriorly under direct visualization. The length of the osteotomy depends on the need for more distal femoral reconstruction. The limb is internally rotated, and multiple drill holes are made posteriorly along the line of the intended osteotomy. Distally, a reciprocating saw facilitates a beveled or chamfered resection. A wide osteotome is taken from anterior to posterior, and the osteotomy is complete. On removal of the cemented prosthesis, the polymethylmethacrylate is removed using a combination of hand tools, high-speed burrs, and ultrasonic devices. The ETO facilitates cement removal under direct visualization.

Several other techniques have been advocated for cement removal. One method is the controlled perforation technique, using strategically placed 8-mm controlled perforations on the anterolateral aspect of the femur. These perforations are used to visualize and guide high-speed burrs and hand tools. Another approach uses strategically placed windows. End-cutting burrs or reamers may be used in revision of an uncemented component with a well-formed pedestal. If perforation is a concern, it is advisable to create a controlled 8-mm perforation on the anterolateral aspect of the femur at the level of the pedestal.

After the femoral canal has been cleared of all polymethylmethacrylate and fibrous material, sequential reaming of the femur is performed using flexible, thin-shaft reamers. To accommodate the plasma spray porous coating, the femur should be overreamed by 1.5 mm in the region of the porous coating and 0.5 mm in the distal nonporous-coated portion of the prosthesis. Proximally, the femur is prepared with conical reamers and broaches. The component is placed in 5° to 10° anteversion, and a slot for the keel of the calcar prosthesis is created in the proximal femur. Stem length should extend at least twice the femoral width below the most distal compromised portion of the femur. The extent of porous coating is correlated with the extent of endosteal cavitation and erosions.

Prosthesis Implantation

The selection of monoblock versus modular calcar replacement is based on the degree and amount of mismatch between the proximal and distal femurs. When it is difficult to negotiate the femoral canal with the predetermined anterior bow of the right and left monoblock components, the modular component is a better choice. Modular femoral stems can be allowed to rotate within the femoral canal during the trialing process and to accommodate slightly distorted femoral anatomy. Once the trial prosthesis is seated, the capturing screw is secured to permit the surgeon to appropriately align the stem on the definitive prosthesis. Once satisfactory completion of trial reduction has occurred, the definitive prosthesis is seated. It is generally introduced at approximately 90° anteversion and is rotated into 5° to 10° anteversion as it is driven down the femur until final seating is completed.

If there are concerns about the quality of the femoral bone, a medial strut should be applied. Strut grafts are generally fashioned around the keel of the prosthesis platform. Morcellized allograft is placed between the strut graft and the host bone, and the strut is secured to the host bone with cerclage wires or cables. If patients are undergoing ETO, or if any question regarding the trochanter's integrity needs to be resolved, a trochanteric bolt or claw is used to secure the trochanter to the prosthesis. Cerclage wires or cables are placed distally in patients with ETOs. Morcellized graft can also be supplemented at the osteotomy site.

Wound Closure

Femoral reconstruction is generally accomplished after satisfactory acetabular reconstruction so trial reduction with various head and neck units is now performed. The most appropriate head and neck device that equalizes limb length and provides stability is selected and seated. The gluteus medius, gluteus minimus, and vastus lateralis are now repaired in continuity through drill holes in the greater trochanter using heavy nonabsorbable or bioabsorbable sutures in a running fashion. These are oversewn with interrupted bioabsorbable sutures. The fascia lata is then closed with interrupted bioabsorbable sutures. Subcutaneous tissue and skin are closed in a routine fashion. A bulky dressing is applied, the patient is turned supine, and an abduction orthosis is placed.

Postoperative Regimen

A cast brace is used for 6 to 8 weeks postoperatively in patients with a prior history of dislocation, soft-tissue compromise about the hip, neuromuscular disease resulting in diminished muscle strength, or inability to follow hip precautions secondary to history of Alzheimer's disease or senile dementia. All patients are asked to use walkers or crutches for 6 to 8 weeks with protected weight bearing. Intravenous perioperative antibiotics (a first-generation cephalosporin and gentamicin sulfate) are administered for 48 hours, followed by 5 to 10 days of an oral first-generation cephalosporin. Prophylaxis protocol for deep venous thrombosis is based on both the patient's history and the presence or absence of thromboembolic-related comorbidities. Prophylaxis is typically multifactorial and may include thigh-high compressive stockings, intermittent plantar pulse boots, early mobilization, and aspirin versus incorporation of low molecular weight heparin or warfarin sodium.

———————————————■

■ Avoiding Pitfalls and Complications

Pitfalls and complications can occur at any stage of the process, beginning with the initial patient evaluation. We must decisively differentiate between aseptic and septic failure. Mandatory preoperative radiographs and thorough preoperative planning will ensure that the surgeon has the appropriate array of tools, including prostheses of various lengths, modular and nonmodular components, morcellized and strut allografts, trochanter bolt, plate, and claw options, cerclage wires, cables, and plates. The patient must undergo preadmission testing and pass a thorough assessment by a general medical practitioner before surgery to avoid perioperative medical complications. Extensile exposures should be carefully planned and performed. Careful maneuvers to dislocate the hip at the time of exposure will avoid femur fracture. Controlled removal of the prosthetic device and polymethylmethacrylate or distal pedestal helps prevent femur compromise.

Cautious use of the ETO may facilitate preservation of femoral bone stock. Careful reaming of the femoral canal with overreaming of 1.5 mm for the porous coating facilitates stem insertion and avoids potential fracture. Proximal femoral resection for the calcar replacement must be adequate, with an appropriate amount of bone removed to avoid the possibility of fracturing the greater trochanter. No extra bone should remain about the trochanteric fragment. If this is not appropriately resected, fracture of the trochanter can occur when introducing either the trial or definitive prosthesis. During the reaming process, trialing, and final prosthetic implantation, avoid distal femoral perforation with the reamers, the trial components, or the prosthesis.

Modular devices should be avoided in patients with totally deficient proximal femurs. Fracture of modular stems is a known complication that typically occurs at the taper junction. Reports of modular stem fractures can be accessed via the US Food and Drug Administration MAUDE database (http://www.fda.gov/search/databases.html). In 1999, Biomet introduced a proprietary process of roller hardening of tapers that increased taper strength by a factor of 3.5. No roller-hardened device has fractured to date. However, using the modular calcar replacement in the totally deficient proximal femur is not recommended.

Fatigue fractures of distally fixed, monoblock, extensively coated stems have been reported. Exercise caution when potting any stem in the diaphysis without reconstituting proximal bone stock and support. The reconstructive surgeon must be knowledgeable about the chosen surgical procedure and be prepared to address all potential complications.

————■

■ References

Berry DJ: Total hip arthroplasty in special cases: Total hip arthroplasty in patients with proximal femoral deformity. *Clin Orthop* 1999;369:262-272.

Clarke HD, Damron TA, Trousdale RT, Sim FH, Larson DR: Head and neck replacement prosthesis in revision hip arthroplasty: Experience with a single modern design. *Orthopaedics* 1999;22:313-318.

Emerson RH Jr, Head WC, Higgins LL: A new method of trochanteric fixation after osteotomy in revision total hip arthroplasty with a calcar replacement femoral component. *J Arthroplasty* 2001;16:76-80.

Frndak PA, Mallory TH, Lombardi AV Jr: Translateral surgical approach to the hip. The abductor muscle "split." *Clin Orthop* 1993;295:135-141.

Griffin JB: The calcar femorale redefined. *Clin Orthop* 1982;164:211-214.

Grunig R, Morscher E, Ochsner PE: Three to 7 year results with the uncemented SL femoral revision prosthesis. *Arch Orthop Trauma Surg* 1997;116:187-197.

Harris WH: Revision surgery for failed, nonseptic total hip arthroplasty: The femoral side. *Clin Orthop* 1982;170:8-20.

Harris WH, Allen JR: The calcar replacement femoral component for total hip arthroplasty: Design, uses and surgical technique. *Clin Orthop* 1981;157:215-224.

Head WC, Emerson RH Jr, Higgins LL: A titanium cementless calcar replacement prosthesis in revision surgery of the femur: 13 year experience. *J Arthrop* 2001;16:183-187.

Head WC, Malinin TI, Emerson RH Jr, Mallory TH: Restoration of bone stock in revision surgery of the femur. *Int Orthop* 2000;24:9-14.

Head WC, Wagner RA, Emerson RH Jr, Malinin TI: Revision total hip arthroplasty in the deficient femur with a proximal load-bearing prosthesis. *Clin Orthop* 1994;298:119-126.

Huiskes R: The various stress patterns of press-fit, ingrown, and cemented femoral stems. *Clin Orthop* 1990;261:27-38.

Leinbach IS: Prosthesis replaces entire hip joint. *JAMA* 1969;207:1445-1446.

Lombardi AV Jr, Head WC, Mallory TH, Emerson RH Jr: Principles of reconstruction in revision hip arthroplasty: Technique and results of bone grafts for treatment of femoral and acetabular deficits. *J Orthop Sci* 1997;2:442-446.

Mallory TH: Preparation of the proximal femur in cementless total hip revision. *Clin Orthop* 1988;235:47-60.

Mallory TH, Lombardi AV Jr, Herrington SM: Effect of surgical technique on long-term survivorship, in *Revision Total Hip Arthroplasty*. Philadelphia, PA, Lippincott Williams & Wilkins, 1999.

Mauer SG, Baitner AC, Di Cesare PE: Reconstruction of the failed femoral component and proximal femoral bone loss in revision hip surgery. *J Am Acad Orthop Surg* 2000;8:354-363.

McLaughlin JR, Harris WH: Revision of the femoral component of a total hip arthroplasty with the calcar-replacement femoral component: Results after a mean of 10.8 years postoperatively. *J Bone Joint Surg* 1996;78:331-339.

Shilling JW, Sharkey PF, Hozack WJ, Rothman RH: Femoral revision hip arthroplasty: Modular versus nonmodular femoral component for severe femoral deficiency. *Oper Tech Orthop* 2000;10:133-137.

Stern MD, Goldstein TB: The use of the Leinbach prosthesis in intertrochanteric fractures of the hip. *Clin Orthop* 1977;128:325-331.

Taylor JW, Rorabeck CH: Hip revision arthroplasty: Approach to the femoral side. *Clin Orthop* 1999;369:208-222.

Coding

CPT Codes		Corresponding ICD-9 Codes		
27134	Revision of total hip arthroplasty; both components, with or without autograft or allograft	996.4	996.66	996.77
27138	Revision of total hip arthroplasty; femoral component only, with or without allograft	996.4	996.66	996.77

CPT copyright © 2004 by the American Medical Association. All Rights Reserved.

Chapter 55

Femoral Revision: Uncemented Tapered Fluted Stems

Stephen B. Murphy, MD

Indications

Revision total hip arthroplasty (THA) with uncemented fluted fixation of the femoral component uses two types of implants: those with cylindrical flutes and those with tapered flutes (**Figure 1**). Implants with cylindrical flutes resist varus-valgus, flexion-extension, and rotational forces but do not resist axial forces. These implants, therefore, require proximal metaphyseal fixation to resist axial forces and are contraindicated in patients with an absent or mechanically compromised metaphysis. Implants with tapered flutes resist axial forces and, therefore, can be used in patients with an absent or mechanically compromised metaphysis, provided that the implant has sufficient fatigue resistance.

The indications for these implants in revision THA vary by surgeon. Some use these implants routinely in most patients with compromised proximal femoral metaphyseal bone, whereas others prefer to use them selectively, in circumstances that are not ideal for cemented, extensively coated, uncemented, or modular proximally fixed implants. Such circumstances include patients who have a large-diameter femoral canal, compromised proximal femoral bone stock, deficient intramedullary cancellous bone, and deficient diaphyseal bone.

Contraindications

Tapered fluted stems generally are contraindicated in patients with a strong metaphysis in whom proximal load transfer can be achieved rather than bypassed and in patients with such severe femoral bone loss that insufficient diaphyseal bone is available for tapered flute-bone fixation.

Alternative Treatments

Alternatives to fluted fixation include cemented femoral components, extensively coated femoral components that obtain scratch fit in the diaphysis, structural allograft-implant composites (with or without flutes), and impaction grafting.

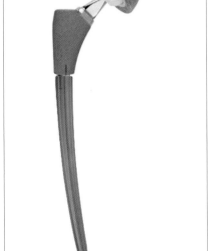

Figure 1 **A** and **B**, Femoral components with tapered flutes.

Table 1 Results of Uncemented Tapered Fluted Fixation

Author(s) (Year)	Number of Hips	Implant Type	Mean Follow-up (Range)	Results
Bohm and Bischel (2001)	129	Wagner (nonmodular, tapered, fluted)	4.8 years	6 stems re-revised
Bircher, et al (2001)	99	Wagner (nonmodular, tapered, fluted)	NA	92% 10-year stem survival 6 of 99 stems with marked subsidence
Kwong, et al (2003)	143	Link MP (modular, tapered, fluted)	3.4 years (2–6)	No failures resulting from aseptic loosening Mean subsidence 2.1 mm (0–11.3)
Murphy and Rodriguez (2004)	35	Link MP (modular, tapered, fluted)	3.5 years (minimum 2 years)	34 of 35 implants osseointegrated

NA = Not applicable

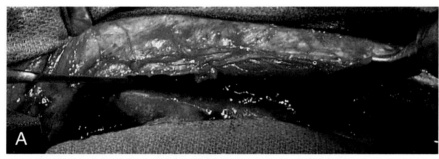
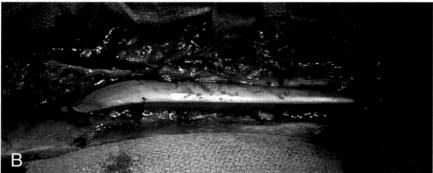

Figure 2 **A** and **B,** The transfemoral exposure is similar to the extended trochanteric osteotomy. Meticulous attention is paid to maintaining the vascularity of the bone flap by minimizing periosteal dissection and maximally preserving the overlying muscle. Long lateral bone flaps facilitate implant and cement removal with minimal bone stock loss. The long flap maximizes surface area of bone apposition to promote bone healing. Because the flap is weakest at the vastus tubercle, care should be taken to avoid stressing that area when the flap is developed and during subsequent retraction during surgery. (Reproduced with permission from Murphy SB, Rodriguez J: Revision total hip arthroplasty with proximal bone loss. *J Arthroplasty* 2004;19(4 suppl 1):115-119.)

Results

Tapered fluted stems reliably osseointegrate to the host bone. In a report of 54 revisions, 34 of 35 hips followed for a minimum of 2 years (mean, 43 months) had osseointegrated; one failed to osseointegrate as a result of bone stock loss that extended below the diaphysis. Postoperative supracondylar fractures requiring secondary internal fixation occurred in only 3 of the 54 hips, highlighting the potential need for prophylactic strut grafts in selected patients. **Table 1** summarizes additional results.

Technique

Exposure

Revision THA with fluted stems can be performed using any one of many exposures, including posterior, anterolateral, transtrochanteric, extended trochanteric, or transfemoral exposures. The exposure can be chosen preoperatively or changed intraoperatively, depending on the anticipated or actual challenges in removing the existing femoral component and cement. The more extensile transfemoral exposure involves bivalving the femur down to the level of the stem tip and leaving the quadriceps, and therefore the blood supply, on the lateral bone flap. This exposure facilitates safe removal of implants and cement with minimal bone stock loss (**Figure 2**) and also may facilitate reaming for and insertion of long fluted tapered stems.

Bone Preparation

The object of bone preparation is to achieve complete implant stability below the metaphyseal level. Therefore, the diaphysis must be precisely prepared to closely match the geometry of the stem. This precision can be achieved using either tapered reamers or very sharp tapered broaches. The bone must be prepared to create a tapered envelope that resists implant subsidence. Prophylactic wires or cable may be passed around the femur before femoral preparation to reduce the risk of fracture.

Prosthesis Implantation

Formal trial reduction before final prosthesis implantation is essential for assessment of stem version, limb length, stability, tissue tension, and impingement. Intraoperative radiographs can be helpful to ensure proper implant size and alignment. Following satisfactory trial reduction, the final implant is inserted. Tapered fluted stems are seated until the tapered flutes are fully engaged and the implant shows no further advancement. If a transtrochanteric, extended trochanteric, or transfemoral exposure is used, wires or cables for bone flap fixation should be passed before final reduction of the hip.

Wound Closure

Capsular repair, if possible, is best achieved prior to trochanteric refixation if the greater trochanter is osteotomized. The desired rigidity of trochanteric fixation depends on the surgical exposure and implant used. If a transfemoral exposure is used in combination with a tapered fluted stem, the goal is to maintain vascularity with fixation primarily at the top and bottom of the bone flap to avoid

strangulation of the blood supply. The vastus lateralis fascia is then closed with a running bioabsorbable suture followed by the fascia lata. Meticulous closure of the subcutaneous tissues promotes isolation of the superficial and deep layers. A running suture in the skin is generally favored over skin staples to promote early sealing of the skin incision.

Postoperative Regimen

Because the femoral component should have immediate intrinsic stability, even before full osseointegration, rehabilitation is determined by the surrounding soft tissues and any concerns about hip joint stability. In patients in whom all or part of the abductors are mobilized and repaired at surgery, protection of the abductors is appropriate. In these patients, 50% weight bearing and avoiding sidelying abduction should be recommended until clinical or radiographic signs of abductor healing or trochanteric union are evident.

———————■

■ Avoiding Pitfalls and Complications

Success following revision using uncemented fluted femoral components depends largely on anticipating and avoiding complications. Choice of exposure is critical. Revision with minimal abductor morbidity and without

trochanteric osteotomy certainly simplifies and accelerates rehabilitation. Conversely, inadvertent fracture of the greater trochanter during revision surgery often results in very limited surface areas of bone apposition and greatly increases the risk of greater trochanteric nonunion. Deliberate, longer trochanteric bone flaps leave a larger surface area of bone apposition and, therefore, improve the likelihood of trochanteric union. Because trochanteric nonunion reduces strength and endurance, increases the incidence of instability, and can cause pain, optimal management of the greater trochanter is paramount.

Maintaining hip joint stability is also critical to optimizing outcome. If a posterior capsule or pseudocapsule is intact, and the greater trochanter is to be mobilized, the joint can be exposed after trochanteric osteotomy using a superior capsulotomy. This procedure leaves the posterior structures undisturbed, conferring immediate postoperative hip joint stability.

Intraoperative and postoperative femoral fracture also should be avoided whenever possible. Prophylactic cerclage wiring is generally worthwhile. More importantly, experience has shown that elderly osteoporotic women with long femoral components are at higher risk for postoperative supracondylar fracture. Distal onlay grafts at the time of reconstruction may be considered in these circumstances.

———————■

References

Berry DJ: Femoral fixation: Distal fixation with fluted, tapered grit-blasted stems. *J Arthroplasty* 2002;17:142-146.

Bircher HP, Riede U, Luem M, Ochsner PE: The value of the Wagner SL revision prosthesis for bridging large femoral defects. *Orthopade* 2001;30:294-303.

Bohm P, Bischel O: Femoral revisions with the Wanger SL revision stem: Evaluation of one hundred twenty-nine revisions followed for a mean of 4.8 years. *J Bone Joint Surg Am* 2001;83:1023-1031.

Kwong LM, Miller AJ, Lubinus P: A modular distal fixation option for proximal bone loss in revision total hip arthroplasty: A 2- to 6-year follow-up study. *J Arthroplasty* 2003;18:94-97.

Murphy SB, Rodriguez J: Revision total hip arthroplasty with proximal bone loss. *J Arthroplasty* 2004;19:115-119.

Coding				
CPT Codes		**Corresponding ICD-9 Codes**		
27134	Revision of total hip arthroplasty; both components, with or without autograft or allograft	996.4	996.66	996.77
27138	Revision of total hip arthroplasty; femoral component only, with or without allograft	996.4	996.66	996.77
Modifier 22	Unusual procedural service			

CPT copyright © 2004 by the American Medical Association. All Rights Reserved.

Chapter 56

Femoral Revision: Impaction Bone Grafting and Cement

Graham A. Gie, FRCSEd
A. J. Timperley, FRCS
Tony D. Lamberton, FRACS

Indications

Femoral impaction grafting may be indicated in patients with pain and functional disability secondary to failed total hip arthroplasty (THA). This technique can be used with patients of any age but is most useful in younger patients, especially in those with significantly compromised bone stock. It also may be used when the host bone cannot provide stable mechanical fixation of an implant, whether cemented or uncemented. Femoral impaction grafting is also suitable for second stage reconstruction after deep infection.

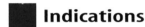

Contraindications

Femoral impaction grafting may not be indicated in elderly patients or in those whose condition is medically compromised. This is especially the case when it is possible to achieve distal fixation and when impaction would require extensive proximal reconstruction of the femur.

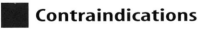

Alternative Treatments

Alternative methods of femoral revision include using cemented components, extensively porous-coated long stem implants, distal fit long-stemmed tapered devices, and proximal femoral allograft reconstruction. Each of these alternatives has been used with success in appropriate situations, but none restores the femoral bone stock in the same way as femoral impaction grafting.

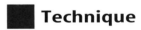

Results

The advantage of impaction grafting over other forms of femoral reconstruction in revision THA is that it restores bone stock in deficient femora as the impacted allograft chips incorporate and subsequently remodel in the host skeleton.

Our results with this technique have been very good, specifically with regard to outcome scores, implant survivorship, and radiologic evidence of bone stock restoration. Survivorship of the stem for all indications is 90.6% in 540 patients with minimum 2-year follow-up. Results of several studies are summarized in **Table 1**.

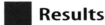

Technique

Preoperative Planning

Patients should be thoroughly screened for previous or current infection, especially if they have undergone previous hip surgery. Patients should also undergo routine testing for inflammatory markers, including C-reactive protein and erythrocyte sedimentation rate.

With clinical suspicion of infection, the hip joint is aspirated preoperatively. If infection exists, or if a high index of suspicion for infection remains, a two-stage procedure is performed. The first stage uses high-dose antibiotics in cement spacers. Antibiotic powder is added to the bone graft during stage two, the impaction grafting procedure.

Preoperative radiographs are analyzed in detail. AP radiographs of the pelvis and femur (showing the entire length of the existing implant) and lateral radiographs are required to detect femoral bone deficiencies and identify other technical concerns before sur-

Table 1   Results of Impaction Grafting Technique

Author(s) (Year)	Number of Hips	Implant Type	Mean Patient Age (Range)	Mean Follow-up (Range)	Results
Gie, et al (1993)	56	Exeter	68 years (46–87)	30 months (18–49)	No revisions for aseptic loosening
Halliday, et al (2003)	226	Exeter	68 years (32–81)	78 months (24–147)	90.5% survivorship for reoperation at 11 years 99.1% survivorship for aseptic loosening at 10 to 11 years
Lamberton, et al (2004)*	540	Exeter	71 years (32–96)	92 months (31–164)	90.4% survivorship for reoperation at 15 years 99.0% survivorship for aseptic loosening at 15 years
Elting, et al (1995)	56	Collarless polished tapered	65 years (35–88)	31 months (24–64)	93% survivorship Harris Hip score average 90 points
Knight and Helming (2000)	31	Collarless polished tapered	70 years (42–97)	31 months (7–46)	87% good to excellent results
Piccaluga, et al (2002)	59	Charnley	65 years (32–88)	57 months (24–144)	93% survivorship for aseptic loosening

Exeter (Stryker, Rutherford, NJ)

*Unpublished data presented at the American Academy of Orthopaedic Surgeons Annual Meeting, 2004.

gery. These views are compared with previous radiographs in an attempt to identify the reason the existing implant failed.

The amount of bone necessary for the reconstructive procedure is estimated, and the number of allograft femoral heads or strut grafts required is ordered from a bone bank. Stainless steel reconstruction meshes may not be necessary to reconstruct the femo-

ral tube, but they should be readily available in the event they are required intraoperatively.

The preoperative radiographs should be carefully templated to determine the size, length, and offset of the femoral stem required for the revision. The definitive stem offset and size are determined intraoperatively.

The location of the distal canal plug is marked 3 to 4 cm beyond the

tip of the femoral stem. This permits the buildup of at least 2 cm of well-packed bone chips in the canal distal to the implant, the hollow centralizer (1 cm), and the cement mantle. For example, with a standard 160-mm length implant, the plug must be at a minimum depth of 19 cm from the tip of the trochanter; with a 220-mm implant, the plug must be at a minimum depth of 250 mm.

A template is used to confirm the position of the plug and to measure the distance to the plug from the tip of the greater trochanter. The diameter of the plug is estimated.

Occasionally, a suitable well-fixed cement plug may be left in situ to act as a canal plug. Before this plug can be used, however, infection must be ruled out, lysis must be absent from the surrounding bone, and the depth of the plug must be measured to ensure that it is sufficient to allow the reconstruction.

Long-stemmed implants should be considered in patients whose cortical bone stock loss is at a level that corresponds to the tip of a conventional-length stem when fracture is present and in patients with extensive bone stock loss. The tip of the stem should bypass any distal femoral lysis by a minimum of one cortical diameter (3 cm). Severe lysis or a fracture should be bypassed by at least two cortical diameters (6 cm).

Exposure

The patient is positioned in the lateral decubitus position and securely supported with a sacral pad and support pads on the anterior superior iliac spine (**Figure 1**). The lower limb is free-draped to provide exposure from the iliac crest to the knee.

We use a posterior approach exclusively because of its versatility and extensibility. A posterolateral incision is made, incorporating or excising the previous scar, if possible. If prior surgeries used the anterolateral approach, or the old scar is unsuitable, then a new incision is made. Limited clearing of subcutaneous fat from the fascia lata is performed in the line of the incision to facilitate closure.

The incision should begin through an area of the fascia lata that was not involved in previous exposures to permit development of the subfascial plane and identification of a good fascial layer to facilitate closure. The gluteus maximus is split in the line of its fibers to expose the supra-acetabular region. The sciatic nerve is identified by palpation and blunt dissection. We do not expose the nerve throughout the surgical field unless the posterior column of the pelvis is deficient and requires augmentation. The ischium, sciatic notch, lower border of the gluteus minimus, and the ilium superior and posterior to the socket should be identified during the course of the exposure.

Before the hip joint is entered and the prosthesis is exposed, a needle is passed through the pseudocapsule and fluid is aspirated for Gram staining and microscopic examination. Should there be an excessive number of neutrophils, or should other organisms be identified, the procedure is limited to débridement as the first stage of a two-stage procedure. Frozen sections of multiple tissue samples may be useful if any doubt remains about the presence of joint infection.

With the hip positioned in slight flexion, adduction, and internal rotation, the tendinous insertion of the gluteus maximus is released from the linea aspera over approximately two thirds of its length to decrease the tension on the femur during dislocation. Using cutting diathermy, the capsule and remnants of the external rotators are released from their attachment to the posterior aspect of the femur along the intertrochanteric ridge, raising a posteriorly based flap. The proximal margin of the flap runs parallel to the inferior border of the gluteus minimus and back to the posterior margin of the acetabulum; the distal margin is

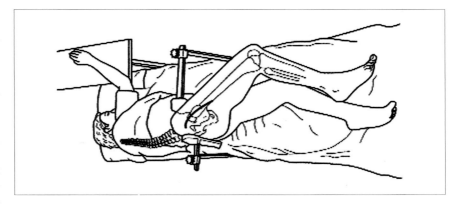

Figure 1 The preferred lateral decubitus positioning using hip immobilizers. The patient is supported by a sacral pad and support pads on the anterior superior iliac spine.

the posterior inferior aspect of the capsule, extending down toward the transverse acetabular ligament.

Stay sutures are placed in the flap and used to reflect it posteriorly, protecting the sciatic nerve. An excessively thick and scarred pseudocapsule is partially excised or thinned to facilitate exposure. The capsular flap can be reattached to the posterior aspect of the femur at the end of surgery.

With further internal rotation, the psoas tendon is usually released from the lesser trochanter and the anterior capsule is released from the anterior aspect of the femur using sharp dissection or diathermy. This release must be performed before the limb is significantly flexed and internally rotated because the anterior wall of the femur is often flimsy from osteolysis and may fracture or avulse during joint dislocation.

After mobilization of the proximal femur, the head of the prosthesis is visible. A bone hook is passed around the neck of the prosthesis to directly achieve dislocation. The femur should not be rotated at this time because it may fracture.

Removal of the Femoral Component

Considerable soft-tissue dissection may be needed to safely remove the femoral component. Once the proximal femur is adequately displayed

with the aid of a femoral elevating retractor, cement is removed from over the shoulder of the prosthesis using a high-speed burr. Any residual bone, soft tissue, or cement around the femoral component should be cleared. The femoral component is then gently extracted. Vigorous attempts at extraction may cause fracture of the femur.

If the femoral component cannot be removed without excessive force, an extended trochanteric osteotomy (ETO) is performed. An ETO does not preclude impaction grafting. At the time of reconstruction, a phantom that bypasses the distal osteotomy site is seated down the femur to the correct level and is used as a template while the osteotomy is reduced and held with cables.

Adequate mobilization and delivery of the proximal femur are essential to permit reconstruction. The proximal part of the greater trochanter must be exposed sufficiently to allow insertion of the guide wire down the medullary canal in the midline axis so that the subsequently formed neomedullary canal is in neutral alignment, avoiding either varus or valgus. This often requires opening the trochanteric overhang laterally by approximately 1 cm to accommodate introduction of instruments in the correct alignment without risking trochanteric fracture.

Cement must be completely removed from the area chosen for impaction grafting. However, the distal cement plug may be left in position and used to occlude the distal canal during reconstruction if the plug is more than 3 cm beyond the most distal lytic area of the femur and is solidly fixed and if there is no infection. All granulomatous tissue and fibrous membrane should be thoroughly débrided, followed by copious irrigation of the canal. Six separate specimens of tissue and membrane from the interfaces should be sent for microbiologic examination.

Femoral impaction grafting restores the femur to a state equivalent to that existing at the time of the primary arthroplasty. If required, the first step is cortical tube restoration with mesh, followed by cancellous restoration with impaction grafting.

The success of impaction grafting depends on adequate physical constraint of the graft material. Any defects in the femur must therefore be repaired before impaction grafting. Malleable stainless steel meshes are secured with monofilament cerclage wires to contain any cortical defects or perforations or periprosthetic fractures. These meshes are placed by reflecting the vastus lateralis anteriorly to expose the femoral defect, with only minimal stripping of soft tissue from the bone.

Cortical strut allografts also may be required in certain situations to augment the diaphysis. For example, when a long-stemmed implant cannot be accommodated within the medullary canal, a standard length stem is used and bypassed with the cortical struts. Uncontained defects in the calcar region are reconstructed later in the procedure.

Prophylactic cerclage wiring is recommended if there is poor-quality bone in the proximal femur or any evidence of longitudinal splitting of cortical bone. Without wiring, vigorous packing during impaction grafting may result in an intraoperative femoral fracture or extension of a crack in the femur. If proximal repair is anticipated later, cerclage wiring will be performed simultaneously.

Preparation of the Graft

Graft preparation is critical to the success of this procedure. We use allograft from fresh frozen femoral heads almost exclusively. Rhesus compatibility is important only if the patient is a rhesus-negative woman of childbearing age. The allograft femoral heads are thawed, and any remaining soft tissue and articular cartilage are then removed using rongeurs.

The femoral heads are passed through a bone mill to generate allograft chips for impaction. The mill permits two sizes of chips to be made. The smaller chips (averaging 3- to 4-mm diameter), are used in the distal canal. Larger chips (8- to 10-mm diameter) are used in the proximal femur. In very ectatic canals, hand-made allograft "croutons" (10- to 12-mm diameter) are made with a rongeur and mixed with smaller chips for packing around the seated phantom.

A standard length reconstruction typically requires two femoral heads, each cut in half to facilitate milling, with three half-heads made into small chips for distal impaction and one half-head milled into large chips for proximal impaction. Therefore, a minimum of two femoral heads should be available for each patient. Additional femoral heads may be needed if indicated in preoperative planning or if the acetabulum also requires grafting.

Note that neither very fine-milled bone nor bone slurry is suitable for impaction grafting because neither have the mechanical properties required for adequate impaction, and their use will lead to graft failure.

Distal Occlusion of the Femur

Before grafting, the medullary canal must be occluded distally to constrain the graft. A canal plug usually is used. The diameter is estimated with preoperative templating and confirmed with canal sounds. The threaded polyethylene plug is screwed onto an intramedullary guide rod. Both are inserted into the medullary canal with a cannulated introducer sleeve coupled to a slap hammer (**Figure 2,** *A*). The plug is advanced to the templated level and the introducer sleeve removed. Calibrations on the introducer sleeve ensure placement at the correct depth. The guide wire remains in situ and cannulated instruments are passed over it during impaction grafting.

To use a retained cement plug, the largest diameter distal impactor that will pass down the canal is introduced to the level of the plug to act as a drill centralizer. The intramedullary drill is passed through the impactor and the cement drilled to a depth of 6 mm. A threaded guide rod can then be passed through the impactor and screwed into the hole drilled in the cement plug (**Figure 2,** *B*).

If it is difficult to securely place the distal canal plug, then the largest plug that passes through the isthmus to the correct depth is used and secured by passing one or two Kirschner wires percutaneously into or immediately below the level of the plug.

Graft Impaction

Cannulated instruments pack the graft in the distal and proximal femur, passing over the guide wire (**Figure 3**). The proximal impactor (phantom) of the templated size is passed over the rod to ensure that it will seat down to the appropriate level to restore limb length. The phantom should easily pass down the guide wire to a depth that comfortably restores the correct limb length. Any sizing adjustments are made at this point.

The rod should not be driven into varus as the impactor is inserted. If this occurs, further development of the posterolateral slot in the trochanter is necessary until neutral alignment of the proximal impactor is achieved. The guide wire should lie freely in the canal proximally and align with the midpoint of the popliteal fossa when viewed from its proximal end (**Figure 4**, *A*).

DISTAL IMPACTION

Before the distal impactors are used to impact the bone chips, it must be determined how far down the canal each size impactor can pass without jamming, which could result in fracture.

A distal impactor one size smaller in diameter than the diameter of the intramedullary plug is selected, and a plastic clip is attached to grooves on the impactor at the level of the greater trochanter to mark the intended depth of insertion (**Figure 4**, *B*). This creates a 2-cm distal bone plug. The impactor should easily pass over the guide wire to the plug without obstruction. The depth on 2-cm withdrawal of this impactor should be 2 cm less than the depth to which the plug was inserted.

Larger-diameter impactors are sequentially introduced as far down the canal as they will pass and similarly marked with a clip (**Figure 4**, *C*). The impactor should not be driven beyond this depth when impacting the bone chips.

The smaller-diameter allograft chips are introduced into the medullary canal around the guide rod using an open-ended 10- or 20-mL syringe. One of the larger impactors is used to manually push the chips down the canal. Using the first impactor (the one that passes down to the plug), bone chips are firmly compacted by hand down the distal plug to the marked depth, creating a loosely packed 2-cm plug.

The impactor should then be connected to the slap hammer for proper impaction. The impaction process continues by introducing and impacting more chips and using progressively larger impactors.

The plug should be tight and not migrate down the canal. Any move-

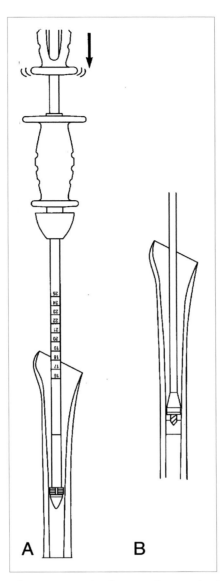

Figure 2 **A** and **B**, diagrams showing distal canal occlusion with the canal plug or a retained cement plug.

ment is indicated in the calibration on the guide wire opposite the tip of the trochanter. If the plug cannot be stabilized, it can be percutaneously transfixed at the correct depth with a Kirschner wire.

Impaction continues until the chip level reaches the distal impaction line, indicated by the most distal groove on the distal impactors (**Figure 4**, *D*). Once this point has been reached, the proximal impactors

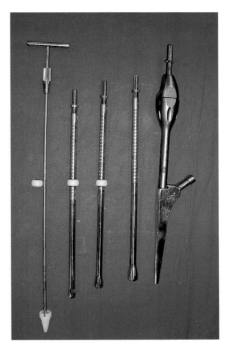

Figure 3 Cannulated femoral impaction instruments used to pack the graft in the distal and proximal femur. (Courtesy of Stryker, Newbury, Berkshire, United Kingdom.)

(phantoms) should be used. The phantom will be driven into the distally impacted bone, giving it some initial stability. It is important not to pack chips beyond the distal impaction line, because this may make it impossible to introduce the phantom.

PROXIMAL IMPACTION

The appropriate proximal impactor (phantom) is mounted on the slap hammer assembly and passed over the guide rod, then driven into the distally impacted bone. This creates enough stability to permit an initial trial reduction using the phantom to confirm that limb length will be restored. The slap hammer is removed, a trial head is placed on the neck of the phantom, and the hip is reduced with the guide wire remaining in situ. The level to which the phantom is inserted is marked on the proximal femur to reference the insertion depth.

Once the proximal femur is marked at the correct level, the phan-

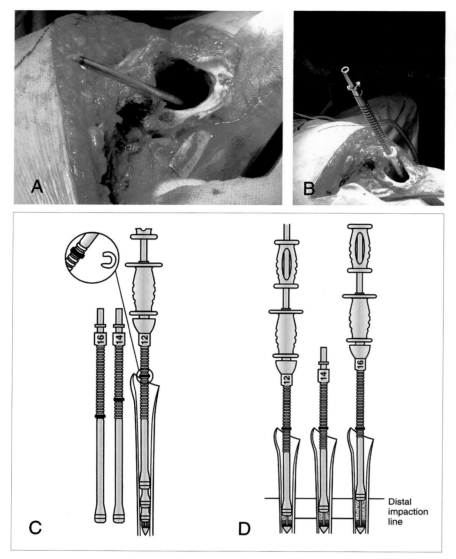

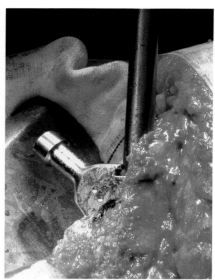

Figure 5 The proximal femur is marked to indicate the position of the phantom proximal impactor.

Figure 4 **A**, A guide wire is positioned freely in the medullary canal, with the canal plug attached distally. **B**, The distal impactor is positioned with depth marker clip in situ. **C**, Correct depth marking of the distal impactors. **D**, Progressive distal impaction is performed until the distal impaction line is reached.

tom is removed. More graft is introduced into the canal in approximately 10-mL increments and initially advanced manually using a distal impactor. The phantom is then repeatedly driven into the graft using the slap hammer.

The slap hammer handle is used to control rotation of the phantom to ensure that the neomedullary canal is formed in the correct amount of anteversion, usually 10° to 15°. Graft is se-

quentially added and vigorously impacted until the canal has been completely filled.

A second trial reduction may be performed with the guide rod still in position. A stability assessment and confirmation of the level to which the femoral component should be inserted can thus be obtained. This position is marked on the proximal femur to reference the depth of insertion and rotation of the definitive implant

(**Figure 5**). Impingement may require further excision of soft tissue or bone. A larger offset femoral stem occasionally may be indicated.

With the phantom seated at the correct depth, reconstruction should now proceed to repair any bone deficiency of the proximal femur. Reconstruction is required if bone loss extends to the level of the lesser trochanter on any aspect, and the graft should be brought up to a level that corresponds to at least the lowest of the three neck markings on the phantom (and therefore on the implant). The stem must be supported up to this level to ensure torsional stability within the femur.

Proximal reconstruction is performed using malleable stainless steel meshes secured with monofilament wires. If the loss of proximal bone in the calcar area extends to but does not involve the lesser trochanter, one of three sizes of acetabular rim mesh usually is easily contoured over the deficient area and held with monofilament wires (**Figure 6**, *A*). Anatomically contoured calcar mesh is available for larger defects (**Figure 6**, *B* and *C*).

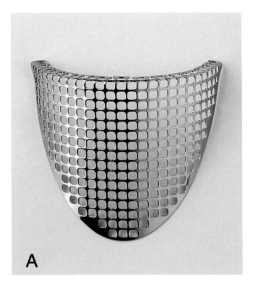
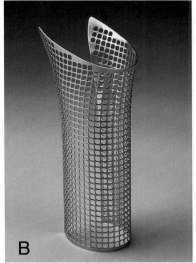
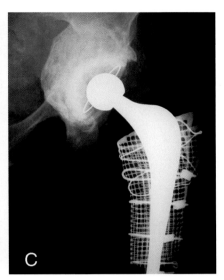

Figure 6   **A**, Rim mesh. **B**, Anatomic calcar mesh. **C**, AP radiograph of the hip showing reconstruction using anatomic calcar mesh. (Courtesy of Stryker, Newbury, Berkshire, United Kingdom.)

The meshes are secured with cerclage wires. An initial wire is passed through a drill hole made in the greater trochanter as far laterally as possible, halfway between the tip and the level of the lesser trochanter. Both cortices are drilled and the wire passed anteriorly and medially around the femoral neck. The wire is threaded through one of the proximal holes in the anterior edge of the mesh, brought back posteriorly, and then threaded through the posterior edge of the mesh before being tightened to its free end. This fixed wire prevents the mesh from moving up or down on the femur.

A second wire is passed around the femur deep to the vastus lateralis just below the lesser trochanter and similarly threaded through the mesh and tightened to itself. A third wire is occasionally necessary, and the calcar mesh may require four wires. Cables may be used distally but are to be avoided proximally because of the potential risk of intra-articular debris from cable fretting.

At this stage the larger-diameter bone chips should be used for final proximal packing. The proximal tamping instruments manually introduce these chips around the seated phantom, and they are then impacted with a mallet (**Figure 7**) until no further chips can be introduced.

When the femur appears to be fully grafted, one final maneuver is performed. Using the slap hammer, the phantom is withdrawn by 2 cm and a final introduction of large allograft chips is made. These chips are packed around the phantom manually, using the proximal tamps. The phantom is then driven into this bone, resulting in further graft impaction. Absolute axial and torsional stability of the phantom should be evident when impaction is complete. Several blows with the slap hammer should result in minimal (less than 1 mm) axial advancement of the phantom, and withdrawal without using the slap hammer should be extremely difficult. A further trial reduction can be performed at this time.

Prosthesis Implantation

Cancellous restoration is now complete, with formation of a neomedullary canal, and the femur is ready to accept the prosthesis (**Figure 8**, *A*). The stem chosen for implantation is the same size as the proximal phantom impactor used for final packing (the phantom being oversized to allow

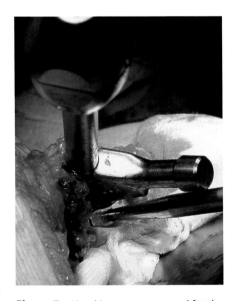

Figure 7   Hand impactors are used for the final proximal impaction. (Courtesy of Stryker, Newbury, Berkshire, United Kingdom.)

for the cement mantle and distal centralizer).

The slap hammer and guide wire are then removed. The phantom remains in position, keeping the graft under compression, until immediately before cement insertion. The canal can be kept dry by placing a No. 14 French gauge suction catheter down the lumen of the phantom.

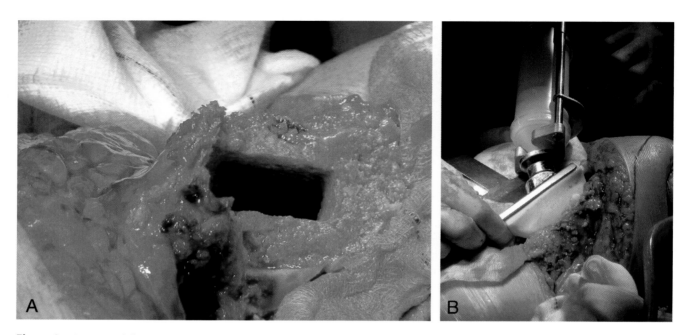

Figure 8 **A**, Neomedullary canal just prior to cementation. **B**, Cement pressurization into the neomedullary canal.

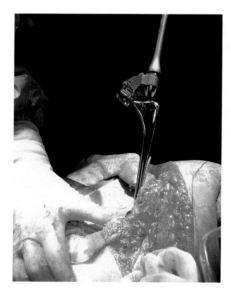

Figure 9 Stem insertion in correct alignment with additional thumb pressurization.

Cementation is performed with the same technique used for a polished tapered primary THA. Bone cement is introduced retrograde after the phantom is removed. We also use a revision cement gun with a tapered nozzle to ensure that the graft is not disrupted. After the canal has been filled, we place a flexible femoral seal over the nozzle,

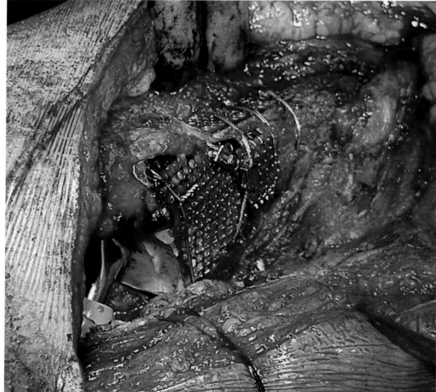

Figure 10 Final reduction with correct neck length modular head.

which is then cut off flush with the seal. The cement gun is reapplied to

the proximal femur and cement is then pressurized into the graft (**Figure 8**, *B*).

Pressurization is maintained until the viscosity of the cement is appropriate for stem insertion. This usually occurs approximately 6 minutes after mixing if room temperature is 68°F (20°C) but may vary by cement manufacturer.

The final component is then mounted on its introducer, ready for insertion with the special "wingless" centralizer fitted to the end of the prosthesis to minimize graft disruption. The stem is inserted to its predetermined position, with strict attention directed to alignment of the stem. The surgeon's thumb is applied to the medial aspect of the femoral neck throughout insertion to occlude cement extrusion from the medullary canal and thus maintain pressurization of the cement (**Figure 9**).When the desired position for the prosthesis is reached, the stem introducer is removed and a seal is applied around the proximal femur to maintain pressure on the cement and graft while the cement polymerizes.

A final trial reduction is then performed with appropriate neck length heads. The appropriate implant is then selected after testing for limb length, range of motion, tissue tension, and stability (**Figure 10**).

Wound Closure

After reduction with the definitive head implanted, the posterior capsule is reattached via drill holes to the posterior aspect of the femur with No. 2 or No. 5 nonabsorbable braided sutures. Routine wound closure is completed over a single deep suction drain.

Postoperative Regimen

The drain is removed 1 day postoperatively, and AP pelvis and full-length femoral radiographs are obtained. If radiographs are satisfactory, the patient is mobilized 1 to 2 days postoperatively. Toe-touch weight bearing is advised in most patients at least for the first 6 weeks, when radiographs are repeated.

In elderly patients with compliance issues, full weight bearing is permitted at an early stage with the use of assistive devices. The risk of a fall outweighs any risk to the reconstruction from full weight bearing.

Clinical and radiographic surveillance continues at 3 months, 6 months, 1 year, and 2 years postoperatively, with follow-up occurring every 2 years thereafter.

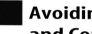

Avoiding Pitfalls and Complications

The potential problems associated with impaction bone grafting, principally femoral fracture and massive subsidence, are well known. Prophylactic wiring, strut allograft reinforcement of femurs with extensive bone loss, and long-stemmed implants have dramatically reduced the fracture rate. The incidence of significant subsidence has been reduced by use of larger bone chips proximally and in capacious canals, better distribution of particle size, tighter impaction of chips within the femoral canal, and the use of longer stems in patients with severe bone stock loss.

Most reported complications resulted from inappropriate surgical technique.

References

Brewster NT, Gillespie WJ, Howie CR, et al: Mechanical considerations in impaction bone grafting. *J Bone Joint Surg Br* 1999;81:118-124.

Eldridge JD, Smith EJ, Hubble MJ, Whitehouse SL, Learmonth ID: Massive early subsidence following femoral impaction grafting. *J Arthroplasty* 1997;12:535-540.

English H, Timperley A, Dunlop D, Gie G: Impaction grafting of the femur in two-stage revision for infected total hip replacement. *J Bone Joint Surg Br* 2002;84:700-705.

Gie GA, Linder L, Ling RS, et al: Impacted cancellous allografts and cement for revision total hip arthroplasty. *J Bone Joint Surg Br* 1993;75:14-21.

Giesen EB, Lamerigts NM, Verdonschot N, et al: Mechanical characteristics of impacted morcellised bone grafts used in revision of total hip arthroplasty. *J Bone Joint Surg Br* 1999;81:1052-1057.

Halliday BR, English HW, Timperley AJ, Gie GA, Ling RS: Femoral impaction grafting with cement in revision total hip replacement: Evolution of the technique and results. *J Bone Joint Surg Br* 2003;6:809-817.

Hostner J, Hultmark P, Karrholm J, Malchau H, Tveit M: Impaction technique and graft treatment in revisions of the femoral component: Laboratory studies and clinical validation. *J Arthroplasty* 2001;16:76-82.

Jazrawi LM, Della Valle CJ, Kummer FJ, Adler EM, Di Cesare PE: Catastrophic failure of a cemented, collarless, polished, tapered cobalt-chromium femoral stem used with impaction bone-grafting: A report of two cases. *J Bone Joint Surg Am* 1999;81:844-847.

Karrholm J, Hultmark P, Carlsson L, Malchau H: Subsidence of a non-polished stem in revisions of the hip using impaction allograft: Evaluation with radiostereometry and dual-energy X- ray absorptiometry. *J Bone Joint Surg Br* 1999;81:135-142.

Knight JL, Helming C: Collarless polished tapered impaction grafting of the femur during revision total hip arthroplasty: Pitfalls of the surgical technique and follow-up in 31 cases. *J Arthroplasty* 2000;15:159-165.

Malkani AL, Voor MJ, Fee KA, Bates CS: Femoral component revision using impacted morcellised cancellous graft: A biomechanical study of implant stability. *J Bone Joint Surg Br* 1996;78:973-978.

Masterson EL, Masri BA, Duncan CP: The cement mantle in the Exeter impaction allografting technique: A cause for concern. *J Arthroplasty* 1997;12:759-764.

Meding JB, Ritter MA, Keating EM, Faris PM: Impaction bone-grafting before insertion of a femoral stem with cement in revision total hip arthroplasty: A minimum two-year follow-up study. *J Bone Joint Surg Am* 1997;79:1834-1841.

Pekkarinen J, Alho A, Lepisto J, Ylikoski M, Ylinen P, Paavilainen T: Impaction bone grafting in revision hip surgery: A high incidence of complications. *J Bone Joint Surg Br* 2000;82:103-107.

Piccaluga F, Gonzalez Della Valle A, Encinas Fernandez JC, Pusso R: Revision of the femoral prosthesis with impaction allografting and a Charnley stem: A 2- to 12-year follow-up. *J Bone Joint Surg Br* 2002;84:544-549.

Ullmark G, Nilsson O: Impacted corticocancellous allografts: Recoil and strength. *Arthroplasty* 1999;14:1019-1023.

Coding

CPT Codes		Corresponding ICD-9 Codes		
27134	Revision of total hip arthroplasty; both components, with or without autograft or allograft	996.4	996.66	996.77
27138	Revision of total hip arthroplasty; femoral component only, with or without allograft	996.4	996.66	996.77

CPT copyright © 2004 by the American Medical Association. All Rights Reserved.

Chapter 57

Femoral Revision: Allograft Prosthetic Composite

Bassam A. Masri, MD, FRCSC
Clive P. Duncan, MD, MSc, FRCSC

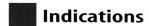 Indications

Allograft prosthetic composites are one option available to the orthopaedic surgeon faced with repairing severe bone loss of the proximal femur, either in the revision setting or following tumor resection. However, this treatment remains controversial, and its precise indications are still not clear despite a growing body of published literature. The technique allows reconstruction of the proximal femur by using a long stem femoral component fixed to a femoral allograft ex vivo, with the composite then secured to the remaining healthy segment of the host femur. Our technique will be discussed in this chapter.

Because of its complexity and potentially high complication rate, this technique should be reserved for patients whose degree of bone loss renders other reconstructive techniques impossible unless a tumor prosthesis is used. Classifying the de-gree of bone loss helps the surgeon decide if a proximal femoral allograft is required. Many classification systems have been devised, but we prefer that of Gross and associates (**Table 1**). This system reserves the technique of proximal femoral allograft prosthetic composite for patients whose circumferential femoral bone loss is more than 5 cm long. With lesser degrees of bone loss, the surgeon can use alternative techniques that may include cemented or uncemented stems or impacted allograft and strut grafts as outlined in **Table 1**.

Using an allograft prosthetic composite in patients with extensive femoral bone loss presents several potential advantages. The union of host femur and proximal femoral allograft creates an opportunity to augment existing bone stock and to provide a strong and durable reconstruction, particularly in the younger patient. Union of the host's greater trochanter and the allograft can improve abductor function, which in turn reduces the risk of postoperative dislocation and allows a more natural gait pattern. If the distal stem of the prosthesis is intentionally not fixed to the host femur by cement or biologic ingrowth, any revision required as a result of infection or graft resorption will be easier to accomplish.

This technique will fulfill its promise of bone stock augmentation

Table 1 Gross and Associates' Classification of Femoral Bone Stock

Classification	Description of Femoral Defect	Treatment Options
Type I	No substantial loss of bone stock	Straightforward cemented or uncemented femoral prosthesis
Type II	Cavitary (intraluminal) loss of bone stock	Proximal porous-coated stem Extensively porous-coated stem Modular uncemented stem Long stem component inserted with cement Cemented stem with impaction grafting
Type III	Contained loss of cortical bone stock	Same as for type II, but with the addition of cortical strut allograft
Type IV	Uncontained loss of cortical bone stock < 5 cm in length. The defect involves the calcar and lesser trochanter but does not extend into the diaphysis	Calcar-replacing implant
Type V	Uncontained loss of cortical bone stock > 5 cm in length	Allograft prosthetic composite Tumor prosthesis

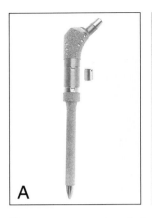
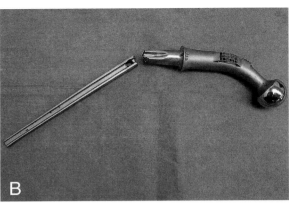

Figure 1 **A,** A modern design tumor prosthesis (or megaprosthesis) is the main alternative to the use of a circumferential proximal femoral allograft. **B,** Fatigue failure of an early design of tumor prosthesis. This stem was removed from a fit 47-year-old man and had been in situ for 20 years after resection of a chondrosarcoma. The use of an allograft prosthetic composite is now favored in the younger patient.

and better function if the surgeon strictly adheres to the principles outlined in this chapter. The technique is technically demanding and unforgiving of error.

Contraindications

This use of an allograft prosthetic composite is contraindicated in patients who have adequate bone stock to permit reconstruction using other methods. Surgeons or institutions lacking familiarity with complex allograft techniques should not attempt this technique but should refer patients to specialized centers.

Surgery and recovery times are lengthy. Most experienced institutions report operations lasting 3 to 6 hours, a significant physiologic challenge for the patient. The recovery period is extensive, requiring protected weight bearing on the affected limb until union at the host-graft interface is achieved. This can take up to 9 months. The procedure is probably not suitable for patients with extensive comorbidities or a limited life expectancy. Alternative treatments may

pose a lesser risk and allow faster recovery.

The presence of active infection precludes use of proximal femoral allografts in a single-stage revision. However, successful use of these allografts has been reported when used in the second part of a staged revision for infection. Therefore, a history of infection is not in itself an absolute contraindication as long as the infection is no longer active.

Alternative Treatments

The use of the proximal femoral allograft is reserved for patients with extensive femoral bone loss. Alternatives to use of this allograft are limited. The principal alternative is the tumor prosthesis or megaprosthesis (**Figure 1**, *A*). This procedure is technically much less demanding, needs a substantially shorter surgical time, and allows a much faster recovery. However, some reports indicate a high late failure rate with these prostheses (**Figure 1**, *B*); thus, these are best reserved for patients who are elderly and less ac-

tive or who have a limited life expectancy because of malignancy.

Results

Most published results using allograft prosthetic composites have come from a small number of specialist institutions. **Table 2** summarizes the results from some of the larger series with intermediate- to long-term follow-up. A number of factors makes it difficult to compare results between different centers. First, there is no standard for reporting femoral deficiencies. The procedure has been performed for a wide range of indications and on patients with varying degrees of bone loss. Second, surgical techniques vary greatly by institution. For example, some use specially designed prostheses whereas others use standard femoral stems. The method of fixation also differs. Some surgeons cement distally while others advocate distal press-fit or rely on step-cut stability at the allograft-host junction and use of a long stem that bypasses the junction without rigid distal fixation. Finally, there is no universally accepted method for reporting of results and no consensus regarding which method should be used to assess postoperative function or what actually constitutes a clinical success.

The results from the different centers show relatively high rates of complications and reoperations, thus confirming that these patients present some of the greatest challenges in reconstructive orthopaedics.

Technique

The preferred technique used at our institution is described in this chapter. Other techniques have been described

Table 2   Medium- to Long-Term Results of Allograft Prosthetic Composite

Author(s) (Year)	Number of Allografts	Mean Follow-up (Range)	Mean Harris Hip Scores (Range)	Results	Complications		
					Infection	Nonunion (%)	Dislocation (%)
Head, et al (1987)	22	28 months (21–40)	65 (30–90)	9 Reoperations (41%), 16 Patients (73%), Good or excellent results	0 (0%)	3 (14%)	5 (23%)
Roberson (1992)	24	48 months (12–96)	82 (55–90)	1 Reoperation (4%), 12 Patients (50%), Good or excellent results	2 (2%)	2 (8%)	1 (4%)
Chandler, et al (1994)	30	22 months (2–46)	78 (38–90)	3 Reoperations (10%)	1 (3%)	1 (3%)	5 (17%)
Gross, et al (1995)	168	58 months (6–138)	66 (21–100)	17 Reoperations (10%)	5 (3%)	7 (4%)	9 (5%)
Haddad, et al (2000)	40	106 months (60–138)	79 (26–96)	13 Reoperations (33%)	2 (5%)	3 (8%)	4 (10%)
Blackley, et al (2001)	63	132 months (112–180)	70 (47–95)	13 Reoperations (21%)	5 (8%)	4 (5%)	4 (6%)

in the literature and are preferred at other centers.

Use of the proximal femoral allograft is technically challenging and requires meticulous preoperative planning. The patient's medical condition should be optimized because of the long time to be spent under anesthesia. The average blood loss during these procedures is approximately 2.5 L. Most institutions use a cell-saver device along with preoperative autologous donation to reduce the need for homologous transfusion. It is also prudent to have tumor prostheses available as a salvage option if the allograft procedure needs to be abandoned.

Good quality radiographs should be obtained preoperatively and should include an AP view of the pelvis as well as full-length AP and lateral views of the femur. Preoperative planning focuses on measuring the extent of femoral bone loss and the length of allograft necessary to reconstruct that deficit and to restore normal limb length and biomechanics around the hip (**Figure 2**). The allograft is ordered before the surgery. It should be longer than the allograft suggested by the preoperative plan to allow for correction of any inaccuracies in measurement discovered intraoperatively.

The allograft diameter should be matched as closely as possible to that of the host femur. A suitable long stem prosthesis to use with the allograft should also be ordered, preferably an implant familiar to the surgeon. A long stem prosthesis with a narrow distal segment is ideal (**Figure 3**) because it allows cementation into the allograft while the narrow distal segment serves as an intramedullary guide within the host femur and does not compromise the step-cut interdigitation at the allograft-host junction.

Fresh bone allografts elicit an immune response from the host that may cause a delay in graft incorporation and lead to resorption of donor bone. The most common way to reduce the immune response is freezing or freeze-drying the graft, with or without irradi-

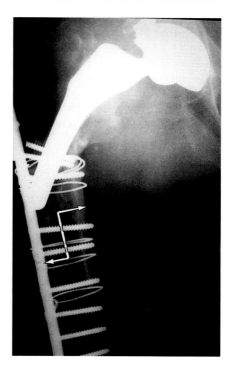

Figure 2   Preoperative AP radiograph of a 47-year-old man with marked proximal bone loss and a periprosthetic fracture (Vancouver classification type B3) treated with an allograft prosthetic composite. The double-headed arrow marks the level of the step-cut determined during preoperative planning.

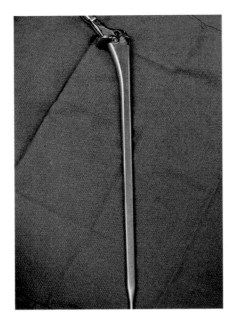

Figure 3 The ideal prosthesis for use with a proximal femoral allograft should have a long, narrow stem, that bypasses the host–allograft junction and avoids the need for excessive reaming of the allograft bone.

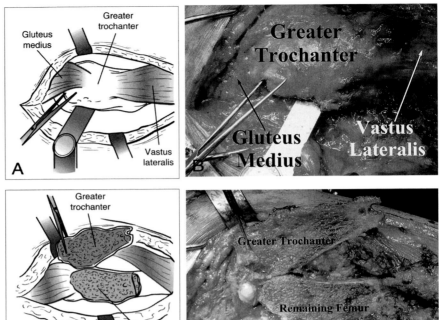

Figure 4 The trochanteric slide approach is commonly used for this procedure. Diagram **(A)** and intraoperative photograph **(B)** show the trochanter osteotomized in the sagittal plane, taking care to preserve the attachments of the glutei muscles proximally and the vastus lateralis distally. Diagram **(C)** and intraoperative photograph **(D)** show the greater trochanter with its attached muscles reflected anteriorly to reveal the remainder of the host femur, which is retained where possible for use as autograft around the allograft prosthetic composite.

ation, to help reduce the risk of viral transmission. This may also reduce graft immunogenicity. Our institution uses grafts with 2.5 megarad (Mrad) irradiation. They are stored at a temperature of -70°C; at this temperature, the shelf life is 5 years.

Exposure

The patient is positioned on his or her side, and the pelvis is secured in a vertical orientation using suitable restraints. The operation requires wide exposure. A transtrochanteric approach is generally chosen because it is extensile and allows reattachment of the host trochanter to the allograft femur, thus restoring abductor function. We prefer the trochanteric slide (**Figure 4**) or an extended trochanteric osteotomy instead of a traditional transverse trochanteric osteotomy because the former preserves the vastus-gluteal muscle sling and is associated with a lower rate of trochanteric escape.

Bone Preparation

The proximal femur is exposed by reflecting the vastus lateralis off the intermuscular septum and retracting it anteriorly. Do not denude the remaining femur of soft tissues because they will be used later in the procedure as a vascularized autograft. In patients whose hips have continuity between the greater trochanter and the lateral cortex of the proximal femur, an extended femoral osteotomy is performed. This procedure allows the lateral femoral cortex, with its intact muscular attachment and blood supply, to be wrapped around the allograft bone, thus not only potentially protecting it from resorption but also allowing better fixation of the greater trochanter to the allograft bone. Remaining usable medial bone is left connected to its muscular attach-

ments so that it can be used as a vascularized autograft to augment the allograft-host junction.

The junction of healthy host bone and deficient femur is identified, and a preliminary transverse osteotomy is made at a slightly higher level than the anticipated final resection level. A step-cut designed to mate with a matching, reciprocal step-cut on the allograft is fashioned in the host femur. The step-cut configuration, although technically much more difficult than a transverse junction, is much more rotationally stable. This technique permits the allograft-host junction, once healed, to transfer most of the load from the allograft to the host bone, thus eliminating the need for cement or a tight press-fit between the femoral stem and the host femur. We prefer not to have a tight press-fit and try to achieve stability of the construct through the step-cut procedure. This can be the most technically demanding portion of the operation.

Acetabular preparation should occur before femoral preparation because alteration of the center of rotation of the hip will impact limb-length measurements. A Steinmann pin or other device inserted in the supra-acetabular region may be used to guide limb-length measurements. An alternate technique compares the relative positions of the medial malleoli before and after reconstruction. All patients must be advised preoperatively that exact limb-length equalization may not be possible.

Graft Preparation

After infection has been excluded and the decision to proceed with the reconstruction is made, preparation of the graft is undertaken by part of the surgical team on a separate table. This occurs while the other team is working on exposure and implant removal (**Figure 5**). The graft is unwrapped, and specimens are obtained for culture. It is then placed in a warm solution of povidone-iodine for defrosting.

The experience of several institutions suggests that optimal results are achieved when the prosthesis is cemented into the allograft but not into the host. Uncemented fixation of the prosthesis within the allograft is not feasible because ingrowth cannot be expected. The prosthesis, therefore, is liable to subside and fail.

When the allograft prosthetic composite has been prepared, the bone surfaces are clean and dry, permitting near-perfect cementing technique. Excellent fixation of the prosthesis within the allograft can be achieved as a result. The medullary canal of the allograft is almost invariably narrower than that of the host; therefore, the surgeon should not try to achieve an interference fit between the prosthesis and the host femur. We believe that this is neither required nor

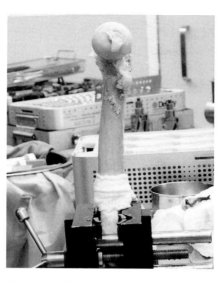

Figure 5 The allograft is prepared on a back table by a separate surgical team while the patient's hip is being exposed and the old prostheses are being removed.

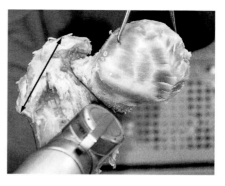

Figure 6 The head and neck are removed in preparation for stem insertion. The double-headed arrow demonstrates where the greater trochanter will also be removed so that the patient's greater trochanter can be attached after insertion of the allograft prosthetic composite.

desirable because it results in use of a stem that is too large for the allograft segment, requiring excessive reaming of the graft, which weakens it. Not all surgeons agree with this philosophy, however, and some aim for a press-fit in the distal femur to improve stability of the host-graft junction. The latter requires use of different prostheses and more reaming of the allograft.

The allograft is prepared by removing any residual soft tissue. An osteotomy of the neck is made, and the femoral head is removed (**Figure 6**). The greater trochanter is also removed so that the host trochanter may be attached, and the graft is then reamed and broached until the selected stem can be easily inserted into the allograft, thus ensuring an adequate cement mantle.

After acetabular reconstruction is completed, the length of the required graft should be measured by inserting the femoral prosthesis into the host femur and then reducing the hip. Traction is applied to the limb until the desired limb length is achieved. The location of the most distal section of the step-cut is determined (about 4 to

5 cm), and the femoral stem is marked at that level. The femoral stem is then removed and placed on top of the allograft so that the collar of the stem and the previously prepared calcar region of the allograft are aligned. This permits identification of the most distal section of the allograft that will mate with the host bone. A transverse cut is made at that level. As a second check, the femoral stem is inserted within the allograft, and the preliminary allograft prosthetic composite is reduced into the acetabulum. Traction is then applied so that limb lengths are reproduced. At this stage of the procedure, the most distal section of the host step-cut should be close to the distal end of the allograft. Having completed these checks, the surgeon creates the step-cut in the allograft (**Figure 7**).

It is better to make the graft too long rather than too short. It is always possible to shorten the graft when fine-tuning the host-allograft junction, but it is impossible to make the composite longer except by leaving the femoral stem proud of the proximal femur. It is also imperative that any preliminary measurements be made with the shortest possible head segment so that minor errors in length can potentially be salvaged with a longer neck.

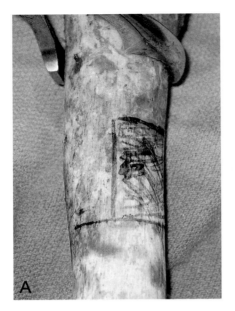

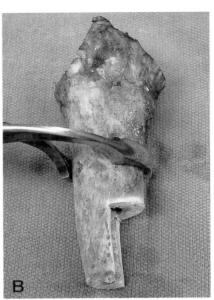

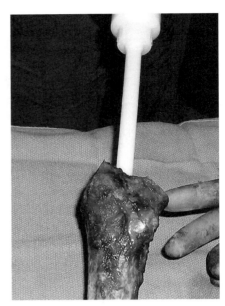

Figure 7 The step-cut is created in the allograft. **A,** The surgeon first marks the step-cut and double checks that the correct segment will be discarded. This photograph shows that an initial transverse cut will be made along the lower horizontal line. Completion of the step-cut will mean that the shaded area will be discarded. **B,** The same allograft after completion of the step-cut.

Figure 8 Cement is injected in a retrograde manner to ensure a complete column of cement.

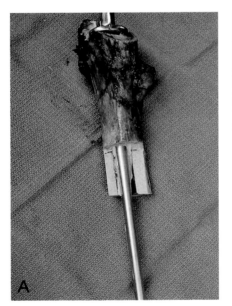

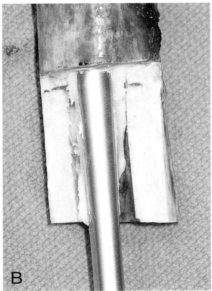

Figure 9 **A,** The allograft prosthetic composite after the cement has cured. **B,** Close-up of the step-cut region where the excess cement has been carefully cleared from the cut bone surfaces so that it does not interfere with union of the junction.

then pressurized to force the cement into the interstices of the endosteal bone. The prosthesis is then inserted cautiously to control the anteversion of the stem within the graft. It is essential that excess cement be cleared from the step-cut so that it does not interfere with healing between the host and graft. To prevent the cement from extruding over the step-cut surface, the surgeon can place a finger cut from a surgical glove over the distal end of the graft and use it to seal the femoral canal. The cement is then pressurized against this seal. As the implant is inserted into the allograft, the finger of the glove can be cut to allow the stem to exit the allograft distally. Before the cement sets, the distal end of the allograft is meticulously cleaned, removing any excess cement that may interfere with graft-host union (**Figure 9**).

When the cement cures, the allograft prosthetic composite is inserted into the host femur and the hip is reduced. Cables are passed around or through the lesser trochanter of the allograft and are later used to reattach

Prosthesis Implantation

Once the step-cut has been made, the graft is taken to the back table and then washed and dried in preparation for cementing. Antibiotic-impregnated cement is injected into the graft canal in retrograde fashion so that the canal is completely filled (**Figure 8**). It is

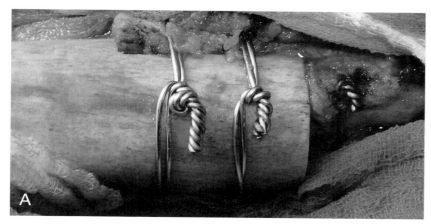

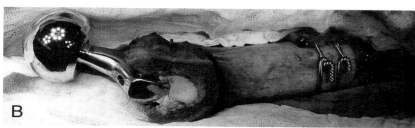

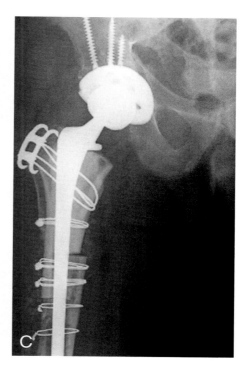

Figure 10 **A,** The step-cut is stabilized using cerclage wires. **B,** The final reconstruction prior to attachment of the patient's greater trochanter. **C,** The postoperative radiograph of the patient shown in Figure 3. The greater trochanter has been reattached using a cable grip system, and the junctional region has been packed with bone graft.

the host's greater trochanter using a cable-clamp device. We use a cable grip to enhance fixation, but we use wires at step-cut or if an extended osteotomy is used (the most common scenario). If an extended osteotomy fragment was created at the time of exposure, the distal portion of the host lateral cortex is fixed to the allograft using cerclage wires, and cables are not used. Although the step-cut is inherently stable, it is further secured with cerclage wires to ensure rigid stability (**Figure 10**). This is important because the long-term function of the entire construct depends on the stability of that junction and not on press-fit, bone ingrowth, or cementation into the host femur. In some hips, particularly with very distal junctions that cannot be made rigid, further rotational stability can be achieved by the addition of allograft struts to the junction. Morcellized bone graft should be packed around the step-cut region to promote host-graft union.

The surgeon should harvest as much autologous bone graft from the field (eg, acetabular reamings) as possible. If the amount is insufficient, morcellized allograft bone can be used in addition. Any remaining vascularized cortical bone that remains from the host femur should be mobilized distally and used to augment the host-allograft junction by wrapping the remaining vascularized host bone around the allograft, carefully incorporating as much of the junction as possible.

Wound Closure

The deep tissues are then closed using heavy bioabsorbable sutures over a suction drain. The subcutaneous tissues are closed using No. 2-0 bioabsorbable sutures, and the skin is closed using staples.

Postoperative Regimen

Our postoperative protocol includes thromboprophylaxis with low molec-

ular weight heparin for at least 10 days and intravenous antibiotics for 5 days or until the intraoperative cultures are reported. Patients are mobilized with toe-touch weight bearing 1 day postoperatively and should maintain this restricted weight-bearing status for at least 3 to 4 months, depending on radiographic evidence of healing at the host-allograft junction. If healing is progressing well at follow-up, weight bearing may be gradually increased so that the patient is at full weight bearing by 5 to 9 months postoperatively. Although we realize that this protocol may be conservative, our technique depends on the healing of the host-allograft junction and not on any fixation of the prosthesis within the distal host bone. A previous review of our experience with distal fixation revealed that the rate of allograft resorption was much higher than that reported by Gross and associates.

Active abduction exercises begin 6 months postoperatively to allow adequate healing of the host greater trochanter to the allograft trochanteric bed.

———————■

■ Avoiding Pitfalls and Complications

The use of allograft prosthetic composites is complex and technically challenging and presents a number of potential pitfalls and complications. The rates of complications reported in the literature vary widely among institutions, possibly reflecting the variety of techniques used.

Infection

Several factors combine to predispose patients to infection. Infection rates described in the literature vary between 3% and 13%. The extent of dissection and intraoperative blood loss, the duration of the operation, graft contamination, preexisting occult infection, and comorbidities are possible etiologic factors. They should be minimized if they cannot be avoided. The operation should be performed by experienced staff to minimize surgical time, soft-tissue dissection, and blood loss. The graft should be prepared by a second surgical team to increase efficiency and minimize surgical time. The graft and host should be screened for infection, and prophylactic antibiotics should be administered, both systemically and from within the cement. The graft and the wound should be copiously irrigated with saline-containing antibiotics.

If infection develops, it should be managed with a standard two-stage revision, an allograft being used in the second stage, if required. Using this technique, eradication of infection has been reported in 80% of cases.

Nonunion of the Host-Allograft Junction

The rate of nonunion of the host-allograft junction described in the literature varies widely, being reported as 3.5% to 23%. A number of factors may predispose to junctional nonunion, and only some of them are under the surgeon's control. The most important factors are the method of distal fixation, the surface area of bone contact, the stability of the junction, and the preservation of favorable biology.

Several methods of distal stem fixation have been tried, including cementing the prosthesis distally into the host femur, distal interference fit, interlocking fixation, and the technique described above that achieves stability through rigid fixation of a step-cut osteotomy. Experience demonstrates that, although cadaver models suggest that distal cementing confers good stability, in the clinical setting this technique results in a higher risk of nonunion, possibly through distraction of the junction or because cement becomes interposed between the two bone surfaces. Achieving an interference fit distally risks overreaming of the allograft and may lead to distraction at the junction, thus predisposing to nonunion. Most reports currently advocate proximal cementing without distal fixation because this technique is less often associated with nonunion. The step-cut produces a large surface area of contact between the two bone surfaces and also provides inherent stability. Both factors help to explain the improved rates of union resulting from this technique. All traces of cement should be meticulously cleaned from the allograft step-cut before insertion in the host femur. The addition of a cortical strut allograft will augment stability. The biology of healing may be optimized by preserving soft-tissue attachments to the host femur fragments, which are used as vascularized bone graft, and by placing additional autograft bone chips and reamings around the region of the junction.

Allograft nonunion may initially be treated with bone grafting with au-tograft if the junction is still mechanically stable. If the junction has lost its stability, the allograft may need to be revised to another allograft prosthetic composite or to a tumor prosthesis.

Trochanteric Nonunion and Escape

Nonunion of the greater trochanter is common, particularly when transverse trochanteric osteotomy is used. Nonunion likely occurs because of the distraction forces applied to the interface and because the blood supply to the healing area arises only from the host trochanter. As long as trochanteric escape does not result, nonunion in itself is not a major problem. However, escape of the trochanter may lead to pain, a limp, and the more serious problem of instability. The risk of this complication may be reduced through use of the trochanteric slide or extended femoral osteotomy, which preserve the trochanteric attachments of both the vastus lateralis and the gluteus medius. The trochanter is thus dynamically pushed into the trochanteric bed by the opposing forces of the abductor muscles and the vastus lateralis muscle. It is important postoperatively to avoid active abduction exercise while the trochanter heals.

Dislocation

One advantage that proximal femoral allografts have over megaprostheses is a potentially lower rate of dislocation because of the greater capacity for soft-tissue attachment to the allograft. Despite this advantage, dislocation rates following the use of allografts are reported to be 5% to 22%. Rates are higher in the presence of trochanteric escape and nonunion. We therefore prefer the trochanteric slide or extended femoral osteotomy. Dislocation rates are also higher if the femoral component is revised alone, leaving the cup in situ, but we do not advocate revision of all acetabular components for this reason. When the acetabular component is revised, use of a large diameter femoral head (**Figure 10**, *B*) or, when necessary, a constrained cup, may be considered. We prefer to reserve constrained components for the truly high-risk patient, or in those instances when satisfactory intraoperative stability cannot be achieved.

Allograft Resorption

Aseptic graft resorption occurs in up to 34% of proximal femoral allografts and is a major drawback to their use. Resorption is typically seen on the periosteal surface and usually begins within the first postoperative year. It may progress over the next 2 to 3 years, but the rate of resorption typically slows over the long term and only rarely causes failure of the reconstruction. Nevertheless, monitoring allograft recipients for resorption is required because these patients are symptom free while this silent complication occurs.

The etiology of resorption is yet to be determined. Potential causes include graft revascularization, host immune response, or graft processing lapses. Because the etiology is uncertain, prevention is difficult. To lessen its consequences, however, use of an allograft with strong cortical bone and minimal reaming are required. Maintaining as much host bone around the allograft as possible may also reduce this risk.

Allograft Fracture

Incorporation of a proximal femoral allograft occurs only at the host-allograft junction, and the remainder of the allograft remains devitalized and inert. It has no potential for remodeling and is therefore at risk of fracture. Reported fracture rates vary from 0% to 18%, and higher rates are reported for reconstructions performed for tumors.

To prevent fractures it is important to avoid drilling the allograft because of its lack of remodeling potential. Weakening the allograft through excessive reaming should also be avoided. Fracture rates are higher in the presence of junctional nonunion. If the allograft fractures and the patient is symptomatic, the allograft needs to be revised to another allograft prosthetic composite or to a tumor prosthesis.

Aseptic Loosening

Long-term failure because of aseptic loosening is a potential complication of our technique as it is for any method of hip reconstruction. The risk can be reduced by optimizing the cementing technique used to secure the femoral stem within the allograft, with particular attention directed to washing and drying the allograft endosteal bone surface, plugging the distal femoral canal, and following retrograde injection with pressurization of the cement into the allograft.

Disease Transmission

The use of allograft tissue always raises concerns about disease transmission, particularly agents such as human immunodeficiency virus. The risks of viral transmission can be reduced to 1 in 1,667,600 by adhering to the standards of the American Association of Tissue Banks and by irradiating the graft with a dose of 2.5 Mrad.

Fungal and bacterial infections have also been reported. The risks for these are reduced by handling the allograft in a sterile fashion during harvesting and preparation and by irradiating the graft.

References

Blackley HR, Davis AM, Hutchison CR, Gross AE: Proximal femoral allografts for reconstruction of bone stock in revision arthroplasty of the hip: A nine- to fifteen-year follow-up. *J Bone Joint Surg Am* 2001;83:346-354.

Chandler H, Clark J, Murphy S, et al: Reconstruction of major segmental loss of the proximal femur in revision total hip arthroplasty. *Clin Orthop* 1994;298:67-74.

Gross AE, Hutchison CR, Alexeeff M, et al: Proximal femoral allografts for reconstruction of bone stock in revision arthroplasty of the hip. *Clin Orthop* 1995;319:151-158.

Haddad FS, Garbuz DS, Masri BA, Duncan CP: Structural proximal femoral allografts for failed total hip arthroplasty (THA): A minimum review of five years. *J Bone Joint Surg Br* 2000;82:830-836.

Haddad FS, Garbuz DS, Masri BA, et al: Femoral bone loss in patients managed with revision hip replacement: Results of circumferential allograft replacement. *Instr Course Lect* 2000;49:147-162.

Haddad FS, Spangehl MJ, Masri BA, Garbuz DS, Duncan CP: Circumferential allograft replacement of the proximal femur: A critical analysis. *Clin Orthop* 2000;371:98-107.

Head WC, Berklacich FM, Malinin TI, Emerson RH: Proximal femoral allografts in revision total hip arthroplasty. *Clin Orthop* 1987;225:22-36.

Roberson JR: Proximal femoral bone loss after total hip arthroplasty. *Orthop Clin North Am* 1992;23:291-302.

Coding

CPT Codes		Corresponding ICD-9 Codes		
27134	Revision of total hip arthroplasty; both components, with or without autograft or allograft	996.4	996.66	996.77
27138	Revision of total hip arthroplasty; femoral component only, with or without allograft	996.4	996.66	996.77
Modifier 22	Unusual procedural services			

CPT copyright © 2004 by the American Medical Association. All Rights Reserved.

Indications

Bone loss after failure of both cemented and uncemented femoral components has been shown to diminish the clinical results of subsequent revisions. As a result, different techniques to restore bone stock to the revision femur have been developed.

Cortical onlay strut allografting, in particular, has become a preferred method of augmenting femoral bone stock in revision femoral hip surgery because of its simplicity and predictability. Bone necrosis alone does not alter the mechanical strength of bone. However, incorporation of autograft or allograft bone produces a porosity that profoundly decreases the strength of the graft (**Figure 1**). Therefore, cortical grafts are strongest initially but are weakened by the revascularizing repair process. Cortical autografts in dogs lose about 40% of their strength from 6 weeks to 6 months. In human autografts, porosity, mechanical strength, and radiographic density do not return to normal for 2 years. Because of this predictable period of graft weakness, the ideal use of allograft bone graft is to supplement the deficient host bone, not to become the primary supporting bone of the surgical construct. Animal models have shown superior strut graft healing and incorporation with rigid fixation to the host bone.

Femoral strut grafts are indicated in revision total hip arthroplasty (THA) for the reconstruction of deficient host bone. Bone graft is added during the revision procedure to address the loss of bone resulting from the implant failure. Its addition will both contribute to more normal bone support for the revision component and reverse the trend of progressive bone loss with revision surgery. Theoretically, this addition will make any subsequent revisions more successful. Strut grafts on the femur can be used to restore bone loss from osteolysis in the setting of a stable femoral component (**Figure 2**).

Loss of proximal bone support with a well-fixed distal implant will place the femoral component at mechanical risk of breakage, the so-called bending cantilever mode of failure. The source of the bone loss is less important than the extent and location of the loss. Osteolysis is the most common source of bone loss, followed by periprosthetic fracture and windows or gutters placed for removal of components or cement. Strut grafts can theoretically be placed anywhere on

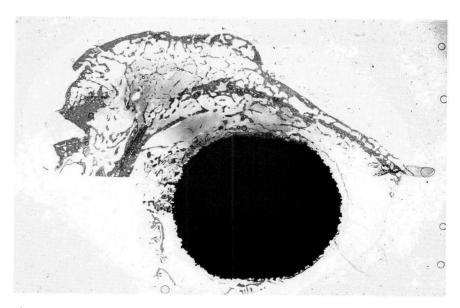

Figure 1 A transverse histologic section of a 32-month human retrieval showing complete incorporation of the strut graft, with the strut graft forming a neocortex for the femur. Note the increased porosity of the graft and the remodeling of both the graft and the host femur.

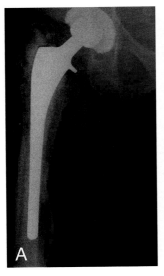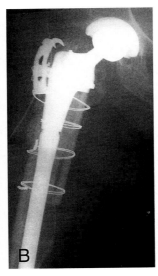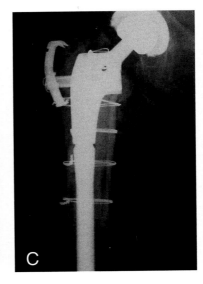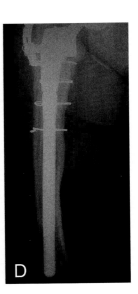

Figure 2   **A,** Preoperative AP radiograph showing a failed cemented stem and bone ingrowth at the acetabulum. Note the subsidence of the femoral component and osteolysis down the medial canal to below the tip. **B,** Postoperative AP radiograph showing reconstruction with a calcar replacement bone ingrowth prosthesis and a medial cortical strut allograft held with doubled cerclage. **C,** AP radiograph at 6 months showing union of the strut graft to the femur. **D,** AP radiograph at 5 years showing complete remodeling of the graft and host femur.

the femoral shaft. As a general rule more grafts are used proximally than distally. The most common indication for use of a strut graft on the proximal medial femur, an area prone to osteolysis, is collapse of the previous failed femoral implant into varus with erosion of the calcar, diminishing the support available to the revision component.

Loss of bone below the lesser trochanter, in the setting of a well-fixed distal stem, can also be an indication for a strut graft on the femur. A strut graft would be indicated especially in an active but heavy patient or where there is a modular femoral stem with an implant junction in the area of bone loss. Such modular implants are weaker than monoblock designs. The advantage of such medial placement of the graft in this construct is that it does not irritate the iliotibial band, which can be irritated by grafts placed on the lateral side of the femur.

Windows and gutters weaken the femur in proportion to their size and location. Such defects in the femoral tube diminish the hoop stresses in the bone. Large defects, defects in ac-

tive heavy patients, and defects near the tip of the femoral component are at the highest risk for producing bone fracture and, therefore, are good indications for strut grafting.

After an extended osteotomy for exposure of the femur, a strut graft can be effective in augmenting the lateral bone stock and should probably be used routinely when fracture of the osteotomy bone piece has occurred. Strut grafts can contribute to the augmentation of bone deficiency, which may have been one of the contributing factors to a periprosthetic fracture, and serve as a source of internal fracture fixation. Although they are principally osteoconductive, all strut grafts, whether freeze dried or fresh frozen, are weakly osteoinductive and thus can contribute to the stimulation of fracture healing. As a general rule, the strut graft alone cannot serve as the sole means of internal fixation. Rather, it should be combined with a longer stem or some type of plate and wire or screw construct to produce the rigid fixation necessary for optimal fracture healing. Inadvertent intraoperative fractures, in which the integ-

rity of the femur is substantially compromised more than can be fixed with a simple wire, can be treated with a strut graft.

Although they are most commonly used on the endosteal surface of the femur, strut grafts can be placed inside the femur itself, in the dilated patulous femur. This use can serve as an alternative to nonstructural bone chips and impaction grafting.

———————■

■ Contraindications

The use of strut grafts to provide structural support of the femoral implant is contraindicated. They can, however, be used to aid in rotational support of the implant as long as axial support on the host bone is sufficient.

Strut grafts can be a source of iliotibial band irritation anywhere on the lateral side of the femur but most commonly have been a clinical problem in the distal femur. Strut grafts add bulk to the thigh; therefore, the combination of the revision femoral component and graft will contribute to tension on the healing incision. Adequate soft-tissue capacity for such bulk needs to be ensured.

All bone grafts derive their healing cells from the surrounding host soft tissues; therefore, strut grafts used in heavily irradiated and thus dysvascular tissues may be less likely to unite. A metal bone plate may be a better option in this setting. Strut grafts should not be used in infected wounds, but they have been successfully used after treatment of the infection.

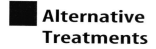

Alternative Treatments

Nonstructural bone chips typically are used in the endosteal canal but also can be used to fill windows and gutters. The graft bone is contained by the cavity and soft tissues and can certainly be used where there is no mechanical weakening of the femur that needs to be treated. The best defects for this technique would be in the midfemoral area, away from the calcar and tip of the stem.

A metal plate with cables or wires can serve the same mechanical function as the strut graft but lacks the capacity to unite to the host bone to restore bone stock. Such plate devices can be combined with the strut graft when needed and are especially useful for fixation of periprosthetic fractures.

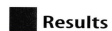

Results

In the revision THA, cortical onlay strut allografts have been reported to be effective in restoring femoral bone stock. Improved bone stock will not always translate into a successful revision implant, but lack of sufficient bone has been known for many years

Table 1 Results of Revision THA Using Strut Grafts

Author(s) (Year)	Number of Hips	Implant Type	Mean Patient Age (Range)	Mean Follow-up (Range)	Results
Emerson, et al (1992)	114	N/A	N/A	25 months	96% union (mean to union, 8.3 months)
Gross, et al (2003)	52	N/A	N/A	57 months	96% union 4% resorbed
Barden, et al (2003)	20	N/A	N/A	56 months	90% union 10% resorbed

N/A = Not applicable

to correlate with a diminished clinical outcome (**Table 1**).

Technique

Exposure

The exposure should anticipate the use of strut grafts. Most revisions will require no special change in hip exposure technique. Strut grafts can be used for anterolateral, transtrochanteric, and posterior approaches. Ideally the graft should be covered with a healthy layer of well-vascularized muscle. If the hip tissues are heavily scarred, a separate soft-tissue transfer to the thigh should be planned. There is no one best technique for this, but a rectus abdominus flap will work very well. Soft-tissue expanders may be used also.

Bone Preparation

Animal models have shown that the remodeling of the strut graft starts in the junction between the graft and the host and that both the underlying host bone and the overlying graft are remodeled. There is no need to remove all of the periosteum, and small gaps fill in well. Large gaps should probably be filled with bone chips. There is no need to decorticate the femoral shaft.

Both fresh frozen and freeze-dried bone can be successfully used. Graft resorption may be less in the fresh frozen grafts as a result of the documented increased antigenicity of these grafts, although resorption is not a common observation. The literature, however, does not support any actual clinical difference between freeze-dried and fresh frozen grafts. The advantage of fresh frozen bone is that the bone is stronger. However, in the setting of bone supplementation, strength is not as important as in clinical settings in which the graft provides more primary implant support or fracture stabilization. The advantage of freeze-dried bone is that it is the least immunogenic and is easily stored at room temperature in peel packs. A selection of grafts can be readily available and easily visualized through the wrapper for shape and sizing purposes. Bone banks typically use tibial bone to make the cortical struts, but other tubular cortical bones can be used. The shape and strength of the tibia are appropriate for most uses, and strut grafts can easily be shaped and sized to fit the clinical circumstance.

For the femur, minimal shaping of the strut graft is required but pointed areas should be rounded, and on occasion, a burr or high-speed cutting tool should be used to adjust the graft for maximal conformity to the host bone. Hip range of motion should be assessed for the proximal medial strut grafts to prevent impingement in flexion that might contribute to hip instability.

Strut grafts have been studied in animal models with and without internal fixation, and they are more successful with fixation. They can be readily fixed with cerclage wires (usually doubled), cables, or screws. Screws are less useful in the presence of an intramedullary stem. There is minute deformation of the graft as the cerclage fixation is applied. Thus, the tightness of the fixation must be tested up and down the graft until all wires are equally tight, and the graft is no longer deforming. This adjustment is more easily done with cerclage wires, but cables probably provide stronger fixation and can be placed using multiple tensioning tools. The choice of wires or cables should probably be de-termined by the strength require-ments of the underlying revision con-struct.

Wound Closure

Bone grafts alone have not been shown to be a cause of increased infec-tion when comparing cases of similar complexity. Patients requiring bone grafting are more complex by defini-tion, and wound complications can ruin an otherwise skillful operation. The original anatomic layers should be individually repaired, and the clo-sure should be tight to limit drainage and promote primary healing. Joint range-of-motion exercise should be started after hemostasis has been achieved and the wound is dry.

Postoperative Regimen

The patient's weight-bearing status should be judged on the overall strength of the graft-host bone-im-plant composite. A protected gait is prudent for 6 to 12 weeks. Progression of weight bearing should depend on the patient's symptoms, radiographic implant stability, and clinical gait pa-rameters determined by balance and strength.

Avoiding Pitfalls and Complications

Care must be taken with tightening of cerclage fixation because overtighten-ing could cause fracture of the host bone. Wire knots should be placed to avoid iliotibial band irritation. Promi-nent parts of the strut should be shaved to avoid tender areas.

References

Barden B, Fitzek SG, Huttegger C, Loer F: Supportive strut grafts for diaphyseal defects in revision hip arthroplasty. *Clin Orthop* 2003;387:148-155.

Emerson RH Jr, Malinin TI, Cuellar AD, Head WC, Peters PC: Cortical strut allografts in the recon-struction of the femur in revision total hip arthroplasty: A basic science and clinical study. *Clin Orthop* 1992;285:35-44.

Gross AE, Wong PKC, Hutchinson CR, King AE: Onlay cortical strut grafting in revision arthroplasty of the hip. *J Arthroplasty* 2003;18(suppl 1):104-106.

Haddad FS, Duncan CP, Berry DJ, et al: Periprosthetic femoral fractures around well-fixed implants: Use of cortical onlay allografts with or without a plate. *J Bone Joint Surg Am* 2002;84:945-950.

Tshmala M, Cox E, DeCock H, Goddeeris BM, Mattheeuws D: Antigenicity of cortical bone allografts in dogs and effect of ethylene oxide-sterilization. *Vet Immunol Immunopathol* 1999;69:47-59.

Coding

CPT Codes		Corresponding ICD-9 Codes		
27134	Revision of total hip arthroplasty; both components, with or without autograft or allograft	996.4 820.22	996.66 821.01	996.77
27138	Revision of total hip arthroplasty; femoral component only, with or without allograft	996.4 820.22	996.66 821.01	996.77
27245	Open treatment of intertrochanteric, peritrochanteric, or subtrochanteric femoral fracture; with intramedullary implant, with or without interlocking screws or cerclage	170.7 733.15 733.22 820.9 996.4	198.5 733.20 733.29 820.22 996.66	733.14 733.21 820.8 821.01 996.77
27506	Open treatment of femoral shaft fracture, with or without external fixation, with insertion of intramedullary implant, with or without cerclage and/or locking screws	733.15 821.01 821.29	820.01 821.10 821.3	821.00 821.11 821.30
Modifier 22	Unusual procedural services			

CPT copyright © 2004 by the American Medical Association. All Rights Reserved.

Bone grafting is included in the CPT code for revision THA. One of the advantages of strut grafting is that is adds less time to the surgery than more extensive allograft techniques.

Chapter 59

Conversion of Failed Hemiarthroplasty

Peter F. Sharkey, MD

 Indications

Unipolar or bipolar hemiarthroplasty has been recommended for numerous hip conditions, including displaced subcapital hip fractures, osteoarthritis, and osteonecrosis. The efficacy of these implants has been established, but some patients have residual pain, a limp, and/or weakness severe enough to warrant revision surgery. It is not uncommon for patients to report "acetabular pain" in the groin or buttocks region after hemiarthroplasty, even when the femoral stem is well fixed and the unipolar or bipolar articulation is functioning as designed.

The reasons or risk factors for residual pain after hemiarthroplasty have not been clearly established. An unresurfaced acetabulum may be associated with pain in some patients. Erosion of the articular cartilage has been proposed as one source of this pain. Conversion of the acetabular portion of the arthroplasty to a fixed socket has been reported to successfully relieve groin or buttock pain in 80% of patients. Residual pain persists in the remainder of these patients, even with radiographic evidence of a well-fixed socket. Failure that results from severe aseptic pain mandates conversion to a total hip arthroplasty (THA). Hemiarthroplasty also can fail as a result of femoral stem loosening; in this situation, revision of the failed construct also can provide pain relief.

The need for revision surgery increases with time, even without loosening of the femoral stem because of the deleterious effects and deterioration of a metal-on-cartilage construct.

Successful conversion of a failed hemiarthroplasty to THA requires careful preoperative planning and skilled surgical technique. The clinical history must be thoughtfully elicited and evaluated. The nature of the pain should be determined. If the patient has severe groin pain or buttocks pain with activity, the status of the bipolar or unipolar articulation must be considered. If the patient was sedentary preoperatively, remains so after surgery, and the pain is associated with rest or occurs at night, then a work-up for infection should follow. An elevated C-reactive protein level and/or erythrocyte sedimentation rate are indications for preoperative hip aspiration. An infected hemiarthroplasty is treated similarly to an infected THA. Generally, pain in the acetabular portion of the hemiarthroplasty presents in the groin or the buttocks region and has a mechanical quality, characterized typically as "start-up" pain and pain with weight bearing. Radiographs may show evidence of joint space narrowing and loss of articular cartilage (**Figure 1**). Thigh or knee pain implicates the femoral component, and radiographs must be studied for subtle signs of femoral component loosening.

Pain and dysfunction after hemiarthroplasty should be quantitated and patient expectations ascertained. Patients who sustain a hip fracture are usually asymptomatic before the injury; therefore, their appreciation of the results of arthroplasty differs from that of a patient who has a long-standing painful osteoarthritis and disability. Additionally, hip fracture is a serious injury associated with loss of function, even with successful treatment. These factors should be considered when evaluating the patient. Unrealistic patient expectations or generalized debilitated status are not predictably corrected with additional surgery.

Examination should include range of motion to elicit pain and determine its location. The wound and surrounding soft tissues are inspected for evidence of infection. Additionally, limb length must be carefully measured. If the length of the operated-on leg is longer, it may be difficult to correct without resulting in hip instability. This possibility must be discussed preoperatively with the patient.

———————■

■ **Contraindications**

Contraindications to conversion of bipolar arthroplasty to THA include patients who have had prior hip fracture and are minimally ambulatory and so debilitated that further surgery is un-

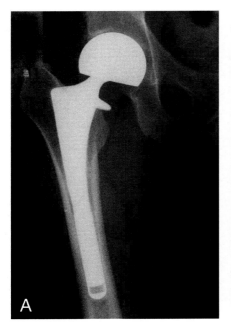
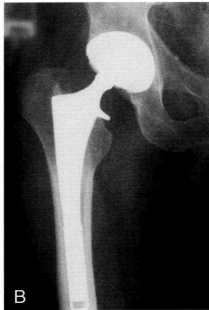

Figure 1 **A,** AP radiograph of a 48-year-old man shows joint space narrowing and loss of articular cartilage after hemiarthroplasty. **B,** Postoperative AP radiograph following conversion to THA.

Table 1 Results of Revision of Hemiarthroplasty to Total Hip Arthroplasty

Author(s) (Year)	Number of Hips	Mean Patient Age (Range)	Mean Follow-up (Range)	Results
Sharkey, et al (1998)	45	65 years (32–85)	34.8 months (24–79.2)	24.4% reoperation rate at latest follow-up Average 50-point improvement in Harris hip score
Bilgen, et al (2000)	15	59 years (30–75)	32 months (12–54)	0% reoperation rate at latest follow-up Average 49.5-point improvement in Harris hip score
Cossey and Goodwin (2001)	46	76.1 years (NA)	12 months (NA)	0% reoperation rate at latest follow-up 88% with complete resolution of symptoms
Sierra and Cabanela (2002)	132	73.1 years (SD = 10)	85.2 months (61.2–183.6)	12.8% overall reoperation rate 70% reported patient satisfaction

NA = Not available

SD = Standard deviation

likely to provide substantial clinical benefit. If the patient's overall medical condition significantly increases the risk of surgical intervention, then alternatives should be explored. Likewise, if severe osteoporosis compromises the quality and likely success of acetabular revision, then the logic of surgical intervention must be carefully considered. The surgeon must scrutinize the patient's history, examination, and radiographs and determine if conversion arthroplasty will positively impact lifestyle and mobility. Infection must always be considered when evaluating a painful arthroplasty and, if present, is a contraindication to routine conversion surgery. Finally, alternative causes of hip pain such as neurologic, soft-tissue related, and other sources, must be excluded before proceeding with surgery.

Alternative Treatments

Nonsurgical treatment for the painful hemiarthroplasty should be considered when the patient is not a surgical candidate. Protected weight bearing with a cane or walker may relieve arthritic symptoms. Nonsteroidal anti-inflammatory drugs may also relieve pain but should be used judiciously in a frail, elderly population. Intra-articular corticosteroid injections may also help and can be used for both therapeutic and diagnostic purposes. Narcotic analgesia for this chronic problem should be considered only when all other options are exhausted.

Results

Results of conversion of hemiarthroplasty to THA can be very gratifying in selected patients. Groin or low buttock pain, which are the chief complaints associated with hemiarthroplasty, can be successfully relieved in about 80% of patients (**Table 1**). Care must be taken to evaluate the femoral side of the articulation as a source of pain. Revision of all components is indicated if the femoral component is suspected of loosening, causing thigh pain, or is malpositioned.

Technique

Exposure

The previous incision or at least part of the previous incision should be used whenever possible. However, the approach used for the hemiarthroplasty need not be repeated. Because the transtrochanteric, posterior, and direct lateral approaches are all effective, selection should be based on surgeon familiarity and experience with revision surgery. The exposure should not be limited to the acetabulum; the femoral component must also be carefully inspected to ensure that it is not only well fixed but also well positioned. The approach should readily allow for extended trochanteric osteotomy, if this technique becomes necessary. In some patients, exposure is made more difficult by severe acetabular protrusio. Forceful dislocation can result in iatrogenic femoral fracture. If the protrusion is moderate, then a "doorway" can be made by removing a small amount of the lateral acetabular rim, and this may facilitate dislocation. In more severe protrusion, dislocation can be performed if the bipolar component can be disassembled in situ either by unlocking the bipolar ring or loosening the femoral head from its modular taper. On rare occasion, it will be necessary to cut the femoral prosthesis at the neck and revise both components.

Femoral stem removal, when necessary, follows established principles of femoral revision (chapter 50). A unique feature of failed Austin Moore–type uncemented hemiarthroplasties is that they may be loose but incarcerated by virtue of bone bridges

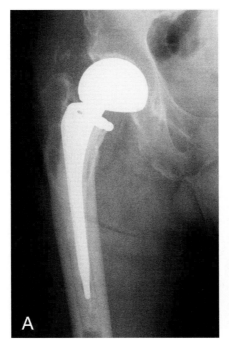
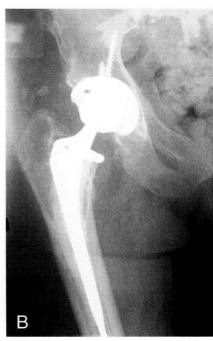

Figure 2 **A,** AP radiograph of a 69-year-old man who has pain despite a well-fixed femoral stem in a bipolar hemiarthroplasty. **B,** The bipolar portion of the prosthesis was converted to a fixed acetabulum, and the femoral head was removed from the modular femoral prosthesis. To achieve stability and equal limb lengths, a standard 32-mm head neck combination was impacted onto the femoral component.

that have grown through macrofenestrations in the implant. These bone bridges must be divided with a mini-osteotome or high-speed cutting instrument before the implant can be extracted safely.

Bone Preparation

Osteopenic bone is likely to be encountered during conversion surgery. Patients often undergo bipolar arthroplasty as a result of hip fracture, a circumstance in which the bone should be expected to be osteoporotic. Pain, immobility, and disability can weaken the bone even further after unsuccessful hemiarthroplasty. The hemiarthroplasty implant creates a stress shielding phenomenon that additionally weakens the acetabular bone. Extreme caution is necessary when reaming the acetabular bone. Usually a thin layer of subchondral bone shields very soft underlying cancellous bone. If the subchondral bone is reamed away, se-

cure fixation will be difficult to obtain. In this population, the acetabulum usually is small. Reaming should begin with small reamers, and caution is needed to maintain 360° of rim bone intact for adequate initial press-fit and stability. The amount of underreaming is individualized both to attain a press-fit and to avoid producing an intraoperative acetabular fracture.

Prosthesis Implantation

Preoperatively, the previous surgical reports should be obtained to determine the type of femoral stem and femoral head replacement component (either bipolar or unipolar) in place. This is particularly true if the femoral stem is well fixed. Once the manufacturer of the femoral stem is identified, the features of the implant should be reviewed to determine whether it is modular and what modular options are available. This information is essential because it will aid in disassembly of the compo-

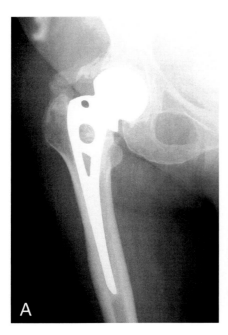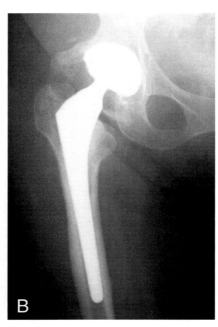

Figure 3   A, Austin Moore–type femoral component with bone growth through the fenestrations. **B,** Revision was successful with minimal bone loss by carefully freeing prosthesis using thin, flexible osteotomes.

Avoiding Pitfalls and Complications

As with all revision surgeries, instability may be a problem after conversion. If the hemiarthroplasty was performed because of subcapital fracture, then the articular capsule will not be contracted, adding to the risk of instability after conversion. Previous surgery can impair or damage the surrounding musculature, increasing the risk for chronic dislocation after conversion. Any instability that is encountered intraoperatively should be addressed. During conversion surgery, offset liners should be available to increase soft-tissue tension and used if needed. Additionally, a constrained socket is useful in the event that instability cannot be controlled without unreasonable lengthening of the lower extremity or overtensioning the soft tissue with a lateral offset femoral prosthesis.

A large (greater than 32 mm) femoral head diameter may prove helpful to improve hip stability and can be considered, if feasible. If the stem is monoblock, not being converted, or large-diameter heads are not be available, limb-length equality may not be possible. Patients should not be promised that surgery will equalize limb length because this is not the primary goal of the surgery.

Preoperatively and intraoperatively, the femoral stem is carefully evaluated for loosening; if the stem is loose, revision of the stem is indicated. In addition, if the patient has significant thigh pain accompanying the groin pain, revision of the stem should be considered. Unfortunately, revision of a well-fixed stem is sometimes necessary and often determined intraoperatively if instability is present or the femoral stem is significantly malpositioned. Revision stems should be readily available during conversion surgery, even if the stem appears to be

nents and facilitate reconstruction of the hip if only the acetabular portion of the hemiarthroplasty is revised. A full set of head sizes and neck lengths is necessary to handle all contingencies of conversion surgery (**Figure 2**). Radiographs should be inspected for acetabular erosion, polyethylene wear, osteolysis, heterotopic ossification, and femoral bone loss.

In general, an uncemented socket is preferred for conversion surgery of a hemiarthroplasty. The socket should have means for secondary fixation, including screw holes. Underreaming the socket may improve fixation. Care must be taken during reaming to avoid penetrating the subcortical bone, exposing weak cancellous bone and creating a situation in which protrusio may occur. The surgeon should be prepared to cement the socket if fixation cannot be achieved with an uncemented implant.

Wound Closure
Wound closure should be performed routinely using a technique familiar to the surgeon. Closure in layers with the skin closed with staples and a compressive dressing is generally acceptable. However, in selected patients with poor soft-tissue quality, nylon suture can be considered for skin closure.

Postoperative Regimen
The postoperative regimen depends on the surgical reconstruction. If a severe protrusion requires bone grafting with cage reconstruction, then 6 weeks to 3 months of 10% weight bearing may be required. Likewise, if femoral reconstruction is performed in conjunction with an acetabular repair, then partial weight bearing also may be necessary, depending on initial component stability. Postoperatively early mobilization is emphasized along with thromboembolic prophylaxis. I prefer to use indomethacin or radiation routinely to prevent heterotopic ossification. Generally, after 6 weeks to 3 months of physical therapy, patients can ambulate pain free without assistive devices.

———————————■

well fixed preoperatively. Revision of the stem is more likely with non-modular stems.

If a traditional Austin Moore prosthesis is being converted to a THA, care must be taken to address bone bridges through the fenestrations of the prosthesis. These bone bridges can inhibit implant removal. To remove the implant without significantly damaging the femoral bone, thin osteotomes or thin bone-cutting power tools often can be used to free the implant (**Figure 3**).

If a bipolar implant has been in place for a long time, polyethylene wear may have occurred and osteolysis encountered. In this situation, the possibility of osteolysis should be anticipated, and bone graft options must be available at the time of surgery, if needed. If osteolysis is noted, a thorough synovectomy with débridement of all granulomatous tissue is performed before bone grafting.

——————■

References

Bilgen O, Karaeminogullari O, Kulecioglu A: Results of conversion of total hip prosthesis performed following painful hemiarthroplasty. *J Int Med Res* 2000;28:307-312.

Cossey AJ, Goodwin ML: Failure of Austin Moore hemiarthroplasty: Total hip replacement as a treatment strategy. *Injury* 2002;33:19-21.

Dalldorf PG, Banas MP, Hicks DG, Pellegrini VD Jr: Rate of degeneration of human acetabular cartilage after hemiarthroplasty. *J Bone Joint Surg Am* 1995;77:877-882.

Floren M, Lester DK: Outcomes of total hip arthroplasty and contralateral bipolar hemiarthroplasty: A case series. *J Bone Joint Surg Am* 2003;85:523-526.

Ravikumar KJ, Marsh G: Internal fixation versus hemiarthroplasty versus total hip arthroplasty for displaced subcapital fractures of femur: 13 year results of a prospective randomized study. *Injury* 2000;31:793-797.

Sharkey PF, Rao R, Hozack WJ, Rothman RH, Carey C: Conversion of the hemiarthroplasty to total hip arthroplasty: Can groin pain be eliminated? *J Arthroplasty* 1998;13:627-630.

Sierra RJ, Cabanela ME: Conversion of failed hip hemiarthroplasties afer femoral neck fractures. *Clin Orthop* 2002;399:129-139.

Torisu T, Izumi H, Fujikawa Y, Masumi S: Bipolar hip arthroplasty without acetabular bone grafting for dysplastic osteoarthritis: Results after 6-9 years. *J Arthroplasty* 1995;10:15-27.

Coding

CPT Codes		Corresponding ICD-9 Codes		
27132	Conversion of previous hip surgery to total hip arthroplasty, with or without autograft or allograft	715.15 718.25 996.77	715.25 996.4	715.35 996.66
27134	Revision of total hip arthroplasty; both components, with or without autograft or allograft	715.15 718.25 996.77	715.25 996.4	715.35 996.66
Modifier 52	Reduced Services (Under certain circumstances a service or procedure is partially reduced or eliminated at the physician's discretion. Under these circumstances the service provided can be identified by its usual procedure number and the addition of the modifier "52," signifying that the service is reduced. This provides a means of reporting reduced services without disturbing the identification of the basic service.)			

CPT copyright © 2004 by the American Medical Association. All Rights Reserved.

Chapter 60

Greater Trochanter and Abductor Mechanism Problems After Total Hip Arthroplasty

Richard A. Berger, MD

Indications

The abductor mechanism has two main functions: (1) it provides stability for the hip joint to prevent dislocation; and (2) it provides the co-contraction force needed to stabilize the hip in single-leg stance. A dysfunctional abductor mechanism can result in instability, dislocation, and/or a limp. Abductor and greater trochanteric problems also are frequently associated with lateral hip pain. Unfortunately, trochanter and abductor mechanism problems are often difficult to remedy, and frequently the results are less than satisfactory.

Abductor and trochanteric problems fall into three broad categories: (1) trochanteric fracture in the perioperative period and acute trochanteric fracture; (2) trochanteric escape and trochanteric nonunion; and (3) dysfunctional abductor muscle mechanism, usually resulting from denervation of the abductors, poor healing of detached abductors, or chronic scarring as a result of multiple procedures or infection.

The main indications for surgical treatment of greater trochanteric and abductor mechanism problems in total hip arthroplasty (THA) are abductor weakness with associated abductor limp, hip instability related to abductor deficiency, and pain related to trochanteric nonunion or soft-tissue deficiency in the greater trochanteric region.

Surgery should be considered only when there is a reasonable likelihood that such intervention will improve the patient's symptoms. Successful fixation of a fracture or nonunion of the greater trochanter can improve abductor gait, restore hip stability, and reduce pain. However, repeat fixation is not always successful; therefore, the surgeon needs to weigh the likelihood of success against the risks of surgery. Successful reattachment of unhealed or avulsed abductor muscles may improve hip stability and gait to some degree, but clinically there may be only moderate improvement and pain relief is unpredictable.

───────■

Contraindications

Few areas of hip reconstruction require more careful judgment than the decision to perform further surgery to resolve greater trochanteric or abductor problems. Results are unpredictable and frequently disappointing. Surgery is contraindicated unless substantial benefit is likely to be provided. Surgery for pain relief frequently is disappointing, and surgery to improve hip stability or reduce a limp should be considered only if substantial improvement in the patient's anatomic problem is likely. A satisfactory result is less likely in patients with severely scarred tissues, longstanding problems, severely retracted abductor mechanisms, and/or a markedly damaged greater trochanteric area.

Reoperation should be avoided when the abductor dysfunction problem is neurogenic because this problem cannot be resolved through mechanical reattachment of the abductor mechanism. Abductor dysfunction may be related to neuropathy of the central cord, lumbar plexus, or superior gluteal nerve division or dysfunction. Centrally, the abductors can be weakened by central or lateral stenosis. Abductor dysfunction also can be caused by lumbar plexopathy. For these patients there is no remedy other than addressing the spine pathology. A superior gluteal nerve injury may occur because of traction or from surgical dissection greater than 5 cm proximal to the tip of the trochanter. No remedy currently exists for this problem; some cases will resolve spontaneously. Electromyelographic investigation can be used to help determine the innervation of the abductor mechanism. MRI can provide information on abductor muscle atrophy and continuity to the greater trochanter.

───────■

Alternative Treatments

Abductor and greater trochanteric dysfunction that causes a limp may be treated nonsurgically with an abductor strengthening program. Patient compliance with such a program leads to gradual improvement in many cases. Using a cane in the opposite hand dramatically improves gait in most patients with abductor mechanism problems and often resolves the problem satisfactorily.

Hip instability related to abductor problems or trochanteric nonunion may require surgical treatment. If the abductor problems cannot be addressed or resolved, other interventions to improve hip stability should be considered, including conversion to constrained implants or use of extra-large femoral heads or bipolar or tripolar constructs.

Lateral hip pain associated with abductor or trochanteric problems often is not completely ameliorated by surgical treatment directed at the abductor mechanism or trochanter because of scarring or deficient bone and soft tissue in this sensitive area. However, pain often can be improved by removing broken or loose trochanteric cables, wires, or internal fixation devices. Injection of corticosteroids into the trochanteric bursa also helps reduce lateral hip pain in some patients.

Technique

Acute Greater Trochanter Fracture

Trochanteric fracture in the perioperative period is relatively common and may occur intraoperatively, with small portions of the abductor being avulsed during surgery. Complete fracture of the greater trochanter also can occur intraoperatively, most commonly in the varus trochanter that overhangs the femoral canal. Trochanteric fractures also may occur in the initial perioperative period because of the normal weakening of the abductor bed from femoral preparation or related to a combination of disuse osteoporosis and the pull of the abductors on a weakened proximal femur.

Exercising caution during THA in at-risk patients, particularly those with a varus greater trochanter, can prevent many problems. Care to remove the capsule laterally facilitates entering the trochanteric bed with reamers and broaches without creating undue stress on the trochanter. The varus greater trochanter is more problematic in uncemented femoral fixation because of the shape of the prosthesis, but it can be problematic with cemented fixation as well. The key to prevention of fractures is to ream or broach into the trochanteric bed without applying undue lateral pressure on the medial aspect of the trochanter, particularly in patients with osteoporotic bone.

Avulsion of the posterior greater trochanter can occur when an anterolateral approach is used (especially when testing hip stability in flexion and internal rotation) because of the pull of the piriformis. Conversely, with the posterolateral approach, these avulsions can occur on the anterior trochanter when testing hip stability in full extension and external rotation. Therefore, particularly in patients with osteoporotic bone, hip stability testing must be done gently to avoid avulsing a portion of the trochanter.

Intraoperative trochanteric fractures can be classified as a simple, minimal avulsion of part of the trochanter or a complete trochanteric fracture. If the avulsion is quite small (defined as less than 10% to 15% of the trochanter), it can simply be tacked down with sutures during closure. However, if a major portion of the trochanter is fractured, additional fixation must be used. Numerous techniques are available for fixing the trochanter. A claw system is the easiest and most popular way to fix trochanteric fractures. However, the claw works only if the trochanteric segment is large enough to be captured by the proximal tines. When the trochanteric fragment is too small to be held by the claw, other methods must be used. These include wire, wire and mesh, or other suture techniques, such as a Krackow stitch with the abductor mechanism tied into the trochanter through drill holes. Suturing techniques may be preferable in a very thin patient for whom a claw or claw plate may cause irritation and pain that may lead to a second surgical intervention.

Postoperative trochanteric fractures commonly occur in the initial postoperative period. If the trochanter is nondisplaced or minimally displaced (less than 5 to 8 mm) and the abductor mechanism is intact, nonsurgical treatment with protected ambulation and assistive devices can be used. Serial radiographs should be obtained as part of follow-up. When there is complete discontinuity of the abductor mechanism, surgical repair typically is desirable, regardless of the degree of trochanteric displacement. A fracture that is displaced more than 1 cm usually is best treated surgically because a displaced trochanter compromises abductor function because of mechanical disadvantage.

Whatever form of fixation is selected, there should be minimal stress on the abductors when the trochanter is brought down to the trochanteric bed. This usually is not a problem with intraoperative fractures, fractures identified early postoperatively, and acute fractures because the abductors have not yet retracted and scarred proximally.

After the trochanter has been fixed and abductor mechanism continuity has been restored, it is important to protect the repair. In severe cases it is useful to use an abduction orthosis. Limiting active abduction in the first 6 to 8 weeks and requiring ambulation with arm support also protects the abductors and promotes healing.

Late trochanteric fractures can occur for many reasons, including a direct blow on the trochanter in a fall, but they are more commonly associated with severe disuse osteoporosis of the trochanteric fragment or with trochanteric osteolysis. Late fractures that result from trauma but with a good reaming base should be treated in the same way as a perioperative trochanteric fracture. However, in patients with severe stress shielding or trochanteric osteolysis, where bone quality is severely compromised, additional measures are often required. Many minimally displaced greater trochanteric fractures associated with osteolysis can be treated nonsurgically until healing occurs, then the problems leading to osteolysis can be corrected surgically. In these circumstances, greater trochanteric repair or refixation should be considered only when (1) marked migration that compromises abductor function has occurred; and (2) the likelihood of successful reattachment is sufficient to justify the surgical risk. The trochanter can be fixed with wires, a claw and cables, or a claw plate (**Figure 1**). The trochanter must be repaired to a viable trochanteric bed. With significant disuse osteoporosis or trochanteric osteolysis, this often requires advancing the trochanter distally, in some cases down to the diaphyseal portion of the femoral cortex. Details on performing this procedure are described in the next section.

Late Trochanteric Escape and Trochanteric Nonunion

Patients with late trochanteric escape or trochanteric nonunion usually have proximal retraction of the greater trochanter with scarring and shortening of the abductor mechanism. Many patients are best treated nonsurgically

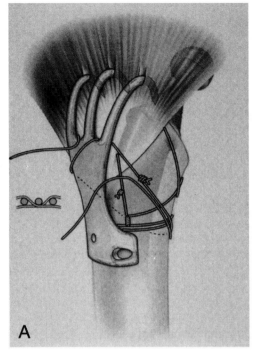 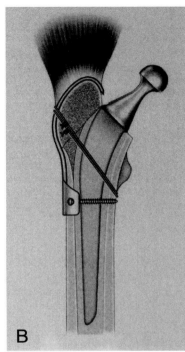

Figure 1 Fixation with the trochanteric claw plate. **A,** The double oblique cerclage wire around the trochanteric claw plate. **B,** Lateral view of the femur showing the cerclage wire and distal fixation of the plate with 4.5-mm screws. (Reproduced with permission from Hamadouche M, Zniber B, Dumaine V, Kerboull M, Courpied JP: Reattachment of the ununited greater trochanter following total hip arthroplasty. *J Bone Joint Surg Am* 2003;85:1330-1337.)

because of the unpredictable results of surgical repair. If surgical treatment is selected, in many cases it is necessary to release part of the abductors to bring the trochanteric fragment back to the trochanteric bed with minimal soft-tissue tension. This usually requires releasing the anterior portion of the abductors where it inserts on the fascia and into the wing of the ilium. In extreme cases, such as longstanding trochanteric escape, complete proximal release of the abductors to allow them to slide distally may be required (**Figure 2**).

This procedure is easiest to perform by beginning at the edge of the acetabulum, working underneath the abductors, and peeling the abductors from the ilium anteriorly to posteriorly. The abductors must be released from the crest of the ilium as well, which is done by making a counterincision along the wing of the ilium, ei-

ther from underneath the abductors on the ilium or from the superficial aspect of the abductors on the ilium. The entire abductor is released so that the trochanter can be advanced distally to be apposed to healthy bone. When the release is complete, only the neurovascular bundle (the superior gluteal artery, vein, and nerve entering posteriorly through the sciatic notch) is attached to the gluteus medius and minimus. Great care must be taken to avoid injuring the neurovascular structures exiting the sciatic notch because damaging them will result in denervation or devascularization and complete loss of abductor function.

After the abductors are partially or completely released, the trochanter is reattached to the femur on a bed of healthy bone. It is important to remove any soft tissue interposed between the greater trochanter and the

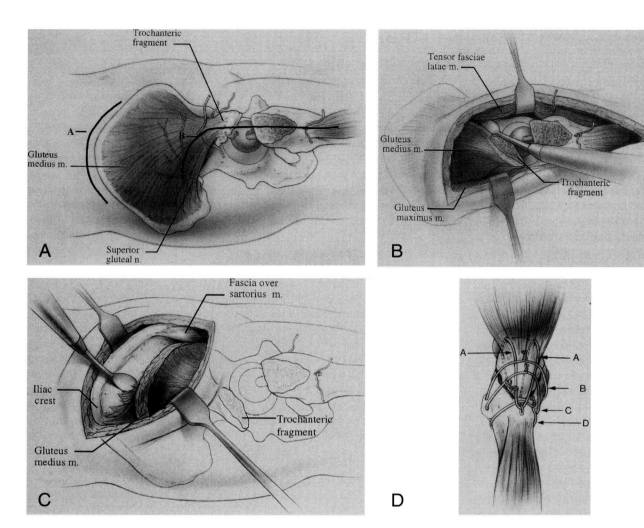

Figure 2 Surgical technique of distal advancement of the abductor muscles off the ilium for reattachment of a migrated greater trochanter fragment nonunion. **A,** The hip is approached through the original incision (B). A curvilinear incision (A) can be used to subperiosteally elevate the abductor muscles off the ilium for trochanteric advancement. **B,** All fibrous tissue and capsule around the joint and above the acetabular rim are removed. A Cobb elevator is used to elevate the abductor muscles off the ilium. The elevation remains subperiosteal to avoid the superior gluteal neurovascular structures that are commonly found within 3 to 5 cm from the top of the greater trochanter. **C,** The abductor muscles are elevated subperiosteally from the ilium until the trochanteric fragment can be advanced freely. **D,** The trochanteric bed is débrided, cancellous bone graft from the exposed ilium is applied, and the trochanteric fragment is reattached with wires (A, B, C, and D) under compression with the hip in neutral abduction. (Reproduced with permission from Chin KR, Brick GW: Reattachment of the migrated ununited greater trochanter after revision hip arthroplasty: The abductor slide technique. *J Bone Joint Surg Am* 2000;82:401-408.)

new trochanteric bed. A claw usually provides good fixation. If a complete abductor release is performed, the abductors do not need to be reapproximated proximally at their origin. Simple closure with the fascia over the abductors holds them in the correct position. An abduction orthosis should be used postoperatively to prevent adduction. The abductors

should be protected for at least 8 to 12 weeks to allow the abductors to heal to the underlying ilium proximally and the trochanter to heal distally. Abductor function generally returns in 3 to 6 months, and most patients can ambulate independently for short distances. When a complete abductor release is performed, a cosmetic indentation just distal to the iliac crest

remains where the abductors were released.

Abductor Muscle Avulsion

Avulsion of the abductor mechanism from the greater trochanter occurs most commonly as a consequence of poor muscle healing after an anterolateral approach to the hip. This problem is most common in elderly women and in patients who have preoperative abductor tears (present in up to 25% of all patients requiring THA). When this occurs, profound abductor weakness may be present with no radiographic findings. This problem is difficult to diagnose and usually is initially believed to be prolonged abductor weakness. Treatment options include nonsurgical management or abductor reattachment. When reattachment is selected, the most effective treatment is a suturing technique using heavy braided nonbioabsorbable sutures or tape to provide firm fixation of the abductors onto the greater trochanter. Many patients regain some abductor strength, although it usually does not return to normal. After abductor repair, protection with a spica cast or hip abduction orthosis is advised for 6 to 12 weeks.

Avoiding Pitfalls and Complications

One common pitfall is to encourage overly optimistic patient expectation about the results of surgery for greater trochanteric and abductor problems. Patients should be cautioned about the unpredictable results of most repeat surgeries for these problems and the low likelihood that repeat surgery will completely ameliorate lateral hip pain over the trochanter. Patients with longstanding problems with trochanteric bone deficiency, poor bone quality, and/or trochanteric retraction are less likely to achieve satisfactory results.

Inadequate fixation of the fractured or avulsed trochanter can lead to early trochanteric escape. Emphasis should be placed on using a fixation method that securely captures and holds the frequently osteoporotic trochanter while avoiding trochanteric devascularization.

In all procedures, the superior gluteal nerve and vessels must be carefully protected to maintain abductor viability and function.

Postoperatively, adequate protection of the repair, with limited weight bearing, and abductor orthosis or a spica cast can be valuable to prevent early mechanical overload of the abductor or trochanteric fixation.

Trochanteric fixation devices may cause irritation and require subsequent removal. This procedure should be performed only after the trochanter has completely healed, preferably no earlier than 9 to 12 months postoperatively.

References

Bernard AA, Brooks S: The role of trochanteric wire revision after total hip replacement. *J Bone Joint Surg Br* 1987;69:352-354.

Chen WM, McAuley JP, Engh CA Jr, Hopper RH Jr, Engh CA: Extended slide trochanteric osteotomy for revision total hip arthroplasty. *J Bone Joint Surg Am* 2000;82:1215-1219.

McCarthy JC, Bono JV, Turner RH, Kremchek T, Lee J: The outcome of trochanteric reattachment in revision total hip arthroplasty with a cable grip system: Mean 6-year follow-up. *J Arthroplasty* 1999;14:810-814.

Silverton CD, Jacobs JJ, Rosenberg AG, et al: Complications of a cable grip system. *J Arthroplasty* 1996;11:400-404.

Weber M: Berry DJ: Abductor avulsion after primary total hip arthroplasty: Results of repair. *J Arthroplasty* 1997;12:202-206.

Younger TI, Bradford MS, Magnus RE, Paprosky WG: Extended proximal femoral osteotomy: A new technique for femoral revision arthroplasty. *J Arthroplasty* 1995;10:329-338.

Coding

CPT Codes		Corresponding ICD-9 Codes	
27246	Closed treatment of greater trochanteric fracture, without manipulation	820.2	733.82
27248	Open treatment of greater trochanteric fracture, with or without internal or external fixation	820.2	733.82

Chapter 61

Hip Arthroscopy

Joseph C. McCarthy, MD

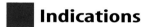

Indications

Patients who are candidates for hip arthroscopy should have functionally limiting symptoms and reproducible physical findings. Hip pain caused by an intra-articular lesion in the adult can present as pain in the anterior groin, anterior thigh, buttock, greater trochanter, or medial knee. Mechanical symptoms such as clicking, catching, locking, or giving way are also common. Restricted range of motion either from pain or a perceived mechanical block is further indication of an intra-articular etiology. Physical examination findings can include any or all of the following: (1) a positive McCarthy sign (ie, with both hips fully flexed, pain is reproduced by extending the affected hip, first in external rotation, then in internal rotation); (2) inguinal pain with flexion, adduction, and internal rotation of the hip; and (3) anterior inguinal pain with ipsilateral resisted straight leg raising. Signs and symptoms may be preceded by a traumatic event, such a fall or twisting injury, or may have an insidious onset. Pain is generally exacerbated with activity and does not respond to ice, rest, nonsteroidal anti-inflammatory drugs, and physical therapy. Nonsurgical treatment may be successful for muscle strains or other extra-articular problems; however, it does resolve an acetabular labral or chondral tear.

Labral Tears

Labral tears represent the most common cause for mechanical hip symptoms such as clicking, catching, locking, or giving way (**Figure 1**). Acetabular labral lesions occur anteriorly in most reported series, especially in patients who have sustained occult trauma or have intractable hip pain related to sports participation. Labral tears accompanied by chondral lesions also can be associated with occult trauma. The inciting event is often a pivoting maneuver during an athletic activity such as tennis, karate, hockey, football, or soccer. Patients who sustain minor trauma without dislocation almost invariably have anterior tears accompanied by mechanical symptoms and intractable pain. Labral tears secondary to trauma are generally isolated to one region, depending on the direction and extent of trauma.

Intractable hip pain is evaluated with plain radiographs, arthrography, bone scintigraphy, CT, and MRI, but these studies often have little diagnostic yield. Plain radiographs may demonstrate calcified loose bodies or osteoarthritis but overall have very poor diagnostic yield for intra-articular pathology, including the cartilage changes associated with early stages of osteoarthritis. The addition of contrast in conjunction with CT and MRI increases the diagnostic yield of intra-articular hip pathology, principally in

detecting labral lesions. Specialized imaging studies, including high-contrast or gadolinium-enhanced MR arthrography, have improved the diagnostic sensitivity for labral injuries (**Figure 2**).

Arthrography may somewhat increase the diagnostic yield. In a study correlating radiographic findings with hip arthroscopy findings, my colleagues and I reported that the most commonly overlooked cause of pain was acetabular labral lesions. Acetabular labral tears detected arthroscopically correlated significantly with anterior inguinal pain (r = 1, P = 0.00), painful clicking episodes (r = 0.809, P = 0.00), transient locking (r = 0.370, P = 0.00), or giving way (r = 0.320, P = 0.0024), and with the physical findings of a positive hip extension sign (r = 0.676, P = 0.00). In another series, hip arthrography was

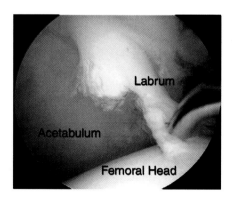

Figure 1 An anterior acetabular labral tear.

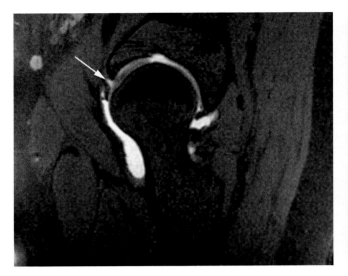

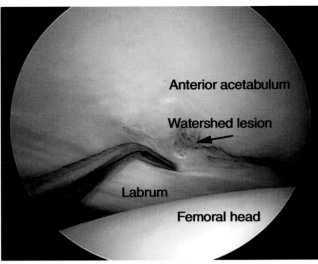

Figure 2 A gadolinium-enhanced MR arthrogram demonstrating a labral tear (arrow).

Figure 3 A watershed lesion (arrow) is seen at the labrochondral junction in the anterior portion of the acetabulum.

positive in 44 of 50 patients with a suspected acetabular labral tear. However, only 12 of 55 patients underwent hip arthroscopy with no mention of arthrographic correlation to intraoperative findings.

Labral tears can be classified according to location, morphology, and associated articular changes. With respect to location, tears can be anterior, posterior, or superior (lateral). Hypertrophy of the anterior labrum associated with impingement on the anterior acetabulum is common in dysplasia and results in the classic mechanical symptoms. Tears associated with mild dysplasia typically occur anteriorly but also can be more diffuse with higher degrees of dysplasia or more advanced osteoarthritis. In a report of 436 patients who underwent hip arthroscopy, 250 (54.8%) had labral tears at the articular margin of the labrum. Almost all labral lesions (234) (93.6%) were located in the anterior quadrant of the acetabulum. Posterior labral pathology was more commonly associated with a discrete episode of hip trauma, typically involving impact loading of the extremity. A total of 73% of patients with labral tears had associated acetabular chondral le-

sions, and 94% of those were in the same region as the labral tear. The results of this study suggest that disruption of the labrum along the articular margin may contribute to delamination of the articular cartilage adjacent to the labral lesion, causing more global labral and articular cartilage degeneration.

Chondral Lesions

Acetabular chondral lesions may occur in association with loose bodies, posterior dislocation, osteonecrosis, slipped capital femoral epiphysis, dysplasia, and osteoarthritis; however, these lesions are often also seen in association with labral tears. Because these injuries are most frequently associated with labral tears, they are usually located in the anterior acetabulum. The severity of the chondral lesion can be graded according to Outerbridge criteria and is highly correlated with surgical outcome. In one series, Outerbridge grade III or IV lesions were more common in patients with labral tears or fraying than in patients with a normal labrum ($P = 0.0144$). The severity of chondral lesions increased from

46% to 75% ($P = 0.0021$) when fraying of the labrum was present.

The most common chondral lesion is the "watershed" lesion in which the torn labrum is separated from the articular surface at the labrocartilage junction (**Figure 3**). Watershed lesions are often associated with an acetabular cyst resulting from pressure of the joint fluid beneath an area of delaminated cartilage with repetitive loading. These anterior cysts may be visualized on plain radiographs in the absence of joint space narrowing or other degenerative changes. Acetabular cysts associated with labral tears and chondral injuries are the result of, not the cause of, mechanical symptoms.

Loose Bodies

Calcified loose bodies are typically readily identified on radiographs, but CT or MRI, with or without contrast, can be more sensitive. Mechanical symptoms such as locking or catching can corroborate clinical suspicion. Arthroscopy establishes the diagnosis and provides simultaneous treatment using a minimally invasive technique. Isolated or multiple (2 to 300) fragments, as seen in synovial chondromatosis, are possible.

Synovial Conditions

Treatment of synovial chondromatosis consists of arthroscopic removal of loose bodies (between 5 and 300). They often require morcellization, especially those clustered within the fovea. Articular damage can be addressed and synovectomy performed at the same time. Although recurrence has been reported in up to 14% of patients, a second arthroscopy may be beneficial in the absence of advanced chondral destruction.

Arthroscopic débridement of the synovium can be useful in the management of inflammatory conditions such as pigmented villonodular synovitis without a prolonged rehabilitation period. Rheumatoid arthritis accompanied by intense joint pain that has been unresponsive to prolonged nonsurgical treatment may benefit from arthroscopic intervention with lavage, synovial biopsy and/or partial synovectomy, and treatment of intra-articular cartilage lesions. Surgical outcomes depend on the stage of articular cartilage involvement.

Crystalline diseases such as gout or pseudogout can produce extreme hip joint pain that is often undetected unless it coexists with a labral or chondral injury. Arthroscopic treatment consists of copious lavage and mechanical removal of crystals that are diffusely distributed throughout the synovium and embedded within the articular cartilage. Concurrent synovial biopsy can be helpful for medical management.

Patients with Ehler-Danlos syndrome may have associated hip pain and instability. In combination with medical diagnosis, arthroscopic treatment consists of skin and synovial biopsy to further define disease classification. Thermal capsular shrinkage also has been used judiciously with favorable short-term results.

Following Total Hip Arthroplasty

A patient with a painful total hip arthroplasty (THA) usually can be diagnosed clinically (eg, limb-length discrepancy, abductor weakness), radiographically (eg, component loosening, malposition, trochanteric nonunion), or by special studies (eg, bone scintigraphy, aspiration arthrography for subtle loosening or sepsis). However, arthroscopy may be warranted to establish a diagnosis in a patient with a negative work-up or a history of failed surgical treatment. In addition, intra-articular third bodies such as broken wires or loose screws can be removed arthroscopically, and dense scar tissue tethering the hip flexors can be resected.

Following Trauma

Even minor trauma involving the hip joint can result in hematoma, chondral loose bodies, and labral tears. Foreign bodies, such as bullet fragments that produce intra-articular symptoms, can be removed arthroscopically. Dislocations and fracture-dislocations can result in loose bodies, labral injuries, or shear damage to the chondral surfaces of the femoral head or acetabulum that are not often visualized on MRI. Pipkin fractures can result in displaced bone or cartilage from the femoral head or a ruptured ligamentum teres. The articular lesions resulting from these injuries can be addressed arthroscopically.

Contraindications

Joint conditions amenable to medical management, such as arthralgias associated with hepatitis or colitis or hip pain referred from other sources such as a compression fracture of L1, should be ruled out prior to surgery. Periarticular conditions such as stress fractures of the femoral neck, insuffi-

ciency fractures of the pubis or ischium, and transient osteoporosis are also best treated by nonendoscopic means.

Osteonecrosis and synovitis in the absence of mechanical symptoms do not warrant arthroscopy. Acute skin lesions or ulceration, especially in the vicinity of portal placement, would exclude arthroscopy. Sepsis with accompanying osteomyelitis or abscess formation requires open surgery. Certain conditions that limit the potential for hip distraction such as ankylosis, dense heterotopic bone formation, or significant protrusio also dissuade arthroscopy.

Morbid obesity also is a relative contraindication for arthroscopy not only because of distraction limitations but also because of the requisite length of instruments necessary to access and maneuver within the deeply recessed joint. In my opinion, advanced osteoarthritis is also a contraindication for arthroscopy.

Alternative Treatments

Patients with moderate dysplasia who present with pain and instability and a center-edge angle of Wiberg of less than 16° should be evaluated for a periacetabular osteotomy.

Developmental or acquired abnormalities of the acetabulum and proximal femur can result in a decreased anterior offset of the femoral head. These so-called "pistol grip" deformities, best seen on a true lateral radiograph, may result in an impingement of the femoral neck against the anterior acetabulum in hyperextension and lateral rotation (CAM effect). Similarly, a retroverted acetabulum may also result in contact stresses to the anterior articular structures. More research is needed to determine the benefits of removing bone from the

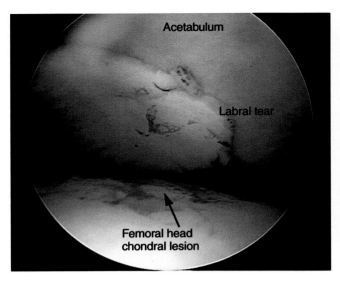

Figure 4 A stage 2 labral tear with a lesion of the adjacent femoral head (arrow).

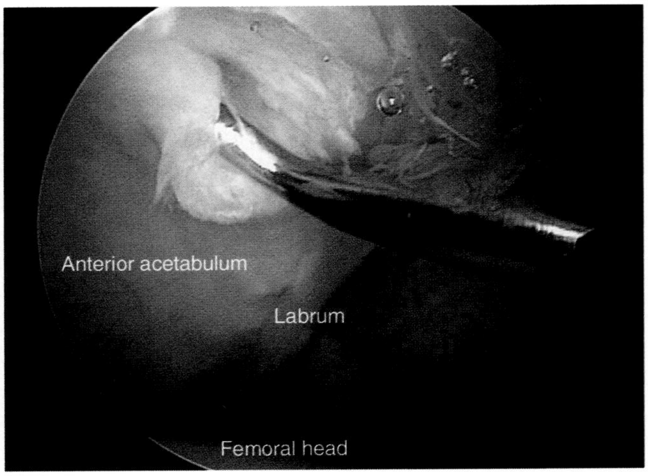

Figure 5 A stage 3B labral tear and associated chondral flap.

anterior femoral head-neck junction to correct impingement that may damage the labrum and adjacent acetabular cartilage.

Results

My colleagues and I presented a four-stage classification system correlated with outcome in a report on 62 patients with labral tears (**Table 1**). Stage 0 is characterized by a contusion of the labrum with adjacent synovitis (1 patient). Stage 1 is a discrete, labral-free margin tear with intact femoral and acetabular articular cartilage. Of the patients (10 hips) with a stage 1 tear, all but one patient had a good to excellent result (91%). This single patient required an iliopsoas release with V-Y lengthening of the iliotibial band 9 months after arthroscopy for recurrent painful snapping hip.

Stage 2 is a labral tear with focal articular damage to the subjacent femoral head but with intact acetabular articular cartilage (**Figure 4**). In 9 of the 11 hips (82%) with this type of tear, good to excellent outcomes re-

sulted when the tear was resected. Two patients (18%) required further surgical intervention secondary to recurrent symptoms and eventually underwent open synovectomy, capsulectomy, and release of the reflected rectus femoris tendon.

Stage 3 involves a labral tear with an adjacent focal acetabular articular cartilage lesion, with or without femoral head articular cartilage chondromalacia. These tears are classified into two subgroups, depending on the size of the acetabular cartilage defect. Stage 3A lesions involve less than 1 cm of acetabular articular cartilage, and stage 3B lesions (**Figure 5**) involve more than 1 cm of acetabular cartilage. Patients with stage 3 labral tears did not fair nearly as well as those with the previous two types, with the extent of the acetabular cartilage erosion directly impacting the result. Stage 3A labral tears (21 hips) were associated with a good to excellent result in 15 patients (71%). Two patients underwent open synovectomy, anterior capsulectomy, and rectus femoris release. Within the stage 3B group (10 hips), results were good to excellent in four hips (40%), fair in three hips (30%), and poor in two hips (22%). Two pa-

tients required additional surgical intervention.

Stage 4 tears involve diffuse acetabular labral damage and associated diffuse chondral articular cartilage changes in the joint (9 hips). At a minimum of 2 years following hip arthroscopy, outcomes were directly correlated with the stage of labral injury. Outcomes for patients with stage 4 labral tears directly correlated with the extent of hip joint osteoarthritis. If articular cartilage involvement was diffuse on the femoral head and acetabulum, regardless of the appearance on plain radiographs, the symptomatic improvement following arthroscopy was transient. Seven of the nine patients (78%) had a poor result at follow-up, and of these three (43%) required THA within 2 years of arthroscopy.

The above findings are similar to results reported by Farjo and associates in which 10 of 14 patients had good results in the absence of osteoarthritis, whereas only 3 of 14 had a good result in the presence of osteoarthritis. Byrd and Jones also reported a significant improvement in a modified Harris hip score for patients with labral tears or loose bodies but only a

14-point improvement in the presence of osteoarthritis.

■ Technique

Hip arthroscopy allows a comprehensive evaluation of labral and chondral anatomy in all quadrants of the joint, but more importantly it provides a means for treating myriad intra-articular lesions, including labral tears and chondral lesions. The procedure is performed on an outpatient basis under general or regional anesthesia.

Patient Positioning

Proper positioning and portal placement are critical to patient safety and surgical outcome. Positioning of the patient, in either a supine or lateral decubitus position with distraction, is a matter of surgeon preference; however, the femoral head must be distracted from the acetabulum between 7 and 10 mm to allow a complete view of the articular surfaces (**Figure 6**). The actual force required to distract the femoral head from the acetabulum varies considerably by individual and has been reported to range from 25 to 200 lb (approximately 112 to 900 N). In most patients the procedure can be performed with 50 lb (225 N) or less of distraction force. Most importantly, the duration of distraction should be limited to less than 2 hours.

The lateral decubitus position, as popularized by Glick, is my preferred position for hip arthroscopy because it provides access to the hip joint via paratrochanteric portals, which allows visualization and instrumentation of the anterior aspect of the joint where intra-articular pathology is most prevalent.

Portal Placement

Accurate portal placement is essential for optimal visualization and operative success. The greater trochanter

Table 1   Results of Hip Arthroscopy for Labral Tears

Author(s) (Year)	Number of Patients	Mean Follow-up	Complications	Results
McCarthy, et al (2003)	62	24 months	1 transient lateral femoral cutaneous nerve palsy	91% excellent result for labral tear without chondral injury
Byrd and Jones (2000)	38	24 months	1 neurapraxia of lateral femoral cutaneous nerve 1 focal myositis (same patient)	Modified Harris hip score improved by 31 points if no chondral damage
Fitzgerald (1995)	64	53 months	1 meralgia paresthetica	89% improved (16 of 64 had chondral cartilage damage)
Farjo, et al (1999)	28	34 months	2 sciatic and 1 pudendal transient nerve palsies	71% good result if no osteoarthritis on radiograph
Santori and Villar(2000)	58	42 months	NR	67% improved (28 of 58 had chondral damage)

NR = Not reported

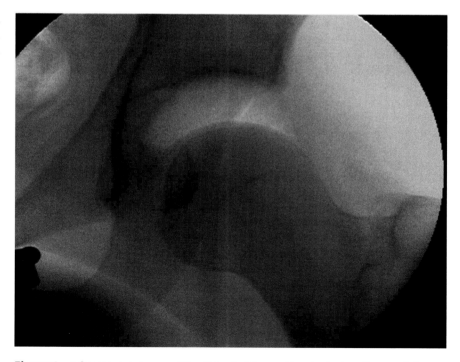

Figure 6   A fluoroscopic image of the distracted femoral head prior to arthroscopic instrumentation.

serves as the reference for each of the paratrochanteric portals. The anterior paratrochanteric portal is placed 2 cm anterior and 1 cm proximal to the anterosuperior "corner" of the greater trochanter.

In the same manner as described for the anterior portal, the joint is entered with the trocar at about the intertrochanteric line. The capsule is relatively thin at its insertion on the anterior femoral neck. However, because of the relative obliquity of the trocar to the joint capsule and the anteversion of the femoral neck, an arthroscope that is directed too anteriorly and inserted too deeply risks injury to the femoral neurovascular bundle. This portal allows visualization of the femoral head, the anterior neck, and the anterior intrinsic capsular folds. The synovial tissues beneath the zona orbicularis and the anterior labrum are easily seen and lesions addressed from this portal as well.

The posterior paratrochanteric portal corresponds directly with the anterior paratrochanteric portal. The entry site is 2 cm posterior to the tip of the greater trochanter at the level of the anterior paratrochanteric portal. The trocar is advanced with the femur in a neutral or slightly internally rotated position because the external rotation of the hip places the posterior margin of the greater trochanter precariously close to the sciatic nerve. Despite the potential hazard with this portal, it affords an excellent view of the posterior aspect of the femoral head, the posterior labrum, posterior capsule, the ligament of Weitbrecht, and the inferior edge of the ischiofemoral ligament.

Arthroscopic treatment of labral tears involves judicious débridement back to a stable base and to healthy-appearing tissue while preserving the capsular labral tissue. The labrum is an important anatomic structure; therefore, overresection should be avoided. If there are associated full-thickness chondral defects, the subchondral bone is drilled or treated with a microfracture technique to enhance fibrocartilage formation.

Postoperative Regimen

Hip arthroscopy is done as an outpatient procedure. Patients can bear weight as tolerated and usually require crutches for 3 to 5 days. Formal physical therapy is not encouraged for the first 6 weeks while joint effusion is present. Patients may walk, swim, or ride a stationary bike as comfort allows during the first 6 weeks. Physical therapy protocols for high-demand patients such as competitive athletes begin early with water and flexibility exercises. Cutting and pivoting can be initiated as soon as the postoperative effusion has dissipated, followed by more sport-specific activities.

Avoiding Pitfalls and Complications

When a patient presents with a symptomatic loose body or labral tear, the surgeon must choose between open arthrotomy and arthroscopy. In most cases, I believe arthroscopy can be performed with a lower complication risk than an arthrotomy. Nevertheless, arthroscopy has its own potential risks. Hip arthroscopy is subject to the joint's unique anatomic constraints, attendant technical considerations, and permanent or transient complications. Although described in the literature, I have not seen complications such as sciatic or femoral palsy, osteonecrosis, compartment syndrome, broken instruments, pulmonary embolus, or death in my patients. Fewer than 2% of patients have experienced transient peroneal or pudendal nerve effects. Two patients with meralgia parasthetica reported resolution within 2 weeks. Mild chondral scuffing occurred in only 1% of patients. All of the above complications have been associated with difficult or protracted distraction.

Avoiding complications involves achieving sufficient distraction (7 to 10 mm), using dedicated hip instruments, and exercising precise surgical skill. Judicious patient selection is essential; only those patients with mechanical symptoms that persist despite nonsurgical treatment and positive findings on physical examination should be considered.

Hip arthroscopy involves a steep learning curve. Visiting high-volume centers, attending instructional courses, and practicing in bioskills laboratories contribute to technical proficiency. Meticulous attention to positioning, distraction time, and portal placement are essential. Complication rates between 0.5% and 5% are reported in the literature, most often related to distraction. Improvements in technique and instrumentation have made hip arthroscopy an efficacious way to diagnose and treat a variety of intra-articular problems.

Acknowledgment

The author would like to thank Jo-Ann Lee, MS, for her assistance in preparation of the manuscript

---

References

Byrd JW, Jones KS: Prospective analysis of hip arthroscopy with 2-year follow-up. *Arthroscopy* 2000;16:578-587.

Farjo LA, Glick JM, Sampson TG: Hip arthroscopy for acetabular labral tears. *Arthroscopy* 1999;15:132-137.

Fitzgerald RH Jr: Acetabular labrum tears: Diagnosis and treatment. *Clin Orthop* 1995;311:60-68.

Glick JM, Sampson TG, Gordon RB, Behr JT, Schmidt E: Hip arthroscopy by the lateral approach. *Arthroscopy* 1987;3:4-12.

McCarthy J, Noble P, Aluisio FV, et al: Anatomy, pathologic features, and treatment of acetabular labral tears. *Clin Orthop* 2003;406:38-47.

McCarthy JC, Noble PC, Schuck MR, Wright J, Lee J: The role of labral lesions to development of early degenerative hip disease. *Clin Orthop* 2001;393:25-37.

Newberg AH, Newman JS: Imaging the painful hip. *Clin Orthop* 2003;406:19-28.

Santori N, Villar RN: Acetabular labral tears: Result of arthroscopic partial limbectomy. *Arthroscopy* 2000;16:11-15.

Coding

CPT Codes		Corresponding ICD-9 Codes		
29860	Arthroscopy, hip, diagnostic, with or without synovial biopsy (separate procedure)	711.15 716.15	711.45 732.1	711.95 732.7
29861	Arthroscopy, hip, surgical; with removal of loose body or foreign body	716.15	732.1	732.7
29862	Arthroscopy, hip, surgical; with débridement/shaving of articular cartilage (chondroplasty), abrasion arthroplasty, and/or resection of labrum	716.15	732.1	732.7
29863	Arthroscopy, hip, surgical; with synovectomy	716.15	732.1	732.7

CPT copyright © 2004 by the American Medical Association. All Rights Reserved.

Coding for arthroscopic hip surgery needs to evolve as the number and complexity of conditions treated arthroscopically evolves. Presently coding is limited to diagnostic arthroscopy with or without synovial biopsy, operative arthroscopy with synovectomy, operative arthroscopy with removal of loose or foreign body, and operative arthroscopy with débridement of cartilage, chondroplasty, and/or labral resection. Medicare and some other third-party payors currently do not allow billing of an arthroscopic procedure performed in conjunction with an open procedure.

Chapter 62

Developmental Dysplasia of the Hip: Pelvic Osteotomies

Robert T. Trousdale, MD

Indications

Osteotomies about the hip should be limited to young patients who have symptomatic hip dysplasia without excessive proximal migration of the center of rotation, a reasonably well-preserved range of motion, and no more than mild to moderate secondary degenerative changes of the articular surface. Prognosis is poor for patients with severe secondary osteoarthritic changes of the dysplastic hip. In most patients with hip dysplasia, the primary anomaly is located on the acetabular side of the joint, and pelvic osteotomy thus permits correction of this abnormality. Femoral os-

teotomy should be added to the pelvic procedure when marked, concurrent femoral anatomic abnormalities are present. Femoral osteotomy is rarely indicated as an isolated procedure in the treatment of the dysplastic hip.

Dysplastic hips share a spectrum of anatomic anomalies, present to a greater or lesser extent depending on the severity of the dysplasia. On the pelvic side, the true acetabulum is shallow, the hip center is usually lateralized, the hip socket typically has excessive anteversion, and the deficiency is most typically located anteriorly and superiorly (**Figure 1**). Occasionally (approximately 18% to 40% of the time) the socket is retroverted

and the head is poorly covered posteriorly (**Figure 2**). On the femoral side, the head usually is small, the neck has excessive acetabular anteversion and may be short, the neck-shaft angle is increased, and the greater trochanter is displaced proximally. Retrotorsion problems of the acetabulum and/or femur can lead to anterior impingement problems in flexion. Most of these conditions lead to a decrease in hip contact area. Lateralization of the hip center increases the body-weight lever arm, resulting in transmittal of high forces across the limited surface area. These increased contact pressures may eventually lead to articular cartilage changes. The probability of sec-

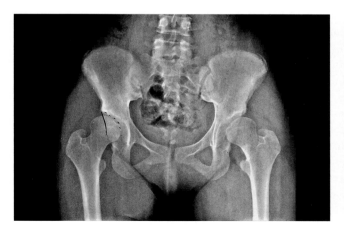

Figure 1   AP pelvic radiograph of patient with classic dysplastic hip. The acetabulum is shallow, and the hip center is lateralized with anterior and superior deficiency. Note the excessive acetabular anteversion with the anterior wall (dotted line) covering much less of the femoral head than the posterior wall (solid line).

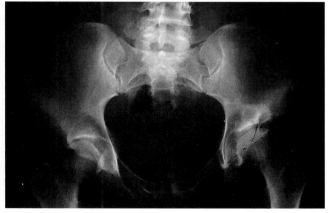

Figure 2   AP pelvic radiograph of dysplastic left hip with a retroverted acetabulum. Note that the posterior wall (solid line) crosses over the anterior wall (dotted line) prior to meeting the lateral edge of the sourcil.

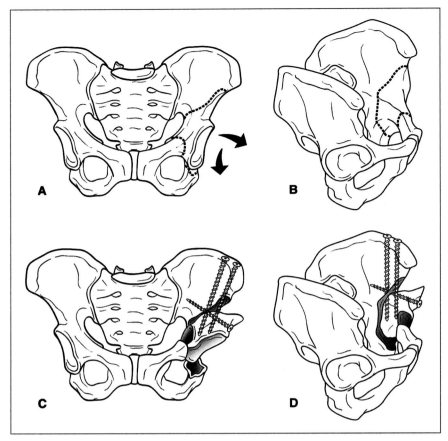

Figure 3 Diagrams demonstrating locations of osteotomies before (**A** and **B**) and after (**C** and **D**) correction and three-screw fixation. (Figures 3 A and B are adapted with permission from the Mayo Foundation, Rochester, MN.)

ticular cartilage from further degenerative change.

Contraindications

Contraindications to reorientation osteotomy include severe arthritis, marked out-of-round femoral head or acetabulum, severe obesity, or patient age older than 50 to 60 years.

Alternative Treatments

Patients with dysplasia who are asymptomatic or have minimal symptoms probably should be treated nonsurgically. The natural history of the dysplasia should be discussed with the patient, and radiographs obtained every few years to monitor the development of osteoarthritis. Treatment with nonsteroidal anti-inflammatory agents and avoiding high-impact activities are reasonable initial recommendations. Surgical intervention should be reserved for patients with persistent symptoms that limit daily activities in combination with substantial structural abnormalities of the joint. Surgical options include arthroscopy, arthrodesis, resection arthroplasty, osteotomy, and total hip arthroplasty (THA). Pelvic realignment osteotomy is the procedure of choice for most symptomatic young patients with dysplasia. THA should be reserved for patients with marked articular cartilage loss. Arthroscopy may be considered for mildly dysplastic hips with major mechanical symptoms related to either loose bodies or labral tears, but little data have been published on the long-term outcomes of this procedure in this patient subgroup.

Before arthroscopy is recommended to patients with hip symp-

ondary osteoarthritis of the hip developing is in part determined by the severity of the dysplasia.

Patients with hip dysplasia typically have activity-related groin pain that is in part secondary to subluxation of the femoral head and can be reproduced with forced hyperextension and external rotation of the hip. Catching, locking, or giving way may be indications of associated labral and/or chondral pathology. Patients with excessive retroversion of the acetabulum will commonly have groin pain secondary to impingement. This is usually reproduced with flexion internal rotation of the hip. Plain radiographs, including AP and lateral views as well as a false profile view, are the first steps in the imaging evaluation. MRI, with or without gadolinium enhancement, and CT are not routinely necessary but may be helpful in evaluating hip pain in the absence of associated marked structural anomalies. MRI and CT scans permit further evaluation of suspected intra-articular pathology such as labral tears, loose bodies, chondral defects, or synovial disease.

In symptomatic patients with hip dysplasia, increased joint congruity after reorientation of the osteotomized fragment permits more normal load transmission through a broader surface area subjected to less pressure. Some pelvic osteotomies also medialize the hip center of rotation, thus lessening joint reactive forces. These changes can reduce pain, improve function, and possibly protect the ar-

Table 1 Results of the Bernese Periacetabular Osteotomy in Dysplastic Hips

				Results			
Author(s) (Year)	Number of Osteotomies (Patients)	Mean Patient Age (Range)	Mean Follow-up (Range)	Number (%) of Combined/ Subsequent Osteotomies	Number (%) of Conversions to THA (Patients)	Clinical Results	Major Complications*
Siebenrock, et al (1999)	71 (60)	29.3 years (13–56)	11.3 years (10.0–13.8)	16/5 (23/7)	12[†] (17)	73% Good to excellent	13
Trousdale, et al (1995)	42 (42)	37 years (11–56)	4 years (2–8)	10/3 (24/7)	6 (14)	Harris hip score 62 to 86	3
Crockarell, et al (1999)	21 (19)	21 years (17–43)	3.2 years (2.0–4.3)	4/1 (20/5)	1 (5)	Harris hip score 62 to 86	9
Matta, et al (1999)	66 (58)	33.6 years (19–51)	4 years (2–10)	10/0 (15)	5[‡] (8)	77% Good to excellent	16
Trumble, et al (1999)	123 (115)	32.9 years (14–54)	4.3 years (2–10)	33/6[§] (27/5)	7 (6)	83% Good to excellent	8

*Includes neurovascular injury, intra-articular osteotomies, loss of correction, resubluxation, nonunion, infection or symptomatic heterotopic ossification
[†]Second osteotomies in 6 patients and fusion in 1 patient
[‡]Three more patients awaiting hip reconstruction
[§]Femoral osteotomy or trochanteric advancement

toms, marked structural anomalies such as retrotorsion of the acetabulum and femoral offset problems should be ruled out. Both may be subtle but can be detected on proper radiographic evaluation. Arthroscopy is unlikely to provide long-term relief in the presence of these structural abnormalities.

Arthrodesis and resection arthroplasty should be reserved for the rare dysplastic patient who is not a candidate for osteotomy or THA.

───■

Pelvic Osteotomies

Many types of pelvic osteotomies have been described for the treatment of hip dysplasia. Reconstructive osteotomy is intended to restore more normal hip anatomy and biomechanics, improve symptoms, and perhaps prevent secondary osteoarthritis. Salvage osteotomy is performed to relieve pain when articular surface congruity cannot be restored because of marked anatomic anomaly.

The Bernese periacetabular osteotomy, developed by Ganz and associates, is the reconstructive pelvic osteotomy currently preferred by many surgeons (**Figure 3**). This osteotomy is indicated for patients with hip symptoms including mechanical overload, impingement (secondary to retroverted acetabula), or instability resulting from improper acetabular coverage. It requires only one incision with a series of straight, relatively reproducible extra-articular cuts. It permits large corrections of the osteotomized fragment in all directions, including lateral rotation, anterior rotation, medialization of the hip joint, correction of version abnormalities, and medialization of the hip center of rotation. The posterior column of the pelvis is left intact so minimal internal fixation is required. Early ambulation with no external immobilization is possible. The vascularity of the acetabular fragment is preserved, and the joint can be opened and examined without further risk of devascularizing the osteotomized fragment. The shape of the true pelvis is not markedly altered, thus permitting the potential for normal vaginal delivery. This procedure can also be performed without violation of the abductor mechanism, which facilitates rehabilitation and recovery.

───■

Results

Preliminary surgical outcomes for pelvic osteotomy were first reported by Ganz and associates and others in a mixed group of 63 patients (75 hips), with and without secondary degenerative changes. Results described marked improvements in pain and ex-

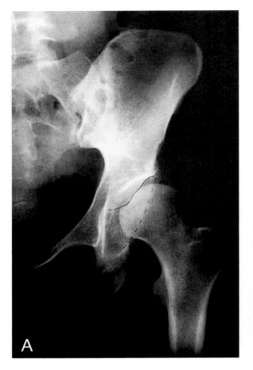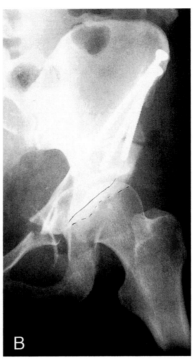

Figure 4   Preoperative (**A**) and postoperative (**B**) AP radiographs of a patient with symptomatic classic hip dysplasia. Note in the postoperative radiograph that the contact area has markedly improved and the hip center has been medialized.

cellent femoral head coverage in both coronal and sagittal planes. Intermediate follow-up data are now becoming available (**Table 1**).

Most reports note a marked reduction in patient symptoms and improvement in coverage of the femoral head. Several factors are associated with less favorable outcomes, including patient age at the time of the procedure, moderate to severe preoperative hip arthritis, associated labral lesions, and poor correction of the acetabular fragment. The status of the articular cartilage prior to osteotomy is of paramount importance.

The Bernese periacetabular osteotomy is a successful operation in terms of pain relief in patients with moderate degenerative changes of the hip but is less satisfactory in patients with more advanced degeneration. The most difficult part of this procedure is determining the amount of correction needed for each patient; sub-

optimal correction is directly related to poor results. Previous surgery does not preclude a satisfactory outcome. Periacetabular osteotomy may alter the natural history of hip dysplasia, but longer follow-up studies are necessary to assess its effectiveness in preventing degenerative changes.

Technique

Exposure

Osteotomy techniques are described extensively in the literature and continue to evolve. Most surgeons use an approach that spares the abductor muscles, usually through the inner aspect of the pelvis, and include partial osteotomy of the ischium, complete osteotomy of the pubic bone, and biplane osteotomy of the ilium, maintaining the continuity of the posterior column.

Bone Preparation

Once the osteotomies are completed, the periacetabular fragment is mobilized. The most challenging aspect of this procedure is ensuring proper correction. The periacetabular segment is typically displaced medially, rotated anteriorly and laterally (maintaining proper anteversion), and provisionally fixed with two smooth pins. A true AP radiograph of the pelvis is obtained intraoperatively to assess correction, which is considered to be satisfactory when the acetabular roof is horizontal, the femoral head is congruous, the anterior rim covers less of the femoral head than the posterior rim, the rims meet at the lateral edge of the sourcil, ensuring proper acetabular anteversion, the femoral head is medialized within 5 to 15 mm of the ilioischial line, and Shenton's line is near normal (**Figures 4** and **5**).

The acetabular fragment is then fixed with three long, fully threaded cortical screws. Some institutions are beginning to use computer assistance to facilitate the osteotomies and maximize the correction. I routinely open the joint to evaluate for labral or chondral pathology and check for femoral acetabular impingement between the anterior femoral neck and the anterior acetabulum. Torn labral fragments are excised or repaired, depending on the status of the labrum. The prominent anteroinferior iliac spine is trimmed and inserted as bone graft in the gap created anteriorly by the transverse iliac osteotomy before repairing the sartorius and rectus femoral muscle origins that were removed during exposure.

Wound Closure

The deep fascia is closed with interrupted sutures and skin closure is routine. A deep drain is used for 24 hours.

Postoperative Regimen

Postoperative epidural anesthesia is used for pain control for 48 hours. The

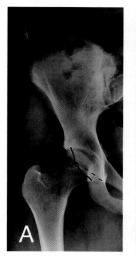
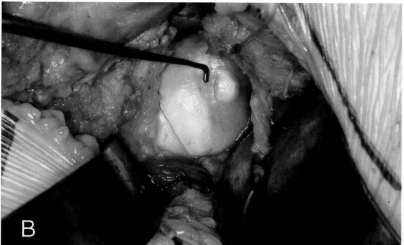
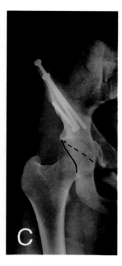

Figure 5 **A,** Preoperative AP radiograph of a young patient with severe right groin pain reproduced with flexion and internal rotation and a retroverted acetabulum. Note that the posterior wall (solid line) crosses the anterior wall (dotted line) prior to meeting the sourcil. **B,** Intraoperative photograph showing a ridge in the femoral head-neck junction where impingement occurs on the acetabular rim. **C,** Postoperative AP radiograph after a "reverse" periacetabular osteotomy that corrected acetabular anteversion. Note that the posterior wall (solid line) covers more of the femoral head than the anterior wall (dotted line), and both meet at the lateral edge of the sourcil.

patient is mobilized the day after surgery, and partial weight bearing begins and is maintained for the first 4 to 6 weeks postoperatively. Thereafter, weight bearing as tolerated, abduction exercises, water exercises, and stationary bike activities are encouraged. Union of the iliac osteotomy is usually complete by 6 to 8 weeks postoperatively. Most patients do not use ambulatory aids and can begin resuming activities as tolerated by the third month after surgery.

Avoiding Pitfalls and Complications

Pelvic osteotomies are complex procedures. The surgeon's overall experience and expertise are important factors affecting the incidence of complications. The learning curve is long, and the potential complication rate is high. Training with surgeons who routinely perform this procedure and practice in the anatomy laboratory are recommended.

Nerve dysfunction is a potential complication. The lateral femoral cutaneous nerve or some of its branches are frequently injured during the anterior approach to the hip joint. As many as 75% of patients note paresthesias in the lateral aspect of the thigh, but most of these do not require treatment. Femoral nerve palsies have been reported with the less commonly used direct anterior approach or in patients who have had previous surgeries. This procedure can be performed with intraoperative electromyographic monitoring. In one series, transient sciatic nerve palsy developed in five patients. Most vascular complications during this operation have been related to the ilioinguinal approach; in the same series, femoral or iliac artery thrombosis developed in seven patients, resulting in one limb loss.

Inadvertent extension of the osteotomy can occur. Intra-articular extension of the ischial osteotomy has been reported to occur, especially in hips with marked proximal femoral head migration and a lax inferior capsule. Such extension does not cause articular incongruity, but it can interrupt the blood supply to the acetabu-lum and contribute to necrosis of the osteotomized fragment. Intra-articular extension of the vertical limb of the iliac osteotomy can create an incongruent joint after correction, leading to secondary arthritis. The iliac osteotomy also can be extended accidentally through the posterior column into the sciatic notch, thus destabilizing the pelvic ring.

Nonunion of the pubic or (less commonly) ischial osteotomy may result from large interfragmentary gaps, suboptimal position, or iliopsoas tendon interposition. Most pubic nonunions are asymptomatic radiologic findings. Bone grafting and plate fixation rarely are required for iliac or ischial nonunions. Heterotopic ossification has been almost eradicated by using modified anterior approaches that leave the adductors inviolate. If heterotopic ossification does occur, it is usually asymptomatic. Bone excision can be attempted in patients with limited motion. Overcorrection of the osteotomized fragment can lead to anterior or lateral impingement symptoms or posterior subluxation of the femoral head.

Femoral head subluxation can also result from neglected associated marked femoral deformity. Anterior femoral acetabular impingement can be a sign of excessive anterior correction or retroversion of the acetabular fragment, but it can also be a complication for patients with appropriate correction. If this problem is recognized during surgery, the fragment can be repositioned or the anterior femoral neck just inferior to the femoral head articular surface can be trimmed.

————■

■ References

Crockarell J Jr, Trousdale RT, Cabanela ME, Berry DJ: Early experience and results with the periacetabular osteotomy: The Mayo Clinic experience. *Clin Orthop* 1999;363:45-53.

Ganz R, Klaue K, Vinh TS, Mast JW: A new periacetabular osteotomy for the treatment of hip dysplasias: Technique and preliminary results. *Clin Orthop* 1988;232:26-36.

Hussell JG, Mast JW, Mayo KA, Howie DW, Ganz R: A comparison of different surgical approaches for the periacetabular osteotomy. *Clin Orthop* 1999;363:64-72.

Hussell JG, Rodriguez JA, Ganz R: Technical complications of the Bernese periacetabular osteotomy. *Clin Orthop* 1999;363:81-92.

Matta JM, Stover MD, Siebenrock K: Periacetabular osteotomy through the Smith-Petersen approach. *Clin Orthop* 1999;363:21-32.

Murphy SB, Ganz R, Muller ME: The prognosis in untreated dysplasia of the hip: A study of radiographic factors that predict the outcome. *J Bone Joint Surg Am* 1995;77:985-989.

Myers SR, Eijer H, Ganz R: Anterior femoroacetabular impingement after periacetabular osteotomy. *Clin Orthop* 1999;363:93-99.

Pring ME, Trousdale RT, Cabanela ME, Harper ME: Intraoperative electromyographic monitoring during periacetabular osteotomy. *Clin Orthop* 2002;400:158-164.

Siebenrock KA, Schöll E, Lottenbach M, Ganz R: Bernese periacetabular osteotomy. *Clin Orthop* 1999;363:9-20.

Tönnis D, Heinecke A: Acetabular and femoral anteversion: Relationship with osteoarthritis of the hip. *J Bone Joint Surg Am* 1999;81:1747-1770.

Trousdale RT, Cabanela ME, Berry DJ, Wenger DE: Magnetic resonance imaging pelvimetry before and after a periacetabular osteotomy. *J Bone Joint Surg Am* 2002;84:552-556.

Trousdale RT, Ekkernkamp A, Ganz R, Wallrichs SL: Periacetabular and intertrochanteric osteotomy for the treatment of osteoarthritis in dysplastic hips. *J Bone Joint Surg Am* 1995;77:73-85.

Trumble SJ, Mayo KA, Mast JW: The periacetabular osteotomy: Minimum 2 year follow-up in more than 100 hips. *Clin Orthop* 1999;363:54-63.

Coding

CPT Codes		Corresponding ICD-9 Codes		
27122	Acetabuloplasty; resection, femoral head (eg, Girdlestone procedure)	716.15 718.8	718.2 733/14	718.6 905.06
27140	Osteotomy and transfer of greater trochanter of femur (separate procedure)	732.1 736.32	733.81 781.2	736.31
27146	Osteotomy, iliac, acetabular or innominate bone	343.9 733.81 754.3 754.32	718.25 741.0 754.30 754.33	718.35 741.9 754.31 754.35
27147	Osteotomy, iliac, acetabular or innominate bone; with open reduction of hip	343.9 741.0 754.31	718.25 741.9 754.32	718.35 754.30 754.33
27151	Osteotomy, iliac, acetabular or innominate bone; with femoral osteotomy	343.9 741.0 754.31 733.35	718.25 741.9 754.32	718.35 754.30 754.33
27156	Osteotomy, iliac, acetabular or innominate bone; with femoral osteotomy and with open reduction of hip	343.9 741.0 754.31 733.35	718.25 741.9 754.32	718.35 754.30 754.33
27158	Osteotomy, pelvis, bilateral (eg, congenital malformation)	343.9	741.0	741.9
27165	Osteotomy, intertrochanteric or subtrochanteric including internal or external fixation and/or cast	715.15 732.1 736.32 754.32 755.61	715.25 733.81 754.30 754.33 755.62	715.35 736.31 754.31 754.35 755.63
27284	Arthrodesis, hip joint (including obtaining graft)	715.15 718.2 718.8 808.49 808.8	715.25 718.4 808.0 808.53 808.9	715.35 718.6 808.43 808.59 905.6
27286	Arthrodesis, hip joint (including obtaining graft); with subtrochanteric osteotomy	714.9 715.35 718.6 808.43 808.59	715.15 718.2 718.8 808.49 808.8	715.25 718.4 808.0 808.53 808.9
29860-3	Arthroscopy, hip, diagnostic, with or without synovial biopsy (separate procedure)	711.15 716.15	711.45 732.1	711.95 732.7

CPT copyright © 2004 by the American Medical Association. All Rights Reserved.

Chapter 63

Hip Arthrodesis

Stuart L. Weinstein, MD
Donald S. Garbuz, MD
Clive P. Duncan, MD, MSc, CRCSC

Indications

Hip arthrodesis was widely used to treat end-stage hip osteoarthritis before the development of total hip arthroplasty (THA). However, arthrodesis was largely abandoned in the 1930s in favor of motion-sparing procedures such as cup arthroplasty. Its popularity further eroded in the early 1970s as THA gained acceptance. Patients are aware of the success rates associated with THA, making hip arthrodesis a less attractive option. In addition, orthopaedic surgeons often have little experience with hip arthrodesis because of the limited number of surgeries performed each year.

Despite the high success rate of THA, concerns remain about its long-term durability in patients younger than 40 years of age. Revision rates as high as 45% have been reported in younger patients, but may be considerably less with uncemented implants and alternative bearing surfaces. Even with uncertainties about the long-term durability of THA, many young patients continue to choose THA because of its predictable pain relief, rapid recovery time, and excellent functional outcome.

Arthrodesis should be considered in selected symptomatic adolescents or adults younger than 40 years of age with monoarticular end-stage hip osteoarthritis and resultant pain. The ideal candidate is a manual laborer who wants to return to work. Patients should be free of low back pain, ipsilateral knee pain, and contralateral hip pain or pathology. Radiographs of these areas should be normal. Patients undergoing arthrodesis for osteonecrosis also should have MRI of the contralateral hip to rule out silent disease. Patients who do not meet all the indications for hip arthrodesis should be considered for alternative procedures such as resurfacing or THA.

Patients must have realistic expectations about the outcome of arthrodesis. Talking with other patients who have successfully undergone arthrodesis is helpful so that the patient can see that arthrodesis relieves hip pain, restores functional capacity, and allows for return to vigorous physical activity, including heavy manual labor. Should disabling low back pain, ipsilateral knee pain, or contralateral hip pain eventually develop, converting the arthrodesis to a THA may be an option. Patients must make an informed choice, with a clear realization of the limitations imposed by hip arthrodesis as well as the potential benefits and restrictions that may occur should it become necessary to convert the arthrodesis to a THA.

Contraindications

Hip arthrodesis is contraindicated in patients with contralateral hip pathology, symptoms in the lumbar spine, or evidence of knee pathology or instability on the ipsilateral side.

Nonambulatory children and some young adults with cerebral palsy, severe joint destruction, and degenerative joint disease are best treated with hip resection arthroplasty.

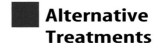 Alternative Treatments

Alternative treatments include nonsurgical measures, resection arthroplasty, osteotomy, hemiresurfacing, and THA.

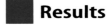 Results

Most long-term studies report that patients are satisfied with the results of arthrodesis and lead active lives without hip pain. Several reports on the long-term durability of arthrodesis (**Table 1**) indicate that most patients return to manual labor for as long as

Table 1 Long-Term Results of Hip Arthrodesis

Author(s) (Year)	Number of Hips	Mean Patient Age (Range)	Mean Follow-up (Range)	Results
Callaghan, et al (1985)	28	25 years (10–58)	37 years (17–50)	61% low back pain 57% ipsilateral knee pain 28% contralateral hip pain
Sponseller, et al (1984)	53	14 years (3–35)	38 years	57% low back pain 45% ipsilateral knee pain 17% contralateral knee pain

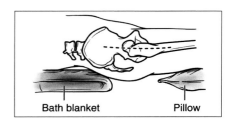

Figure 1 The patient is positioned on bath blankets from the shoulders to the pelvis to elevate the pelvis from the operating table. The patient's limbs are supported by pillows or bath blankets to maintain alignment and to ensure that they are the same level from the operating table. The incision extends 5 to 8 cm proximal and distal to the greater trochanter.

30 years. At long-term (approximately 20 years) follow-up, the most common complaints were low back pain and ipsilateral knee pain. However, 65% of these patients were uncertain whether they would choose the procedure again. Furthermore, patients are now rarely willing to accept the functional limitations that occur 10 to 15 years after hip fusion.

Both surgeon and patient must understand the functional and long-term limitations of a successful hip arthrodesis. Patients typically have a short leg and walk more slowly postoperatively. Most patients have a pain-free hip but still have more limitations on their activities than individuals who have not had arthrodesis. The most common complaints occur with activities that require hip flexion, such as sitting, bending, and putting on shoes and socks. Prolonged sitting in confined spaces such as theaters and airplanes is particularly troublesome, and some patients, especially women, have difficulty with sexual activity. Hip arthrodesis can be a successful and durable operation, but patients must anticipate its limitations.

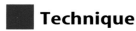

Technique

Numerous surgical techniques are used to achieve hip fusion. Most modern techniques are designed to provide high fusion rates and minimize the need for postoperative immobilization. Another critical consideration is preservation of the hip abductors because future conversion to THA will be desired in a substantial number of patients.

One goal in performing hip arthrodesis is to ensure that as much normal hip architecture as possible is preserved in the event conversion to THA is necessary. Proper positioning of the leg in relation to the pelvis is important to prevent or delay the onset of back and knee symptoms. Gait analysis shows that increased transverse and sagittal rotation of the pelvis, increased knee flexion throughout the stance phase, and increased motion of the contralateral hip compensate for the loss of hip motion. The optimal position of fusion has not been established, but generally the hip should be fused in 20° to 30° of flexion, neutral to slight adduction, and 10° of external rotation. Abduction and internal rotation must be avoided. Some drift into adduction has been reported in fusions performed in younger patients; therefore, with these patients it is best to attempt a neutral position with reference to abduction and adduction.

Cobra Plating Technique (Iowa)

The goal of hip arthrodesis is to achieve a solid bony union sufficient to satisfy patients' high functional demands. This is accomplished through maximal bony contact and rigid internal fixation. It is also important to prevent shortening the limb in the event that conversion to THA becomes necessary. Patient positioning during surgery is critical so that the surgeon can assess the appropriate positioning of the limb in relation to the pelvis.

EXPOSURE

The patient should be placed in a supine position with both hips properly prepared and draped. Bath blankets are placed under the middle of the patient's back to elevate the pelvis (**Figure 1**). Both lower extremities are prepared and draped free to allow visualization of the anterosuperior iliac spine on the contralateral side and to allow mobility of the opposite hip to check for appropriate limb positioning.

A longitudinal 5- to 8-cm skin incision is made proximal and distal to the greater trochanter. Dissection is carried down to the interval between the tensor fasciae latae and the gluteus maximus. After the anterior and posterior borders of the gluteus medius are identified, a trochanteric osteotomy is performed, using either an osteotome or an oscillating saw, taking great care to prevent injury to the medial femoral circumflex vessels (**Figure 2**). Injury to the vessels may result in loss of blood supply to the femoral head.

The hip joint capsule is incised in a T shape, with one limb along the acetabular margin anteriorly and a perpendicular incision toward the an-

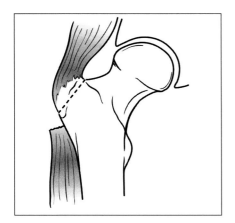

Figure 2 After identification of the anterior and posterior borders of the gluteus medius, retractors are inserted and a trochanteric osteotomy is performed using either an osteotome or an oscillating saw. It is important to prevent injury to the medial femoral circumflexed vessels.

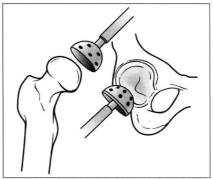

Figure 3 The femoral head is denuded of all cartilage and shaped to fit the acetabulum using a combination of straight and curved osteotomes and/ or a concave hemispheric reamer. The acetabulum is prepared by removing all cartilage down to bleeding bone, usually by using a convex hemispheric reamer.

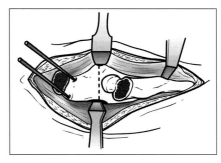

Figure 4 A pelvic osteotomy, similar to that of the Chiari procedure, is used when the acetabulum is shallow and the hip has been subluxated. The osteotomy extends from the sciatic notch to the anteroinferior spine just above the acetabulum.

terosuperior surface of the femoral head and neck. Again, care must be taken to avoid injury to the medial femoral circumflex vessels. Once the capsule has been incised, the femoral head can be dislocated anteriorly.

BONE PREPARATION

The femoral head is denuded of all cartilage and shaped to fit the acetabulum. This can be done with a combination of straight and curved osteotomes and/or a concave hemispheric reamer (**Figure 3**). The extremity must not be shortened significantly; therefore, it is important to avoid shortening the proximal femur in patients with osteonecrosis or loss of femoral head height secondary to Legg-Calvé-Perthes disease or slipped capital femoral epiphysis. In patients with significant osteonecrosis, a power drill can be used to burr or fenestrate the femoral head.

The acetabulum is prepared by removing all cartilage down to bleeding bone with a convex hemispheric reamer (**Figure 3**). A good bleeding surface on the acetabular side is extremely important to promote healing. Fenestrating the femoral head is preferred to the significant shortening

that may be needed to reach bleeding bone, particularly in patients with osteonecrosis. Any marrow from the reaming should be saved for later use as supplemental graft.

If the acetabulum is shallow and the hip has been subluxated, a pelvic osteotomy similar to the Chiari procedure is performed. The osteotomy extends from the sciatic notch to the anteroinferior spine just above the acetabulum (**Figure 4**), although the actual angle of the osteotomy is less important than it is in the Chiari procedure. The sciatic notch is carefully exposed, with subperiosteal dissection using a Cobb elevator and sponges. Once the notch is identified and a cobra retractor placed in it, the posterior cortex can be cut with a large right-angled Kerrison rongeur to ensure the osteotomy enters the notch at the appropriate point. The osteotomy is generally performed with osteotomes, although an oscillating saw may be used. The intrapelvic structures must be protected, and in some patients exposing the inner side of the pelvis subperiosteally may be helpful. The osteotomy should be displaced medially enough to provide adequate coverage superior to the femoral head and neck.

After the femoral head and acetabulum are prepared and pelvic osteotomy (if necessary) is completed, the limb is placed into 25° to 30° of flexion, 5° to 10° of adduction, and 10° of external rotation; the limb is then held in position. A padded roll can be placed under the thigh to elevate the hip approximately 10° to 15°. This elevation, combined with the normal 15° of hip flexion present with normal lordosis, should place the hip in the appropriate degree of flexion. A long, sterile goniometer can be used to compare the position of the femur to the pelvis. With the opposite limb draped free, the hip can be hyperflexed to remove all lumbar lordosis and assess the degree of hip flexion in the operative hip. We suggest using fluoroscopy to assess abduction and adduction. The entire pelvis must be viewed, with the field encompassing both proximal femurs.

Internal Fixation

A cobra plate is then appropriately contoured. A distal bend must be made in the cobra plate so that when it is applied to the distal femur it does not abduct the hip. The cobra plate is then attached to the distal ilium (above the osteotomy, if one has been made) and an AO tensioner is applied to the femur distal to the plate to apply appropriate compression (**Figure 5**).

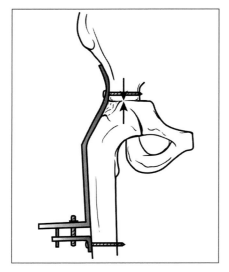

Figure 5 The cobra plate requires a distal bend so that the hip is not abducted when the plate is applied to the distal femur. The plate is subsequently attached to the distal ilium.

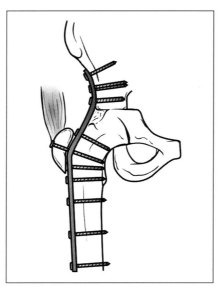

Figure 6 Cortical screws are drilled, tapped, and inserted. The greater trochanter is attached over the plate with a screw and washer. Any residual reamings are then packed in the gaps between the plate and the proximal femur.

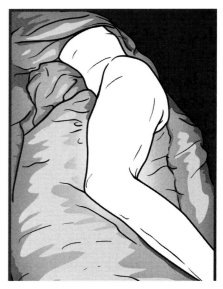

Figure 7 The patient is positioned in the lateral decubitus position with the affected hip facing up on a deflatable bean bag positioner. The lateral positioning needs to be precise; therefore, an AP radiograph is obtained to confirm alignment of the center of the sacrum with the symphysis pubis.

The remaining cortical screws are then drilled, tapped, and inserted. Finally, the greater trochanter is attached over the plate with a screw and washer. Any residual reaming materials are then packed into the gaps between the plate and the proximal femur (**Figure 6**).

WOUND CLOSURE

A drain is placed, and the wound is closed.

POSTOPERATIVE REGIMEN

The patient can begin toe-touch weight bearing as tolerated beginning the first postoperative day. An orthotic can be used for the first 6 weeks after surgery if there is any question about the stability of fixation or patient compliance with postoperative instructions. Toe-touch weight bearing is maintained for approximately 6 weeks, and then the patient is reassessed clinically and radiographically. If satisfactory progress toward fusion is evident, weight bearing can be gradually increased over the next 6 to 10 weeks. Most patients do not require external walking aids by 4 to 5 months postoperatively.

Cobra Plating Technique (Vancouver)

The Vancouver technique is a modification of the original cobra plate compression technique described by Castle and Schneider. This technique avoids the need for pelvic osteotomy because the socket is medialized and the plate contoured to the pelvis and femur.

EXPOSURE

The patient is placed in the lateral position with the affected hip facing up (**Figure 7**). The contralateral limb is flexed to help reduce spinal lordosis. An AP radiograph is obtained to confirm the position of the pelvis before the procedure begins.

A straight lateral incision is centered over the greater trochanter and curved slightly posteriorly (**Figure 8**, *A*). The femoral shaft is exposed by elevating the vastus lateralis. A classic greater trochanteric osteotomy is then performed, and the trochanteric fragment is elevated and retracted proximally (**Figure 8**, *B*). An anterior cap-

sulectomy is performed to ensure that the posterior capsule is preserved so that the extraosseous blood supply to the femoral head is not disrupted.

BONE PREPARATION

The hip is dislocated anteriorly (**Figure 9**, *A*), and the acetabulum and femoral head are prepared. The acetabulum is reamed with hemispheric reamers and medialized to the level of the inner pelvis. The femoral head is reamed with an oversized female reamer. Matching reamers, formerly used for resurfacing THA, are used (**Figure 9**, *B* through *D*) so that a very tight cancellous bone to cancellous bone contact area is achieved.

INTERNAL FIXATION

The limb is now positioned in 20° of flexion, 5° of external rotation, and 10° of adduction. Note that the adduction usually will be decreased by 10° once the outrigger compression device is applied. A cobra plate is selected, and benders are used to shape the plate to fit the outer table of the pelvis and the lateral aspect of the femur. The plate is initially fixed to the acetabulum with a central proximal screw. At this point, gentle compression is applied distally and an intraoperative radiograph is obtained to confirm the desired degree of adduction (femur relative to pelvis). At this point adduction should be 10° to 20° so that once compression is complete the limb will be in neutral adduction (ie, equivalent to 10° adduction of femoral shaft to pelvis). If the radiographs confirm appropriate positioning, the remaining proximal screws are inserted followed by compression with the AO compression device (**Figure 10**, *A*). Screws are then inserted through the plate into the femoral shaft. The greater trochanter is then reattached in its anatomic position using cancellous screws with washers (**Figure 10**, *B*).

POSTOPERATIVE REGIMEN

The patient is placed on crutches for 3 months postoperatively, with toe-touch weight bearing during the first 6 weeks followed by progression to full weight bearing by 3 months postoperatively. Union is expected by 4 months postoperatively, and patients generally can expect to return to work by 6 to 12 months after surgery.

Anterior Plating Technique

This technique, described by Beaule and associates, has the same advantages as other modern hip arthrodesis techniques: rigid internal fixation, medialization of the construct, and maximal bone contact, but it also completely spares the abductors and minimizes deformity of the pelvis, both important technical considerations for patients who may later require conversion to THA.

EXPOSURE

The patient is placed in the supine position, and a modified Smith-Peterson

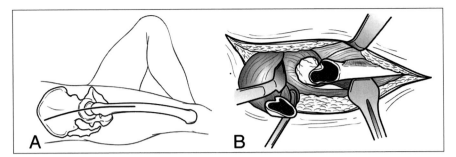

Figure 8 A slightly curved lateral incision is made (**A**), and the femur and capsule are exposed by elevation of the vastus lateralis and greater trochanter (**B**).

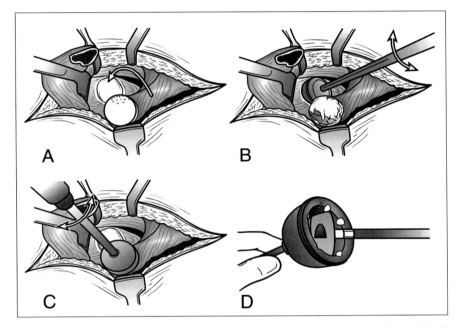

Figure 9 The hip is dislocated anteriorly (**A**) after which the acetabulum and femoral head are prepared with closely matching reamers (**B** and **C**). These reamers date from the first era of surface replacement (**D**).

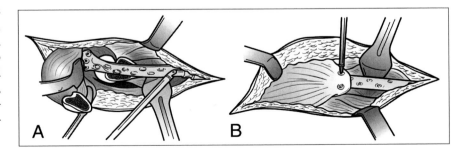

Figure 10 Initial fixation is with a proximal screw in the cobra head, and initial compression is with the distal outrigger (**A**) followed by radiographic confirmation of plate placement and limb alignment. The proximal screws are then inserted, compression is completed, the remaining screws inserted, and the greater trochanter accurately repositioned and fixed (**B**).

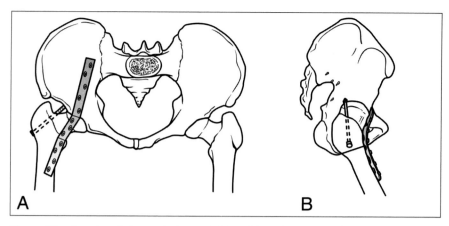

Figure 11 Anterior plating technique. AP **(A)** and lateral **(B)** views of the pelvis with optimal position of plate and lateral lag screw. (Reproduced with permission from Beaule PE, Matta JM, Mast JW: Hip arthrodesis: Current indications and techniques. *J Am Acad Orthop Surg* 2002;10:249-258.)

approach is used, including exposure of the inner aspect of the pelvis. The sartorius and two heads of the rectus are released from the origin. The vastus lateralis is elevated to expose the femur.

BONE PREPARATION AND PLATING

After denuding the femoral head and acetabulum, a 6.5-mm lag screw is inserted from the lateral aspect of the greater trochanter into the supra-acetabular region. A 12- or 14-hole low-contact dynamic compression plate is molded to the anterior contour of the femur, pelvic brim, and proximal femur (**Figure 11**). The plate typically is fixed to the pelvis first. Compression is obtained by use of the tensioning device on the femur. The plate is then further secured to the femur with standard screws.

WOUND CLOSURE

Routine wound closure in layers is performed.

POSTOPERATIVE REGIMEN

The patient is allowed weight bearing of approximately 30 lb for 10 weeks. After 12 weeks, if there is radiographic evidence of union, the patient is allowed full weight bearing. In the original series, the rate of union was 83%, and patient satisfaction was high.

———————————■

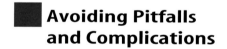

Avoiding Pitfalls and Complications

A major pitfall of hip arthrodesis is malunion, but this can be avoided by

strict adherence to surgical technique and the use of intraoperative radiographs. For surgeons with little prior experience with this procedure, supine positioning of the patient may assist in precise limb positioning.

Nonunion can occur but has decreased in incidence with use of modern techniques of internal fixation. Rates of union with modern techniques have been reported to be between 85% and 95%. If nonunion occurs, and infection has been ruled out, repeat arthrodesis with an iliac crest bone graft is the preferred treatment.

Patient satisfaction is the main goal of surgery. In the short term, a well-informed patient and a successful arthrodesis will usually result in a satisfied patient. A detailed discussion about outcomes and functional limitations should be part of the patient's informed consent process.

In the long term, difficulties are usually encountered in adjacent joints. Low back pain and ipsilateral knee pain are seen in more than half of all patients at long-term follow-up. In these patients, conversion to THA is appropriate. Conversion most predictably will relieve back pain and, to a lesser extent, relieve ipsilateral knee or contralateral hip pain. The outcome following THA will largely depend on the adequacy of the abductors, making it critically important to protect the abductors and the greater trochanter during the procedure.

———————————■

References

Beaule PE, Matta JM, Mast JW: Hip arthrodesis: Current indications and techniques. *J Am Acad Orthop Surg* 2002;10:249-258.

Callaghan JJ, Brand RA, Pedersen DR: Hip arthrodesis: A long-term follow-up. *J Bone Joint Surg Am* 1985;67:1328-1335.

Callaghan JJ, McBeath AA: Arthrodesis, in Callaghan JJ, Rosenberg AG, Rubash HE (eds): *The Adult Hip.* New York, NY, Lippincott-Raven, 1998, pp 749-759.

Duncan CP, Spangehl M, Beauchamp C, McGraw R: Hip arthrodesis: An important option for advanced disease in the young adult. *Can J Surg* 1995;38(suppl 1):S39-S45.

Fulkerson JP: Arthrodesis for disabling hip pain in children and adolescents. *Clin Orthop* 1977;128:296-302.

Karol LA, Halliday SE, Gourineni P: Gait and function after intra-articular arthrodesis of the hip in adolescents. *J Bone Joint Surg Am* 2000;82:561-569.

Kilgus DJ, Amstutz HC, Wolgin MA, Dorsey FJ: Joint replacement for ankylosed hips. *J Bone Joint Surg* 1990;72:45-54.

Schneider R: Hip arthrodesis with the cobra head plate and pelvic osteotomy. *Reconstr Surg Traumatol* 1974;14:1-37.

Sponseller PD, McBeath AA, Perpich M: Hip arthrodesis in young patients: Long- term follow-up study. *J Bone Joint Surg Am* 1984;66:853-859.

Strathy GM, Fitzgerald RH Jr: Total hip arthroplasty in the ankylosed hip: A ten year follow up. *J Bone Joint Surg Am* 1988;70:963-966.

Coding

CPT Codes		Corresponding ICD-9 Codes		
27284	Arthrodesis, hip joint (including obtaining graft)	715.15 718.25 718.85 808.49 808.8	715.25 718.45 808.0 808.53 808.9	715.35 718.65 808.43 808.59 905.6
27286	Arthrodesis, hip joint (including obtaining graft); with subtrochanteric osteotomy	715.15 718.25 718.85 808.49 808.8	715.25 718.45 808.0 808.53 808.9	715.35 718.65 808.43 808.59 905.6

Intertrochanteric Femoral Osteotomies for Developmental and Posttraumatic Conditions

Richard F. Santore, MD

Indications

Intertrochanteric or proximal femoral osteotomy has an enduring role in reconstructive surgery of the hip. The original, and ongoing, indication is to induce healing of femoral neck nonunion by valgus repositioning of the upper fragment. This repositioning is designed to convert the high shear forces of a vertical nonunion of the femoral neck into the compressive forces of a more horizontal repositioning (**Figure 1**). Marti demonstrated

that posttraumatic osteonecrosis of the femoral head, in the absence of segmental collapse and secondary osteoarthritis, is not a contraindication to valgus osteotomy. Posttraumatic deformity remains another principal indication, as do limb-length inequality, certain cases of acquired varus deformity resulting from Legg-Calvé-Perthes disease, apparent varus as a result of slipped capital femoral epiphysis, and certain cases of osteonecrosis and osteoarthritis secondary to hip dysplasia. Repositioning below a suc-

cessful hip arthrodesis also is an indication.

Rotational osteotomy of the pelvis for hip dysplasia has assumed the role once played by intertrochanteric osteotomy. The latter is now used as a complement to rotational pelvic osteotomy in approximately one in ten patients. Indications for its use in this role include limb-length adjustment, resetting the rotation arc of the limb, or combined valgus and limb lengthening in patients who have Legg-Calvé-Perthes disease with a high-

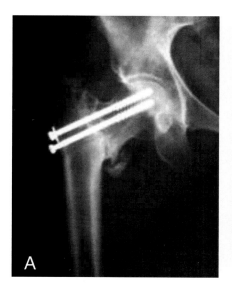

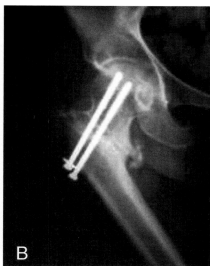

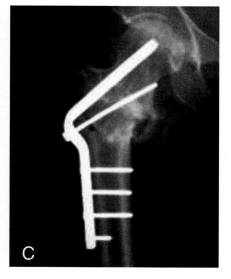

Figure 1 **A,** AP view of the right hip of a physically active 60-year-old woman shows a nonunion of a femoral neck fracture 6 months following closed reduction and internal fixation. The affected leg is 2.5 cm shorter than the normal, opposite leg. **B,** AP view with the hip in adduction to simulate the effect of a valgus intertrochanteric osteotomy. **C,** AP view obtained 3 months following valgus intertrochanteric osteotomy without wedge resection. The osteotomy healed, and limb lengths are equal.

Table 1 Result of Valgus Intertrochanteric Osteotomy for Femoral Neck Fracture Nonunion and Malunion

Author(s) (Year)	Number of Patients	Mean Patient Age (Range)	Mean Follow-up (Range)	Results
Marti, et al (1989)	50	53 years (19–76)	7 years (3–13)	78% good to excellent results 7 conversions to THA (14% failure rate)
Anglen (1997)	13	Mean: NR (18–59 years)	25 months (9-42)	100% fracture healing 92% return to full weight bearing 88% return to previous employment
Bartonieck, et al (2003)	15	54 years (29–84)	5.5 years (2–10)	100% improved Harris hip scores 93% fracture healing with no complications

riding greater trochanter, or varus and limb shortening associated with hip dysplasia on the acetabular side. In most cases, pelvic and intertrochanteric osteotomies are done under the same anesthesia. I recommend performing the intertrochanteric osteotomy then the pelvic osteotomy because with this sequence the final position of the acetabular segment is more easily modified intraoperatively based on fluoroscopic information.

Inclusion criteria for a valgus osteotomy include the following: (1) patient comfort in adduction, which replicates the postoperative position of the femoral head; (2) reduced lateral impingement and/or improvement in the joint space on an AP view of the hip in adduction; (3) an improved or normal horizontal relationship between the tip of the greater trochanter and the center of the femoral head in adduction; and (4) at least 15° of passive adduction on physical examination. In patients with osteonecrosis, valgus and flexion are indicated when there is a small anterolateral necrotic segment that is partially extruded by adduction.

Criteria for varus osteotomy include the following: (1) improved patient comfort in abduction, which rep-

licates the postoperative position of the femoral head; (2) excellent joint congruency on an AP radiograph with the hip in abduction; (3) a rotationally controlled AP radiograph that demonstrates a femoral neck-shaft angle of at least 145°.

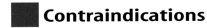

■ Contraindications

Contraindications include marked osteoporosis, active history of tobacco use, marked stiffness in the hip, absence of a "position of comfort," depression, and osteomyelitis. Advanced osteoarthritis, though a contraindication to rotational pelvic and varus intertrochanteric osteotomies, is not an absolute contraindication to a salvage Bombelli-type valgus/extension osteotomy for arthritic changes secondary to hip dysplasia.

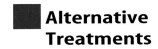

■ Alternative Treatments

The main surgical alternative to an osteotomy of upper femur is total hip

arthroplasty (THA). The technology and reliability of THA are improving over time. However, every new technology is not necessarily reliable, and serious caveats to THA remain in the young patient, particularly when biologic solutions are reasonable. In the subset of dysplasia indications, the principal alternative is a rotational pelvic osteotomy, which should be done whenever possible. Also, hip arthroscopy can be a reasonable alternative in patients with mechanical hip symptoms and mild dysplasia or mild impingement.

A number of nonsurgical alternatives are available as well, including (1) activity modification to exclude vigorous and high-impact activities; (2) weight loss to a target body mass index of 22, if possible; (3) use of impact-absorbing shoes and/or inserts, heel inserts, or shoe modification to lengthen the short side; (3) change in occupation; (4) use of cane or crutch on the contralateral side; and (5) use of nonnarcotic analgesics and glucosamine sulfate and chondroitin sulfate. The use of nonsteroidal anti-inflammatory drugs (NSAIDs) has become controversial. I believe that all NSAIDs should be used with caution when prescribed for long-term use. Patients frequently ask for an exercise program that is kind to the hip. I recommend swimming, including the use of floatation devices for the legs as done by wheelchair athletes, to avoid any exercise-induced strain on the hip.

■ Results

Several studies have demonstrated that valgus-producing intertrochanteric osteotomy can produce a high rate of union in femoral neck fracture nonunion (**Table 1**).

A study of patients with intertrochanteric malunion or nonunion that had collapsed into varus reported healing in 14 of 15 patients treated by valgus osteotomy with a high-angle (120°) blade plate.

In an early study on the use of intertrochanteric osteotomy, a 78% success rate was reported at 11- to 22-year follow-up of 68 hips in 55 patients with slipped capital femoral epiphysis who were treated with triplane osteotomy. Another study of patients with grade II slips treated by Bombelli-type triplane osteotomy reported that at follow-up 2 to 10 years later, all patients remained pain free postoperatively, and 39% had an increase in total range of motion.

The results over time for osteonecrosis are much less favorable. Although short-term results were favorable, in one study good to excellent results were reported in only 58% of patients at an average of 8.2 years after intertrochanteric osteotomy. Another group of investigators reported a steady rate of conversion to THA in the 10 years after intertrochanteric osteotomy for osteonecrosis. Although 73% of patients in their study were still satisfied at 5 years, only 60% of hips had been converted to THA by 8 years postoperatively.

Several authors have demonstrated that a small necrotic segment is a favorable factor in ultimate success after osteotomy. Sugioka and associates reported a 78% success rate in 474 hips treated with up to 180° of rotation using his unique osteotomy. They, too, correlated success with size of lesion and early Ficat stage on presentation. For reasons not well understood, these results have been difficult to replicate outside of Japan, and the popularity of this approach has diminished in recent years.

A widely cited report from 1980 on the use of intertrochanteric osteotomy for sequelae of dysplasia consisting of 263 patients at one institution, and a 1970s Swiss multicenter study of 2,200 patients, reported excellent long-term results in 30% of patients and satisfactory results in an-

other 30%. The rest required conversion to THA. Varus osteotomy for coxa valga subluxans (ie, moderate hip dysplasia associated with a congruent hip and a valgus femoral neck-shaft angle [>144°] of the upper femur) and valgus osteotomy for superolateral overload (Bombelli type) are associated with roughly a 70% likelihood of a good outcome at 10 years. The results of successful THA generally provide significantly superior pain relief and restoration of near-normal function compared with a successful intertrochanteric osteotomy. Unfortunately, almost all of the published series combine the results of varus and valgus osteotomies and fail to distinguish an osteotomy done for prearthritic pain from one done as a salvage for established arthritis. Most of these studies were conducted before the widespread use of THA.

————————■

■ Technique

The patient is supine on a radiolucent table, and fluoroscopy is used. Careful preoperative planning on tracing paper, copies of the radiographs, or a computer-based planning tool is indicated.

Exposure
Exposure consists of longitudinal opening of the tensor and gluteal myofascia in the line of the skin incision and anterior elevation of the vastus lateralis. Proximally, the interval between the anterior edge of the abductors and the tensor can be opened to access the hip joint if intra-articular exposure is needed, such as if an osteophyte must be removed or an impingement zone on the femoral neck must be resected.

Varus Osteotomy
Varus osteotomies generally are done with 90° plates, whereas valgus os-

teotomies are done with high-angle plates of 110°, 120°, or 130°. Varus osteotomies shorten the limb, which can be exploited to advantage in patients whose limbs are long on the operative side. In patients with equal limb lengths, an open wedge technique without wedge resection minimizes shortening. The apparent and real components of the medial shift of the femoral shaft should be controlled in accordance with plans for future THA stem insertion needs. Several offsets are available in most commonly used blade plate devices to help control this variable. Varus of more than 20° is indicated in exceptional circumstances only. Interfragmentary compression with a tensioning device after insertion of the blade plate contributes to stability of the osteosynthesis.

Valgus Osteotomy
The geometric changes produced by valgus osteotomies lend themselves to lengthening, which is a benefit in patients with a short operative limb. Up to 3 cm of lengthening can be achieved by a 30° to 40° valgus intertrochanteric osteotomy without wedge resection. Conversely, full wedge resection is required, and use of additional segmental parallel wedge resections must be anticipated, to avoid unintended limb lengthening after valgus osteotomy in patients whose limbs are not short preoperatively. In all osteotomies, lack of attention and failure to discuss limb length issues with patients preoperatively can dramatically affect patient satisfaction.

Some degree of deliberate lateralization of the femoral shaft distal to the osteotomy is desirable in most valgus osteotomies and is achieved by using a blade length that is longer than the seating chisel tract in the femoral head. The difference between the depth of chisel insertion and the blade length represents the lateralization of the shaft. The degree of lateralization is determined as a part of preoperative planning for future THA and is verified by fluoroscopy at the time of surgery. The degree of valgus achieved is based on the angle of insertion of the chisel relative to the femoral shaft and the angle of the blade plate.

Intraoperatively, the fluoroscopic image of the upper femur after plate insertion should look virtually identical to that of the preoperative plan. Before final anchoring the side plate to the femoral shaft, the surgeon should ensure that the patella is pointing toward the ceiling in the provisional position to prevent unintended external rotation of the foot. A deliberate change in rotation occasionally is part of the preoperative plan but must be achieved before screws are placed into the femur. I strongly discourage the use of compression screw devices for angulation osteotomies; these devices fail to provide rotational control of the proximal fragment of the femur and fail to prevent femoral shaft displacement.

Wound Closure

Closure consists of repairing the vastus lateralis tendon to its site of origin on the vastus tubercle to cover the plate with muscle and tendon. Repair of the tensor fascia lata is the same as that for hip fracture surgery.

Postoperative Regimen

Ambulation with two crutches in a normal, heel-to-toe gait pattern begins on the first postoperative day. Partial weight bearing is encouraged, approximating the weight of the leg. Weight bearing as tolerated is permitted at postoperative week 5, with progression to a single crutch by approximately week 10. A single crutch or cane is then used until the patient no longer limps. Gait support is longer following open wedge osteotomies than for closing wedge osteotomies. Swimming pool-based activities are encouraged as soon as the patient can safely enter and exit the pool, usually 6 to 8 weeks postoperatively.

Radiographs are reviewed at weeks 6 and 12 and at 6 months and 1 year. Abductor weakness can be anticipated for up to 1 year after varus osteotomy and may be permanent in as many as 30% of patients. If weakness is permanent, advancement of the greater trochanter at the time of hardware removal can be very helpful. In these situations, the surgeon must advise the patient preoperatively about how abductor weakness affects limb length and can cause a limp. Hardware is removed any time after 1 year if radiographs show unequivocal evidence of mature bone healing and if normal gait is present. Hardware removal is important for three reasons: (1) bone strength is never normal under the plate; (2) the plate invariably is a source of some degree of hardware bursitis, and patients always feel better after the device is removed; and (3) if hardware is removed well before future THA, the risks of intraoperative fracture and postoperative infection are probably much less.

Planning Total Hip Arthroplasty After Femoral Osteotomy

The results of intertrochanteric osteotomy cannot be assumed to offer definitive, lifelong pain relief or protection from the eventual progression to end-stage osteoarthritis. In anticipation of the eventual need for THA, the intertrochanteric osteotomy should be performed in a way that facilitates conversion to THA. The trajectory for insertion of the femoral stem is an important consideration when the osteotomy fragments are displaced in several planes. Significant displacement can be performed as needed to correct a developmental or posttraumatic deformity, as long as the anticipated shape of the fully remodeled femur is compatible with stem insertion. For this reason, it is helpful to plan the level of osteotomy to be at the upper border of the lesser trochanter. At the time of THA, deformities above this level can be corrected by resecting the femoral neck down to this level as long as there is clearance for the greater trochanter.

Avoiding Pitfalls and Complications

Access to the contralateral ankle during the surgery can help the surgeon intraoperatively assess the effect of the osteotomy on limb length. Preparing the entire operative leg free allows for evaluation of hip range of motion and rotation of the osteosynthesis.

Straight leg raising should be discouraged for the first few months to minimize forces on the osteotomy site. I use formal physical therapy sparingly in part because few physical therapists are familiar with the rehabilitation requirements and concerns following a hip osteotomy.

References

Anglen JO: Intertrochanteric osteotomy for failed internal fixation of femoral neck fracture. *Clin Orthop* 1997;341:175-182.

Bartonicek J, Skala-Rosenbaum J, Dousa P: valgus intertrochanteric osteotomy for malunion and non-union of trochanteric fractures. *J Orthop Trauma* 2003;17:606-612.

Ferguson GM, Cabanela ME, Ilstrup DM: Total hip arthroplasty after failed intertrochanteric osteotomy. *J Bone Joint Surg Br* 1994;76:252-257.

Jacobs MA, Hungerford DS, Krackow KA: Intertrochanteric osteotomy for avascular necrosis of the femoral head. *J Bone Joint Surg Br* 1989;71:200-204.

Marti RK, Schuller HM, Raaymakers EL: Intertrochanteric osteotomy for non-union of the femoral neck. *J Bone Joint Surg Br* 1989;71:782-787.

Millis M, Murphy S, Poss R: Osteotomies about the hip for the prevention and treatment of osteoarthritis. *J Bone Joint Surg Am* 1995;77:626-647.

Sugioka Y, Hotokebuchi T, Tsutsui H: Transtrochanteric anterior rotational osteotomy for idiopathic and steroid-induced necrosis of the femoral head: Indications and long-term results. *Clin Orthop* 1992;277:111-120.

Trousdale RT, Ekkernkamp A, Ganz R, Wallrichs SL: Periacetabular and intertrochanteric osteotomy for the treatment of osteoarthrosis in dysplastic hips. *J Bone Joint Surg Am* 1995;77:73-85.

Coding

CPT Codes		Corresponding ICD-9 Codes		
27165	Intertrochanteric osteotomy (varus/valgus/flexion/extension)	718.65 732.2 733.82 736.81 781.2	719.55 733.42 736.31 754.32 V54.0	732.1 733.81 736.32 754.33
27465	Intertrochanteric shortening (when shortening is a deliberate objective of the procedure)	733.81	736.81	
27466	Intertrochanteric lengthening (when lengthening is a deliberate objective of the procedure)	733.81	736.81	
27140	Trochanteric lateralization or advancement	732.1	781.2	

CPT copyright © 2004 by the American Medical Association. All Rights Reserved.

Chapter 65

Femoral-Acetabular Management of Impingement Problems

Reinhold Ganz, MD

Indications

Open débridement is indicated primarily for young patients with symptomatic hip impingement resulting from structural problems of the femur and/or acetabulum. Femoral-acetabular impingement can result from local or circumferential acetabular overlap or from such femoral problems as nonspherical femoral heads, an insufficiently narrowed anterior femoral head-neck junction, and similar problems produced by Legg-Calvé-Perthes disease. Other conditions, including synovial chondromatosis and cartilaginous exostosis, also can be treated successfully with surgical dislocation. More recently, use of this technique has been expanded to include a new generation of surgical treatments, such as relative femoral neck lengthening, safe subcapital reorientation of a slipped capital femoral epiphysis, varus osteotomies of the femoral neck (eg, for caput valgum), and anterior or posterior rotational osteotomies of the femoral neck for osteonecrosis or femoral head defects.

Surgical hip dislocation allows inspection of the damage pattern and dynamic proof that the damage was caused by femoral-acetabular impingement. Impingement can be the result of morphologic abnormalities of the acetabulum and/or proximal femur; however, most patients have a combination of both. The speed of the destructive process is determined by the force with which the critical motion is executed. Acetabular causes of impingement produce a pincer mechanism, whereas femoral causes produce a cam abutment mechanism. Early surgical intervention may slow the progression of hip degeneration, suggesting that a delay in surgical treatment or an initial course of nonsurgical treatment is not recommended in this group of symptomatic young patients.

On the acetabular side, local or global overlap can be addressed by resection osteochondroplasty of the excessive rim or by reorientation of a retroverted acetabulum using a periacetabular osteotomy (PAO). The approach selected depends on the depth of the posterior wall and the status of the acetabular articular cartilage in the area of anterior overlap. The quality of the acetabular cartilage is evaluated preoperatively with magnetic resonance arthrography. For PAO to be considered, the posterior rim must be located clearly medial to the femoral head center. In addition, the amount of retroversion should not be so great that it precludes correction of acetabular version. For all other situations, overlap excision osteochondroplasty is preferred.

On the femoral side, clearance can be improved by resection osteochondroplasty of the nonspherical portion of the femoral head or the prominent anterior neck. Infrequently, correction of the proximal femur using a valgus or flexion intertrochanteric osteotomy also may be necessary. Relative femoral neck lengthening with trochanteric advancement is another option that improves clearance.

Contraindications

Joint débridement and reconstruction is contraindicated in patients with end-stage osteoarthritis or in patients whose structural problems cannot be corrected. Advanced patient age (ie, older than 50 to 55 years) may be a relative contraindication, depending on the severity of the secondary osteoarthritic changes and whether the patient will accept an unpredictable result. The predictability of joint salvage surgery decreases as the severity of secondary osteoarthritic changes increases.

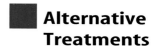 Alternative Treatments

Alternative treatments for patients with secondary cartilage damage, labral tears, and impingement problems include hip arthroscopy, surgical débridement through other approaches, or total hip arthroplasty (THA). THA should be reserved for patients with end-stage osteoarthritic changes. Furthermore, most authors would agree that THA should be avoided for as long as possible in young, active patients.

Hip arthroscopy is being used with increasing frequency; unfortunately, the keyhole view achieved during arthroscopy provides only limited access to the joint, which prevents full appreciation of the pathogenic process within the joint and ultimately limits treatment options. Unlimited access to the entire joint is possible only with complete surgical dislocation. Therefore, when hip arthroscopy is being considered, the surgeon must understand that the labral alterations in femoral-acetabular impingement do not represent the entire problem. Removal of a damaged labrum is only palliative; it does not address the cause of the disease.

Hip arthroscopy may be indicated in the treatment of femoral-acetabular impingement if the process is very localized and accessible or when degeneration is too advanced to justify an open technique. Hip arthroscopy may improve with time, but currently its limitations make treating the more global abnormalities that exist in most patients difficult and often inadequate. It is especially difficult to determine arthroscopically whether the amount of trimming is sufficient to guarantee impingement-free motion. Given these limitations and the ongoing need for better understanding of the various morphologies, I recommend open techniques for most patients with impingement.

Results

My colleagues and I observed approximately 1,000 surgical dislocations of the hip in which femoral-acetabular impingement resulted in lesions at the periphery of the joint that acted as initiators for early degenerative diseases. The causes of impingement were primary or secondary morphologic aberrations of the joint. These observations provided the impetus for the development of novel surgical modalities of treatment that focus on removal or reorientation of bone that creates femoral-acetabular impingement. Thus far, these new modalities have helped relieve symptoms and improve function in most young, active patients. However, these procedures are less likely to be successful in patients with extensive damage to articular cartilage. Our preliminary results were further improved when the anatomic rim was restored by repairing the débrided labrum with anchor sutures. Early recognition of femoral-acetabular impingement and timely intervention at early stages of the disease are likely to have a considerable impact on the natural history of the disease, delaying the onset of end-stage osteoarthritis in this group of young, active patients.

My colleagues and I published our early experience with surgical dislocation in 2001. Since then, there has been marked improvement in patients' pain and function scores. The outcome for dislocation is also reliable in patients with posttraumatic retrotorsion problems, exostosis, and intra-articular synovial disease.

Technique

Exposure

Surgical dislocation is the technique of exposure used for all procedures described in this chapter. I have performed this technique nearly 1,000 times without causing osteonecrosis. Routine monitoring of femoral head perfusion intraoperatively is possible using laser Doppler flowmetry.

The patient is placed in a lateral decubitus position, and either a Kocher-Langenbeck or Gibson approach is used to expose the vastus lateralis muscle, the greater trochanter, and the gluteus medius muscle. I prefer the latter because it avoids splitting the gluteus maximus muscle and poses less risk of an unsightly deformity of the subcutaneous fatty tissue posterior to the incision.

Using a trochanteric flip approach (**Figure 1**, *A*), the hip capsule is exposed between the piriformis and gluteus minimus muscles (**Figure 1**, *B*). After a Z- or T-shaped capsulotomy (**Figure 1**, *C*), the femoral head is dislocated anteriorly with flexion and external rotation. The leg is brought over the front of the operating table and placed in a sterile bag (**Figure 2**). Full dislocation is facilitated by incision of the round ligament using specially curved scissors. In a routine procedure, the integrity of all external rotator muscles (including the piriformis) is maintained, allowing full protection of the ramus profundus of the medial femoral circumflex artery, including the most peripheral anastomosis with the inferior gluteal artery. In hips with scarring from previous surgery or trauma or when the sciatic nerve is double-barreled around the piriformis muscle, the sciatic nerve may be less mobile; in these instances, careful dissection and mobilization of the nerve and/or release of the piriformis tendon may help to avoid stretching the nerve during dislocation.

Complete visualization of the acetabulum is possible with the use of three retractors (**Figure 3**). The posterior border becomes visible when the knee is elevated by an assistant who applies axial pressure, bringing the femoral head posterior to the acetabulum. The femoral head is easily visualized when the knee is lowered. A blunt retractor placed around the femoral neck, along with rotation of the leg, facilitate visualization of the posterior contour of the femoral head. The retinaculum covering the terminal branches of the ramus profundus is

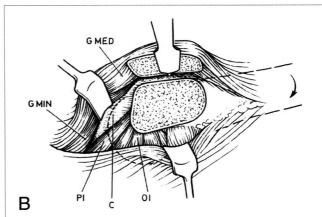

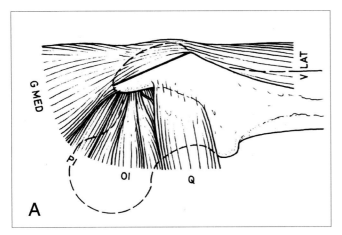

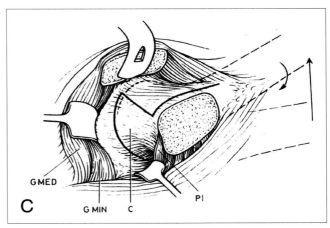

Figure 1 **A,** The right hip in the lateral decubitus position. Trochanteric osteotomy with the gluteus medius (G MED) and vastus lateralis (V LAT) attached to the trochanteric fragment. PI = piriformis, OI = obturator externus, Q = quadratus femoris. **B,** With an anterior flip of the trochanteric fragment and external rotation of the femur (arrow), the capsule (C) is exposed between the gluteus minimus (G MIN) and the piriformis (PI). OI = obturator internus. **C,** With further external rotation and flexion of the femur (arrows), the anterosuperior circumference of the capsule is exposed using three retractors. The Z-shaped capsulotomy runs anteriorly along the capsular insertion on the femur and posteriorly along the acetabular rim. The connecting incision is parallel to the femoral neck and starts at the anterosuperior contour of the osteotomy basis of the trochanter. (Reproduced with permission from Ganz R, Gill TJ, Gautier E, et al: Surgical dislocation of the adult hip: A technique with full access to femoral head and acetabulum without the risk of avascular necrosis. *J Bone Joint Surg Br* 2001;83:1119-1124.)

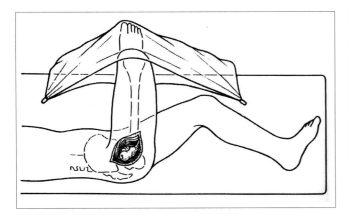

Figure 2 For anterior subluxation and dislocation of the hip joint, the leg is brought over the front of the operating table and placed in a sterile bag. (Reproduced with permission from Ganz R, Gill TJ, Gautier E, et al: Surgical dislocation of the adult hip: A technique with full access to femoral head and acetabulum without the risk of avascular necrosis. *J Bone Joint Surg Br* 2001;83:1119-1124.)

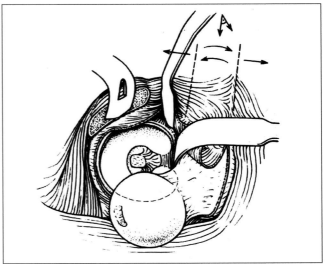

Figure 3 With manipulation of the femur (arrows) and the use of three retractors, the entire the acetabulum can be exposed. (Reproduced with permission from Ganz R, Gill TJ, Gautier E, et al: Surgical dislocation of the adult hip: A technique with full access to femoral head and acetabulum without the risk of avascular necrosis. *J Bone Joint Surg Br* 2001;83:1119-1124.)

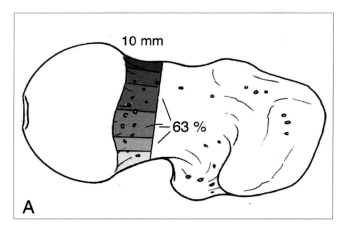
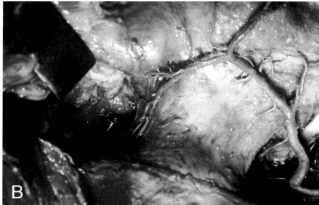

Figure 4 **A,** More than 60% of the vessels penetrating the femoral head are located in a 10-mm zone at the superior femoral head-neck junction. **B,** The posterior aspect of the femoral neck has no vessels penetrating the femoral head.

clearly visible as a mobile layer of connective tissue on the posterosuperior aspect of the femoral neck. The terminal vessels penetrate the femoral head about 2 mm below the lateral border of the cartilage (**Figure 4**, *A*). However, there are no vessels feeding the femoral head at the posterior neck and anterior to the retinaculum (**Figure 4**, *B*). During exposure, the cartilage must be constantly irrigated to prevent drying.

Dynamic Assessment of Impingement

Limitations in hip motion should be assessed before dislocation. This assessment, along with preoperative imaging studies, allow the surgeon to identify the types and location of the impingement, both of which are key for surgical decision making. The status of the synovial membrane is assessed with preoperative MR arthrography and intraoperative visualization; the amount of synovial fluid in the joint is an indicator of the inflammation present.

Impingement most commonly occurs with flexion and internal rotation, but it also may occur in flexion adduction or flexion abduction. With coxa valga, and especially if the posteroinferior rim of the acetabulum is

prominent, impingement is possible in extension and external rotation.

With the leg in flexion and external rotation and placed in a sterile bag on the side of the operating table as described earlier, the femoral head can be subluxated. This step allows the impingement lesion to be identified and regional damage to be débrided through a localized osteoplasty of the femoral head and neck. Unyielding hips or hips with larger abnormalities require full dislocation. Average time from skin incision to complete surgical dislocation is 30 minutes; blood loss is 300 mL or less.

Following joint débridement, the stump of the round ligament on the femoral head is resected, and the joint is assessed for fragments that may be lost within the socket. After reduction, the capsule is repaired but not tightened because tightening may create tension on the retinacular vessels, leading to decreased perfusion to the femoral head. The greater trochanter is reattached using two or three 3.5-mm cortical screws.

Postoperatively, continuous passive motion is used for the first week to prevent adhesions between the capsule and the femoral side of the osteochondroplasty. Ambulation with guarded weight bearing is allowed for 8 weeks. The trochanteric osteotomy

needs 8 weeks to heal, and restoration of full abductor function takes another 3 to 4 weeks. With relative lengthening of the femoral neck, additional intertrochanteric osteotomy, or femoral neck osteotomy, restricted weight bearing should be extended to 12 weeks. No special postoperative treatment is required. Patients generally do well with self-directed home physical therapy to restore motion and muscle strength. No regular medication or other treatment to prevent ectopic ossification is used.

Acetabular Resection Osteoplasty

Surgical dislocation of the hip joint not only allows complete evaluation of the articular cartilage and the labrum but also allows for control of version and socket depth. Together, information obtained from the preoperative imaging studies and surgical dislocation provide an accurate idea about how much of the acetabular rim has to be or can be resected. Testing the structures with a nerve hook or probe follows to determine whether partial or complete excision of the labrum is needed and to assess the quality of the articular cartilage and determine whether it is detached from subchondral bone. Palpation helps to confirm whether the labrum is thin over a bony

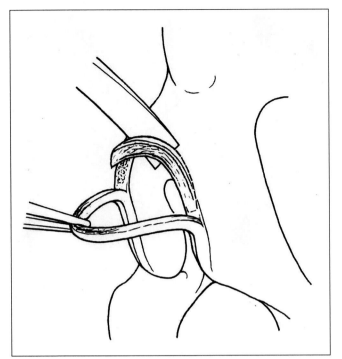

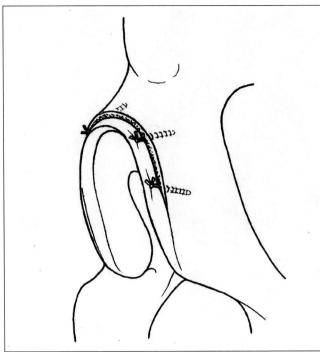

Figure 5 Technique of rim débridement preserving the labrum. The labrum is taken down, and the excessive rim with the damaged cartilage is resected using a 10-mm curved osteotome. (Reproduced with permission from Lavigne M, Parvizi J, Beck M, et al: Anterior femoro-acetabular impingement: Part 1. Techniques of joint preserving surgery. *Clin Orthop* 2004;418:61-66.)

Figure 6 Refixation of the labrum using nonabsorbable sutures on bone anchors. The distance between anchors is 1.5 to 2 cm. (Reproduced with permission from Lavigne M, Parvizi J, Beck M, et al: Anterior femoro-acetabular impingement: Part 1. Techniques of joint preserving surgery. *Clin Orthop* 2004;418:61-66.)

apposition of the rim, a fact that should already be known from the preoperative imaging studies.

In patients with anterior overlap (with or without retroversion but fulfilling the criteria mentioned above), a controlled resection of the excessive rim is indicated. If, as is commonly the case, the labrum shows substantial areas of integrity, it is mobilized from the osseous rim and preserved for later refixation. Complete excision of the labrum is reserved for hips in which the labrum is fully destroyed or have excessively thinned labrum, making refixation technically impossible.

The osteoplasty is done using a 10-mm curved osteotome (**Figure 5**). The osteotome is held slightly angled to the acetabular plane, and the rim is resected in small increments, interrupted by reduction of the femoral head and repeated checks of the clear-

ance. If possible, the area of cartilage damage is included in the resection up to a stable cutting edge of cartilage. The amount of rim resection is limited by the individual coverage. Destabilization of the femoral head must be avoided. Healthy labrum is refixed to the new rim using suture anchors 1.5 to 2 cm apart and nonabsorbable sutures (**Figure 6**).

Refixation of the labrum is best performed with the femoral head dislocated. The refixed labrum should be flush with the cartilage surface. Whether labrum length is excessive after trimming of the rim depends on the final circumference of the acetabular rim relative to the circumference before the procedure. In most cases, the labrum is slightly long but does not require shortening or excision. The stability of the labrum fixation is tested only after trimming the femoral

side, and the resolution of impingement is confirmed by repeated passive motion just before closure of the capsule.

Young patients with impingement resulting from acetabular retroversion associated with normal anatomy of the proximal femur may be candidates for reverse PAO. As described earlier, there should be no posterior overlap, and preoperative MR arthrography should confirm the integrity of the acetabular cartilage in the area of anterior overlap. In general, patients with these indications are typically very young and female, whereas in males acetabular retroversion without a femoral abnormality is rare. Reverse PAO with reorientation of the acetabulum into anteversion of about 15° requires slight modification from the PAO performed for a patient with classic dysplasia. Specifically, lat-

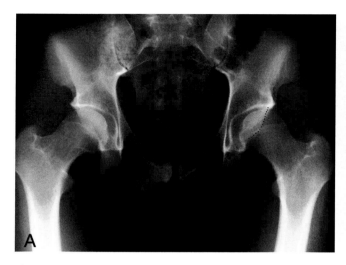
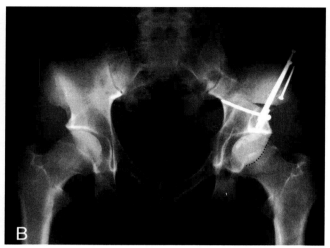

Figure 7 A, Preoperative AP radiograph of the pelvis shows pincer impingement caused by retroversion of the proximal third of the acetabulum. The dotted line shows the crossover sign of the acetabular rims (posterior rim). **B,** Postoperative AP radiograph after a reverse PAO decreased anterior coverage. The posterior border of the acetabulum is now more prominent over the femoral head (dotted line), and the anterior border covers the femoral head less than before. The crossover sign has disappeared.

eral overlap must be avoided (**Figure 7**).

Head Contouring Osteochondroplasty

Nonspherical extension of the femoral head covered by hyaline cartilage leading to cam impingement is rather common, particularly in male patients. In most cases, anterior nonspherical extension of the femoral head with a normal lateral waist between the femoral head and neck is seen. Lateral femoral head extensions, which appear as a pistol-grip deformity on radiographs also have an anterior extension. The latter is a more crucial finding for impingement than the visible lateral contour because more clear space is needed for flexion than for abduction. At dislocation, there is often a clear demarcation between the area of normal femoral head cartilage and the cartilage area that is subjected to cam impingement. Fraying and fissures on the surface of the hyaline cartilage occurs as a result of repetitive jamming against the acetabular cartilage.

Femoral head osteochondroplasty is performed using a 10-mm

curved osteotome, beginning at the demarcation line and proceeding toward the femoral head-neck junction, staying rather superficial in the femoral head (**Figure 8**). Osteochondroplasty in the anterior aspect can be performed without special attention to vasculature; however, great care is needed when making the cuts at the anterolateral sector of the retinaculum. The vessel perforations into the epiphyseal bone in this area have to be protected. At a more posterior aspect of the femoral head-neck junction, no vessels penetrate the femoral head. At the critical posterosuperior area with the retinaculum clearly visible, pieces of bone are removed by fracturing them with the osteotome, first bending them distally to break their base and then turning them up at their soft-tissue attachment. The pieces of cartilage and bone are then sharply dissected from the retinaculum tissue. Circumferential shaping of the head is possible with this technique, although such extensive recontouring is rarely necessary.

In some hips, the abnormality is characterized by more a lack of anterolateral offset between the femoral

head and neck than a femoral bump. This lack in offset may be associated with secondary bone apposition as a reaction to the chronic impingement. It is seen mainly in female patients with predominantly acetabular causes of impingement.

At the end of the procedure, special templates are used to check the sphericity of the remaining femoral head (**Figure 9**). The femoral head is then relocated, and motion is tested to ensure it is free of impingement. If necessary, further excisional osteoplasty can be performed. Before closure of the capsule, the femoral head is dislocated again, and the new, sharp edge on the femoral head cartilage created by the osteotome is smoothed with a scalpel. Bone wax is applied to the bleeding cancellous bone surface to prevent the capsule from adhering to the surface of the femoral neck.

The final check of motion includes external rotation in full extension with visual evaluation of the posteroinferior joint. Because mechanically increased joint motion may result in new areas of impingement, especially at the posteroinferior joint

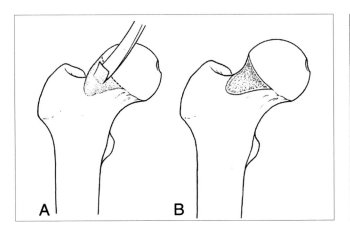

Figure 8 **A,** A nonspherical extension of the femoral head is tapered down to the size of the true femoral neck using a 10-mm curved osteotome. **B,** The result of this resection should not be a wedge removed from the femoral neck but should show a smooth waist between the femoral head and neck. The cancellous surface is sealed with wax to avoid scar fixation of the capsule up to the cartilage border. (Reproduced with permission from Lavigne M, Parvizi J, Beck M, et al: Anterior femoro-acetabular impingement: Part 1. Techniques of joint preserving surgery. *Clin Orthop* 2004;418:61-66.)

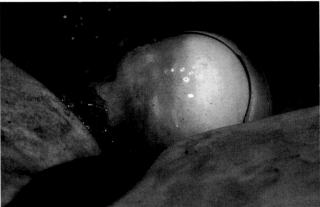

Figure 9 Intraoperative photograph showing transparent templates used to control nonsphericity of the femoral head and define the line of trimming.

area, this step must not be missed. If there is a problem, the impingement in this area also must be addressed (eg, by trimming the posterosuperior rim and/or the trochanteric bone).

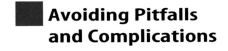

Avoiding Pitfalls and Complications

Little morbidity is associated with this surgical dislocation, and the number of complications has slightly decreased since our first publication in 2001. Pitfalls include the potential for osteonecrosis. However, my colleagues and I reported that this risk is quite low and has been further minimized with the advent of laser Doppler flowmetry. Fracture of the femoral neck is a possibility if too much of the femoral neck is resected, but I have not seen this problem in more than 1,000 patients. Trochanteric nonunion also is a potential problem, but most patients who undergo this surgery are young with excellent healing potential. Therefore, I believe that the chance of nonunion is relatively small if adequate fixation with two or three screws is obtained. The remaining unknowns are associated with fixing a torn labrum and addressing hyaline articular cartilage problems. In the future, grafting of hyaline articular cartilage may be possible and may permit these techniques to be used patients with more severe secondary degenerative changes.

■ References

Beck M, Parvizi J, Boutier V, et al: Anterior femoro-acetabular impingement: Part 2. Clinical midterm results. *Clin Orthop* 2004;418:67-73.

Ganz R, Gill TJ, Gautier E, et al: Surgical dislocation of the adult hip: A technique with full access to femoral head and acetabulum without the risk of avascular necrosis. *J Bone Joint Surg Br* 2001;83:1119-1124.

Ganz R, MacDonald SJ: Indications and modern techniques of proximal femoral osteotomies in the adult. *Sem Arthroplasty* 1997;8:38-50.

Ganz R, Parvizi J, Beck M, et al: Femoro-acetabular impingement: An important cause of early osteoarthritis of the hip. *Clin Orthop* 2003;417:112-120.

Gautier E, Ganz K, Krügel N, Gill TJ, Ganz R: Anatomy of the medial femoral circumflex artery and its surgical implications. *J Bone Joint Surg Br* 2000;82:679-683.

Lavigne M, Parvizi J, Beck M, et al: Anterior femoro-acetabular impingement: Part 1. Techniques of joint preserving surgery. *Clin Orthop* 2004;418:61-66.

Leunig M, Fraitzl CR, Ganz R: Frühe Schädigung des acetabulären Knorpels bei der Epiphysiolysis capitis femoris. *Orthopade* 2002;31:894-899.

Leunig M, Werlen S, Ungersböck A, Ito K, Ganz R: Evaluation of the acetabular labrum by MR arthrography. *J Bone Joint Surg Br* 1997;79:230-234.

Locher S, Werlen S, Leunig M, Ganz R: Arthro-MRI mit radiärer Schnittsequenz zur Darstellung der präradiologischen Hüftpathologie. *Z Orthop* 2002;140:1-5.

Nötzli HP, Siebenrock KA, Hempfing A, Ramseier LE, Ganz R: Perfusion of the femoral head during surgical dislocation of the hip: Monitoring by laser-Doppler flowmetry. *J Bone Joint Surg Br* 2002;84:300-304.

Reynolds D, Lucas L, Klaue K: Retroversion of the acetabulum: A cause of hip pain. *J Bone Joint Surg Br* 1999;81:281-288.

Sevitt S, Thompson RG: The distribution and anastomoses of arteries supplying the head and neck of the femur. *J Bone Joint Surg Br* 1965;47:560-573.

Siebenrock KA, Ganz R: Osteochondroma of the femoral neck. *Clin Orthop* 2002;394:211-218.

Siebenrock KA, Schöniger R, Ganz R: Anterior femoro-acetabular impingement due to retroversion and its treatment by periacetabular osteotomy. *J Bone Joint Surg Am* 2003;85:278-286.

Chapter 66

Osteonecrosis of the Femoral Head: Early Stage Disease

Michael A. Mont, MD
Phillip S. Ragland, MD

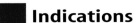 Indications

Nonsurgical Treatment

Early osteonecrosis of the femoral head is more likely to be treated successfully with head-preserving procedures (eg, core decompression, various bone grafting techniques, osteotomies) than is postcollapse disease. In some cases, nonsurgical treatment is appropriate for asymptomatic patients with small precollapse lesions. These lesions are often diagnosed in the contralateral hip after evaluation of a symptomatic hip, and some are incidental findings on radiographic examination of other organ systems, such as a lower abdominal/pelvic evaluation to rule out kidney stones. Surgical treatment of asymptomatic patients remains controversial. The literature has reported that less than 50% of asymptomatic hips progress to end-stage disease requiring total hip arthroplasty (THA). There is a lack of well-designed prospective studies to determine how many asymptomatic hips with small lesions respond successfully to nonsurgical treatment.

Protected weight bearing with various assistive devices such as a cane, a single crutch, or two crutches has not been found to be effective. Some authors report that these methods result in more than an 80% failure rate at a mean follow-up of 34 months. Thus, protected weight bearing should be considered a radical instead of a conservative measure given the natural history of untreated disease. A more appropriate indication for protected weight bearing may be in patients with advanced disease in whom head-preserving procedures are contraindicated. In this situation, this modality may relieve symptoms temporarily until the patient decides to undergo THA. Assistive devices for ambulation also may be useful preoperatively for patients who eventually undergo a head-preserving procedure. Theoretically, this intervention could slow the rate of collapse and alleviate pain.

Anecdotal information on the value of noninvasive and nonsurgical treatment recently has been reported. Pharmacologic agents have been used to target the pathophysiologic mechanism of the disease. For example, the effectiveness of lipid-lowering agents has been tested in patients with systemic lupus erythematosus and high serum cholesterol and lipids. Antihypertensive agents could be used in patients with renal hypertension. Many patients have inherited coagulation disorders, and some have genetic defects that led to hypofibrinolysis or thrombophilia. Anticoagulation therapy has been used for these patients. Other recent studies report the efficacy of ditridonates for treatment of early-stage disease. None of these pharmacologic agents has been studied prospectively, and all should be considered experimental at this time. Nonsurgical modalities have no role in treating postcollapse lesions in which the femoral head has undergone early collapse and therefore been biomechanically compromised.

Other nonsurgical modalities used to treat osteonecrosis include electrical stimulation, ultrasound, and hyperbaric oxygen. Electrical stimulation may be a useful modality in early-stage disease, but it is not currently approved by the US Food and Drug Administration. Hyperbaric oxygen not only is ineffective but also impractical.

Surgical Treatment

Groin pain is the primary indication for surgery in patients with documented osteonecrosis. Imaging studies are the principal tools for planning surgical treatment of patients with osteonecrosis. Specifically, MRI in conjunction with AP and frog-lateral radiographs easily confirm the diagnosis. Four primary radiographic factors are useful for determining whether surgical treatment is necessary: (1) the state of the femoral head (pre- or postcollapse); (2) the size of the lesion; (3) the amount of femoral head depression; and (4) the extent of acetabular involvement. Bone scans are unnecessary and may miss up to 30% of lesions. CT or tomography is not necessary in most patients unless

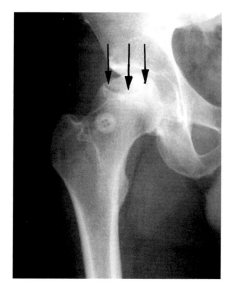

Figure 1 AP radiograph showing stage III lesions with a crescent sign (arrows) indicating subchondral fracture and collapse.

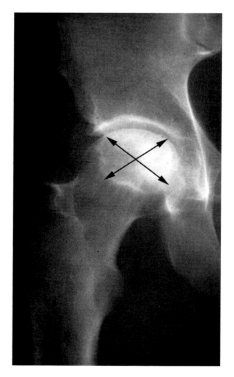

Figure 3 AP radiograph showing an easily identifiable large lesion (arrows).

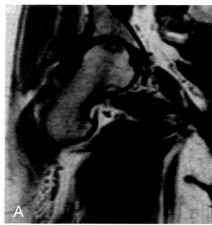 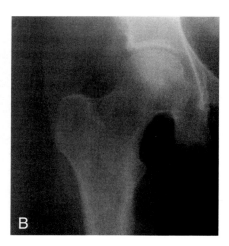

Figure 2 Stage I osteonecrosis of the femoral head in a young symptomatic patient. These images show a small lesion visible on MRI (**A**) but not apparent on plain radiography (**B**).

a crescent sign have the best prognosis. A crescent sign results from a subchondral fracture and indicates that the femoral head is at risk of impending or present biomechanical compromise (**Figure 1**).

The size of the lesion is easily delineated by plain radiographs in stage II or III Ficat disease. In some cases, it may be more difficult to estimate the size of the lesion on plain radiographs, especially in early-stage disease (**Figure 2**). In these patients, the lesions can be well characterized by MRI. In our experience, it is important only to differentiate between small- to medium-sized lesions from large lesions (**Figure 3**). The size of the lesion is easily delineated from radiographs (in patients with radiographic-evident osteonecrosis) or from MRI scans. Measurements of the exact amount of femoral head involvement are less important than qualitatively knowing whether a lesion is small to medium sized or large (approximately 30% of the femoral head involved) (**Figure 4**). Patients with large lesions have the worst prognosis.

The radiographic appearance (ie, shape, lesion size) of the femoral head is the principal factor in determining whether surgical treatment is necessary. However, demographic factors such as age also may influence the

choice of treatment. Patients with certain diagnoses and risk factors (eg, systemic lupus erythematosus, corticosteroids) may have a poorer prognosis for femoral head preservation than other patients with osteonecrosis.

———————————■

■ Alternative Treatments

Many options are available to treat osteonecrosis in its early stages; most are discussed below. The other main treatment options are nonsurgical treatment, consisting of analgesics and, if needed for pain relief, a cane or crutches. THA is an established, effective treatment for late-stage disease.

Head-Preserving Procedures

Head-preserving procedures typically require healthy femoral and acetabular chondral surfaces. Some procedures are performed without intraoperatively assessing the femoral head cartilage (ie, core decompression, vascularized fibular grafting). In these cases, other imaging studies or tests might be considered. For example, if core decompression is being considered for a precollapse medium- to large-sized lesion, CT or tomography can be used to

subtle collapse of the femoral head is suspected.

Patients in early-stage radiographic disease (precollapse) without

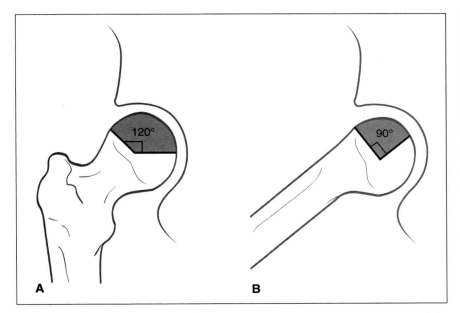

Figure 4 The arc of area involved is determined by drawing a line from the center of the femoral head to the joint line along the outer margins of the lesion in both the AP (**A**) and lateral (**B**) views. Hips with a total arc of area (A + B) greater than 200° have a poor prognosis. In this figure, total arc of area would be 120° + 90° = 210°.

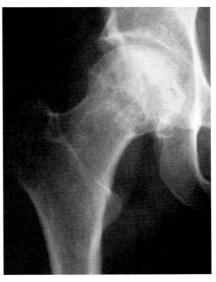

Figure 6 AP radiograph of a patient with stage II osteonecrosis of the femoral head in which cartilage is preserved.

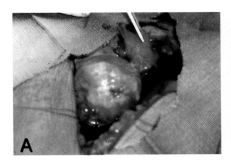

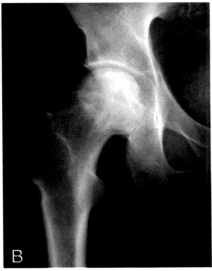

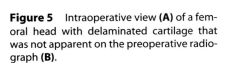

Figure 5 Intraoperative view (**A**) of a femoral head with delaminated cartilage that was not apparent on the preoperative radiograph (**B**).

identify any collapse of the femoral head because core decompression yields a poor prognosis in most patients with any femoral head collapse. Hip arthroscopy can provide information about cartilage changes, but a role for diagnostic or therapeutic arthroscopy for osteonecrosis has not been defined. Intraoperative inspection of the

femoral head is important when considering bone grafting or resurfacing. If a bone grafting procedure is planned but the femoral head cartilage is found to be delaminated (**Figure 5**), femoral head resurfacing or THA may be more appropriate. Likewise, a hip believed to be collapsing on preoperative evaluation might be considered for a head-

preserving procedure (ie, bone grafting) if the cartilage is pristine on intraoperative inspection (**Figure 6**). Additionally, intraoperative assessment of the acetabulum is necessary when considering a limited femoral head resurfacing. If there is too much acetabular cartilage damage, a limited procedure should be avoided.

Arthroplasty

Femoral head depression of more than 2 mm has negative prognostic implications for all femoral head-preserving procedures (eg, core decompression, bone grafting, osteotomy). Femoral collapse of more than 2 mm often indicates that the cartilage surface is disrupted. Additionally, patients with radiographically apparent osteoarthritis involving the acetabulum should not undergo head-preserving procedures (**Figure 7**). Patients with femoral head collapse of more than 2 mm or acetabular cartilage damage typically are candidates for THA. Bone- or cartilage-sparing procedures would be expected to be less efficacious in older patients. In addition, patients who are medically

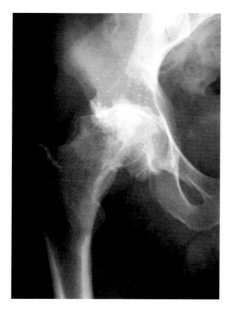

Figure 7 AP radiograph of a patient with stage IV osteonecrosis showing acetabular involvement, femoral head collapse, and loss of joint interval. Standard THA is the only option.

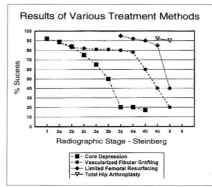

Figure 8 Head-sparing procedures are more effective in early-stage disease.

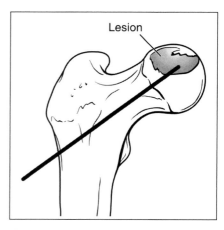

Figure 9 A 3.2-mm pin can be used to establish core tracks percutaneously through the femoral neck. This is accomplished from a lateral approach under fluoroscopic guidance.

compromised may be more appropriately treated with one definitive procedure such as THA rather than procedures that may be temporizing and possibly require another procedure in a short period of time.

▪ Techniques

Core Decompression

Core decompression is most efficacious in hips with small- or medium-sized precollapse lesions (**Figure 8**). Multiple studies have reported worse results with this procedure in patients with larger lesions or femoral head collapse. Core decompression reduces the intraosseous hypertension that is found in the bone compartment of the femoral head. This procedure may effect an alteration in the natural history of the disease. The technique has many variables. Historically, an 8- to 10-mm cannula is drilled into the lesion, with or without the addition of supplementary bone grafting. We prefer to use multiple small drill holes

(3.2 mm), which also produce the same decrease in intraosseous pressure.

Core decompression can be performed with the patient in either the supine or lateral decubitus position using a standard or fracture table. A 3.2- to 3.5-mm Steinmann pin is inserted laterally and percutaneously under fluoroscopic guidance and advanced until it abuts the lateral cortex of the femoral metaphysis opposite the superior portion of the lesser trochanter (**Figure 9**). The femur is penetrated, and then the pin is advanced through the femoral neck, into the femoral head, and to the lesion. It is important to ensure that the chondral surface of the femoral head is not penetrated. While advancing the pin, lateral fluoroscopic views should be obtained to ensure that the pin remains in the medullary canal of the femoral neck. The number of passes is determined by the size of the lesion. For small lesions, we make two passes through the lesion, and for medium- to large-sized lesions, we make three passes. All passes are done through the original entry hole in the femur to avoid creating multiple subtrochanteric stress risers. Once the drilling is completed, the pin is removed and the wound is closed.

We usually advise a limited (5-week) period of protected weight bearing (one crutch or cane) postop-

eratively. The results of this technique have been variable, with satisfactory results ranging from 40% to 90%.

Osteotomies

Femoral osteotomy for osteonecrosis is based on the concept of rotating the involved segment away from the weight-bearing surface of the joint. We use both uniplanar (varus and valgus) and multiplanar (transtrochanteric) osteotomies (**Figure 10**).

The results of osteotomy vary, ranging from 60% to 90% at 5- to 12-year follow-up in several large series. The best results have been reported with small- or medium-sized lesions. Osteotomy currently is used less often in the United States because of its variable results and because it deforms the proximal femur, which may make future THA much more difficult.

Vascularized Bone Grafting

With this procedure, a vascularized pedicle of bone (usually the fibula) is transplanted through a core track and anastomosed with the local blood supply to bolster the collapsing femoral head (**Figure 11**). The goal is to provide mechanical support and potentially introduce a vascular supply and mesenchymal cells to the area. How-

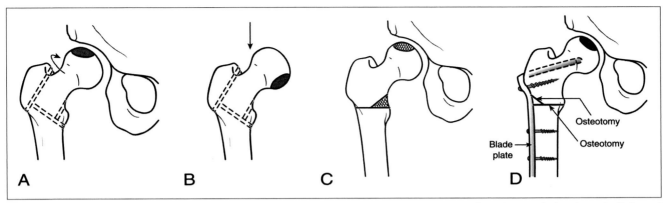

Figure 10 Transtrochanteric (**A** and **B**) and rotational (**C** and **D**) osteotomies shift the lesion away from the weight-bearing axis. (Adapted from Etienne G, Mont M, Ragland PS: The diagnosis and treatment of nontraumatic osteonecrosis of the femoral head. *Instr Course Lect* 2004;53:67-85.)

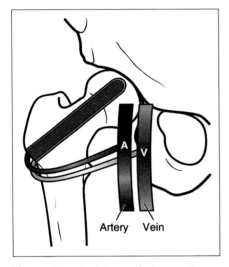

Figure 11 Grafting technique using a vascularized fibular graft (A = femoral stem, U = femoral vein).

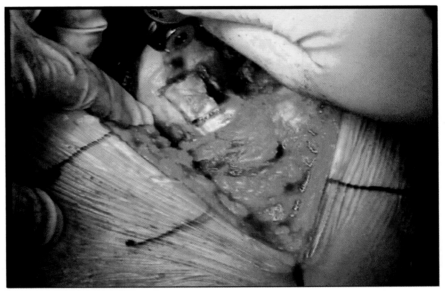

Figure 12 Intraoperative photograph showing the trapdoor window created at the femoral head-neck junction.

ever, the technique can be difficult and requires a team member with microvascular expertise to harvest and anastomose the graft. This procedure can be used for all stages of the disease up to the point of severe head depression and/or acetabular changes. Results vary widely, from 10% to 90% in large series at 4- to 8-year follow-up.

Nonvascularized Bone Grafting
Nonvascularized bone grafting is best performed at earlier stages in patients with early-stage disease, before the femoral head or acetabular cartilage is damaged. The acetabular and femoral cartilage must be inspected and palpated at the time of surgery. If the femoral cartilage is not intact (ie, delamination has occurred) or is not of good quality, other procedures must be considered.

Nonvascularized bone grafting was first used when autograft or allograft material was implanted in the femoral head for structural support. More recently, a number of techniques have become popular in which graft is introduced either through a trapdoor in the femoral head cartilage or through the femoral head-neck junction (**Figure 12**). **Table 1** shows the results of several recent series at 4- to 11-year follow-up in patients whose lesions were associated with minimal femoral head collapse and no acetabular involvement.

To perform nonvascularized cancellous bone grafting, we currently use an anterolateral approach. The hip is dislocated and a 2 × 2 cm cortical window is created in the superior as-

Table 1   Results of Bone Grafting Techniques

Author(s) (Year)	Number of Hips	Type of Procedure	Mean Follow-up (Range)	Clinical Success Rate (%)
Yoo, et al (1992)	81	V	5.2 years (3–10.8)	91%
Urbaniak, et al (1996)	646	V	1–17 years	83%
Buckley, et al (1991)	20	C	8 years (2–19)	90%
Nelson and Clark (1993)	52	C	6 years (2–12)	77%
Itoman and Yamamoto (1983)	38	W	9 years (2–15)	61%
Scher and Jakim (1993)	45	T, O	5.5 years (2.7–10.5)	87%
Rosenwasser, et al (1994)	15	W	12 years (10–15)	81%
Meyers, et al (1983)	9	T	3 years (1–9)	89%
Mont, et al	24	T	4.7 years (2.5–5)	83%
Mont, et al (2003)	21	W	4 years (3–4.7)	86%

V = Vascularized fibular graft; T = Trapdoor, nonvascularized bone graft; W = Window in femoral neck, nonvascularized bone graft; O = With ancillary osteotomy; C = Nonvascularized bone grafting through a core track

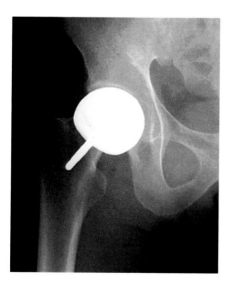

Figure 13   AP radiograph showing the results of hemiresurfacing by a bone-preserving procedure, which may be considered when the acetabulum is not involved.

pect of the femoral neck at the femoral head-neck junction. The dead bone is removed, and the excavated area is filled with autogenous bone graft, bone graft substitute, and, in some cases, pins. Patients are kept at 20% weight bearing for 6 weeks at which time they are advanced to 50% weight bearing, followed by full weight bearing at 3 months.

Limited Femoral Resurfacing Arthroplasty
Limited femoral resurfacing is used in patients who have large lesions with severe femoral head collapse. The goal is to use the resurfacing component to replace dead bone but to avoid touching the acetabular side (**Figure 13**). The best results have been reported

before acetabular changes occur. Thus, limited femoral head resurfacing should be used in early-stage disease because of the risks for acetabular changes after collapse. The results of this procedure have been highly variable, with some surgeons reporting an 80% to 90% success rate at 7 years, whereas others report much higher failure rates. Some patients may have persistent groin pain, which is thought to be due to contact by the metal resurfacing component on the acetabular cartilage.

Surgical Indications Treatment Algorithm

A suggested surgical indications treatment algorithm is presented in **Table 2**. For early-stage disease (ie, small- or medium-sized lesions without a crescent sign), core decompression is appropriate. For medium- and large-sized lesions before femoral head collapse, various bone grafting procedures or osteotomies may be appropriate, depending on the size of the lesion. When there is cartilage damage but no acetabular damage, hemiresurfacing can be used. Finally, when there is acetabular damage, THA (resurfacing or standard) is appropriate. As new procedures and various biologic agents (growth and differentiation factors) are evaluated, this algorithm may change to yield more effective outcomes.

Avoiding Pitfalls and Complications

Core Decompression
Selecting the proper point of entry on the femur is a key consideration

in avoiding the most important complication: subtrochanteric fracture. Aligning the drill hole with the upper third of the lesser trochanter and then drawing an imaginary line from the top of the lesser trochanter to the lateral cortex typically will result in the appropriate entry site into metaphyseal bone, and away from the diaphysis. Entry into diaphyseal bone can result in a subtrochanteric fracture. Penetrating the femoral head also should be avoided because it may be associated with chondrolysis. Reviewing AP and lateral fluoroscopic images of the femoral head intraoperatively is helpful to ensure that the drill is not inserted any closer than 5 to 10 mm from the top of the femoral head. Multiple entry points also should be avoided when drilling to avoid any stress riser than could lead to a femoral fracture.

Osteotomies

These can be difficult procedures and should be performed only by surgeons who have specific training in the technique. Appropriate preoperative planning is necessary to verify the area of the femoral head to be rotated out of the weight-bearing zone. In addition, adequate fixation of the osteotomy site and good coaptation of the bone surfaces are necessary to avoid nonunion. Patients should not be allowed to bear full weight until there is radiographic evidence of bridging of the osteotomy site.

Vascularized Bone Grafting

As with core decompression, the importance of the entry site in the metaphyseal area is of key importance in preventing complications. Entry that is too low in the diaphyseal area may result in subtrochanteric hip fracture. Head penetration also must be avoided. In some patients who might have cartilage delamination, these

Table 2 Surgical Indications Treatment Algorithm

Ficat and Arlet Stage	Description	Treatment Modalities
I	Asymptomatic	Nonsurgical
	Symptomatic	Core decompression, bone grafting, osteotomies
II	Small, medium lesion	Core decompression, bone grafting, osteotomies
II	Large lesion	Bone grafting
III	Large lesion (head depression >2 mm)	Bone grafting, hemiresurfacing, or THA
IV	Acetabular osteoarthritis	THA

procedures may be combined with arthroscopy to confirm that the cartilage is still intact.

Nonvascularized Bone Grafting

As with other procedures, penetrating the femoral head can be avoided by visualizing the entire femoral head either fluoroscopically or by dislocating the hip. All dead bone should be removed and replaced with new bone graft or other graft materials that are placed into a bed of bleeding bone to ensure appropriate healing.

The trapdoor should not be more than 50% of the diameter of the femoral neck to prevent an unduly large stress riser, which could lead to a femoral neck fracture. Fortunately, this complication is rare if proper surgical technique and postoperative weight-bearing precautions are observed. The trapdoor should be firmly secured with bioabsorbable pins or another type of fixation to ensure healing.

Weight bearing must be limited the first 6 to 12 weeks postoperatively because of the stress riser that is created at the femoral head-neck junction during the procedure.

Limited Femoral Resurfacing

Patients must have an appropriate amount of acetabular cartilage before a limited resurfacing procedure can be done. Early failure rates and high risk for persistent groin pain are associated with this procedure if performed in a patient with cartilage delamination on the acetabular side. Proper alignment of the initial entry pin with the center of the femoral neck also is important, as is appropriate seating of the femoral component and avoiding femoral neck notching. Marking the proper location of the trial femoral component before the actual component is seated is helpful to ensure that the component is not left proud, which could lead to a stress riser and ultimately a fracture.

Acknowledgments

The authors would like to thank Colleen Kazmarek for her editorial assistance.

References

Buckley PD, Gearen PF, Petty RW: Structural bone-grafting for early atraumatic avascular necrosis of the femoral head. *J Bone Joint Surg Am* 1991;73:1357-1364.

Lieberman JR, Berry DJ, Mont MA, et al: Osteonecrosis of the hip: Management in the 21st century. *Instr Course Lect* 2003;52:337-355.

Mont MA, Einhorn TA, Sponseller PD, Hungerford DS: The trapdoor procedure using autogenous cortical and cancellous bone grafts for osteonecrosis of the femoral head. *J Bone Joint Surg Br* 1998;80:56-62.

Mont MA, Hungerford DS: Current concepts review: Non-traumatic avascular necrosis of the femoral head. *J Bone Joint Surg Am* 1995;77:459-474.

Mont MA, Jones LC, Einhorn TA, et al: Osteonecrosis of the femoral head: Potential treatment with growth and differentiation factors. *Clin Orthop* 1998;355S:314-335.

Mont MA, Ragland PS, Etienne G: Outcome of non-vascularized bone grafting for osteonecrosis of the femoral head. *Clin Orthop* 2003;417:84-92.

Nelson LN, Clark CR: Efficacy of Phemister bone grafting in nontraumatic aseptic necrosis of the femoral head. *J Arthroplasty* 1993;8:253-258.

Rosenwasser MP, Garino JP, Kiernan HA, Michelsen CB: Long-term follow-up of thorough débridement and cancellous bone grafting of the femoral head for avascular necrosis. *Clin Orthop* 1994;306:17-27.

Santore RF: Intertrochanteric osteotomy for osteonecrosis. *Semin Arthroplasty* 1991;2:208-213.

Scher MA, Jakim I: Intertrochanteric osteotomy and autogenous bone-grafting for avascular necrosis of the femoral head. *J Bone Joint Surg Am* 1993;75:1119-1133.

Steinberg ME, Mont MA: Osteonecrosis, in Chapman MW (ed): *Chapman's Orthopaedic Surgery*, ed 3. Philadelphia, PA, Lippincott-Williams & Wilkins, 2001, p 3263.

Urbaniak JR, Harvey EJ: Revascularization of the femoral head in osteonecrosis. *J Am Acad Orthop Surg* 1998;6:44-54.

Yoo MC, Chung DW, Hahn CS: Free vascularized fibula grafting for the treatment of osteonecrosis of the femoral head. *Clin Orthop* 1992;277:128-138.

Coding

CPT Codes		Corresponding ICD-9 Codes
20955	Bone graft with microvascular anastomosis; fibula	773.42
27066	Excision of bone cyst or benign tumor; deep, with or without autograft	773.42
27067	Excision of bone cyst or benign tumor; with autograft requiring separate incision	773.42
27130	Arthroplasty, acetabular and proximal femoral prosthetic replacement (total hip arthroplasty), with or without autograft or allograft	773.42
27165	Osteotomy, intertrochanteric or subtrochanteric including internal or external fixation and/or cast	773.42
27284	Arthrodesis, hip joint (including obtaining graft)	773.42
27286	Arthrodesis, hip joint (including obtaining graft); with subtrochanteric osteotomy	773.42

CPT copyright © 2004 by the American Medical Association. All Rights Reserved.

Index